A Guide to

Psychiatric Mental Health Nursing, 6th Edition

The **6th Edition** leads the way in evidence and innovation with a new streamlined design, state-of-the-art content and new and updated special features!

STREAMLINED, STUDENT FRIENDLY DESIGN

- Each chapter begins with a Chapter Outline, Chapter Objectives, Key Terms, and Core Concepts.

- Each chapter closes with New! Bulleted Summaries followed by Review Questions and References organized into three categories: Classic, Contemporary, and Internet.

---

29 CHAPTER

Mood Disorders

CHAPTER OUTLINE

OBJECTIVES
HISTORICAL PERSPECTIVE
EPIDEMIOLOGY
TYPES OF MOOD DISORDERS
DEPRESSIVE DISORDERS
APPLICATION OF THE NURSING PROCESS
TO DEPRESSIVE DISORDERS

BIPOLAR DISORDER (MANIA)
APPLICATION OF THE NURSING PROCESS
TO BIPOLAR DISORDER (MANIA)
TREATMENT MODALITIES FOR MOOD
DISORDERS
SUMMARY AND KEY POINTS
REVIEW QUESTIONS

KEY TERMS

bipolar disorder
cognitive therapy
cyclothymic
disorder
delirious mania
dysthymic disorder
hypomania

melancholia
postpartum depression
premenstrual
dysphoric disorder
psychomotor
retardation
tyramine

CORE CONCEPTS

depression
mania
mood

OBJECTIVES

After reading this chapter, the student will be able to:

1. Recount historical perspectives of mood disorders.
2. Discuss epidemiological statistics related to mood disorders.
3. Describe various types of mood disorders.
4. Identify predisposing factors in the development of mood disorders.
5. Discuss implications of depression related to developmental stage.
6. Identify symptomatology associated with mood disorders and use this information in client assessment.
7. Formulate nursing diagnoses and goals of care for clients with mood disorders.
8. Identify topics for client and family teaching relevant to mood disorders.
9. Describe appropriate nursing interventions for behaviors associated with mood disorders.
10. Describe relevant criteria for evaluating nursing care of clients with mood disorders.
11. Discuss various modalities relevant to treatment of mood disorders.

Depression is likely the oldest and still one of the most frequently diagnosed psychiatric illnesses. Symptoms of depression have been described almost as far back as there is evidence of written documentation.

An occasional bout with the "blues," a feeling of sadness or downheartedness, is common among healthy people and considered to be a normal response to everyday disappointments in life. These episodes are short-lived as the individual adapts to the loss, change, or failure (real or perceived) that has been experienced. Pathological depression occurs when adaptation is ineffective.

519

CLASSICAL REFERENCES

Beck, A.T., Rush, A.J., Shaw, B.F., & Emery, G. (1979). *Cognitive theory of depression.* New York: Guilford Press.
Freud, S. (1957). *Mourning and melancholia*, Vol. 14 (standard ed.). London: Hogarth Press. (Original work published 1917.)
Seligman, M.E.P. (1973). Fall into helplessness. *Psychology Today*, 7, 43–48.

SUMMARY AND KEY POINTS

- Depression is one of the oldest recognized psychiatric illnesses that is still prevalent today. It is so common, in fact, that it has been referred to as the "common cold of psychiatric disorders."
- The cause of depressive disorders is not entirely known. A number of factors, including genetics, biochemical influences, and psychosocial experiences likely enter into the development of the disorder.
- Secondary depression occurs in response to other physiological disorders.
- Symptoms of depression occur along a continuum according to the degree of severity from transient to

- Genetic influences have been strongly implicated in the development of bipolar disorder. Various other physiological factors, such as biochemical and electrolyte alterations, as well as cerebral structural changes, have been implicated. Side effects of certain medications may also induce symptoms of mania. No single theory can explain the etiology of bipolar disorder, and it is likely that the illness is caused by a combination of factors.
- Symptoms of mania may be observed on a continuum of three phases, each identified by the degree of severity: phase I, hypomania; phase II, acute mania; and phase III, delirious mania.
- The symptoms of bipolar disorder may occur in children

REVIEW QUESTIONS

Self-Examination/Learning Exercise

Situation: Margaret, age 68, was brought to the emergency department of a large regional medical center by her sister-in-law, who stated, "She does nothing but sit and stare into space. I can't get her to eat or anything!" On assessment, it was found that 6 months ago Margaret's husband of 45 years had died of a massive myocardial infarction. They had no children and had been inseparable. Since her husband's death, Margaret has visited the cemetery every day, changing the flowers often on his grave. She has not removed any of his clothes from the closet or chest of drawers. His shaving materials still occupy the same space in the bathroom. Over the months, Margaret has become more and more socially isolated. She refuses invitations from friends, preferring instead to make her daily trips to the cemetery. She has lost 15 pounds and her sister-in-law reports that there is very little food in the house. Today she said to her sister-in-law, "I don't really want to live anymore. My life is nothing without Frank." Her sister-in-law became frightened and, with forceful persuasion, was able to convince Margaret she needed to see a doctor. Margaret is admitted to the psychiatric unit.

Based on the above situation, select the answer that is most appropriate for each of the following questions:

Test Your Critical Thinking Skills

Alice, age 29, had been working in the typing pool of a large corporation for 6 years. Her immediate supervisor recently retired and Alice was promoted to supervisor, in charge of 20 people in the department. Alice was flattered by the promotion but anxious about the additional responsibility of the position. Shortly after the promotion, she overheard two of her former coworkers saying, "Why in the world did they choose her? She's not the best one for the job. I know *I* certainly won't be able to respect her as a boss!" Hearing these comments added to Alice's anxiety and self-doubt.

Shortly after Alice began her new duties, her friends and coworkers noticed a change. She had a great deal of energy and worked long hours on her job. She began to speak very loudly and rapidly. Her roommate noticed that Alice slept very little, yet seldom appeared tired. Every night she would go out to bars and dances. Sometimes she brought men she had just met home to the apartment, something she had never done before. She bought lots of clothes and make-up and had her hair restyled in a more youthful look. She failed to pay her share of the rent and bills but came home with a brand new convertible. She lost her temper and screamed at her roommate to "Mind your own business!" when asked to pay her share.

She became irritable and work, and several of her subordinates reported her behavior to the corporate manager. When the manager confronted Alice about her behavior, she lost control, shouting, cursing, and striking out at anyone and anything that happened to be within her reach. The security officers restrained her and took her to the emergency department of the hospital, where she was admitted to the psychiatric unit. She had no previous history of psychiatric illness.

The psychiatrist assigned a diagnosis of Bipolar I disorder and wrote orders for olanzapine (Zyprexa) 15 mg PO STAT, olanzapine 15 mg PO qd, and lithium carbonate 600 mg qid.

Answer the following questions related to Alice:

1. What are the most important considerations with which the nurse who is taking care of Alice should be concerned?
2. Why was Alice given the diagnosis of Bipolar I disorder?
3. The doctor should order a lithium level drawn after 4 to 6 days. For what symptoms should the nurse be on the alert?
4. Why did the physician order olanzapine in addition to the lithium carbonate?

- **Test Your Critical Thinking Skills** boxes appear at the end of DSM-IV chapters and feature case studies and exercises designed to stimulate problem solving.

- **Appendices feature New!** Controlled drug and pregnancy categories, all DSM-IV-TR classifications, NANDA diagnoses and behaviors, guidelines for mental health assessment, answers to the end-of-chapter review questions, and a glossary.

EASY TO READ AND UNDERSTAND

- **New!** Patient Outcomes in the Care Plans presented as measurable short- and long-term goals.

- **New!** Nursing Case Studies and Care Plans now appear at the end of the disorder chapters.

Table 29–2   Care Plan for the Depressed Client

NURSING DIAGNOSIS: COMPLICATED GRIEVING
RELATED TO: Real or perceived loss, bereavement overload
EVIDENCED BY: Denial of loss, inappropriate expression of anger, idealization of or obsession with lost object, inability to carry out activities of daily living.

Outcome Criteria	Nursing Interven
Short-Term Goals	1. Determine the stage of grief in w
● The client will express anger about the loss.	client is fixed. Identify behaviors a with this stage.
● The client will verbalize behaviors associated with normal grieving.	2. Develop a trusting relationship client. Show empathy, conce unconditional positive regard. B and keep all promises.
Long-Term Goal	3. Convey an accepting attitude, an the client to express feelings open
● The client will be able to recognize his or her own position in the grief process, while progressing at own pace toward resolution.	4. Encourage the client to express a not become defensive if the initia sion of anger is displaced on the

---

CHAPTER 29 ● MOOD DISORDERS **555**

CASE STUDY AND SAMPLE CARE PLAN

NURSING HISTORY AND ASSESSMENT

Sam is a 45-year-old white man admitted to the psychiatric unit of a general medical center by his family physician, Dr. Jones, who reported that Sam had become increasingly despondent over the last month. His wife reported that he had made statements such as, "Life is not worth living," and "I think I could just take all those pills Dr. Jones prescribed at one time; then it would all be over." Sam says he loves his wife and children and does not want to hurt them, but feels they no longer need him. He states, "They would probably be better off without me." His wife appears to be very concerned about his condition, though in his despondency, he seems oblivious to her feelings. His mother (a widow) lives in a neighboring state, and he sees her infrequently. His father was an alcoholic and physically abused Sam and his siblings. He admits that he is

b. **Long-Term Goal:**
  ● Sam will not harm himself during his hospitalization.

2. **Complicated Grieving** related to unresolved losses (job promotion and unsatisfactory parent–child relationships) evidenced by anger turned inward on self and desire to end his life.
  a. **Short-Term Goal:**
  ● Sam will verbalize anger toward boss and parents within 1 week.
  b. **Long-Term Goal:**
  ● Sam will verbalize his position in the grief process and begin movement in the progression toward resolution by discharge from treatment.

PLANNING/IMPLEMENTATION

Risk for suicide

SPECIAL FEATURES AND STATE-OF-THE-ART CONTENT

- **New** and **Updated!** Research articles support evidence–based nursing practice.

- **New** and **Updated!** Information on **psychotropic drugs** appears throughout the text, within the **medication tables**, and in the chapter on psychopharmacology.

- **New!** Clinical Pearl boxes throughout the text provide helpful tips regarding clinically relevant information.

IMPLICATIONS OF RESEARCH FOR EVIDENCE-BASED PRACTICE

Peden, A.R., Rayens, M.K., Hall, L.A., & Grant, E. (2004). Negative Thinking and the Mental Health of Low-Income Single Mothers. *Journal of Nursing Scholarship, (36)*4, 337–344.

Description of the Study: The aims of this study were to: (1) examine the prevalence of a high level of depressive symptoms in low-income, si 6 years of age, (2) evaluate sociodemographic characteri stressors, negative thinking, (3) determine whether negati of self-esteem and chronic toms. Single mothers are a p clinical depression because poverty, low self-esteem, and

---

TABLE 29–6   Medications Used in the Treatment of Bipolar Mania

Classification: Generic (Trade) Name	Daily Adult Dosage Range (mg)	Side Effects
Antimanic		
Lithium carbonate (Eskalith, Lithane; Lithobid)	Acute mania: 1800–2400 Maintenance: 900–1200	Drowsiness, dizziness, headache, dry mouth, thirst, GI upset, nausea and vomiting, fine hand tremors, hypotension, arrhythmias, polyuria, weight gain.
Anticonvulsants		
Clonazepam (Klonopin)	0.75–16	Nausea and vomiting, somnolence, dizziness, blood
Carbamazepine (Tegretol)	200–1200	dyscrasias, diplopia, headache, prolonged bleeding time
Valproic acid (Depakene; Depakote)	500–1500	(with valproic acid), risk of severe rash (with
Gabapentin (Neurontin)	900–1800	lamotrigine), decreased efficacy with oral contraceptives
Lamotrigine (Lamictal)	100–200	(with topiramate).
Topiramate (Topamax)	50–400	
Oxcarbazepine (Trileptal)	600–1200	
Calcium Channel Blocker		
Verapamil (Calan; Isoptin)	80–320	Drowsiness, dizziness, hypotension, bradycardia, nausea, constipation
Antipsychotics		
Chlorpromazine (Thorazine)	75–400	Drowsiness, dizziness, dry mouth, constipation, increased
Olanzapine (Zyprexa)	5–20	appetite, weig
Aripiprazole (Abilify)	10–30	headache (ari
Quetiapine (Seroquel)	400–800	extrapyramida
Risperidone (Risperdal)	1–6	
Ziprasidone (Geodon)	40–160	

CLINICAL PEARL

All antidepressants have varying potentials to cause discontinuation syndromes. Symptoms such as dizziness, headache, nausea, cramping, sweating, malaise, paresthesia, and rebound depression or hypomania have occurred. All antidepressant medication should be tapered gradually to prevent withdrawal symptoms.

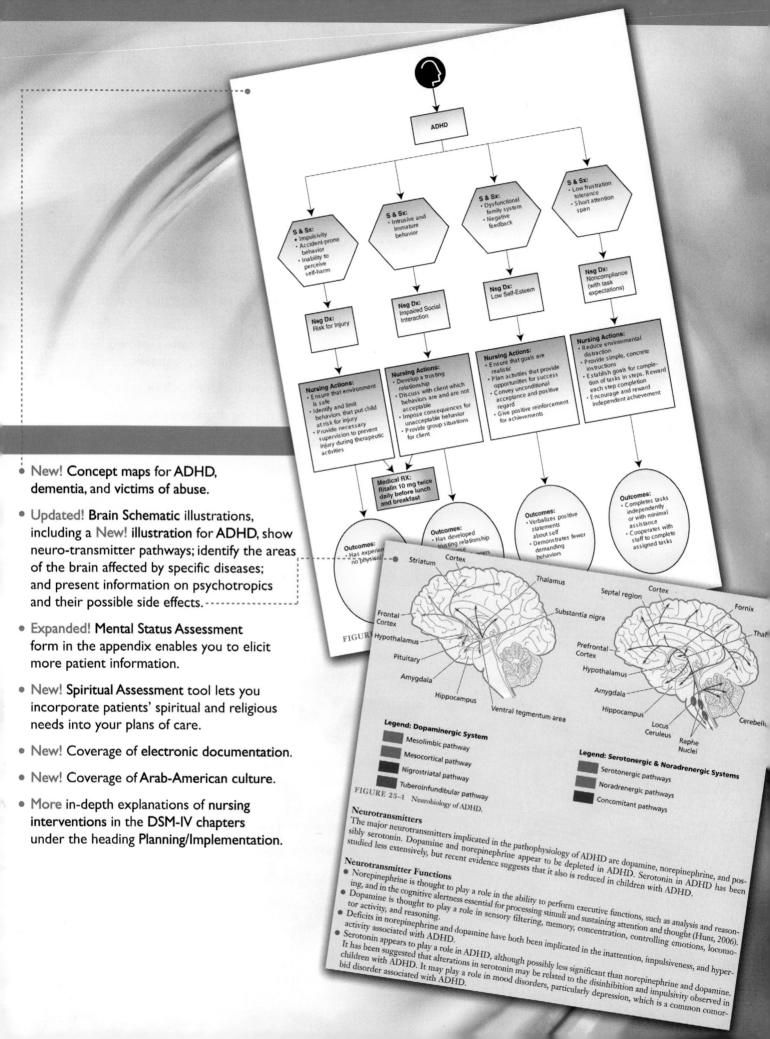

- **New! Concept maps** for ADHD, dementia, and victims of abuse.

- **Updated! Brain Schematic** illustrations, including a **New!** illustration for ADHD, show neuro-transmitter pathways; identify the areas of the brain affected by specific diseases; and present information on psychotropics and their possible side effects.

- **Expanded! Mental Status Assessment** form in the appendix enables you to elicit more patient information.

- **New! Spiritual Assessment** tool lets you incorporate patients' spiritual and religious needs into your plans of care.

- **New!** Coverage of **electronic documentation**.

- **New!** Coverage of **Arab-American culture**.

- **More** in-depth explanations of nursing interventions in the DSM-IV chapters under the heading **Planning/Implementation**.

FIGURE 25–1 Neurobiology of ADHD.

Legend: Dopaminergic System
- Mesolimbic pathway
- Mesocortical pathway
- Nigrostriatal pathway
- Tuberoinfundibular pathway

Legend: Serotonergic & Noradrenergic Systems
- Serotonergic pathways
- Noradrenergic pathways
- Concomitant pathways

Neurotransmitters

The major neurotransmitters implicated in the pathophysiology of ADHD are dopamine, norepinephrine, and possibly serotonin. Dopamine and norepinephrine appear to be depleted in ADHD. Serotonin in ADHD has been studied less extensively, but recent evidence suggests that it also is reduced in children with ADHD.

Neurotransmitter Functions
- Norepinephrine is thought to play a role in the ability to perform executive functions, such as analysis and reasoning, and in the cognitive alertness essential for processing stimuli and sustaining attention and thought (Hunt, 2006).
- Dopamine is thought to play a role in sensory filtering, memory, concentration, controlling emotions, locomotor activity, and reasoning.
- Deficits in norepinephrine and dopamine have both been implicated in the inattention, impulsiveness, and hyperactivity associated with ADHD.
- Serotonin appears to play a role in ADHD, although possibly less significant than norepinephrine and dopamine. It has been suggested that alterations in serotonin may be related to the disinhibition and impulsivity observed in children with ADHD. It may play a role in mood disorders, particularly depression, which is a common comorbid disorder associated with ADHD.

Electronic Learning and Teaching Tools

BONUS! CD-ROM in the back of the book

- Electronic Test Bank with 400 NCLEX-style questions (including the new alternate formats) can be customized by chapter and NCLEX descriptors.

- Student Workbook featuring...

  - Hundreds of Learning Activities.

  - Over 50 Psychotropic Drug Monographs to print and carry to clinical.

  - More than 20 sample Client Education Teaching Guides to photocopy and use as client/family handouts.

  - Medication Assessment Tool for levels of anxiety.

  - Table for assigning nursing diagnoses to client behaviors.

  - Care Plans.

  - And more!

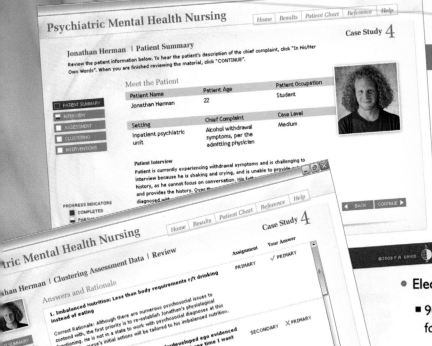

FOR INSTRUCTORS UPON ADOPTION

Instructor's Resource Disk

- Instructors Guide...

  - Chapter Focus/Objectives

  - Key Terms

  - Chapter Outline/Lecture Notes

  - Case Studies

  - Clinical Exercises and Learning Activities

- Electronic Test Bank reflecting the latest NCLEX test plan...

  - 900 NCLEX-style questions, including 100 new alternate format questions.

  - Rationales and page numbers/chapter references for both correct and incorrect answers.

- PowerPoint presentation for each chapter.

- Sample Client Teaching Guides.

- 5 brand-new Case Studies.

FREE! Online resources at DavisPlus

http://davisplus.fadavis.com

- Hundreds of interactive learning activities, many of which can be printed and emailed.

- **Concept Map Creator.**

- **Concept Map Care Plans** from the text.

- **Additional Care Plans** not in the text.

- Over 50 psychotropic drug monographs from *Davis's Drug Guide for Nurses.*

- Animated drug pathways.

- Neurobiological brain images.

- And more!

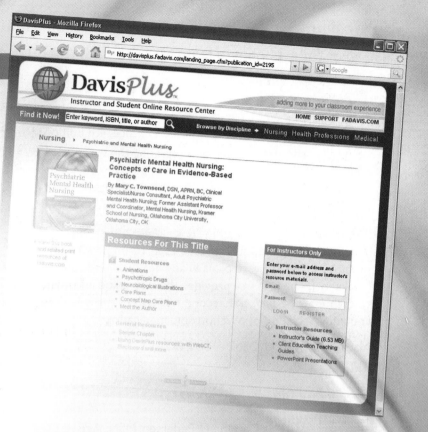

Online at DavisPlus

- All of the content from the **Instructor's Resource Disk.**

- **Resources for Online Courses**—Material from the Student CD, DavisPlus, and Instructor's Resource Disk combined into a single file for easy importation into either **Blackboard** or **Blackboard Campus Edition.**

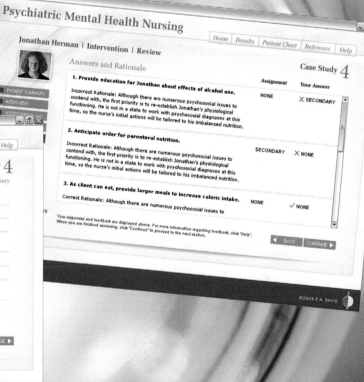

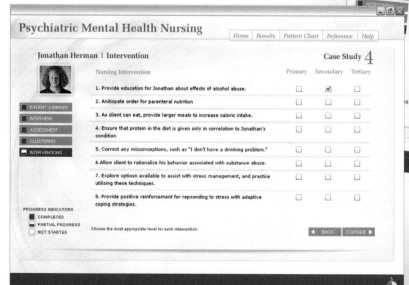

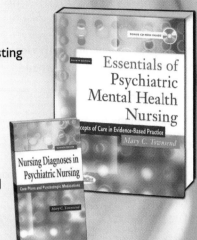
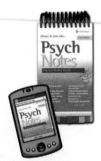
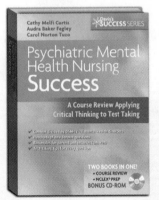
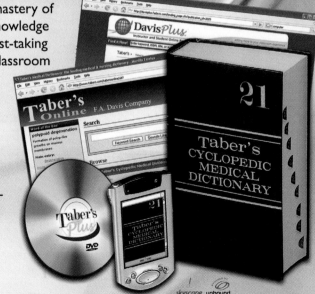

SIXTH EDITION

Psychiatric Mental Health Nursing

Concepts of Care in Evidence-Based Practice

Mary C. Townsend, DSN, APRN, BC

Clinical Specialist/Nurse Consultant
Adult Psychiatric Mental Health Nursing

Former Assistant Professor and
Coordinator, Mental Health Nursing
Kramer School of Nursing
Oklahoma City University
Oklahoma City, Oklahoma

F. A. DAVIS COMPANY • Philadelphia

F. A. Davis Company
1915 Arch Street
Philadelphia, PA 19103
www.fadavis.com

Printed in the United States of America

Last digit indicates print number: 10 9 8 7 6 5 4 3 2

Publisher, Nursing: Robert G. Martone
Senior Developmental Editor: William F. Welsh
Director of Content Development: Darlene D. Pedersen
Project Editor: Padraic J. Maroney
Art and Design Manager: Carolyn O'Brien

As new scientific information becomes available through basic and clinical research, recommended
treatments and drug therapies undergo changes. The author(s) and publisher have done everything
possible to make this book accurate, up to date, and in accord with accepted standards at the time of
publication. The author(s), editors, and publisher are not responsible for errors or omissions or for
consequences from application of the book, and make no warranty, expressed or implied, in regard to the
contents of the book. Any practice described in this book should be applied by the reader in accordance
with professional standards of care used in regard to the unique circumstances that may apply in each
situation. The reader is advised always to check product information (package inserts) for changes and
new information regarding dose and contraindications before administering any drug. Caution is
especially urged when using new or infrequently ordered drugs.

Library of Congress Cataloging-in-Publication Data

Townsend, Mary C., 1941-
  Psychiatric mental health nursing: concepts of care in evidence-based practice /
Mary C. Townsend. — 6th ed.
      p. ; cm.
  Includes bibliographical references and index.
  ISBN-13: 978-0-8036-1917-3
  ISBN-10: 0-8036-1917-0
1. Psychiatric nursing.   I. Title.
  [DNLM: 1. Psychiatric Nursing—methods.   2. Evidence-Based Medicine.   3. Mental
Disorders—nursing.   4. Psychotherapy—methods.   WY 160 T749p 2009]
  RC440.T693 2009   616.89'0231—dc22

THIS BOOK IS DEDICATED TO

FRANCIE

God made sisters for sharing laughter

and wiping tears

Consultants

Angeline Curtis, BSN, MS, APRN, BC
Clinical Nurse Specialist, Mental Health Service Line
VA Medical Center
Decatur, Georgia

Janine Graf-Kirk, RN, BC, MA
Professor and Course Coordinator for Psychiatric
    Mental Health Nursing
Trinitas School of Nursing
Elizabeth, New Jersey

Dottie Irvin, DNS, APRN, BC
Associate Professor
St. John's College
Springfield, Illinois

Phyllis M. Jacobs, RN, MSN
Assistant Professor; Director, Undergraduate
    Nursing Program
Wichita State University School of Nursing
Wichita, Kansas

Carol T. Miller, APRN-PMH, BC
Assistant Professor
Frederick Community College
Frederick, Maryland

Darlene D. Pedersen, MSN, APRN, BC
Director and Psychotherapist, PsychOptions
Philadelphia, Pennsylvania

Kathy Whitley, RN, MSN, FNP-C
Associate Professor, Nursing
Patrick Henry Community College
Martinsville, Virginia

Mara Lynn Williams, RN, BC
Program Director, Psychiatry
Intrepid USA Healthcare Services
Montgomery, Alabama

Reviewers

Teresa S. Burckhalter, MSN, RN, BC
Nursing Faculty
Technical College of the Lowcountry
Beaufort, South Carolina

Elaine Coke, RN, MSN, MBA, HCA, CCRN
Faculty Instructor
Keiser University
Fort Lauderdale, Florida

Angela Luciani, RN, BScN, MN
Nursing Instructor
Nunavut Arctic College
Iqaluit, Nunavut, Canada

Patricia Jean Hedrick Young, EdD, RN, C
Nursing Instructor
The Washington Hospital School of Nursing
Washington, Pennsylvania

Acknowledgments

Robert G. Martone, Publisher, Nursing, F. A. Davis Company, for your sense of humor and continuous optimistic outlook about the outcome of this project.

William F. Welsh, Senior Developmental Editor, Nursing, F. A. Davis Company, for all your help and support in preparing the manuscript for publication.

Cherie R. Rebar, Chair, Associate of Science Nursing Program, Kettering College of Medical Arts, and Golden M. Tradewell, Chair, Department of Nursing, Southern Arkansas University, for your assistance in preparing test questions to accompany this textbook.

Berta Steiner, Director of Production, Bermedica Production Ltd., for your support and competence in the final editing and production of the manuscript.

The nursing educators, students, and clinicians, who provide critical information about the usability of the textbook, and offer suggestions for improvements. Many changes have been made based on your input.

To those individuals who critiqued the manuscript for this edition and shared your ideas, opinions, and suggestions for enhancement. I sincerely appreciate your contributions to the final product.

My daughters, Kerry and Tina, for all the joy you have provided me and all the hope that you instill in me. I'm so thankful that I have you.

My grandchildren, Meghan and Matthew, for showing me what life is truly all about. I am blessed by your very presence.

My furry friends, Bucky, Chiro, and Angel, for the pure pleasure you bring into my life every day that you live.

My husband, Jim, who gives meaning to my life in so many ways. You are the one whose encouragement keeps me motivated, whose support gives me strength, and whose gentleness gives me comfort.

TO THE INSTRUCTOR

There is a saying that captures the spirit of our times—the only constant is change. The twenty-first century continues to bring about a great deal of change in the health care system in general and to nursing in particular. The body of knowledge in nursing continues to grow and expand as rapidly as nursing undergoes change. Nurses must draw upon this research base to support the care that they provide for their clients. This sixth edition of *Psychiatric Mental Health Nursing: Concepts of Care in Evidence-Based Practice* strives to present a holistic approach to evidenced-based psychiatric nursing practice.

Just what does this mean? Research in nursing has been alive for decades. But over the years there has always existed a significant gap between research and practice. Evidence-based nursing has become a common theme within the nursing community. It has been defined as a process by which nurses make clinical decisions using the best available **research evidence,** their **clinical expertise,** and **client preferences.** Nurses are accountable to their clients to provide the highest quality of care based on knowledge of what is considered best practice. Change occurs so rapidly that what is considered best practice today may not be considered so tomorrow, based on newly acquired scientific data.

Included in this sixth edition are a number of research studies that support psychiatric nursing interventions. As nurses, we are bombarded with new information and technological content on a daily basis. Not all of this information yields knowledge that can be used in clinical practice. It is our hope that the information in this new edition will serve to further the movement toward evidence-based practice in psychiatric nursing. There is still a long way to go, and research utilization is the foundation from which to advance the progression. Psychiatric nurses must become involved in nursing research, in disseminating research findings, and in implementing practice changes based on current evidence.

Well into the first decade of the new century, there are many new challenges to be faced. In 2002, President George W. Bush established the New Freedom Commission on Mental Health. This commission was charged with the task of conducting a comprehensive study of the United States mental health service delivery system. They were to identify unmet needs and barriers to services and recommend steps for improvement in services and support for individuals with serious mental illness. In July 2003, the commission presented its final report to the President. The Commission identified the following barriers: fragmentation and gaps in mental health care for children, adults with serious mental illness, and the elderly; and high unemployment and disability for people with serious mental illness. The report also pointed out that the fact that the U.S. has failed to identify mental health and suicide prevention as national priorities has put many lives at stake. The Commission outlined the following goals and recommendations for mental health reform:

- To address mental health with the same urgency as physical health
- To align relevant Federal programs to improve access and accountability for mental health services
- To ensure appropriate care is available for every child with a serious emotional disturbance and every adult with a serious mental illness
- To protect and enhance the rights of people with mental illness
- To improve access to quality care that is culturally competent
- To improve access to quality care in rural and geographically remote areas
- To promote mental health screening, assessment, and referral services
- To accelerate research to promote recovery and resilience, and ultimately to cure and prevent mental illness
- To advance evidence-based practices using dissemination and demonstration projects, and create a public-private partnership to guide their implementation
- To improve and expand the workforce providing evidence-based mental health services and supports
- To promote the use of technology to access mental health care and information

If these proposals become reality, it would surely mean improvement in the promotion of mental health and the care of mentally ill individuals. Many nurse leaders see this period of health care reform as an opportunity for nurses to expand their roles and assume key positions in education, prevention, assessment, and referral. Nurses are, and will continue to be, in key positions to assist individuals with mental illness to remain as independent as possible, to manage their illness within the community setting, and to strive to minimize the number of hospitalizations required.

In 2020, the ten leading causes of mortality throughout the world are projected to include heart disease; cerebrovascular disease; pulmonary disease; lower respiratory infections; tracheal, bronchial and lung cancers; traffic accidents; tuberculosis; stomach cancer; HIV/AIDS; and suicide. Behavior is an important element in prevention of these causes of mortality and in their treatment. In 2020, the three leading causes of disability throughout the world are projected to include heart disease, major depression, and traffic accidents. Behavior is once again an important underpinning of these three contributors of disability, and behavioral and social science research can lower the impact of these causes of morbidity and mortality. Many of these issues are addressed in this new edition.

CONTENT AND FEATURES NEW TO THIS EDITION

New content on Spiritual Concepts (Chapter 6). Important information on assessing the spiritual needs of clients and planning for this aspect of their care has been included. Additional cultural concepts related to **Arab Americans** has also been included.

A Brief Mental Status Evaluation Tool has been included in Chapter 9.

New content on Electronic Documentation (Chapter 9).

New medications that have become available since the last edition are included in Chapter 21, as well as in the relevant diagnosis chapters.

New content related to the neurobiology of Attention-Deficit/Hyperactivity Disorder (ADHD) (Chapter 25). Illustrations of the neurotransmitter pathways and discussion of areas of the brain affected and the medications that target those areas are presented.

Three new Concept Map Care Plans are included: ADHD (Chapter 25); Dementia (Chapter 26); and **Victims of Abuse** (Chapter 36) for a total of 16 in the text.

New content on Fetal Alcohol Syndrome (Chapter 27).

Boxes called "Clinical Pearls" have been included in selected chapters. These boxes present important facts relevant to clinical care of psychiatric clients.

A comprehensive guide for conducting the Mental Status Assessment has been included (Appendix B).

Twenty-two sample client teaching guides (Appendix G).

Nursing interventions are now included under "Planning/Implementation" section of the text. In the diagnosis chapters, nursing interventions have been identified by nursing diagnosis and included within the text portion of the chapter. **Short- and long-term goals are included for each. Nursing care plans are included for selected nursing diagnoses.** Nursing care plans have been retained in other chapters as presented in previous editions.

Case studies with sample care plans are included in the diagnosis chapters.

Chapter summaries are presented as "key points" that emphasize important facts associated with each chapter.

NANDA Taxonomy II from the *NANDA Nursing Diagnoses: Definitions & Classification 2007–2008* **(NANDA International).** Used throughout the text.

FEATURES THAT HAVE BEEN RETAINED

The major conceptual framework of stress-adaptation has been retained for its ease of comprehensibility and workability in the realm of psychiatric nursing. This framework continues to emphasize the multiple causation of mental illness while accepting the increasing biological implications in the etiology of certain disorders.

Selected research studies with implications for evidence-based practice. (In all relevant clinical chapters.)

The concept of holistic nursing is retained in the sixth edition. The author has attempted to ensure that the physical aspects of psychiatric/mental health nursing are not overlooked. In all relevant situations, the mind/body connection is addressed.

Nursing process is retained in the sixth edition as the tool for delivery of care to the individual with a psychiatric disorder or to assist in the primary prevention or exacerbation of mental illness symptoms. The six steps of the nursing process, as described in the *ANA Nursing: Scope and Standards of Practice* (2004), are used to provide guidelines for the nurse. These standards of care are included for the *DSM-IV-TR* diagnoses, as well as the aging individual, victims of abuse, the bereaved individual, and in forensic nursing practice. Other examples are included in several of the therapeutic approaches. The six steps include:

Assessment: Data collection, under the format of *Background Assessment Data: Symptomatology*, which provides extensive assessment data for the nurse to draw upon when performing an assessment. Several assessment tools are also included.

Diagnosis:	Analysis of the data is included from which nursing diagnoses common to specific psychiatric disorders are derived.
Outcome Identification:	Outcomes are derived from the nursing diagnoses and stated as measurable goals.
Planning:	Plans of care are presented (either within the text, in care plan format, or both) with selected nursing diagnoses for all *DSM-IV-TR* diagnoses, as well as for the elderly client, the elderly homebound client, the primary caregiver of the client with a chronic mental illness, forensic clients in trauma care and correctional institutions, and the bereaved individual. *Critical Pathways of Care* are included for clients in alcohol withdrawal, schizophrenic psychosis, depression, manic episode, PTSD, and anorexia nervosa. The planning standard also includes tables that list topics for educating clients and families about mental illness. **Also included: 22 concept map care plans for all major psychiatric diagnoses.**
Implementation:	The interventions that have been identified in the plan of care are included along with rationale for each. Case studies at the end of each *DSM-IV-TR* chapter assist the student in the practical application of theoretical material. Also included as a part of this particular standard is Unit Three of the textbook: ***Therapeutic Approaches in Psychiatric Nursing Care.*** This section of the textbook addresses psychiatric nursing intervention in depth, and frequently speaks to the differentiation in scope of practice between the basic level psychiatric nurse and the advanced practice level psychiatric nurse. Advanced practice nurses with prescriptive authority will find the extensive chapter on psychopharmacology particularly helpful.
Evaluation:	The evaluation standard includes a set of questions that the nurse may use to assess whether the nursing actions have been successful in achieving the objectives of care.

Tables that list topics for client education. (Clinical chapters).

Assigning nursing diagnoses to client behaviors. (Appendix E).

Internet references with web site listings for information related to psychiatric disorders (Clinical chapters).

Taxonomy and diagnostic criteria from the *DSM-IV-TR (2000)*. **Used throughout the text.**

Web site. **The F. A. Davis/Townsend website with additional nursing care plans that do not appear in the text, links to psychotropic medications, concept map care plans, and neurobiological content and illustrations.**

ADDITIONAL EDUCATIONAL RESOURCES

Faculty may also find the following teaching aids that accompany this textbook helpful:

Instructor's Resource Disk (IRD). **This IRD contains:**

- Approximately 900 multiple choice questions **(including new format questions reflecting the latest NCLEX blueprint). Most of these questions have been written at the analysis and synthesis levels.**
- Lecture outlines **for all chapters**
- Learning activities **for all chapters (including answer key)**
- Answers to the Critical Thinking Exercises **from the textbook**
- PowerPoint Presentation **to accompany all chapters in the textbook**

All chapters throughout the text have been updated and revised to reflect today's health care reformation and to provide information based on the latest current state of the discipline of nursing. It is my hope that the revisions and additions to this sixth edition continue to satisfy a need within psychiatric/mental health nursing practice. Many of the changes reflect feedback that I have received from users of the previous editions. To those individuals I express a heartfelt thanks. I welcome comments in an effort to retain what some have called the "user friendliness" of the text. I hope that this sixth edition continues to promote and advance the commitment to psychiatric/mental health nursing.

MARY C. TOWNSEND

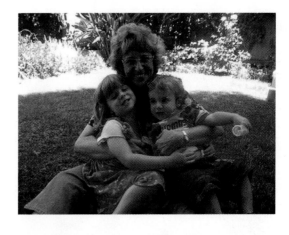

UNIT THREE
THERAPEUTIC APPROACHES IN PSYCHIATRIC NURSING CARE

CHAPTER **14**
Relaxation Therapy **220**

CHAPTER **15**
Assertiveness Training **230**

CHAPTER **16**
Promoting Self-Esteem **241**

CHAPTER 22
Electroconvulsive Therapy 336

CHAPTER 23
Complementary Therapies 344

CHAPTER 24
Client Education 361

CHAPTER 28
Schizophrenia and Other Psychotic Disorders 489

CHAPTER 32
Issues Related to Human Sexuality 619

CHAPTER 33
Eating Disorders 647

CHAPTER 34
Personality Disorders 666

UNIT FIVE

PSYCHIATRIC/MENTAL HEALTH NURSING OF SPECIAL POPULATIONS

CHAPTER 35
The Aging Individual 698

CHAPTER 36
Victims of Abuse or Neglect 726

CHAPTER 37
Community Mental Health Nursing 746

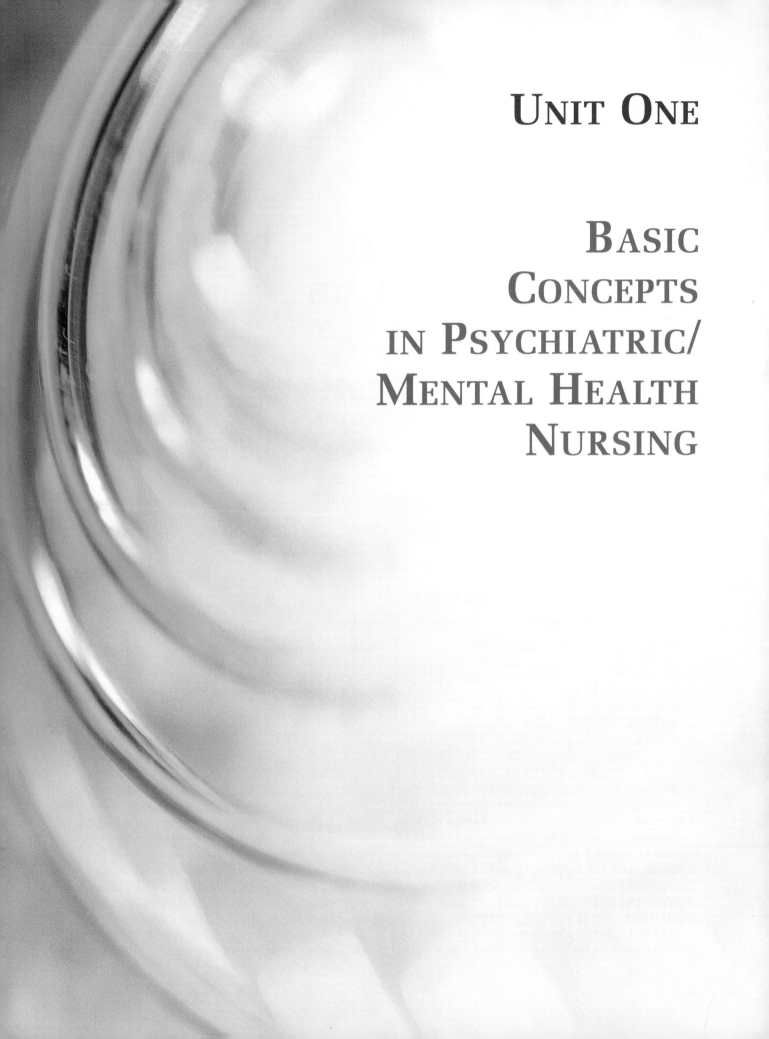

UNIT ONE

BASIC CONCEPTS IN PSYCHIATRIC/ MENTAL HEALTH NURSING

1
CHAPTER

The Concept of Stress Adaptation

CHAPTER OUTLINE

KEY TERMS

"fight or flight syndrome"
general adaptation
   syndrome
precipitating event
predisposing factors

CORE CONCEPTS

adaptation
maladaptation
stressor

OBJECTIVES

After reading this chapter, the student will be able to:

1. Define *adaptation* and *maladaptation*.
2. Identify physiological responses to stress.
3. Explain the relationship between stress and "diseases of adaptation."
4. Describe the concept of stress as an environmental event.
5. Explain the concept of stress as a transaction between the individual and the environment.
6. Discuss adaptive coping strategies in the management of stress.

Psychologists and others have struggled for many years to establish an effective definition of the term stress. This term is used loosely today and still lacks a definitive explanation. Stress may be viewed as an individual's reaction to any change that requires an adjustment or response, which can be physical, mental, or emotional. Responses directed at stabilizing internal biological processes and preserving self-esteem can be viewed as healthy adaptations to stress.

Roy (1976) defined adaptive response as behavior that maintains the integrity of the individual. Adaptation is viewed as positive and is correlated with a healthy response. When behavior disrupts the integrity of the individual, it is perceived as maladaptive. Maladaptive responses by the individual are considered to be negative or unhealthy.

Various twentieth-century researchers contributed to several different concepts of stress. Three of these concepts include stress as a biological response, stress as an environmental event, and stress as a transaction between the individual and the environment. This chapter includes an explanation of each of these concepts.

CORE CONCEPT

Stressor
A biological, psychological, social, or chemical factor that causes physical or emotional tension and may be a factor in the etiology of certain illnesses.

STRESS AS A BIOLOGICAL RESPONSE

In 1956, Hans Selye published the results of his research concerning the physiological response of a biological system to a change imposed on it. Since his initial publication, he has revised his definition of stress, calling it "the state manifested by a specific syndrome which consists of all the nonspecifically-induced changes within a biologic system" (Selye, 1976). This syndrome of symptoms has come to be known as the **"fight or flight syndrome."** Schematics of these biological responses, both initially and with sustained stress, are presented in Figures 1–1

and 1–2. Selye called this general reaction of the body to stress the **general adaptation syndrome.** He described the reaction in three distinct stages:

1. **Alarm Reaction Stage.** During this stage, the physiological responses of the "fight or flight syndrome" are initiated.
2. **Stage of Resistance.** The individual uses the physiological responses of the first stage as a defense in the attempt to adapt to the stressor. If adaptation occurs, the third stage is prevented or delayed. Physiological symptoms may disappear.
3. **Stage of Exhaustion.** This stage occurs when there is a prolonged exposure to the stressor to which the body has become adjusted. The adaptive energy is depleted, and the individual can no longer draw from the resources for adaptation described in the first two stages. Diseases of adaptation (e.g., headaches, mental disorders, coronary artery disease, ulcers, colitis) may occur. Without intervention for reversal, exhaustion ensues, and in some cases even death (Selye, 1956, 1974).

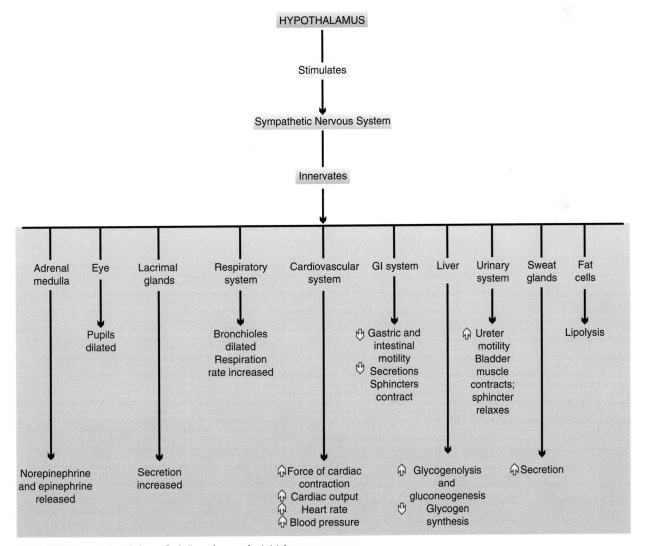

FIGURE 1–1 The "fight or flight" syndrome: the initial stress response.

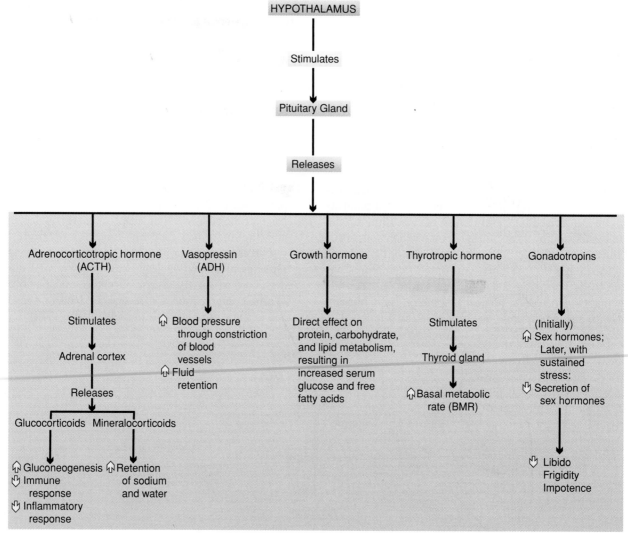

FIGURE 1–2   The "fight or flight" syndrome: the sustained stress response.

This "fight or flight" response undoubtedly served our ancestors well. Those *Homo sapiens* who had to face the giant grizzly bear or the saber-toothed tiger as part of their struggle for survival must have used these adaptive resources to their advantage. The response was elicited in emergency situations, used in the preservation of life, and followed by restoration of the compensatory mechanisms to the preemergent condition (homeostasis).

Selye performed his extensive research in a controlled setting with laboratory animals as subjects. He elicited the physiological responses with physical stimuli, such as exposure to heat or extreme cold, electric shock, injection of toxic agents, restraint, and surgical injury. Since the publication of his original research, it has become apparent that the "fight or flight" syndrome of symptoms occurs in response to psychological or emotional stimuli, just as it does to physical stimuli. The psychological or emotional stressors are often not resolved as rapidly as some physical stressors, and therefore the body may be depleted of its adaptive energy more readily than it is from physical stressors. The "fight or flight" response may be inappropriate, even dangerous, to the lifestyle of today, in which stress has been described as a psychosocial state that is pervasive, chronic, and relentless. It is this chronic response that maintains the body in the aroused condition for extended periods of time that promotes susceptibility to diseases of adaptation.

 CORE CONCEPT

Adaptation
Adaptation is said to occur when an individual's physical or behavioral response to any change in his or her internal or external environment results in preservation of individual integrity or timely return to equilibrium.

STRESS AS AN ENVIRONMENTAL EVENT

A second concept defines stress as the "thing" or "event" that triggers the adaptive physiological and psychological responses in an individual. The event creates change in the life pattern of the individual, requires significant adjustment in lifestyle, and taxes available personal resources. The change can be either positive, such as outstanding personal achievement, or negative, such as being fired from a job. The emphasis here is on *change* from the existing steady state of the individual's life pattern.

Miller and Rahe (1997) have updated the original Social Readjustment Rating Scale devised by Holmes and Rahe in 1967. Just as in the earlier version, numerical values are assigned to various events, or changes, that are common in people's lives. The updated version reflects an increased number of stressors not identified in the original version. In the new study, Miller and Rahe found that women react to life stress events at higher levels than men, and unmarried people gave higher scores than married people for most of the events. Younger subjects rated more events at a higher stress level than did older subjects. A high score on the Recent Life Changes Questionnaire (RLCQ) places the individual at greater susceptibility to physical or psychological illness. The questionnaire may be completed considering life stressors within a 6-month or 1-year period. Six-month totals equal to or greater than 300 life change units (LCUs) or 1-year totals equal to or greater than 500 LCU are considered indicative of a high level of recent life stress, thereby increasing the risk of illness for the individual. The RLCQ is presented in Table 1–1.

It is unknown whether stress overload merely predisposes a person to illness or actually precipitates it, but there does appear to be a causal link (Pelletier, 1992). Life changes questionnaires have been criticized because they do not consider the individual's perception of the event. Individuals differ in their reactions to life events, and these variations are related to the degree to which the change is perceived as stressful. These types of instruments also fail to consider the individual's coping strategies and available support systems at the time when the life change occurs. Positive coping mechanisms and strong social or familial support can reduce the intensity of the stressful life change and promote a more adaptive response.

STRESS AS A TRANSACTION BETWEEN THE INDIVIDUAL AND THE ENVIRONMENT

This definition of stress emphasizes the *relationship* between the individual and the environment. Personal characteristics and the nature of the environmental event are considered. This illustration parallels the modern concept of the etiology of disease. No longer is causation viewed solely as an external entity; whether or not illness occurs depends also on the receiving organism's susceptibility. Similarly, to predict psychological stress as a reaction, the properties of the person in relation to the environment must be considered.

Precipitating Event

Lazarus and Folkman (1984) define *stress* as a relationship between the person and the environment that is appraised by the person as taxing or exceeding his or her resources and endangering his or her well being. A **precipitating event** is a stimulus arising from the internal or external environment and is perceived by the individual in a specific manner. Determination that a particular person/environment relationship is stressful depends on the individual's cognitive appraisal of the situation. *Cognitive appraisal* is an individual's evaluation of the personal significance of the event or occurrence. The event "precipitates" a response on the part of the individual, and the response is influenced by the individual's perception of the event. The *cognitive response* consists of a primary appraisal and a secondary appraisal.

The Individual's Perception of the Event

Primary Appraisal

Lazarus and Folkman (1984) identify three types of primary appraisal: irrelevant, benign-positive, and stressful. An event is judged *irrelevant* when the outcome holds no significance for the individual. A *benign-positive* outcome is one that is perceived as producing pleasure for the individual. *Stress* appraisals include harm/loss, threat, and challenge. *Harm/loss* appraisals refer to damage or loss already experienced by the individual. Appraisals of a *threatening* nature are perceived as anticipated harms or losses. When an event is appraised as *challenging*, the individual focuses on potential for gain or growth, rather than on risks associated with the event. Challenge produces stress even though the emotions associated with it (eagerness and excitement) are viewed as positive, and coping mechanisms must be called upon to face the new encounter. Challenge and threat may occur together when an individual experiences these positive emotions along with fear or anxiety over possible risks associated with the challenging event.

When stress is produced in response to harm/loss, threat, or challenge, a secondary appraisal is made by the individual.

Secondary Appraisal

This secondary appraisal is an assessment of skills, resources, and knowledge that the person possesses to

TABLE 1-1	The Recent Life Changes Questionnaire			
Life Change Event	**LCU**	**Life Change Event**		**LCU**
Health		**Home and Family**		
An injury or illness which:		Major change in living conditions		42
Kept you in bed a week or more, or sent you to the hospital	74	Change in residence:		
Was less serious than above	44	Move within the same town or city		25
Major dental work	26	Move to a different town, city, or state		47
Major change in eating habits	27	Change in family get-togethers		25
Major change in sleeping habits	26	Major change in health or behavior of family member		55
Major change in your usual type/amount of recreation	28	Marriage		50
Work		Pregnancy		67
Change to a new type of work	51	Miscarriage or abortion		65
Change in your work hours or conditions	35	Gain of a new family member:		
Change in your responsibilities at work:		Birth of a child		66
More responsibilities	29	Adoption of a child		65
Fewer responsibilities	21	A relative moving in with you		59
Promotion	31	Spouse beginning or ending work		46
Demotion	42	Child leaving home:		
Transfer	32	To attend college		41
Troubles at work:		Due to marriage		41
With your boss	29	For other reasons		45
With coworkers	35	Change in arguments with spouse		50
With persons under your supervision	35	In-law problems		38
Other work troubles	28	Change in the marital status of your parents:		
Major business adjustment	60	Divorce		59
Retirement	52	Remarriage		50
Loss of job:		Separation from spouse:		
Laid off from work	68	Due to work		53
Fired from work	79	Due to marital problems		76
Correspondence course to help you in your work	18	Divorce		96
Personal and Social		Birth of grandchild		43
Change in personal habits	26	Death of spouse		119
Beginning or ending school or college	38	Death of other family member:		
Change of school or college	35	Child		123
Change in political beliefs	24	Brother or sister		102
Change in religious beliefs	29	Parent		100
Change in social activities	27	**Financial**		
Vacation	24	Major change in finances:		
New, close, personal relationship	37	Increased income		38
Engagement to marry	45	Decreased income		60
Girlfriend or boyfriend problems	39	Investment and/or credit difficulties		56
Sexual difficulties	44	Loss or damage of personal property		43
"Falling out" of a close personal relationship	47	Moderate purchase		20
An accident	48	Major purchase		37
Minor violation of the law	20	Foreclosure on a mortgage or loan		58
Being held in jail	75			
Death of a close friend	70			
Major decision regarding your immediate future	51			
Major personal achievement	36			

SOURCE: Miller and Rahe (1997), with permission.

deal with the situation. The individual evaluates by considering the following:

● Which coping strategies are available to me?
● Will the option I choose be effective in this situation?
● Do I have the ability to use that strategy in an effective manner?

The interaction between the primary appraisal of the event that has occurred and the secondary appraisal of available coping strategies determines the quality of the individual's adaptation response to stress.

Predisposing Factors

A variety of elements influence how an individual perceives and responds to a stressful event. These **predisposing factors** strongly influence whether the response is adaptive or maladaptive. Types of predisposing factors include genetic influences, past experiences, and existing conditions.

Genetic influences are those circumstances of an individual's life that are acquired through heredity. Examples include family history of physical and psychological conditions (strengths and weaknesses) and temperament (behavioral characteristics present at birth that evolve with development).

Past experiences are occurrences that result in learned patterns that can influence an individual's adaptation response. They include previous exposure to the stressor or other stressors, learned coping responses, and degree of adaptation to previous stressors.

Existing conditions incorporate vulnerabilities that influence the adequacy of the individual's physical, psychological, and social resources for dealing with adaptive demands. Examples include current health status, motivation, developmental maturity, severity and duration of the stressor, financial and educational resources, age, existing coping strategies, and a support system of caring others.

This transactional model of stress/adaptation will serve as a framework for the process of nursing in this text. A graphic display of the model is presented in Figure 1–3.

CORE CONCEPT

Maladaptation

Maladaptation occurs when an individual's physical or behavioral response to any change in his or her internal or external environment results in disruption of individual integrity or in persistent disequilibrium.

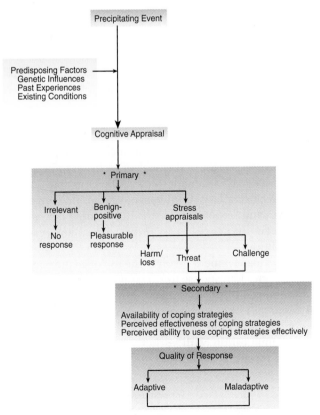

FIGURE 1–3 Transactional model of stress/adaptation.

STRESS MANAGEMENT*

The growth of stress management into a multimillion-dollar-a-year business attests to its importance in our society. Stress management involves the use of coping strategies in response to stressful situations. Coping strategies are adaptive when they protect the individual from harm (or additional harm) or strengthen the individual's ability to meet challenging situations. Adaptive responses help restore homeostasis to the body and impede the development of diseases of adaptation.

Coping strategies are considered maladaptive when the conflict being experienced goes unresolved or intensifies. Energy resources become depleted as the body struggles to compensate for the chronic physiological and psychological arousal being experienced. The effect is a significant vulnerability to physical or psychological illness.

Adaptive Coping Strategies

Awareness

The initial step in managing stress is awareness—to become aware of the factors that create stress and the feelings associated with a stressful response. Stress can be controlled only when one recognizes that it is being experienced. As one becomes aware of stressors, he or she can omit, avoid, or accept them.

Relaxation

Individuals experience relaxation in different ways. Some individuals relax by engaging in large motor activities, such as sports, jogging, and physical exercise. Still others use techniques such as breathing exercises and progressive relaxation to relieve stress. (A discussion of relaxation therapy can be found in Chapter 14.)

Meditation

Practiced 20 minutes once or twice daily, meditation has been shown to produce a lasting reduction in blood pressure and other stress-related symptoms (Davis, Eshelman, & McKay, 2008). Meditation involves assuming a comfortable position, closing the eyes, casting off all other thoughts, and concentrating on a single word, sound, or phrase that has positive meaning to the individual. The technique is described in detail in Chapter 14.

Interpersonal Communication with Caring Other

As previously mentioned, the strength of one's available support systems is an existing condition that significantly influences the adaptiveness of coping with stress.

---

*Techniques of stress management are discussed at greater length in Unit 3 of this text.

Sometimes just "talking the problem out" with an individual who is empathetic is sufficient to interrupt escalation of the stress response. Writing about one's feelings in a journal or diary can also be therapeutic.

Problem Solving

An extremely adaptive coping strategy is to view the situation objectively (or to seek assistance from another individual to accomplish this if the anxiety level is too high to concentrate). After an objective assessment of the situation, the problem-solving/decision-making model can be instituted as follows:

- Assess the facts of the situation.
- Formulate goals for resolution of the stressful situation.
- Study the alternatives for dealing with the situation.
- Determine the risks and benefits of each alternative.
- Select an alternative.
- Implement the alternative selected.
- Evaluate the outcome of the alternative implemented.
- If the first choice is ineffective, select and implement a second option.

Pets

Studies show that those who care for pets, especially dogs and cats, are better able to cope with the stressors of life (Allen, Blascovich, & Mendes, 2002; Barker et al., 2005). The physical act of stroking or petting a dog or cat can be therapeutic. It gives the animal an intuitive sense of being cared for and at the same time gives the individual the calming feeling of warmth, affection, and interdependence with a reliable, trusting being. One study showed that among people who had had heart attacks, pet owners had one-fifth the death rate of those who did not have pets (Friedmann & Thomas, 1995). Another study revealed evidence that individuals experienced a statistically significant drop in blood pressure in response to petting a dog or cat (Whitaker, 2000).

Music

It is true that music can "soothe the savage beast." Creating and listening to music stimulate motivation, enjoyment, and relaxation. Music can reduce depression and bring about measurable changes in mood and general activity.

SUMMARY AND KEY POINTS

- Stress has become a chronic and pervasive condition in the United States today.
- Adaptive behavior is viewed as behavior that maintains the integrity of the individual, with a timely return to equilibrium. It is viewed as positive and is correlated with a healthy response.

- When behavior disrupts the integrity of the individual or results in persistent disequilibrium, it is perceived as maladaptive. Maladaptive responses by the individual are considered to be negative or unhealthy.
- A stressor is defined as a biological, psychological, social, or chemical factor that causes physical or emotional tension and may be a factor in the etiology of certain illnesses.
- Hans Selye identified the biological changes associated with a stressful situation as the "fight or flight syndrome."
- Selye called the general reaction of the body to stress the "general adaptation syndrome," which occurs in three stages: the alarm reaction stage, the stage of resistance, and the stage of exhaustion.
- When individuals remain in the aroused response to stress for an extended period of time, they become susceptible to diseases of adaptation, some examples of which include headaches, mental disorders, coronary artery disease, ulcers, and colitis.
- Stress may also be viewed as an environmental event. This results when a change from the existing steady state of the individual's life pattern occurs.
- When an individual experiences a high level of life change events, he or she becomes susceptible to physical or psychological illness.
- Limitations of this concept of stress include failure to consider the individual's perception of the event, coping strategies, and available support systems at the time when the life change occurs.
- Stress is more appropriately expressed as a transaction between the individual and the environment that is appraised by the individual as taxing or exceeding his or her resources and endangering his or her well being.
- The individual makes a cognitive appraisal of the precipitating event to determine the personal significance of the event or occurrence.
- Primary cognitive appraisals may be irrelevant, benign-positive, or stressful.
- Secondary cognitive appraisals include assessment and evaluation by the individual of skills, resources, and knowledge to deal with the stressful situation.
- Predisposing factors influence how an individual perceives and responds to a stressful event. They include genetic influences, past experiences, and existing conditions.
- Stress management involves the use of adaptive coping strategies in response to stressful situations in an effort to impede the development of diseases of adaptation.
- Examples of adaptive coping strategies include developing awareness, relaxation, meditation, interpersonal communication with caring other, problem solving, pets, music, and others.

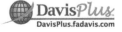

REVIEW QUESTIONS

Self-Examination/Learning Exercise

Select the answer that is most appropriate for questions 1 through 4.

1. Sondra, who lives in Maine, hears on the evening news that 25 people were killed in a tornado in south Texas. Sondra experiences no anxiety upon hearing of this stressful situation. This is most likely because Sondra:

   a. Is selfish and does not care what happens to other people.
   b. Appraises the event as irrelevant to her own situation.
   c. Assesses that she has the skills to cope with the stressful situation.
   d. Uses suppression as her primary defense mechanism.

2. Cindy regularly develops nausea and vomiting when she is faced with a stressful situation. Which of the following is most likely a predisposing factor to this maladaptive response by Cindy?

   a. Cindy inherited her mother's "nervous" stomach.
   b. Cindy is fixed in a lower level of development.
   c. Cindy has never been motivated to achieve success.
   d. When Cindy was a child, her mother pampered her and kept her home from school when she was ill.

3. When an individual's stress response is sustained over a long period, the endocrine system involvement results in which of the following?

   a. Decreased resistance to disease.
   b. Increased libido
   c. Decreased blood pressure.
   d. Increased inflammatory response.

4. Management of stress is extremely important in today's society because:

   a. Evolution has diminished human capability for "fight or flight."
   b. The stressors of today tend to be ongoing, resulting in a sustained response.
   c. We have stress disorders that did not exist in the days of our ancestors.
   d. One never knows when one will have to face a grizzly bear or saber-toothed tiger in today's society.

5. Match each of the following situations to its correct component of the Transactional Model of Stress/Adaptation.

   __c__ 1. Mr. T is fixed in a lower level of development.   a. Precipitating stressor

   __d__ 2. Mr. T's father had diabetes mellitus.   b. Past experiences

   __b__ 3. Mr. T has been fired from his last five jobs.   c. Existing conditions

   __a__ 4. Mr. T's baby was stillborn last month.   d. Genetic influences

6. Match the following types of primary appraisals to their correct definition of the event as perceived by the individual.

   _____ 1. Irrelevant   a. Perceived as producing pleasure

   _____ 2. Benign-positive   b. Perceived as anticipated harms or losses

   _____ 3. Harm/loss   c. Perceived as potential for gain or growth

   _____ 4. Threat   d. Perceived as having no significance to the individual.

   _____ 5. Challenge   e. Perceived as damage or loss already experienced

R E F E R E N C E S

Allen, K., Blascovich, J., & Mendes, W.B. (2002). Cardiovascular reactivity and the presence of pets, friends, and spouses: The truth about cats and dogs. *Psychosomatic Medicine, 64,* 727–739.

Barker, S.B., Knisely, J.S., McCain, N.L., & Best, A.M. (2005). Measuring stress and immune response in healthcare professionals following interaction with a therapy dog: A pilot study. *Psychological Reports, 96,* 713–729.

Davis, M.D., Eshelman, E.R., & McKay, M. (2008). *The relaxation and stress reduction workbook* (6th ed.). Oakland, CA: New Harbinger Publications.

Friedmann, E., & Thomas, S.A. (1995). Pet ownership, social support, and one-year survival after acute myocardial infarction in the cardiac arrhythmia suppression trial. *American Journal of Cardiology, 76*(17), 1213.

Miller, M.A., & Rahe, R.H. (1997). Life changes scaling for the 1990s. *Journal of Psychosomatic Research, 43*(3), 279–292.

Pelletier, K.R. (1992). *Mind as healer, mind as slayer: A holistic approach to preventing stress disorders.* New York: Dell.

Whitaker, J. (2000). Pet owners are a healthy breed. *Health & Healing, 10*(10), 1–8.

C L A S S I C A L   R E F E R E N C E S

Holmes, T., & Rahe, R. (1967). The social readjustment rating scale. *Journal of Psychosomatic Research, 11,* 213–218.

Lazarus, R.S., & Folkman, S. (1984). *Stress, appraisal and coping.* New York: Springer.

Roy, C. (1976). *Introduction to nursing: An adaptation model.* Englewood Cliffs, NJ: Prentice-Hall.

Selye, H. (1956). *The stress of life.* New York: McGraw-Hill.

Selye, H. (1974). *Stress without distress.* New York: Signet Books.

Selye, H. (1976). *The stress of life* (rev. ed.). New York: McGraw Hill.

Mental Health/Mental Illness: Historical and Theoretical Concepts

CHAPTER OUTLINE

OBJECTIVES

HISTORICAL OVERVIEW OF PSYCHIATRIC CARE

MENTAL HEALTH

MENTAL ILLNESS

PSYCHOLOGICAL ADAPTATION TO STRESS

MENTAL HEALTH/MENTAL ILLNESS CONTINUUM

THE *DSM-IV-TR* MULTIAXIAL EVALUATION SYSTEM

SUMMARY AND KEY POINTS

REVIEW QUESTIONS

KEY TERMS

anticipatory grieving
bereavement overload
defense mechanisms
   compensation
   denial
   displacement
   identification
   intellectualization
   introjection
   isolation
   projection
   rationalization

reaction formation
regression
repression
sublimation
suppression
undoing
humors
mental health
mental illness
neurosis
psychosis
"ship of fools"

CORE CONCEPTS

anxiety
grief

OBJECTIVES

After reading this chapter, the student will be able to:

1. Discuss the history of psychiatric care.
2. Define *mental health* and *mental illness*.
3. Discuss cultural elements that influence attitudes toward mental health and mental illness.
4. Describe psychological adaptation responses to stress.
5. Identify correlation of adaptive/maladaptive behaviors to the mental health/mental illness continuum.

The consideration of mental health and mental illness has its basis in the cultural beliefs of the society in which the behavior takes place. Some cultures are quite liberal in the range of behaviors that are considered acceptable, whereas others have very little tolerance for behaviors that deviate from the cultural norms.

A study of the history of psychiatric care reveals some shocking truths about past treatment of mentally ill individuals. Many were kept in control by means that today could be considered less than humane.

This chapter deals with the evolution of psychiatric care from ancient times to the present. **Mental health** and **mental illness** are defined, and the psychological adaptation to stress is explained in terms of the two major responses: anxiety and grief. A mental health/mental illness continuum and the *Diagnostic and Statistical Manual of Mental Disorders, 4th edition, Text Revision (DSM-IV-TR),* multiaxial evaluation system are presented.

HISTORICAL OVERVIEW OF PSYCHIATRIC CARE

Primitive beliefs regarding mental disturbances took several views. Some thought that an individual with mental illness had been dispossessed of his or her soul and that the only way wellness could be achieved was if the soul returned. Others believed that evil spirits or supernatural or magical powers had entered the body. The "cure" for these individuals involved a ritualistic exorcism to purge the body of these unwanted forces. This often consisted of brutal beatings, starvation, or other torturous means. Still others considered that the mentally ill individual may have broken a taboo or sinned against another individual or God, for which ritualistic purification was required or various types of retribution were demanded. The correlation of mental illness to demonology or witchcraft led to some mentally ill individuals being burned at the stake.

The position of these ancient beliefs evolved with increasing knowledge about mental illness and changes in cultural, religious, and sociopolitical attitudes. The work of Hippocrates, about 400 B.C., began the movement away from belief in the supernatural. Hippocrates associated insanity and mental illness with an irregularity in the interaction of the four body fluids—blood, black bile, yellow bile, and phlegm. He called these body fluids **humors,** and associated each with a particular disposition. Disequilibrium among these four humors was thought to cause mental illness, and it was often treated by inducing vomiting and diarrhea with potent cathartic drugs.

During the Middle Ages (A.D. 500 to 1500), the association of mental illness with witchcraft and the supernatural continued to prevail in Europe. During this period, many severely mentally ill people were sent out to sea on sailing boats with little guidance to search for their lost rationality. The expression **"ship of fools"** was derived from this operation.

During the same period in the Middle Eastern Islamic countries, however, a change in attitude began to occur, from the perception of mental illness as the result of witchcraft or the supernatural to the idea that these individuals were actually ill. This notion gave rise to the establishment of special units for the mentally ill within general hospitals, as well as institutions specifically designed to house the insane. They can likely be considered the first asylums for the mentally ill.

Colonial Americans tended to reflect the attitudes of the European communities from which they had immigrated. Particularly in the New England area, individuals were punished for behavior attributed to witchcraft. In the 16th and 17th centuries, institutions for the mentally ill did not exist in the United States, and care of these individuals became a family responsibility. Those without family or other resources became the responsibility of the communities in which they lived and were incarcerated in places where they could do no harm to themselves or others.

The first hospital in America to admit mentally ill clients was established in Philadelphia in the middle of the 18th century. Benjamin Rush, often called the father of American psychiatry, was a physician at the hospital. He initiated the provision of humanistic treatment and care for the mentally ill. Although he included kindness, exercise, and socialization, he also employed harsher methods such as bloodletting, purging, various types of physical restraints, and extremes of temperatures, reflecting the medical therapies of that era.

The 19th century brought the establishment of a system of state asylums, largely the result of the work of Dorothea Dix, a former New England schoolteacher, who lobbied tirelessly on behalf of the mentally ill population. She was unfaltering in her belief that mental illness was curable and that state hospitals should provide humanistic therapeutic care. This system of hospital care for the mentally ill grew, but the mentally ill population grew faster. The institutions became overcrowded and understaffed, and conditions deteriorated. Therapeutic care reverted to custodial care. These state hospitals provided the largest resource for the mentally ill until the initiation of the community health movement of the 1960s (see Chapter 37).

The emergence of psychiatric nursing began in 1873 with the graduation of Linda Richards from the nursing program at the New England Hospital for Women and Children in Boston. She has come to be known as the first American psychiatric nurse. During her career, Richards was instrumental in the establishment of a number of psychiatric hospitals and the first school of psychiatric nursing at the McLean Asylum in Waverly, Massachusetts, in 1882. The focus in this school, and those that followed, was "training" in how to provide custodial care for clients in psychiatric asylums—training that did not include the study of psychological concepts. Significant change did not occur until 1955, when incorporation of psychiatric nursing into their curricula became a requirement for all undergraduate schools of nursing.

Nursing curricula emphasized the importance of the nurse-patient relationship and therapeutic communication techniques. Nursing intervention in the somatic therapies (e.g., insulin and electroconvulsive therapy) provided impetus for the incorporation of these concepts into nursing's body of knowledge.

With the apparently increasing need for psychiatric care in the aftermath of World War II, the government passed the National Mental Health Act of 1946. This legislation provided funds for the education of psychiatrists, psychologists, social workers, and psychiatric nurses. Graduate-level education in psychiatric nursing was established during this period. Also significant at this time was the introduction of antipsychotic medications, which made it possible for psychotic clients to more readily participate in their treatment, including nursing therapies.

Knowledge of the history of psychiatric/mental health care contributes to the understanding of the concepts presented in this chapter and those in Chapter 3, which describe the theories of personality development according to various 19th-century and 20th-century leaders in the psychiatric/mental health movement. Modern

American psychiatric care has its roots in ancient times. A great deal of opportunity exists for continued advancement of this specialty within the practice of nursing.

MENTAL HEALTH

A number of theorists have attempted to define the concept of mental health. Many of these concepts deal with various aspects of individual functioning. Maslow (1970) emphasized an individual's motivation in the continuous quest for self-actualization. He identified a "hierarchy of needs," the lower ones requiring fulfillment before those at higher levels can be achieved, with self-actualization being fulfillment of one's highest potential. An individual's position within the hierarchy may reverse from a higher level to a lower level based on life circumstances. For example, an individual facing major surgery who has been working on tasks to achieve self-actualization may become preoccupied, if only temporarily, with the need for physiological safety. A representation of this needs hierarchy is presented in Figure 2–1.

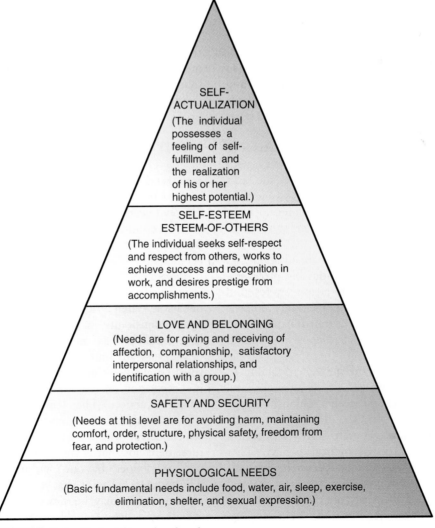

FIGURE 2–1 Maslow's hierarchy of needs.

Maslow described self-actualization as being "psychologically healthy, fully human, highly evolved, and fully mature." He believed that "healthy," or "self-actualized," individuals possessed the following characteristics:

- An appropriate perception of reality
- The ability to accept oneself, others, and human nature
- The ability to manifest spontaneity
- The capacity for focusing concentration on problem solving
- A need for detachment and desire for privacy
- Independence, autonomy, and a resistance to enculturation
- An intensity of emotional reaction
- A frequency of "peak" experiences that validates the worthwhileness, richness, and beauty of life
- An identification with humankind
- The ability to achieve satisfactory interpersonal relationships
- A democratic character structure and strong sense of ethics
- Creativeness
- A degree of nonconformance

Jahoda (1958) has identified a list of six indicators that she suggests are a reflection of mental health:

1. **A Positive Attitude Toward Self.** This includes an objective view of self, including knowledge and acceptance of strengths and limitations. The individual feels a strong sense of personal identity and a security within the environment.
2. **Growth, Development, and the Ability to Achieve Self-actualization.** This indicator correlates with whether the individual successfully achieves the tasks associated with each level of development (see Erikson, Chapter 3). With successful achievement in each level the individual gains motivation for advancement to his or her highest potential.
3. **Integration.** The focus here is on maintaining an equilibrium or balance among various life processes. Integration includes the ability to adaptively respond to the environment and the development of a philosophy of life, both of which help the individual maintain anxiety at a manageable level in response to stressful situations.
4. **Autonomy.** This refers to the individual's ability to perform in an independent, self-directed manner. The individual makes choices and accepts responsibility for the outcomes.
5. **Perception of Reality.** Accurate reality perception is a positive indicator of mental health. This includes perception of the environment without distortion, as well as the capacity for empathy and social sensitivity—a respect and concern for the wants and needs of others.

6. **Environmental Mastery.** This indicator suggests that the individual has achieved a satisfactory role within the group, society, or environment. It suggests that he or she is able to love and accept the love of others. When faced with life situations, the individual is able to strategize, make decisions, change, adjust, and adapt. Life offers satisfaction to the individual who has achieved environmental mastery.

The American Psychiatric Association (APA, 2003) defines mental health as:

A state of being that is relative rather than absolute. The successful performance of mental functions shown by productive activities, fulfilling relationships with other people, and the ability to adapt to change and to cope with adversity.

Robinson (1983) has offered the following definition of mental health:

a dynamic state in which thought, feeling, and behavior that is age-appropriate and congruent with the local and cultural norms is demonstrated. (p. 74)

For purposes of this text, and in keeping with the framework of stress/adaptation, a modification of Robinson's definition of mental health is considered. Thus, *mental health* is viewed as the successful adaptation to stressors from the internal or external environment, evidenced by thoughts, feelings, and behaviors that are age-appropriate and congruent with local and cultural norms.

MENTAL ILLNESS

A universal concept of mental illness is difficult, because of the cultural factors that influence such a definition. However, certain elements are associated with individuals' perceptions of mental illness, regardless of cultural origin. Horwitz (2002) identifies two of these elements as (1) incomprehensibility and (2) cultural relativity.

Incomprehensibility relates to the inability of the general population to understand the motivation behind the behavior. When observers are unable to find meaning or comprehensibility in behavior, they are likely to label that behavior as mental illness. Horwitz states, "Observers attribute labels of mental illness when the rules, conventions, and understandings they use to interpret behavior fail to find any intelligible motivation behind an action." The element of *cultural relativity* considers that these rules, conventions, and understandings are conceived within an individual's own particular culture. Behavior that is considered "normal" and "abnormal" is defined by one's cultural or societal norms. Therefore, a behavior that is recognized as mentally ill in one society may be viewed as "normal" in another society, and vice versa. Horwitz identified a number of cultural aspects of mental illness, which are presented in Box 2–1.

In the *DSM-IV-TR* (American Psychiatric Association [APA], 2000), the APA defined mental illness or a mental disorder as

a clinically significant behavioral or psychological syndrome or pattern that occurs in a person and that is associated with present distress (e.g., a painful symptom) or disability (i.e., impairment in one or more important areas of functioning), or with a significantly increased risk of suffering death, pain, disability, or an important loss of freedom . . . and is not merely an expectable and culturally sanctioned response to a particular event (e.g., the death of a loved one). (p. xxxi)

For purposes of this text, and in keeping with the framework of stress/adaptation, *mental illness* will be characterized as maladaptive responses to stressors from the internal or external environment, evidenced by thoughts, feelings, and behaviors that are incongruent with the local and cultural norms, and interfere with the individual's social, occupational, and/or physical functioning.

PSYCHOLOGICAL ADAPTATION TO STRESS

All individuals exhibit some characteristics associated with both mental health and mental illness at any given point in time. Chapter 1 described how an individual's response to stressful situations was influenced by his or her personal perception of the event and a variety of predisposing factors, such as heredity, temperament, learned response patterns, developmental maturity, existing coping strategies, and support systems of caring others.

Anxiety and grief have been described as two major, primary psychological response patterns to stress. A variety of thoughts, feelings, and behaviors are associated with each of these response patterns. Adaptation is determined by the degree to which the thoughts, feelings, and behaviors interfere with an individual's functioning.

CORE CONCEPT

Anxiety
A diffuse apprehension that is vague in nature and is associated with feelings of uncertainty and helplessness.

Anxiety

Feelings of anxiety are so common in our society that they are almost considered universal. Anxiety arises from the chaos and confusion that exists in the world today. Fears of the unknown and conditions of ambiguity offer

BOX 2–1 Cultural Aspects of Mental Illness

1. Usually members of the lay community, rather than a psychiatric professional, initially recognize that an individual's behavior deviates from the societal norms.
2. People who are related to an individual or who are of the same cultural or social group are less likely to label an individual's behavior as mentally ill than someone who is relationally or culturally distant. Relatives (or people of the same cultural or social group) try to "normalize" the behavior; that is, they try to find an explanation for the behavior.
3. Psychiatrists see a person with mental illness most often when the family members can no longer deny the illness and often when the behavior is at its worst. The local or cultural norms define pathological behavior.
4. Individuals in the lowest social class usually display the highest amount of mental illness symptoms. However, they tend to tolerate a wider range of behaviors that deviate from societal norms and are less likely to consider these behaviors as indicative of mental illness. Mental illness labels are most often applied by psychiatric professionals.
5. The higher the social class, the greater the recognition of mental illness behaviors. Members of the higher social classes are likely to be self-labeled or labeled by family members or friends. Psychiatric assistance is sought near the first signs of emotional disturbance.
6. The more highly educated the person, the greater the recognition of mental illness behaviors. However, even more relevant than the *amount* of education is the *type* of education. Individuals in the more humanistic types of professions (lawyers, social workers, artists, teachers, nurses) are more likely to seek psychiatric assistance than professionals such as business executives, computer specialists, accountants, and engineers.
7. In terms of religion, Jewish people are more likely to seek psychiatric assistance than are Catholics or Protestants.
8. Women are more likely than men to recognize the symptoms of mental illness and seek assistance.
9. The greater the cultural distance from the *mainstream* of society (i.e., the fewer the ties with *conventional* society), the greater the likelihood of negative response by society to mental illness. For example, immigrants have a greater distance from the mainstream than the native born, blacks greater than whites, and "bohemians" greater than bourgeoisie. They are more likely to be subjected to coercive treatment, and involuntary psychiatric commitments are more common.

SOURCE: Adapted from Horwitz (2002).

a perfect breeding ground for anxiety to take root and grow. Low levels of anxiety are adaptive and can provide the motivation required for survival. Anxiety becomes problematic when the individual is unable to prevent the anxiety from escalating to a level that interferes with the ability to meet basic needs.

Peplau (1963) described four levels of anxiety: mild, moderate, severe, and panic. It is important for nurses to be able to recognize the symptoms associated with each level to plan for appropriate intervention with anxious individuals.

TABLE 2–1	Levels of Anxiety			
Level	Perceptual Field	Ability to Learn	Physical Characteristics	Emotional/Behavioral Characteristics
Mild	Heightened perception (e.g., noises may seem louder; details within the environment are clearer) Increased awareness Increased alertness	Learning is enhanced	Restlessness Irritability	May remain superficial with others. Rarely experienced as distressful. Motivation is increased.
Moderate	Reduction in perceptual field. Reduced alertness to environmental events (e.g., someone talking may not be heard; part of the room may not be noticed)	Learning still occurs, but not at optimal ability. Decreased attention span. Decreased ability to concentrate.	Increased restlessness. Increased heart and respiration rate. Increased perspiration. Gastric discomfort. Increased muscular tension. Increase in speech rate, volume, and pitch.	A feeling of discontent. May lead to a degree of impairment in interpersonal relationships as individual begins to focus on self and the need to relieve personal discomfort.
Severe	Greatly diminished; only extraneous details are perceived, or fixation on a single detail may occur. May not take notice of an event even when attention is directed by another	Extremely limited attention span. Unable to concentrate or problem-solve. Effective learning cannot occur.	Headaches Dizziness Nausea Trembling Insomnia Palpitations Tachycardia Hyperventilation Urinary frequency Diarrhea	Feelings of dread, loathing, horror Total focus on self and intense desire to relieve the anxiety.
Panic	Unable to focus on even one detail within the environment. Misperceptions of the environment common (e.g., a perceived detail may be elaborated and out of proportion)	Learning cannot occur. Unable to concentrate. Unable to comprehend even simple directions.	Dilated pupils Labored breathing Severe trembling Sleeplessness Palpitations Diaphoresis and pallor Muscular incoordination Immobility or purposeless hyperactivity Incoherence or inability to verbalize	Sense of impending doom. Terror Bizarre behavior, including shouting, screaming, running about wildly, clinging to anyone or anything from which a sense of safety and security is derived. Hallucinations; delusions. Extreme withdrawal into self.

- **Mild Anxiety.** This level of anxiety is seldom a problem for the individual. It is associated with the tension experienced in response to the events of day-to-day living. Mild anxiety prepares people for action. It sharpens the senses, increases motivation for productivity, increases the perceptual field, and results in a heightened awareness of the environment. Learning is enhanced and the individual is able to function at his or her optimal level.
- **Moderate Anxiety.** As the level of anxiety increases, the extent of the perceptual field diminishes. The moderately anxious individual is less alert to events occurring in the environment. The individual's attention span and ability to concentrate decrease, although he or she may still attend to needs with direction. Assistance with problem solving may be required. Increased muscular tension and restlessness are evident.

- **Severe Anxiety.** The perceptual field of the severely anxious individual is so greatly diminished that concentration centers on one particular detail only or on many extraneous details. Attention span is extremely limited, and the individual has much difficulty completing even the simplest task. Physical symptoms (e.g., headaches, palpitations, insomnia) and emotional symptoms (e.g., confusion, dread, horror) may be evident. Discomfort is experienced to the degree that virtually all overt behavior is aimed at relieving the anxiety.
- **Panic Anxiety.** In this most intense state of anxiety, the individual is unable to focus on even one detail in the environment. Misperceptions are common, and a loss of contact with reality may occur. The individual may experience hallucinations or delusions. Behavior may be characterized by wild and desperate actions or

extreme withdrawal. Human functioning and communication with others is ineffective. Panic anxiety is associated with a feeling of terror, and individuals may be convinced that they have a life-threatening illness or fear that they are "going crazy" or losing control (APA, 2000). Prolonged panic anxiety can lead to physical and emotional exhaustion and can be a life-threatening situation.

A synopsis of the characteristics associated with each of the four levels of anxiety is presented in Table 2–1.

Behavioral Adaptation Responses to Anxiety

A variety of behavioral adaptation responses occur at each level of anxiety. Figure 2–2 depicts these behavioral responses on a continuum of anxiety ranging from mild to panic.

Mild Anxiety. At the mild level, individuals employ any of a number of coping behaviors that satisfy their needs for comfort. Menninger (1963) described the following types of coping mechanisms that individuals use to relieve anxiety in stressful situations:

- Sleeping
- Eating
- Physical exercise
- Smoking
- Crying
- Pacing
- Foot swinging
- Fidgeting
- Yawning
- Drinking
- Daydreaming
- Laughing
- Cursing
- Nail biting
- Finger tapping
- Talking to someone with whom one feels comfortable

Undoubtedly there are many more responses too numerous to mention here, considering that each individual develops his or her own unique ways to relieve anxiety at the mild level. Some of these behaviors are more adaptive than others.

Mild-to-Moderate Anxiety. Sigmund Freud (1961) identified the ego as the reality component of the personality that governs problem solving and rational thinking. As the level of anxiety increases, the strength of the ego is tested, and energy is mobilized to confront the threat. Anna Freud (1953) identified a number of **defense mechanisms** employed by the ego in the face of threat to biological or psychological integrity. Some of these ego defense mechanisms are more adaptive than

others, but all are used either consciously or unconsciously as a protective device for the ego in an effort to relieve mild to moderate anxiety. They become maladaptive when they are used by an individual to such a degree that there is interference with the ability to deal with reality, with effective interpersonal relations, or with occupational performance. Maladaptive use of defense mechanisms promotes disintegration of the ego. The major ego defense mechanisms identified by Anna Freud are discussed here and summarized in Table 2–2.

1. **Compensation** is the covering up of a real or perceived weakness by emphasizing a trait one considers more desirable.

    Example:

    (a) A handicapped boy who is unable to participate in sports compensates by becoming a great scholar. (b) A young man who is the shortest among members of his peer group views this as a deficiency and compensates by being overly aggressive and daring.

2. **Denial** is the refusal to acknowledge the existence of a real situation or the feelings associated with it.

    Example:

    (a) A woman has been told by family doctor that she has a lump in her breast. An appointment is made for her with a surgeon; however, she does not keep the appointment and goes about her activities of daily living with no evidence of concern. (b) Individuals continue to smoke cigarettes even though they have been told of the health risk involved.

3. **Displacement** is the transferring of feelings from one target to another that is considered less threatening or neutral.

    Example:

    (a) A man who is passed over for promotion on his job says nothing to his boss but later belittles his son for not making the basketball team. (b) A boy who is teased and hit by the class bully on the playground comes home after school and kicks his dog.

4. **Identification** is an attempt to increase self-worth by acquiring certain attributes and characteristics of an individual one admires.

    Example:

    (a) A teenage girl emulates the mannerisms and style of dress of a popular female rock star. (b) The young son of a famous civil rights worker adopts his father's attitudes and behaviors with the intent of pursuing similar aspirations.

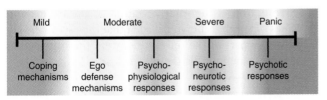

FIGURE 2–2 Adaptation responses on a continuum of anxiety.

TABLE 2–2	Ego Defense Mechanisms		
Defense Mechanism	**Example**	**Defense Mechanism**	**Example**
Compensation Covering up a real or perceived weakness by emphasizing a trait one considers more desirable.	A physically handicapped boy is unable to participate in football, so he compensates by becoming a great scholar.	**Rationalization** Attempting to make excuses or formulate logical reasons to justify unacceptable feelings or behaviors.	John tells the rehab nurse, "I drink because it's the only way I can deal with my bad marriage and my worse job."
Denial Refusing to acknowledge the existence of a real situation or the feelings associated with it.	A woman drinks alcohol every day and cannot stop, failing to acknowledge that she has a problem.	**Reaction Formation** Preventing unacceptable or undesirable thoughts or behaviors from being expressed by exaggerating opposite thoughts or types of behaviors	Jane hates nursing. She attended nursing school to please her parents. During career day, she speaks to prospective students about the excellence of nursing as a career.
Displacement The transfer of feelings from one target to another that is considered less threatening or that is neutral.	A client is angry with his physician, does not express it, but becomes verbally abusive with the nurse.	**Regression** Retreating in response to stress to an earlier level of development and the comfort measures associated with that level of functioning.	When 2–year-old Jay is hospitalized for tonsillitis he will drink only from a bottle, even though his mom states he has been drinking from a cup for 6 months.
Identification An attempt to increase self-worth by acquiring certain attributes and characteristics of an individual one admires	A teenager who required lengthy rehabilitation after an accident decides to become a physical therapist as a result of his experiences.	**Repression** Involuntarily blocking unpleasant feelings and experiences from one's awareness	An accident victim can remember nothing about his accident.
Intellectualization An attempt to avoid expressing actual emotions associated with a stressful situation by using the intellectual processes of logic, reasoning, and analysis	S's husband is being transferred with his job to a city far away from her parents. She hides anxiety by explaining to her parents the advantages associated with the move.	**Sublimation** Rechanneling of drives or impulses that are personally or socially unacceptable into activities that are constructive	A mother whose son was killed by a drunk driver channels her anger and energy into being the president of the local chapter of Mothers Against Drunk Drivers.
Introjection Integrating the beliefs and values of another individual into one's own ego structure	Children integrate their parents' value system into the process of conscience formation. A child says to friend, "Don't cheat. It's wrong."	**Suppression** The voluntary blocking of unpleasant feelings and experiences from one's awareness	Scarlett O'Hara says, "I don't want to think about that now. I'll think about that tomorrow."
Isolation Separating a thought or memory from the feeling, tone, or emotion associated with it.	A young woman describes being attacked and raped, without showing any emotion.	**Undoing** Symbolically negating or canceling out an experience that one finds intolerable	Joe is nervous about his new job and yells at his wife. On his way home he stops and buys her some flowers.
Projection Attributing feelings or impulses unacceptable to one's self to another person	Sue feels a strong sexual attraction to her track coach and tells her friend, "He's coming on to me!"		

5. **Intellectualization** is an attempt to avoid expressing actual emotions associated with a stressful situation by using the intellectual processes of logic, reasoning, and analysis.

[**Example:**]

(a) A man whose brother is in a cardiac intensive care unit following a severe myocardial infarction (MI) spends his allotted visiting time in discussion with the nurse, analyzing test results and making a reasonable determination about the pathophysiology that may have occurred to induce the MI. (b) A young psychology professor receives a letter from his fiancée breaking off their engagement. He shows no emotion when discussing this with his best friend. Instead he analyzes his fiancée's behavior and tries to reason why the relationship failed.

6. **Introjection** is the internalization of the beliefs and values of another individual such that they symbolically become a part of the self to the extent that the feeling of separateness or distinctness is lost.

[**Example:**]

(a) A small child develops her conscience by internalizing what the parents believe is right and wrong.

The parents literally become a part of the child. The child says to a friend while playing, "Don't hit people. It's not nice!" (b) A psychiatric client claims to be the Son of God, drapes himself in sheet and blanket, "performs miracles" on other clients, and refuses to respond unless addressed as Jesus Christ.

7. **Isolation** is the separation of a thought or a memory from the feeling tone or emotions associated with it (sometimes called emotional isolation).

   Example:

   (a) A young woman describes being attacked and raped by a street gang. She displays an apathetic expression and no emotional tone. (b) A physician is able to isolate her feelings about the eventual death of a terminally ill cancer client by focusing her attention instead on the chemotherapy that will be given.

8. **Projection** is the attribution of feelings or impulses unacceptable to one's self to another person. The individual "passes the blame" for these undesirable feelings or impulses to another, thereby providing relief from the anxiety associated with them.

   Example:

   (a) A young soldier who has an extreme fear of participating in military combat tells his sergeant that the others in his unit are "a bunch of cowards." (b) A businessperson who values punctuality is late for a meeting and states, "Sorry I'm late. My assistant forgot to remind me of the time. It's so hard to find good help these days."

9. **Rationalization** is the attempt to make excuses or formulate logical reasons to justify unacceptable feelings or behaviors.

   Example:

   (a) A young woman is turned down for a secretarial job after a poor performance on a typing test. She claims, "I'm sure I could have done a better job on a word processor. Hardly anyone uses an electric typewriter anymore!" (b) A young man is unable to afford the sports car he wants so desperately. He tells the salesperson, "I'd buy this car but I'll be getting married soon. This is really not the car for a family man."

10. **Reaction formation** is the prevention of unacceptable or undesirable thoughts or behaviors from being expressed by exaggerating opposite thoughts or types of behaviors.

    Example:

    (a) The young soldier who has an extreme fear of participating in military combat volunteers for dangerous front-line duty. (b) A secretary is sexually attracted to her boss and feels an intense dislike toward his wife. She treats her boss with detachment and aloofness while performing her secretarial duties and is overly courteous, polite, and flattering to his wife when she comes to the office.

11. **Regression** is the retreating to an earlier level of development and the comfort measures associated with that level of functioning.

    Example:

    (a) When his mother brings his new baby sister home from the hospital, 4-year-old Tommy, who had been toilet trained for more than a year, begins to wet his pants, cry to be held, and suck his thumb. (b) A person who is depressed may withdraw to his or her room, curl up in a fetal position on the bed, and sleep for long periods of time.

12. **Repression** is the involuntary blocking of unpleasant feelings and experiences from one's awareness.

    Example:

    (a) A woman cannot remember being sexually assaulted when she was 15 years old. (b) A teenage boy cannot remember driving the car that was involved in an accident in which his best friend was killed.

13. **Sublimation** is the rechanneling of drives or impulses that are personally or socially unacceptable (e.g., aggressiveness, anger, sexual drives) into activities that are more tolerable and constructive.

    Example:

    (a) A teenage boy with strong competitive and aggressive drives becomes the star football player on his high school team. (b) A young unmarried woman with a strong desire for marriage and a family achieves satisfaction and success in establishing and operating a daycare center for preschool children.

14. **Suppression** is the voluntarily blocking of unpleasant feelings and experiences from one's awareness.

    Example:

    (a) Scarlett O'Hara says, "I'll think about that tomorrow." (b) A young woman who is depressed about a pending divorce proceeding tells the nurse, "I just don't want to talk about the divorce. There's nothing I can do about it anyway."

15. **Undoing** is the act of symbolically negating or canceling out a previous action or experience that one finds intolerable.

Examples:

(a) A man spills some salt on the table, then sprinkles some over his left shoulder to "prevent bad luck." (b) A man who is anxious about giving a presentation at work yells at his wife during breakfast. He stops on his way home from work that evening to buy her a dozen red roses.

Moderate-to-Severe Anxiety. Anxiety at the moderate-to-severe level that remains unresolved over an extended period of time can contribute to a number of physiological disorders. The *DSM-IV-TR* (APA, 2000) describes these disorders as "the presence of one or more specific psychological or behavioral factors that adversely affect a general medical condition." The psychological factors may exacerbate symptoms of, delay recovery from, or interfere with treatment of the medical condition. The condition may be initiated or exacerbated by an environmental situation that the individual perceives as stressful. Measurable pathophysiology can be demonstrated.

The *DSM-IV-TR* states:

Psychological and behavioral factors may affect the course of almost every major category of disease, including cardiovascular conditions, dermatological conditions, endocrinological conditions, gastrointestinal conditions, neoplastic conditions neurological conditions, pulmonary conditions, renal conditions, and rheumatological conditions. (p. 732)

Severe Anxiety. Extended periods of repressed severe anxiety can result in psychoneurotic patterns of behaving. **Neurosis** is no longer a separate category of disorders in the *DSM-IV-TR* (APA, 2000). However, the term is still used in the literature to further describe the symptomatology of certain disorders. Neuroses are psychiatric disturbances, characterized by excessive anxiety that is expressed directly or altered through defense mechanisms. It appears as a symptom, such as an obsession, a compulsion, a phobia, or a sexual dysfunction (Sadock & Sadock, 2007). The following are common characteristics of people with neuroses:

1. They are aware that they are experiencing distress.
2. They are aware that their behaviors are maladaptive.
3. They are unaware of any possible psychological causes of the distress.
4. They feel helpless to change their situation.
5. They experience no loss of contact with reality.

The following disorders are examples of psychoneurotic responses to anxiety as they appear in the *DSM-IV-TR*. They are discussed in this text in Chapters 30 and 31.

1. **Anxiety Disorders.** Disorders in which the characteristic features are symptoms of anxiety and avoidance behavior (e.g., phobias, obsessive-compulsive disorder, panic disorder, generalized anxiety disorder, and posttraumatic stress disorder).
2. **Somatoform Disorders.** Disorders in which the characteristic features are physical symptoms for which there is no demonstrable organic pathology. Psychological factors are judged to play a significant role in the onset, severity, exacerbation, or maintenance of the symptoms (e.g., hypochondriasis, conversion disorder, somatization disorder, pain disorder).
3. **Dissociative Disorders.** Disorders in which the characteristic feature is a disruption in the usually integrated functions of consciousness, memory, identity, or perception of the environment (e.g., dissociative amnesia, dissociative fugue, dissociative identity disorder, and depersonalization disorder).

Panic Anxiety. At this extreme level of anxiety, an individual is not capable of processing what is happening in the environment, and may lose contact with reality. **Psychosis** is defined as a loss of ego boundaries or a gross impairment in reality testing (APA, 2000). Psychoses are serious psychiatric disturbances characterized by the presence of delusions or hallucinations and the impairment of interpersonal functioning and relationship to the external world. The following are common characteristics of people with psychoses:

- They experience minimal distress (emotional tone is flat, bland, or inappropriate).
- They are unaware that their behavior is maladaptive.
- They are unaware of any psychological problems.
- They are exhibiting a flight from reality into a less stressful world or into one in which they are attempting to adapt.

Examples of psychotic responses to anxiety include the schizophrenic, schizoaffective, and delusional disorders. They are discussed at length in Chapter 28.

 CORE CONCEPT

Grief
Grief is a subjective state of emotional, physical, and social responses to the loss of a valued entity.

Grief

Most individuals experience intense emotional anguish in response to a significant personal loss. A loss is anything that is perceived as such by the individual. Losses may be real, in which case they can be substantiated by others (e.g., death of a loved one, loss of personal possessions), or they may be perceived by the individual alone, unable to be shared or identified by others (e.g., loss of the feeling of femininity following mastectomy). Any situation that creates change for an individual can be identified as a loss. Failure (either real or perceived) also can be viewed as a loss.

The loss, or anticipated loss, of anything of value to an individual can trigger the grief response. This period of characteristic emotions and behaviors is called *mourning*. The "normal" mourning process is adaptive and is characterized by feelings of sadness, guilt, anger, helplessness, hopelessness, and despair. Indeed, an absence of mourning after a loss may be considered maladaptive.

Stages of Grief

Kübler-Ross (1969), in extensive research with terminally ill patients, identified five stages of feelings and behaviors that individuals experience in response to a real, perceived, or anticipated loss:

Stage 1—Denial. This is a stage of shock and disbelief. The response may be one of "No, it can't be true!" The reality of the loss is not acknowledged. Denial is a protective mechanism that allows the individual to cope in an immediate time frame while organizing more effective defense strategies.

Stage 2—Anger. "Why me?" and "It's not fair!" are comments often expressed during the anger stage. Envy and resentment toward individuals not affected by the loss are common. Anger may be directed at the self or displaced on loved ones, caregivers, and even God. There may be a preoccupation with an idealized image of the lost entity.

Stage 3—Bargaining. During this stage, which is usually not visible or evident to others, a "bargain" is made with God in an attempt to reverse or postpone the loss. "If God will help me through this, I promise I will go to church every Sunday and volunteer my time to help others." Sometimes the promise is associated with feelings of guilt for not having performed (or having the perception of not having performed) satisfactorily, appropriately, or sufficiently.

Stage 4—Depression. During this stage, the full impact of the loss is experienced. The sense of loss is intense, and feelings of sadness and depression prevail. This is a time of quiet desperation and disengagement from all association with the lost entity. It differs from *pathological* depression, which occurs when an individual becomes fixed in an earlier stage of the grief process. Rather, stage four of the grief response represents advancement toward resolution.

Stage 5—Acceptance. The final stage brings a feeling of peace regarding the loss that has occurred. It is a time of quiet expectation and resignation. The focus is on the reality of the loss and its meaning for the individuals affected by it.

All individuals do not experience each of these stages in response to a loss, nor do they necessarily experience them in this order. Some individuals' grieving behaviors may fluctuate, and even overlap, between stages.

Anticipatory Grief

When a loss is anticipated, individuals often begin the work of grieving before the actual loss occurs. Most people re-experience the grieving behaviors once the loss occurs, but having this time to prepare for the loss can facilitate the process of mourning, actually decreasing the length and intensity of the response. Problems arise, particularly in anticipating the death of a loved one, when family members experience **anticipatory grieving** and the mourning process is completed prematurely. They disengage emotionally from the dying person, who may then experience feelings of rejection by loved ones at a time when this psychological support is so necessary.

Resolution

The grief response can last from weeks to years. It cannot be hurried, and individuals must be allowed to progress at their own pace. In the loss of a loved one, grief work usually lasts for at least a year, during which the grieving person experiences each significant "anniversary" date for the first time without the loved one present.

Length of the grief process may be prolonged by a number of factors. If the relationship with the lost entity had been marked by ambivalence or if there had been an enduring "love-hate" association, reaction to the loss may be burdened with guilt. Guilt lengthens the grief reaction by promoting feelings of anger toward the self for having committed a wrongdoing or behaved in an unacceptable manner toward that which is now lost, and perhaps the grieving person may even feel that his or her behavior has contributed to the loss.

Anticipatory grieving is thought to shorten the grief response in some individuals who are able to work through some of the feelings before the loss occurs. If the loss is sudden and unexpected, mourning may take longer than it would if individuals were able to grieve in anticipation of the loss.

Length of the grieving process is also affected by the number of recent losses experienced by an individual and whether he or she is able to complete one grieving process before another loss occurs. This is particularly true for elderly individuals who may be experiencing numerous losses, such as spouse, friends, other relatives, independent functioning, home, personal possessions, and pets, in a relatively short time. Grief accumulates, and this represents a type of **bereavement overload**, which for some individuals presents an impossible task of grief work.

Resolution of the process of mourning is thought to have occurred when an individual can look back on the relationship with the lost entity and accept both the pleasures and the disappointments (both the positive and the negative aspects) of the association (Bowlby & Parkes, 1970). Disorganization and emotional pain have been experienced and tolerated. Preoccupation with the lost entity has been replaced with energy and the desire to pursue new situations and relationships.

Maladaptive Grief Responses

Maladaptive responses to loss occur when an individual is not able to satisfactorily progress through the stages of grieving to achieve resolution. These responses usually occur when an individual becomes fixed in the denial or anger stage of the grief process. Several types of grief responses have been identified as pathological. They include responses that are prolonged, delayed or inhibited, or distorted. The *prolonged* response is characterized by an intense preoccupation with memories of the lost entity for *many years after the loss has occurred*. Behaviors associated with the stages of denial or anger are manifested, and disorganization of functioning and intense emotional pain related to the lost entity are evidenced.

In the *delayed or inhibited* response, the individual becomes fixed in the denial stage of the grieving process. The emotional pain associated with the loss is not experienced, but anxiety disorders (e.g., phobias, hypochondriasis) or sleeping and eating disorders (e.g., insomnia, anorexia)

may be evident. The individual may remain in denial for many years until the grief response is triggered by a reminder of the loss or even by another, unrelated loss.

The individual who experiences a *distorted* response is fixed in the anger stage of grieving. In the distorted response, all the normal behaviors associated with grieving, such as helplessness, hopelessness, sadness, anger, and guilt, are exaggerated out of proportion to the situation. The individual turns the anger inward on the self, is consumed with overwhelming despair, and is unable to function in normal activities of daily living. Pathological depression is a distorted grief response (see Chapter 29).

MENTAL HEALTH/MENTAL ILLNESS CONTINUUM

Anxiety and grief have been described as two major, primary responses to stress. In Figure 2–3, both of these responses are presented on a continuum according to degree of symptom severity. Disorders as they appear in the *DSM-IV-TR* are identified at their appropriate placement along the continuum.

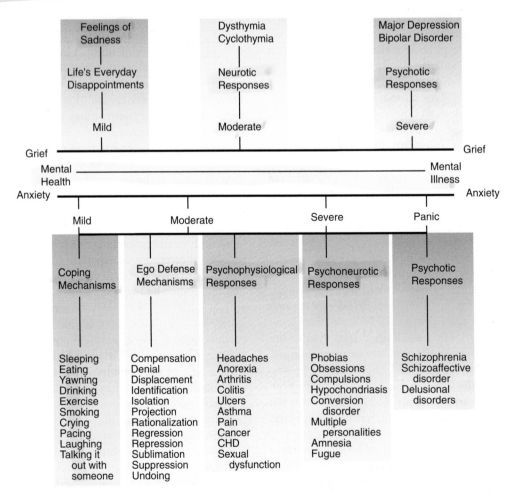

FIGURE 2–3 Conceptualization of anxiety and grief responses along the mental health/mental illness continuum.

THE *DSM-IV-TR* MULTIAXIAL EVALUATION SYSTEM

The APA endorses case evaluation on a multiaxial system, "to facilitate comprehensive and systematic evaluation with attention to the various mental disorders and general medical conditions, psychosocial and environmental problems, and level of functioning that might be overlooked if the focus were on assessing a single presenting problem." Each individual is evaluated on five axes. They are defined by the *DSM-IV-TR* in the following manner:

Axis I—Clinical Disorders and Other Conditions That May Be a Focus of Clinical Attention. This includes all mental disorders (except personality disorders and mental retardation).

[handwritten: autistic, Pschizophrenic]

[handwritten: Know extremes]

[handwritten: DID] → *[handwritten: Dissociative disorder, Depersonalization]*

Axis II—Personality Disorders and Mental Retardation. These disorders usually begin in childhood or adolescence and persist in a stable form into adult life.

Axis III—General Medical Conditions. These include any current general medical condition that is potentially relevant to the understanding or management of the individual's mental disorder. *[handwritten: Hypothyroidism, Dmellitus]*

Axis IV—Psychosocial and Environmental Problems. These are problems that may affect the diagnosis, treatment, and prognosis of mental disorders named on axes I and II. These include problems related to primary support group, social environment, education, occupation, housing, economics, access to health care services, interaction with the legal system or crime, and other types of psychosocial and environmental problems. *[handwritten: Ø job]*

[handwritten: Current GAF 85/35 or 55/35   whats more severe?   the lger # the better]

Box 2 – 2 Global Assessment of Functioning (GAF) Scale

Consider psychological, social, and occupational functioning on a hypothetical continuum of mental health-illness. Do not include impairment in functioning due to physical (or environmental) limitations.

Code	(**Note:** Use intermediate codes when appropriate, e.g., 45, 68, 72)
100 | 91	**Superior functioning in a wide range of activities, life's problems never seem to get out of hand, is sought out by others because of his or her many positive qualities. No symptoms.**
90 | 81	Absent or minimal symptoms (e.g., mild anxiety before an exam), **good functioning in all areas interested and involved in a wide range of activities, socially effective, generally satisfied with life, no more than everyday problems or concerns** (e.g., an occasional argument with family members).
80 | 71	If symptoms are present, they are transient and expectable reactions to psychosocial stressors (e.g., difficulty concentrating after family argument); **no more than slight impairment in social, occupational, or school functioning** (e.g., temporarily falling behind in schoolwork).
70 | 61	Some mild symptoms (e.g., depressed mood and mild insomnia) **OR some difficulty in social, occupational, or school functioning** (e.g., occasional truancy, or theft within the household), **but generally functioning pretty well, has some meaningful interpersonal relationships.**
60 | 51	Moderate symptoms (e.g., flat affect and circumstantial speech, occasional panic attacks) **OR moderate difficulty in social, occupational, or school functioning** (e.g., few friends, conflicts with peers or co-workers).
50 | 41	Serious symptoms (e.g., suicidal ideation, severe obsessional rituals, frequent shoplifting) **OR any serious impairment in social, occupational, or school functioning** (e.g., no friends, unable to keep a job).
40 | 31	Some impairment in reality testing or communication (e.g., speech is at times illogical, obscure, or irrelevant) **OR major impairment in several areas, such as work or school, family relations, judgment, thinking, or mood** (e.g., depressed man avoids friends, neglects family, and is unable to work; child frequently beats up younger children, is defiant at home, and is failing at school).
30 | 21	**Behavior is considerably influenced by delusions or hallucinations OR serious impairment in communication or judgment** (e.g., sometimes incoherent, acts grossly inappropriately, suicidal preoccupation) **OR inability to function in almost all areas** (e.g., stays in bed all day; no job, home, or friends).
20 | 11	Some degree of hurting self or others (e.g., suicide attempts without clear expectation of death; frequently violent; manic excitement) **OR occasionally fails to maintain minimal personal hygiene** (e.g., smears feces) **OR gross impairment in communication** (e.g., largely incoherent or mute).
10 | 1	Persistent danger of severely hurting self or others (e.g., recurrent violence) **OR persistent inability to maintain minimal personal hygiene OR serious suicidal act with clear expectation of death.**
0	**Inadequate information.**

SOURCE: *Diagnostic and Statistical Manual of Mental Disorders* (4th ed.) *Text Revision.* Washington, DC: American Psychiatric Association (2000). With permission.

TABLE 2–3	Example of a Psychiatric Diagnosis	
Axis I	300.4	Dysthymic Disorder
Axis II	301.6	Dependent Personality Disorder
Axis III	244.9	Hypothyroidism
Axis IV		Unemployed
Axis V	GAF = 65 (current)	

Axis V—Global Assessment of Functioning. This allows the clinician to rate the individual's overall functioning on the Global Assessment of Functioning (GAF) Scale. This scale represents in global terms a single measure of the individual's psychological, social, and occupational functioning. A copy of the GAF Scale appears in Box 2–2.

The *DSM-IV-TR* outline of axes I and II categories and codes is presented in Appendix C. An example of a psychiatric diagnosis presented according to the multiaxial evaluation system appears in Table 2–3.

SUMMARY AND KEY POINTS

- Psychiatric care has its roots in ancient times, when etiology was based in superstition and ideas related to the supernatural.
- Treatments were often inhumane and included brutal beatings, starvation, or other torturous means.
- Hippocrates associated insanity and mental illness with an irregularity in the interaction of the four body fluids (humors)—blood, black bile, yellow bile, and phlegm.
- Conditions for care of the mentally ill have improved, largely because of the influence of leaders such as Benjamin Rush, Dorothea Dix, and Linda Richards, whose endeavors provided a model for more humanistic treatment.
- Maslow identified a "hierarchy of needs" that individuals seek to fulfill on their quest to self-actualization (one's highest potential).
- For purposes of this text, the definition of mental health is viewed as the successful adaptation to stressors from the internal or external environment, evidenced by thoughts, feelings, and behaviors that are age-appropriate and congruent with local and cultural norms.
- In determining mental illness, individuals are influenced by *incomprehensibility* of the behavior. That is, whether or not they are able to understand the motivation behind the behavior.
- Another consideration is *cultural relativity*. The "normality" of behavior is determined by cultural and societal norms.
- For purposes of this text, the definition of mental illness is viewed as maladaptive responses to stressors from the internal or external environment, evidenced by thoughts, feelings, and behaviors that are incongruent with the local and cultural norms, and interfere with the individual's social, occupational, and/or physical functioning.
- Anxiety and grief have been described as two major, primary psychological response patterns to stress.
- Peplau defined anxiety by levels of symptom severity: mild, moderate, severe, and panic.
- Behaviors associated with levels of anxiety include coping mechanisms, ego defense mechanisms, psychophysiological responses, psychoneurotic responses, and psychotic responses.
- Grief is described as a response to loss of a valued entity. Loss is anything that is perceived as such by the individual.
- Kübler-Ross, in extensive research with terminally ill patients, identified five stages of feelings and behaviors that individuals experience in response to a real, perceived, or anticipated loss: denial, anger, bargaining, depression, and acceptance.
- Anticipatory grief is grief work that is begun, and sometimes completed, before the loss occurs.
- Resolution is thought to occur when an individual is able to remember and accept both the positive and negative aspects associated with the lost entity.
- Grieving is thought to be maladaptive when the mourning process is prolonged, delayed or inhibited, or becomes distorted and exaggerated out of proportion to the situation. Pathological depression is considered to be a distorted reaction.
- Psychiatric diagnoses are presented by the American Psychiatric Association on a multiaxial evaluation system. Individuals are evaluated on 5 axes: major mental disorders, personality disorders/developmental level, general medical conditions, psychosocial and environmental problems, and level of functioning.

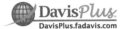 **For additional clinical tools and study aids, visit DavisPlus.**
DavisPlus.fadavis.com

REVIEW QUESTIONS

Self-Examination

Situation: Anna is 72 years old. She has been a widow for 20 years. When her husband had been dead for a year, her daughter gave Anna a puppy, which she named Lucky. Lucky was a happy, lively mutt of unknown origin, and he and Anna soon became inseparable. Lucky lived to a ripe old age of 16, dying in Anna's arms three years ago. Anna's daughter has consulted the community mental health nurse practitioner about her mother, stating, "She doesn't do a thing for herself anymore, and all she wants to talk about is Lucky. She visits his grave every day! She still cries when she talks about him. I don't know what to do!"

Select the answers that are most appropriate for this situation.

1. Anna's behavior would be considered maladaptive because:
   a. It has been more than three years since Lucky died.
   b. Her grief is too intense just over loss of a dog.
   c. Her grief is interfering with her functioning.
   d. People in this culture would not comprehend such behavior over loss of a pet.

2. Anna's grieving behavior would most likely be considered to be:
   a. Delayed
   b. Inhibited
   c. Prolonged
   d. Distorted

3. Anna is most likely fixed in which stage of the grief process?
   a. Denial
   b. Anger
   c. Depression
   d. Acceptance

4. Anna is of the age when she may have experienced many losses coming close together. What is this called?
   a. Bereavement overload
   b. Normal mourning
   c. Isolation
   d. Cultural relativity

5. Anna's daughter has likely put off seeking help for Anna because:
   a. Women are less likely to seek help for emotional problems than men.
   b. Relatives often try to "normalize" the behavior, rather than label it mental illness.
   c. She knows that all old people are expected to be a little depressed.
   d. She is afraid that the neighbors "will think her mother is crazy."

6. On the day that Lucky died, he got away from Anna while they were taking a walk. He ran into the street and was hit by a car. Anna cannot remember any of these circumstances of his death. This is an example of what defense mechanism?
   a. Rationalization
   b. Suppression
   c. Denial
   d. Repression

7. Lucky sometimes refused to obey Anna, and indeed did not come back to her when she called to him on the day he was killed. But Anna continues to insist, "He was the very best dog. He always minded me. He always did everything I told him to do." This represents the defense mechanism of:
   a. Sublimation
   b. Compensation
   c. Reaction Formation
   d. Undoing

8. Anna's maladaptive grief response may be attributed to:

    a. Unresolved grief over loss of her husband.
    b. Loss of several relatives and friends over the last few years.
    c. Repressed feelings of guilt over the way in which Lucky died.
    d. Any or all of the above.

9. For what reason would Anna's illness be considered a neurosis rather than a psychosis?

    a. She is unaware that her behavior is maladaptive.
    b. She exhibits inappropriate affect (emotional tone).
    c. She experiences no loss of contact with reality.
    d. She tells the nurse, "There is nothing wrong with me!"

10. Which of the following statements by Anna might suggest that she is achieving resolution of her grief over Lucky's death?

    a. "I don't cry anymore when I think about Lucky."
    b. "It's true. Lucky didn't always mind me. Sometimes he ignored my commands."
    c. "I remember how it happened now. I should have held tighter to his leash!"
    d. "I won't ever have another dog. It's just too painful to lose them."

Match the following defense mechanisms to the appropriate situation:

_____11. Compensation

    a. Tommy, who is small for his age, is teased at school by the older boys. When he gets home from school, he yells at and hits his little sister.

_____12. Denial

    b. Johnny is in a wheelchair as a result of paralysis of the lower limbs. Before his accident, he was the star athlete on the football team. Now he obsessively strives to maintain a 4.0 grade point average in his courses.

_____13. Displacement

    c. Nancy and Sally are 4 years old. While playing with their dolls, Nancy says to Sally, "Don't hit your dolly. It's not nice to hit people!"

_____14. Identification

    d. Jackie is 4 years old. He has wanted a baby brother very badly, yet when his mother brings the new sibling home from the hospital, Jackie cries to be held when the baby is being fed and even starts to soil his clothing, although he has been toilet trained for 2 years.

_____15. Intellectualization

    e. A young man is late for class. He tells the professor, "Sorry I'm late, but my stupid wife forgot to set the alarm last night!"

_____16. Introjection

    f. Nancy was emotionally abused as a child and hates her mother. However, when she talks to others about her mother, she tells them how wonderful she is and how much she loves her.

_____17. Isolation

    g. Pete grew up in a rough neighborhood where fighting was a way of coping. He is tough and aggressive and is noticed by the football coach, who makes him a member of the team. Within the year he becomes the star player.

_____18. Projection

    h. Fred stops at the bar every night after work and has several drinks. During the last 6 months he has been charged twice with driving under the influence, both times while driving recklessly after leaving the bar. Last night, he was stopped again. The judge ordered rehabilitation services. Fred responded, "I don't need rehab. I can stop drinking anytime I want to!"

_____19. Rationalization

i. Mary tries on a beautiful dress she saw in the store window. She discovers that it costs more than she can afford. She says to the salesperson, "I'm not going to buy it. I really don't look good in this color."

_____20. Reaction Formation

j. Janice is extremely upset when her boyfriend of 2 years breaks up with her. Her best friend tries to encourage her to talk about the breakup, but Janice says, "No need to talk about him anymore. He's history!"

_____21. Regression

k. While jogging in the park, Linda was kidnapped and taken as a hostage by two men who had just robbed a bank. She was held at gunpoint for 2 days until she was able to escape from the robbers. In her account to the police, she speaks of the encounter with no display of emotion whatsoever.

_____22. Repression

l. While Mark is on his way to work a black cat runs across the road in front of his car. Mark turns the car around, drives back in the direction from which he had come, and takes another route to work.

_____23. Sublimation

m. Fifteen-year-old Zelda has always wanted to be a teacher. Ms. Fry is Zelda's history teacher. Zelda admires everything about Ms. Fry and wants to be just like her. She changes her hair and dress style to match that of Ms. Fry.

_____24. Suppression

n. Bart is turned down for a job he desperately wanted. He shows no disappointment when relating the situation to his girlfriend. Instead, he reviews the interview and begins to analyze systematically why the interaction was ineffective for him.

_____25. Undoing

o. Eighteen-year-old Jennifer can recall nothing related to an automobile accident in which she was involved 8 years ago and in which both of her parents were killed.

REFERENCES

American Psychiatric Association. (2003). *American psychiatric glossary* (8th ed.). Washington, DC: American Psychiatric Publishing.

American Psychiatric Association. (2000). *Diagnostic and statistical manual of mental disorders* (4th ed.) *Text revision*. Washington, DC: American Psychiatric Association.

Horwitz, A.V. (2002). The social control of mental illness. Clinton Corners, NY: Percheron Press.

Sadock, B.J., & Sadock, V.A. (2007). *Synopsis of psychiatry: Behavioral sciences/clinical psychiatry* (10th ed.). Baltimore: Lippincott Williams & Wilkins.

Robinson, L. (1983). *Psychiatric nursing as a human experience* (3rd ed.). Philadelphia: W.B. Saunders.

CLASSICAL REFERENCES

Bowlby, J., & Parkes, C.M. (1970). Separation and loss. In E.J. Anthony & C. Koupernik (Eds.), *International yearbook for child psychiatry and allied disciplines: The child and his family*, (Vol. 1). New York: John Wiley & Sons.

Freud, A. (1953). *The ego and mechanisms of defense*. New York: International Universities Press.

Freud, S. (1961). The ego and the id. In *Standard edition of the complete psychological works of Freud*, Vol. XIX. London: Hogarth Press.

Jahoda, M. (1958). *Current concepts of positive mental health*. New York: Basic Books.

Kübler-Ross, E. (1969). *On death and dying*. New York: Macmillan.

Maslow, A. (1970). *Motivation and personality* (2nd ed.). New York: Harper & Row.

Menninger, K. (1963). *The vital balance*. New York: Viking Press.

Peplau, H. (1963). A working definition of anxiety. In S. Burd & M. Marshall (Eds.), *Some clinical approaches to psychiatric nursing*. New York: Macmillan.

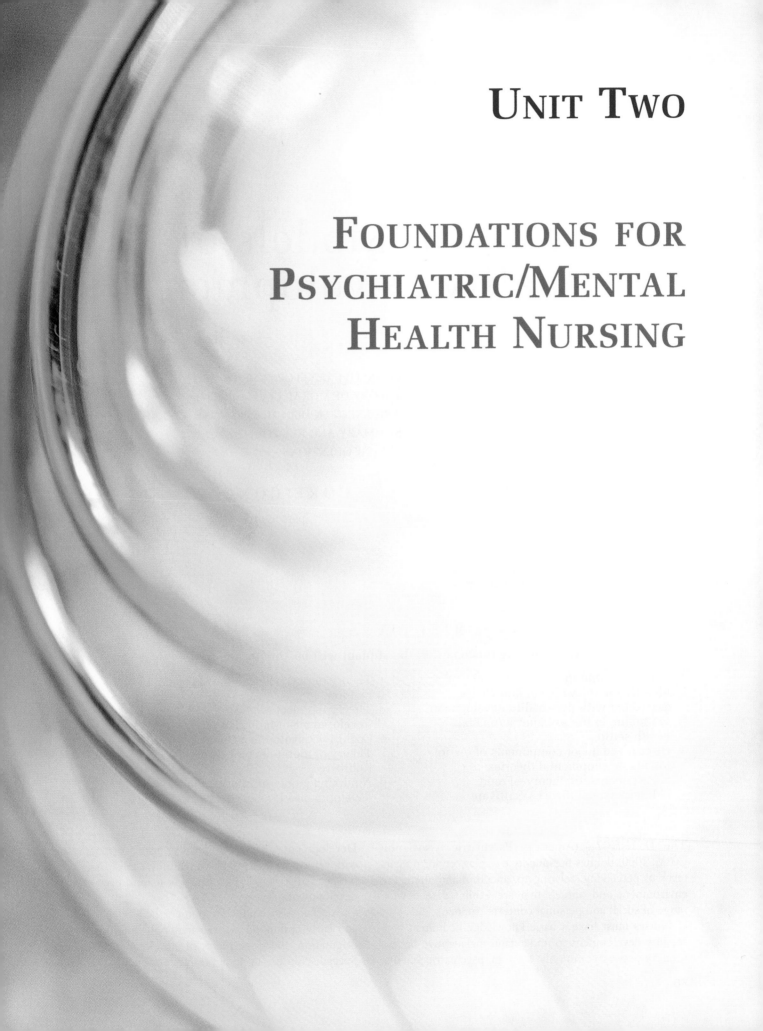

UNIT TWO

FOUNDATIONS FOR PSYCHIATRIC/MENTAL HEALTH NURSING

Theoretical Models of Personality Development

CHAPTER OUTLINE

KEY TERMS

cognitive development
cognitive maturity
counselor
ego
id
libido

psychodynamic nursing
superego
surrogate
symbiosis
technical expert
temperament

CORE CONCEPT

personality

OBJECTIVES

After reading this chapter, the student will be able to:

1. Define *personality*.
2. Identify the relevance of knowledge associated with personality development to nursing in the psychiatric/mental health setting.
3. Discuss the major components of the following developmental theories:
   a. Psychoanalytic theory—Freud
   b. Interpersonal theory—Sullivan
   c. Theory of psychosocial development—Erikson
   d. Theory of object relations development—Mahler
   e. Cognitive development theory—Piaget
   f. Theory of moral development—Kohlberg
   g. A nursing model of interpersonal development—Peplau

The *DSM-IV-TR* (American Psychiatric Association [APA], 2000) defines personality *traits* as "enduring patterns of perceiving, relating to, and thinking about the environment and oneself that are exhibited in a wide range of social and personal contexts" (p. 686).

Nurses must have a basic knowledge of human personality development to understand maladaptive behavioral responses commonly seen in psychiatric clients. Developmental theories identify behaviors associated with various *stages* through which individuals pass, thereby specifying what is appropriate or inappropriate at each developmental level.

Specialists in child development believe that infancy and early childhood are the major life periods for the origination and occurrence of developmental change. Specialists in life-cycle development believe that people continue to develop and change throughout life, thereby suggesting the possibility for renewal and growth in adults.

Developmental stages are identified by age. Behaviors can then be evaluated by whether or not they are recognized as age-appropriate. Ideally, an individual successfully fulfills all the tasks associated with one stage before moving on to the next stage (at the appropriate age). In reality, however, this seldom happens. One reason is related to **temperament**, or the inborn personality characteristics that influence an individual's manner of reacting to the environment, and ultimately his or her developmental progression (Chess & Thomas, 1986). The environment may also influence one's developmental pattern. Individuals who are reared in a dysfunctional family system often have retarded ego development. According to specialists in life-cycle development, behaviors from an unsuccessfully completed stage can be modified and corrected in a later stage.

Stages overlap, and an individual may be working on tasks associated with several stages at one time. When an individual becomes fixed in a lower level of development, with age-inappropriate behaviors focused on fulfillment of those tasks, psychopathology may become evident. Only when personality traits are inflexible and maladaptive and cause either significant functional impairment or subjective distress do they constitute "personality disorders" (APA, 2000). These disorders are discussed in Chapter 34.

CORE CONCEPT

Personality
The combination of character, behavioral, temperamental, emotional, and mental traits that are unique to each specific individual.

PSYCHOANALYTIC THEORY

Freud (1961), who has been called the father of psychiatry, is credited as the first to identify development by stages. He considered the first 5 years of a child's life to be the most important, because he believed that an individual's basic character had been formed by the age of 5.

Freud's personality theory can be conceptualized according to structure and dynamics of the personality, topography of the mind, and stages of personality development.

Structure of the Personality

Freud organized the structure of the personality into three major components: the **id**, **ego**, and **superego**. They are distinguished by their unique functions and different characteristics.

Id

The *id* is the locus of instinctual drives: the "pleasure principle." Present at birth, it endows the infant with instinctual drives that seek to satisfy needs and achieve immediate gratification. Id-driven behaviors are impulsive and may be irrational.

Ego

The *ego*, also called the *rational self* or the "reality principle," begins to develop between the ages of 4 and 6 months. The ego experiences the reality of the external world, adapts to it, and responds to it. As the ego develops and gains strength, it seeks to bring the influences of the external world to bear upon the id, to substitute the reality principle for the pleasure principle (Marmer, 2003). A primary function of the ego is one of mediator, that is, to maintain harmony among the external world, the id, and the superego.

Superego

If the id is identified as the pleasure principle, and the ego the reality principle, the *superego* might be referred to as the "perfection principle." The superego, which develops between ages 3 and 6 years, internalizes the values and morals set forth by primary caregivers. Derived out of a system of rewards and punishments, the superego is composed of two major components: the *ego-ideal* and the *conscience*. When a child is consistently rewarded for "good" behavior, self-esteem is enhanced, and the behavior becomes part of the ego-ideal; that is, it is internalized as part of his or her value system. The conscience is formed when the child is punished consistently for "bad" behavior. The child learns what is considered morally right or wrong from feedback received from parental figures and from society or culture. When moral and ethical principles or even internalized ideals and values are disregarded, the conscience generates a feeling of guilt within the individual. The superego is important in the socialization of the individual because it assists the ego in the control of id impulses. When the superego becomes rigid and punitive, problems with low self-confidence and low self-esteem arise. Examples of behaviors associated with these components of the personality are presented in Box 3–1.

Topography of the Mind

Freud classified all mental contents and operations into three categories: the conscious, the preconscious, and the unconscious.

● The *conscious* includes all memories that remain within an individual's awareness. It is the smallest of the three categories. Events and experiences that are easily

Box 3 – 1   Structure of the Personality

Behavioral Examples

Id	Ego	Superego
"I found this wallet; I will keep the money."	"I already have money. This money doesn't belong to me. Maybe the person who owns this wallet doesn't have any money."	"It is never right to take something that doesn't belong to you."
"Mom and Dad are gone. Let's party!!!!!"	"Mom and Dad said no friends over while they are away. Too risky."	"Never disobey your parents."
"I'll have sex with whomever I please, whenever I please."	"Promiscuity can be very dangerous."	"Sex outside of marriage is always wrong."

remembered or retrieved are considered to be within one's conscious awareness. Examples include telephone numbers, birthdays of self and significant others, the dates of special holidays, and what one had for lunch today. The conscious mind is thought to be under the control of the ego, the rational and logical structure of the personality.

● The *preconscious* includes all memories that may have been forgotten or are not in present awareness but with attention can be readily recalled into consciousness. Examples include telephone numbers or addresses once known but little used and feelings associated with significant life events that may have occurred at some time in the past. The preconscious enhances awareness by helping to *suppress* unpleasant or nonessential memories from consciousness. It is thought to be partially under the control of the superego, which helps to suppress unacceptable thoughts and behaviors.

● The *unconscious* includes all memories that one is unable to bring to conscious awareness. It is the largest of the three topographical levels. Unconscious material consists of unpleasant or nonessential memories that have been *repressed* and can be retrieved only through therapy, hypnosis, or with certain substances that alter awareness and have the capacity to restructure repressed memories. Unconscious material may also emerge in dreams and in seemingly incomprehensible behavior.

Dynamics of the Personality

Freud believed that *psychic energy* is the force or impetus required for mental functioning. Originating in the id, it instinctually fulfills basic physiological needs. Freud called this psychic energy (or the drive to fulfill basic physiological needs such as hunger, thirst, and sex) the **libido**. As the child matures, psychic energy is diverted from the id to form the ego and then from the ego to form the superego. Psychic energy is distributed within these three components, with the ego retaining the largest share to maintain a balance between the impulsive behaviors of the id and the idealistic behaviors of the superego. If an excessive amount of psychic energy is stored in one of these personality components, behavior will reflect that part of the personality. For instance, impulsive behavior prevails when excessive psychic energy is stored in the id. Overinvestment in the ego reflects self-absorbed, or narcissistic, behaviors; an excess within the superego results in rigid, self-deprecating behaviors.

Freud used the terms *cathexis* and *anticathexis* to describe the forces within the id, ego, and superego that are used to invest psychic energy in external sources to satisfy needs. Cathexis is the process by which the id invests energy into an object in an attempt to achieve gratification. An example is the individual who instinctively turns to alcohol to relieve stress. Anticathexis is the use of psychic energy by the ego and the superego to control id impulses. In the example cited, the ego would attempt to control the use of alcohol with rational thinking, such as, "I already have ulcers from drinking too much. I will call my AA counselor for support. I will not drink." The superego would exert control with thinking such as "I shouldn't drink. If I drink, my family will be hurt and angry. I should think of how it affects them. I'm such a weak person." Freud believed that an imbalance between cathexis and anticathexis resulted in internal conflicts, producing tension and anxiety within the individual. Freud's daughter Anna devised a comprehensive list of defense mechanisms believed to be used by the ego as a protective device against anxiety in mediating between the excessive demands of the id and the excessive restrictions of the superego (see Chapter 2).

Freud's Stages of Personality Development

Freud described formation of the personality through five stages of *psychosexual* development. He placed much emphasis on the first 5 years of life and believed that characteristics developed during these early years bore heavily on one's adaptation patterns and personality traits in adulthood. Fixation in an early stage of development will almost certainly result in psychopathology. An outline of these five stages is presented in Table 3–1.

Oral Stage: Birth to 18 Months

During the oral stage, behavior is directed by the id, and the goal is immediate gratification of needs. The focus of energy is the mouth, with behaviors that include sucking, chewing, and biting. The infant feels a sense of attachment and is unable to differentiate the self from the person who is providing the mothering. This includes feelings such as anxiety. Because of this lack of differentiation, a pervasive feeling of anxiety on the part of the mother may be passed on to her infant, leaving the child vulnerable to similar feelings of insecurity. With the beginning of development of the ego at age 4 to 6 months, the infant starts to view the self as separate from the mothering figure. A sense of security and the ability to trust others is derived from the gratification of fulfilling basic needs during this stage.

Anal Stage: 18 Months to 3 Years

The major tasks in the anal stage are gaining independence and control, with particular focus on the excretory function. Freud believed that the manner in which the parents and other primary caregivers approach the task of toilet training may have far-reaching effects on the child in terms of values and personality characteristics. When toilet training is strict and rigid, the child may choose to retain the feces, becoming constipated. Adult retentive personality traits influenced by this type of training include stubbornness, stinginess, and miserliness. An alternate reaction to strict toilet training is for the child to expel feces in an unacceptable manner or at inappropriate times. Far-reaching effects of this behavior pattern include malevolence, cruelty to others, destructiveness, disorganization, and untidiness.

Toilet training that is more permissive and accepting attaches the feeling of importance and desirability to feces production. The child becomes extroverted, productive, and altruistic.

Phallic Stage: 3 to 6 Years

In the phallic stage, the focus of energy shifts to the genital area. Discovery of differences between genders results in a heightened interest in the sexuality of self and others. This interest may be manifested in sexual self-exploratory or group-exploratory play. Freud proposed that the development of the *Oedipus complex* (males) or *Electra complex* (females) occurred during this stage of development. He described this as the child's unconscious desire to eliminate the parent of the same sex and to possess the parent of the opposite sex for him- or herself. Guilt feelings result with the emergence of the superego during these years. Resolution of this internal conflict occurs when the child develops a strong identification with the parent of the same sex and that parent's attitudes, beliefs, and value systems are subsumed by the child.

Latency Stage: 6 to 12 Years

During the elementary school years, the focus changes from egocentrism to more interest in group activities, learning, and socialization with peers. Sexuality is not absent during this period but remains obscure and imperceptible to others. The preference is for same-sex relationships, even rejecting members of the opposite sex.

Genital Stage: 13 to 20 Years

In the genital stage, the maturing of the genital organs results in a reawakening of the libidinal drive. The focus is on relationships with members of the opposite sex and preparations for selecting a mate. The development of sexual maturity evolves from self-gratification to behaviors deemed acceptable by societal norms. Interpersonal relationships are based on genuine pleasure derived from the interaction rather than from the more self-serving implications of childhood associations.

TABLE 3–1	Freud's Stages of Psychosexual Development	
Age	**Stage**	**Major Developmental Tasks**
Birth–18 months	Oral	Relief from anxiety through oral gratification of needs
18 months–3 years	Anal	Learning independence and control, with focus on the excretory function
3–6 years	Phallic	Identification with parent of same sex; development of sexual identity; focus on genital organs
6–12 years	Latency	Sexuality repressed; focus on relationships with same-sex peers
13–20 years	Genital	Libido reawakened as genital organs mature; focus on relationships with members of the opposite sex

Relevance of Psychoanalytic Theory to Nursing Practice

Knowledge of the structure of the personality can assist nurses who work in the mental health setting. The ability to recognize behaviors associated with the id, the ego, and the superego assists in the assessment of developmental level. Understanding the use of ego defense mechanisms is important in making determinations about maladaptive behaviors, in planning care for clients to assist in creating change (if desired) or in helping clients accept themselves as unique individuals.

CLINICAL PEARL: ASSESSING CLIENT BEHAVIORS

ID BEHAVIORS

Behaviors that follow the principle of "if it feels good, do it." Social and cultural acceptability are not considered. They reflect a need for immediate gratification. Individuals with a strong id show little if any remorse for their unacceptable behavior.

EGO BEHAVIORS

These behaviors reflect the rational part of the personality. An effort is made to delay gratification and to satisfy societal expectations. The ego uses defense mechanisms to cope and regain control over id impulses.

SUPEREGO BEHAVIORS

Behaviors that are somewhat uncompromising and rigid. They are based on morality and society's values. Behaviors of the superego strive for perfection. Violation of the superego's standards generates guilt and anxiety in an individual who has a strong superego.

INTERPERSONAL THEORY

Sullivan (1953) believed that individual behavior and personality development are the direct result of interpersonal relationships. Before the development of his own theoretical framework, Sullivan embraced the concepts of Freud. Later, he changed the focus of his work from the *intrapersonal* view of Freud to one with more *interpersonal* flavor in which human behavior could be observed in social interactions with others. His ideas, which were not universally accepted at the time, have been integrated into the practice of psychiatry through publication only since his death in 1949. Sullivan's major concepts include the following:

- *Anxiety* is a feeling of emotional discomfort, toward the relief or prevention of which all behavior is aimed. Sullivan believed that anxiety is the "chief disruptive force in interpersonal relations and the main factor in the development of serious difficulties in living." It arises out of one's inability to satisfy needs or to achieve interpersonal security.
- *Satisfaction of needs* is the fulfillment of all requirements associated with an individual's physiochemical environment. Sullivan identified examples of these requirements as oxygen, food, water, warmth, tenderness, rest, activity, sexual expression—virtually anything that, when absent, produces discomfort in the individual.
- *Interpersonal security* is the feeling associated with relief from anxiety. When all needs have been met, one experiences a sense of total well-being, which Sullivan termed *interpersonal security*. He believed individuals have an innate need for interpersonal security.
- *Self-system* is a collection of experiences, or security measures, adopted by the individual to protect against anxiety. Sullivan identified three components of the self-system, which are based on interpersonal experiences early in life:
  - The *"good me"* is the part of the personality that develops in response to positive feedback from the primary caregiver. Feelings of pleasure, contentment, and gratification are experienced. The child learns which behaviors elicit this positive response as it becomes incorporated into the self-system.
  - The *"bad me"* is the part of the personality that develops in response to negative feedback from the primary caregiver. Anxiety is experienced, eliciting feelings of discomfort, displeasure, and distress. The child learns to avoid these negative feelings by altering certain behaviors.
  - The *"not me"* is the part of the personality that develops in response to situations that produce intense anxiety in the child. Feelings of horror, awe, dread, and loathing are experienced in response to these situations, leading the child to deny these feelings in an effort to relieve anxiety. These feelings, having then been denied, become "not me," but someone else. This withdrawal from emotions has serious implications for mental disorders in adult life.

Sullivan's Stages of Personality Development

Infancy: Birth to 18 Months

During the beginning stage, the major developmental task for the child is the gratification of needs. This is accomplished through activity associated with the mouth, such as crying, nursing, and thumb sucking.

Childhood: 18 Months to 6 Years

At ages 18 months to 6 years, the child learns that interference with fulfillment of personal wishes and desires may result in delayed gratification. He or she learns to accept this and feel comfortable with it, recognizing that delayed gratification often results in parental approval, a more lasting type of reward. Tools of this stage include the mouth, the anus, language, experimentation, manipulation, and identification.

Juvenile: 6 to 9 Years

The major task of the juvenile stage is formation of satisfactory relationships within peer groups. This is accomplished through the use of competition, cooperation, and compromise.

Preadolescence: 9 to 12 Years

The tasks at the preadolescence stage focus on developing relationships with persons of the same sex. One's ability to collaborate with and show love and affection for another person begins at this stage.

Early Adolescence: 12 to 14 Years

During early adolescence, the child is struggling with developing a sense of identity that is separate and independent from the parents. The major task is formation of satisfactory relationships with members of the opposite sex. Sullivan saw the emergence of lust in response to biological changes as a major force occurring during this period.

Late Adolescence: 14 to 21 Years

The late adolescent period is characterized by tasks associated with the attempt to achieve interdependence within the society and the formation of a lasting, intimate relationship with a selected member of the opposite sex. The genital organs are the major developmental focus of this stage.

An outline of the stages of personality development according to Sullivan's interpersonal theory is presented in Table 3–2.

Relevance of Interpersonal Theory to Nursing Practice

The interpersonal theory has significant relevance to nursing practice. Relationship development, which is a major concept of this theory, is a major psychiatric nursing intervention. Nurses develop therapeutic relationships with clients in an effort to help them generalize this ability to interact successfully with others.

Knowledge about the behaviors associated with all levels of anxiety and methods for alleviating anxiety helps nurses to assist clients achieve interpersonal security and a sense of well-being. Nurses use the concepts of Sullivan's theory to help clients achieve a higher degree of independent and interpersonal functioning.

THEORY OF PSYCHOSOCIAL DEVELOPMENT

Erikson (1963) studied the influence of social processes on the development of the personality. He described eight stages of the life cycle during which individuals struggle with developmental "crises." Specific tasks associated with each stage must be completed for resolution of the crisis and for emotional growth to occur. An outline of Erikson's stages of psychosocial development is presented in Table 3–3.

Erikson's Stages of Personality Development

Trust versus Mistrust: Birth to 18 Months

Major Developmental Task. From birth to 18 months, the major task is to develop a basic trust in the mothering figure and learn to generalize it to others.

● Achievement of the task results in self-confidence, optimism, faith in the gratification of needs and desires, and hope for the future. The infant learns to trust when basic needs are met consistently.

TABLE 3–2	Stages of Development in Sullivan's Interpersonal Theory	
Age	**Stage**	**Major Developmental Tasks**
Birth–18 months	Infancy	Relief from anxiety through oral gratification of needs
18 months–6 years	Childhood	Learning to experience a delay in personal gratification without undue anxiety
6–9 years	Juvenile	Learning to form satisfactory peer relationships
9–12 years	Preadolescence	Learning to form satisfactory relationships with persons of same sex; initiating feelings of affection for another person
12–14 years	Early adolescence	Learning to form satisfactory relationships with persons of the opposite sex; developing a sense of identity
14–21 years	Late adolescence	Establishing self-identity; experiencing satisfying relationships; working to develop a lasting, intimate opposite-sex relationship

TABLE 3–3	Stages of Development in Erikson's Psychosocial Theory	
Age	**Stage**	**Major Developmental Tasks**
Infancy (Birth–18 months)	Trust vs. mistrust	To develop a basic trust in the mothering figure and learn to generalize it to others
Early childhood (18 months–3 years)	Autonomy vs. shame and doubt	To gain some self-control and independence within the environment
Late childhood (3–6 years)	Initiative vs. guilt	To develop a sense of purpose and the ability to initiate and direct own activities
School age (6–12 years)	Industry vs. inferiority	To achieve a sense of self-confidence by learning, competing, performing successfully, and receiving recognition from significant others, peers, and acquaintances
Adolescence (12–20 years)	Identity vs. role confusion	To integrate the tasks mastered in the previous stages into a secure sense of self
Young adulthood (20–30 years)	Intimacy vs. isolation	To form an intense, lasting relationship or a commitment to another person, cause, institution, or creative effort
Adulthood (30–65 years)	Generativity vs. stagnation	To achieve the life goals established for oneself, while also considering the welfare of future generations
Old age (65 years–death)	Ego integrity vs. despair	To review one's life and derive meaning from both positive and negative events, while achieving a positive sense of self-worth

● Nonachievement results in emotional dissatisfaction with the self and others, suspiciousness, and difficulty with interpersonal relationships. The task remains unresolved when primary caregivers fail to respond to the infant's distress signal promptly and consistently.

Autonomy versus Shame and Doubt: 18 Months to 3 Years

Major Developmental Task. The major task during the ages of 18 months to 3 years is to gain some self-control and independence within the environment.

● Achievement of the task results in a sense of self-control and the ability to delay gratification, and a feeling of self-confidence in one's ability to perform. Autonomy is achieved when parents encourage and provide opportunities for independent activities.
● Nonachievement results in a lack of self-confidence, a lack of pride in the ability to perform, a sense of being controlled by others, and a rage against the self. The task remains unresolved when primary caregivers restrict independent behaviors, both physically and verbally, or set the child up for failure with unrealistic expectations.

Initiative versus Guilt: 3 to 6 Years

Major Developmental Task. During the ages of 3 to 6 years the goal is to develop a sense of purpose and the ability to initiate and direct one's own activities.

● Achievement of the task results in the ability to exercise restraint and self-control of inappropriate social behaviors. Assertiveness and dependability increase, and the child enjoys learning and personal achievement. The conscience develops, thereby controlling the impulsive behaviors of the id. Initiative is achieved when creativity is encouraged and performance is recognized and positively reinforced.
● Nonachievement results in feelings of inadequacy and a sense of defeat. Guilt is experienced to an excessive degree, even to the point of accepting liability in situations for which one is not responsible. The child may view him- or herself as evil and deserving of punishment. The task remains unresolved when creativity is stifled and parents continually expect a higher level of achievement than the child produces.

Industry versus Inferiority: 6 to 12 Years

Major Developmental Task. The major task for 6- to 12-year-olds is to achieve a sense of self-confidence by learning, competing, performing successfully, and receiving recognition from significant others, peers, and acquaintances.

● Achievement of the task results in a sense of satisfaction and pleasure in the interaction and involvement with others. The individual masters reliable work habits and develops attitudes of trustworthiness. He or she is conscientious, feels pride in achievement, and enjoys play but desires a balance between fantasy and "real world" activities. Industry is achieved when encouragement is given to activities and responsibilities in the school and community, as well as those within the home, and recognition is given for accomplishments.

In the context of nursing, Peplau (1991) relates these four psychological tasks to the demands made on nurses in their relations with clients. She maintains the following:

Nursing can function as a maturing force in society. Since illness is an event that is experienced along with feelings that derive from older experiences but are reenacted in the relationship of nurse to patient, the nurse-patient relationship is seen as an opportunity for nurses to help patients to complete the unfinished psychological tasks of childhood in some degree. (p. 159)

Peplau's psychological tasks of personality development include the four stages outlined in the following paragraphs. An outline of the stages of personality development according to Peplau's theory is presented in Table 3–7.

Learning to Count on Others

Nurses and clients first come together as strangers. Both bring to the relationship certain "raw materials," such as inherited biological components, personality characteristics (*temperament*), individual intellectual capacity, and specific cultural or environmental influences. Peplau relates these to the same "raw materials" with which an infant comes into this world. The newborn is capable of experiencing *comfort* and *discomfort*. He or she soon learns to communicate feelings in a way that results in the fulfillment of comfort needs by the mothering figure who provides love and care unconditionally. However, fulfillment of these dependency needs is inhibited when goals of the mothering figure become the focus, and love and care are contingent on meeting the needs of the caregiver rather than those of the infant.

Clients with unmet dependency needs regress during illness and demonstrate behaviors that relate to this stage of development. Other clients regress to this level because of physical disabilities associated with their illness. Peplau believed that when nurses provide unconditional care, they help these clients progress toward more mature levels of functioning. This may involve the role of "surrogate mother," in which the nurse fulfills needs for the client with the intent of helping him or her grow, mature, and become more independent.

Learning to Delay Satisfaction

Peplau relates this stage to that of toddlerhood, or the first step in the development of interdependent social relations. Psychosexually, it is compared to the anal stage of development, when a child learns that, because of cultural mores, he or she cannot empty the bowels for relief of discomfort at will, but must delay to use the toilet, which is considered more culturally acceptable. When toilet training occurs too early or is very rigid, or when appropriate behavior is set forth as a condition for love and caring, tasks associated with this stage remain unfulfilled. The child feels powerless and fails to learn the satisfaction of pleasing others by delaying self-gratification in small ways. He or she may also exhibit rebellious behavior by failing to comply with demands of the mothering figure in an effort to counter the feelings of powerlessness. The child may accomplish this by withholding the fecal product or failing to deposit it in the culturally acceptable manner.

Peplau cites Fromm (1949) in describing the following potential behaviors of individuals who have failed to complete the tasks of the second stage of development:

● Exploitation and manipulation of others to satisfy their own desires because they are unable to do so independently
● Suspiciousness and envy of others, directing hostility toward others in an effort to enhance their own self-image
● Hoarding and withholding possessions from others; miserliness
● Inordinate neatness and punctuality
● Inability to relate to others through sharing of feelings, ideas, or experiences
● Ability to vary the personality characteristics to those required to satisfy personal desires at any given time

When nurses observe these types of behaviors in clients, it is important to encourage full expression and to

TABLE 3–7	Stages of Development in Peplau's Interpersonal Theory	
Age	**Stage**	**Major Developmental Tasks**
Infancy	Learning to count on others	Learning to communicate in various ways with the primary caregiver in order to have comfort needs fulfilled
Toddlerhood	Learning to delay satisfaction	Learning the satisfaction of pleasing others by delaying self-gratification in small ways
Early childhood	Identifying oneself	Learning appropriate roles and behaviors by acquiring the ability to perceive the expectations of others
Late childhood	Developing skills in participation	Learning the skills of compromise, competition, and cooperation with others; establishment of a more realistic view of the world and a feeling of one's place in it

convey unconditional acceptance. When the client learns to feel safe and unconditionally accepted, he or she is more likely to let go of the oppositional behavior and advance in the developmental progression. Peplau (1991) states:

> Nurses who aid patients to feel safe and secure, so that wants can be expressed and satisfaction eventually achieved, also help them to strengthen personal power that is needed for productive social activities. (p. 207)

Identifying Oneself

"A concept of self develops as a product of interaction with adults" (Peplau, 1991, p. 211). A child learns to structure self-concept by observing how others interact with him or her. Roles and behaviors are established out of the child's perception of the expectations of others. When children perceive that adults expect them to maintain more-or-less permanent roles as infants, they perceive themselves as helpless and dependent. When the perceived expectation is that the child must behave in a manner beyond his or her maturational level, the child is deprived of the fulfillment of emotional and growth needs at the lower levels of development. Children who are given freedom to respond to situations and experiences unconditionally (i.e., with behaviors that are appropriate to their feelings) learn to improve on and reconstruct behavioral responses at their own individual pace. Peplau (1991) states, "The ways in which adults appraise the child and the way he functions in relation to his experiences and perceptions are taken in or introjected and become the child's view of himself" (p. 213).

In nursing, it is important for the nurse to recognize cues that communicate how the client feels about him- or herself and about the presenting medical problem. In the initial interaction, it is difficult for the nurse to perceive the "wholeness" of the client, because the focus is on the condition that has caused him or her to seek help. Likewise, it is difficult for the client to perceive the nurse as a "mother (or father)" or "somebody's wife (or husband)" or as having a life aside from being there to offer assistance with the immediate presenting problem. As the relationship develops, nurses must be able to recognize client behaviors that indicate unfulfilled needs and provide experiences that promote growth. For example, the client who very proudly announces that she has completed activities of daily living independently and wants the nurse to come and inspect her room may still be craving the positive reinforcement associated with lower levels of development.

Nurses must also be aware of the predisposing factors that they bring to the relationship. Attitudes and beliefs about certain issues can have a deleterious effect on the client and interfere not only with the therapeutic relationship but also with the client's ability for growth and development. For example, a nurse who has strong beliefs against abortion may treat a client who has just undergone an abortion with disapproval and disrespect. The nurse may respond in this manner without even realizing he or she is doing so. Attitudes and values are introjected during early development and can be integrated so completely as to become a part of the self-system. Nurses must have knowledge and appreciation of their own concept of self in order to develop the flexibility required to accept all clients as they are, unconditionally. Effective resolution of problems that arise in the interdependent relationship can be the means for both client and nurse to reinforce positive personality traits and modify those more negative views of self.

Developing Skills in Participation

Peplau cites Sullivan's (1953) description of the "juvenile" stage of personality development (ages 6 through 9). During this stage, the child develops the capacity to "compromise, compete, and cooperate" with others. These skills are considered basic to one's ability to participate collaboratively with others. If a child tries to use the skills of an earlier level of development (e.g., crying, whining, demanding), he or she may be rejected by peers of this juvenile stage. As this stage progresses, children begin to view themselves through the eyes of their peers. Sullivan (1953) called this "consensual validation." Preadolescents take on a more realistic view of the world and a feeling of their place in it. The capacity to love others (besides the mother figure) develops at this time and is expressed in relation to one's self-acceptance.

Failure to develop appropriate skills at any point along the developmental progression results in an individual's difficulty with participation in confronting the recurring problems of life. It is not the responsibility of the nurse to teach solutions to problems, but rather to help clients improve their problem-solving skills so that they may achieve their own resolution. This is accomplished through development of the skills of competition, compromise, cooperation, consensual validation, and love of self and others. Nurses can assist clients to develop or refine these skills by helping them to identify the problem, define a goal, and take the responsibility for performing the actions necessary to reach that goal. Peplau (1991) states:

> Participation is required by a democratic society. When it has not been learned in earlier experiences, nurses have an opportunity to facilitate learning in the present and thus to aid in the promotion of a democratic society. (p. 259)

Relevance of Peplau's Model to Nursing Practice

Peplau's model provides nurses with a framework to interact with clients, many of whom are fixed in—or because of illness have regressed to—an earlier level of development. She suggests roles that nurses may assume to assist clients to progress, thereby achieving or resuming their appropriate developmental level. Appropriate developmental progression arms the individual with the ability to confront the recurring problems of life. Nurses serve to facilitate learning of that which has not been learned in earlier experiences.

SUMMARY AND KEY POINTS

● Growth and development are unique with each individual and continue throughout the life span.
● Personality is defined as the combination of character, behavioral, temperamental, emotional, and mental traits that are unique to each specific individual.
● Sigmund Freud, who has been called the father of psychiatry, believed the basic character has been formed by the age of 5.
● Freud's personality theory can be conceptualized according to structure and dynamics of the personality, topography of the mind, and stages of personality development.
● Freud's structure of the personality includes the id, ego, and superego.
● Freud classified all mental contents and operations into three categories: the conscious, the preconscious, and the unconscious.
● Harry Stack Sullivan, author of the Interpersonal Theory of Psychiatry, believed that individual behavior and personality development are the direct result of interpersonal relationships. Major concepts include *anxiety, satisfaction of needs, interpersonal security, and self-system*.
● Erik Erikson studied the influence of social processes on the development of the personality.

● Erikson described eight stages of the life cycle from birth to death. He believed that individuals struggled with developmental "crises," and that each must be resolved for emotional growth to occur.
● Margaret Mahler formulated a theory that describes the separation–individuation process of the infant from the maternal figure (primary caregiver). Stages of development describe the progression of the child from birth to object constancy at age 36 months.
● Jean Piaget has been called the father of child psychology. He believed that human intelligence progresses through a series of stages that are related to age, demonstrating at each successive stage a higher level of logical organization than at the previous stages.
● Lawrence Kohlberg outlined stages of moral development. His stages are not closely tied to specific age groups or the maturational process. He believed that moral stages emerge out of our own thinking and the stimulation of our mental processes.
● Hildegard Peplau provided a framework for "psychodynamic nursing," the interpersonal involvement of the nurse with a client in a given nursing situation.
● Peplau identified the nursing roles of resource person, counselor, teacher, leader, technical expert, and surrogate.
● Peplau describes four psychological tasks that she associates with the stages of infancy and childhood as identified by Freud and Sullivan.
● Peplau believed that nursing is helpful when both the patient and the nurse grow as a result of the learning that occurs in the nursing situation.

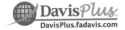 **DavisPlus** **For additional clinical tools**
DavisPlus.fadavis.com **and study aids, visit DavisPlus.**

REVIEW QUESTIONS

Self-Examination/Learning Exercise

Situation: Mr. J. is 35 years old. He has been admitted to the psychiatric unit for observation and evaluation following his arrest on charges that he robbed a convenience store and sexually assaulted the store clerk. Mr. J. was the child of an unmarried teenage mother who deserted him when he was 6 months old. He was shuffled from one relative to another until it was clear that no one wanted him. Social services placed him in foster homes, from which he continuously ran away. During his teenage years he was arrested a number of times for stealing, vandalism, arson, and various other infractions of the law. He was shunned by his peers and to this day has little interaction with others. On the unit, he appears very anxious, paces back and forth, and darts his head from side to side in a continuous scanning of the area. He is unkempt, with poor personal hygiene. He has refused to eat, making some barely audible comment related to "being poisoned." He has shown no remorse for his misdeeds.

Select the answer that is *most* appropriate for this situation.

1. Theoretically, in which level of psychosocial development (according to Erikson) would you place Mr. J.?

   a. Intimacy vs. isolation
   b. Generativity vs. self-absorption
   c. Trust vs. mistrust
   d. Autonomy vs. shame and doubt

2. According to Erikson's theory, where would you place Mr. J. based on his behavior?

   a. Intimacy vs. isolation
   b. Generativity vs. self-absorption
   c. Trust vs. mistrust
   d. Autonomy vs. shame and doubt

3. According to Mahler's theory, Mr. J. did not receive the critical "emotional refueling" required during the rapprochement phase of development. What are the consequences of this deficiency?

   a. He has not yet learned to delay gratification.
   b. He does not feel guilt about wrongdoings to others.
   c. He is unable to trust others.
   d. He has internalized rage and fears of abandonment.

4. In what stage of development is Mr. J. fixed according to Sullivan's interpersonal theory?

   a. Infancy. He relieves anxiety through oral gratification.
   b. Childhood. He has not learned to delay gratification.
   c. Early adolescence. He is struggling to form an identity.
   d. Late adolescence. He is working to develop a lasting relationship.

5. Which of the following describes the psychoanalytical structure of Mr. J.'s personality?

   a. Weak id, strong ego, weak superego
   b. Strong id, weak ego, weak superego
   c. Weak id, weak ego, punitive superego
   d. Strong id, weak ego, punitive superego

6. In which of Peplau's stages of development would you assess Mr. J.?

   a. Learning to count on others
   b. Learning to delay gratification
   c. Identifying oneself
   d. Developing skills in participation

7. In planning care for Mr. J., which of the following would be the primary focus for nursing?

   a. To decrease anxiety and develop trust
   b. To set limits on his behavior

c. To ensure that he gets to group therapy

d. To attend to his hygiene needs

Match the nursing role as described by Peplau with the nursing care behaviors listed on the right:

_____ 8. Surrogate

_____ 9. Counselor

_____ 10. Resource person

a. "Mr. J., please tell me what it was like when you were growing up."

b. "What questions do you have about being here on this unit?"

c. "Some changes will have to be made in your behavior. I care about what happens to you."

REFERENCES

American Psychiatric Association (2000). *Diagnostic and statistical manual of mental disorders* (4th ed.) Text Revision. Washington, DC: American Psychiatric Association.

Marmer, S.S. (2003). Theories of the mind and psychopathology. In R.E. Hales & S.C. Yudofsky (Eds.), *Textbook of clinical psychiatry* (4th ed.). Washington, DC: American Psychiatric Publishing.

Murray, R., & Zentner, J. (2001). *Health promotion strategies through the life span* (7th ed.). Upper Saddle River, NJ: Prentice-Hall.

Peplau, H.E. (1991). *Interpersonal relations in nursing.* New York: Springer, pp. 107–154.

CLASSICAL REFERENCES

Chess, S., & Thomas, A. (1986). *Temperament in clinical practice.* New York: Guilford Press.

Erikson, E. (1963). *Childhood and society* (2nd ed.). New York: WW Norton.

Freud, S. (1961). The ego and the id. *Standard edition of the complete psychological works of Freud,* Vol XIX. London: Hogarth Press.

Fromm, E. (1949). *Man for himself.* New York: Farrar & Rinehart.

Kohlberg, L. (1968). Moral development. In *International encyclopedia of social science.* New York: Macmillan.

Mahler, M., Pine, F., & Bergman, A. (1975). *The psychological birth of the human infant.* New York: Basic Books.

Piaget, J., & Inhelder, B. (1969). *The psychology of the child.* New York: Basic Books.

Sullivan, H.S. (1953). *The interpersonal theory of psychiatry.* New York: WW Norton.

4

C H A P T E R

Concepts of Psychobiology

C H A P T E R   O U T L I N E

OBJECTIVES

THE NERVOUS SYSTEM: AN ANATOMICAL REVIEW

NEUROENDOCRINOLOGY

GENETICS

PSYCHOIMMUNOLOGY

IMPLICATIONS FOR NURSING

SUMMARY AND KEY POINTS

REVIEW QUESTIONS

K E Y   T E R M S

axon
cell body
circadian rhythms
dendrites
genotype
limbic system

neuron
neurotransmitter
phenotype
receptor sites
synapse

C O R E   C O N C E P T S

genetics
neuroendocrinology
psychobiology

O B J E C T I V E S

After reading this chapter, the student will be able to:

1. Identify gross anatomical structures of the brain and describe their functions.
2. Discuss the physiology of neurotransmission in the central nervous system.
3. Describe the role of neurotransmitters in human behavior.
4. Discuss the association of endocrine functioning to the development of psychiatric disorders.
5. Describe the role of genetics in the development of psychiatric disorders.
6. Discuss the correlation of alteration in brain functioning to various psychiatric disorders.
7. Identify various diagnostic procedures used to detect alteration in biological functioning that may be contributing to psychiatric disorders.
8. Discuss the influence of psychological factors on the immune system.
9. Discuss the implications of psychobiological concepts to the practice of psychiatric/mental health nursing.

In recent years, a greater emphasis has been placed on the study of the organic basis for psychiatric illness. This "neuroscientific revolution" began in earnest when the 101st legislature of the United States designated the 1990s as the "decade of the brain." With this legislation came the challenge for studying the biological basis of behavior. Several mental illnesses are now being considered as physical disorders that are the result of malfunctions and/or malformations of the brain.

This is not to imply that psychosocial and sociocultural influences are totally discounted. Such a notion would negate the transactional model of stress/adaptation on which the framework of this textbook is conceptualized.

The systems of biology, psychology, and sociology are not mutually exclusive—they are interacting systems. This is clearly indicated by the fact that individuals experience biological changes in response to various environmental events. Indeed, each of these disciplines may be, at various times, most appropriate for explaining behavioral phenomena.

This chapter focuses on the role of neurophysiological, neurochemical, genetic, and endocrine influences on psychiatric illness. Various diagnostic procedures used to detect alteration in biological function that may contribute to psychiatric illness are identified, and the implications for psychiatric/mental health nursing are discussed.

CORE CONCEPT

Psychobiology
The study of the biological foundations of cognitive, emotional, and behavioral processes.

THE NERVOUS SYSTEM: AN ANATOMICAL REVIEW

The Brain

The brain has three major divisions, subdivided into six major parts:

1. Forebrain
   a. Cerebrum
   b. Diencephalon
2. Midbrain
   a. Mesencephalon
3. Hindbrain
   a. Pons
   b. Medulla
   c. Cerebellum

Each of these structures is discussed individually. A summary is presented in Table 4–1.

Cerebrum

The cerebrum consists of a right and left hemisphere and constitutes the largest part of the human brain. The right and left hemispheres are connected by a deep groove, which houses a band of 200 million **neurons** (nerve cells) called the *corpus callosum*. Because each hemisphere controls different functions, information is processed through the corpus callosum so that each hemisphere is aware of the activity of the other.

The surface of the cerebrum consists of gray matter and is called the *cerebral cortex*. The *gray matter* is so called because the neuron cell bodies of which it is composed look gray to the eye. These gray matter cell bodies are thought to be the actual thinking structures of the brain. Another pair of masses of gray matter called

TABLE 4–1	Structure and Function of the Brain	
Structure	**Primary Function**
I. The Forebrain	
A. Cerebrum	Composed of two hemispheres separated by a deep groove that houses a band of 200 million neurons called the corpus callosum. The outer shell is called the cortex. It is extensively folded and consists of billions of neurons. The left hemisphere appears to deal with logic and solving problems. The right hemisphere may be called the "creative" brain and is associated with affect, behavior, and spatial-perceptual functions. Each hemisphere is divided into four lobes.
1. Frontal lobes	Voluntary body movement, including movements that permit speaking, thinking and judgment formation, and expression of feelings.
2. Parietal lobes	Perception and interpretation of most sensory information (including touch, pain, taste, and body position).
3. Temporal lobes	Hearing, short-term memory, and sense of smell; expression of emotions through connection with limbic system.
4. Occipital lobes	Visual reception and interpretation.
B. Diencephalon	Connects cerebrum with lower brain structures.
1. Thalamus	Integrates all sensory input (except smell) on way to cortex; some involvement with emotions and mood.
2. Hypothalamus	Regulates anterior and posterior lobes of pituitary gland; exerts control over actions of the autonomic nervous system; regulates appetite and temperature.
3. Limbic system	Consists of medially placed cortical and subcortical structures and the fiber tracts connecting them with one another and with the hypothalamus. It is sometimes called the "emotional brain"—associated with feelings of fear and anxiety; anger and aggression; love, joy, and hope; and with sexuality and social behavior.
II. The Midbrain	
A. Mesencephalon	Responsible for visual, auditory, and balance ("righting") reflexes.
III. The Hindbrain	
A. Pons	Regulation of respiration and skeletal muscle tone; ascending and descending tracts connect brain stem with cerebellum and cortex.
B. Medulla	Pathway for all ascending and descending fiber tracts; contains vital centers that regulate heart rate, blood pressure, and respiration; reflex centers for swallowing, sneezing, coughing, and vomiting.
C. Cerebellum	Regulates muscle tone and coordination and maintains posture and equilibrium.

basal ganglia is found deep within the cerebral hemispheres. They are responsible for certain subconscious aspects of voluntary movement, such as swinging the arms when walking, gesturing while speaking, and regulating muscle tone (Scanlon & Sanders, 2006).

The cerebral cortex is identified by numerous folds, called *gyri*, and deep grooves between the folds, called *sulci*. This extensive folding extends the surface area of the cerebral cortex, and thus permits the presence of millions more neurons than would be possible without it (as is the case in the brains of some animals, such as dogs and cats). Each hemisphere of the cerebral cortex is divided into the frontal lobe, parietal lobe, temporal lobe, and occipital lobe. These lobes, which are named for the overlying bones in the cranium, are identified in Figure 4–1.

The Frontal Lobes. Voluntary body movement is controlled by the impulses through the frontal lobes. The right frontal lobe controls motor activity on the left side of the body and the left frontal lobe controls motor activity on the right side of the body. Movements that permit speaking are also controlled by the frontal lobe, usually only on the left side (Scanlon & Sanders, 2006). The frontal lobe may also play a role in the emotional experience, as evidenced by changes in mood and character after damage to this area. The alterations include fear, aggressiveness, depression, rage, euphoria, irritability, and apathy and are likely related to a frontal lobe connection to the **limbic system**. The frontal lobe may also be involved (indirectly through association fibers linked to primary sensory areas) in thinking and perceptual interpretation of information.

The Parietal Lobes. Somatosensory input occurs in the parietal lobe area of the brain. These include touch, pain and pressure, taste, temperature, perception of joint and body position, and visceral sensations. The parietal lobes also contain association fibers linked to the primary sensory areas through which interpretation of sensory-perceptual information is made. Language interpretation is associated with the left hemisphere of the parietal lobe.

The Temporal Lobes. The upper anterior temporal lobe is concerned with auditory functions, while the lower part is dedicated to short-term memory. The sense of smell has a connection to the temporal lobes, as the impulses carried by the olfactory nerves end in this area of the brain (Scanlon & Sanders, 2006). The temporal lobes also play a role in the expression of emotions through an interconnection with the limbic system. The left temporal lobe, along with the left parietal lobe, is involved in language interpretation.

The Occipital Lobes. The occipital lobes are the primary area of visual reception and interpretation. Visual perception, which gives individuals the ability to judge spatial relationships such as distance and to see in three dimensions, is also processed in this area (Scanlon & Sanders, 2006). Language interpretation is influenced by the occipital lobes through an association with the visual experience.

Diencephalon

The second part of the forebrain is the diencephalon, which connects the cerebrum with lower structures of the brain. The major components of the diencephalon

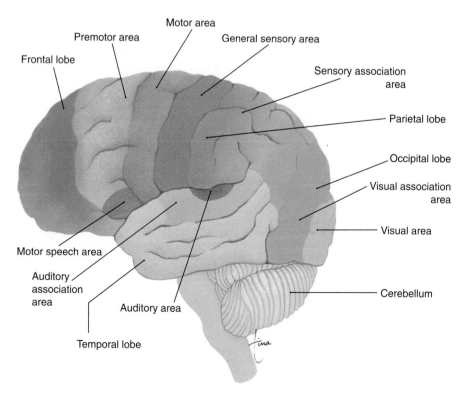

FIGURE 4–1 Left cerebral hemisphere showing some of the functional areas that have been mapped. (From Scanlon, V.C., & Sanders, T: *Essentials of anatomy and physiology*, ed. 5. F.A. Davis, Philadelphia, 2006.)

include the thalamus, the hypothalamus, and the limbic system. These structures are identified in Figures 4–2 and 4–3.

Thalamus. The thalamus integrates all sensory input (except smell) on its way to the cortex. This helps the cerebral cortex interpret the whole picture very rapidly, rather than experiencing each sensation individually. The thalamus is also involved in temporarily blocking minor sensations, so that an individual can concentrate on one important event when necessary. For example, an individual who is studying for an examination may be unaware of the clock ticking in the room, or even of another person walking into the room, because the thalamus has temporarily blocked these incoming sensations from the cortex (Scanlon & Sanders, 2006).

Hypothalamus. The hypothalamus is located just below the thalamus and just above the pituitary gland and has a number of diverse functions.

1. **Regulation of the Pituitary Gland.** The pituitary gland consists of two lobes: the posterior lobe and the anterior lobe.
   a. *The posterior lobe* of the pituitary gland is actually extended tissue from the hypothalamus. The posterior lobe stores antidiuretic hormone (which helps to maintain blood pressure through regulation of water retention) and oxytocin (the hormone responsible for stimulation of the uterus during labor, and the release of milk from the mammary glands). Both of these hormones are produced in the hypothalamus. When the hypothalamus detects the body's need for these hormones, it sends nerve impulses to the posterior pituitary for their release.
   b. *The anterior lobe* of the pituitary gland consists of glandular tissue that produces a number of hormones used by the body. These hormones are regulated by "releasing factors" from the hypothalamus. When the hormones are required by the body, the releasing factors stimulate the release of the hormone from the anterior pituitary and the hormone in turn stimulates its target organ to carry out its specific functions.

2. **Direct Neural Control over the Actions of the Autonomic Nervous System.** The hypothalamus regulates the appropriate visceral responses during various emotional states. The actions of the autonomic nervous system are described later in this chapter.

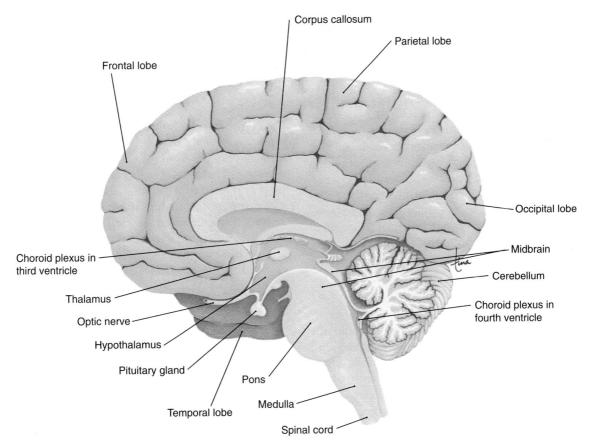

FIGURE 4–2 Midsagittal section of the brain as seen from the left side. This medial plane shows internal anatomy as well as the lobes of the cerebrum. (From Scanlon, V.C., & Sanders, T: *Essentials of anatomy and physiology,* ed. 5. F.A. Davis, Philadelphia, 2006.)

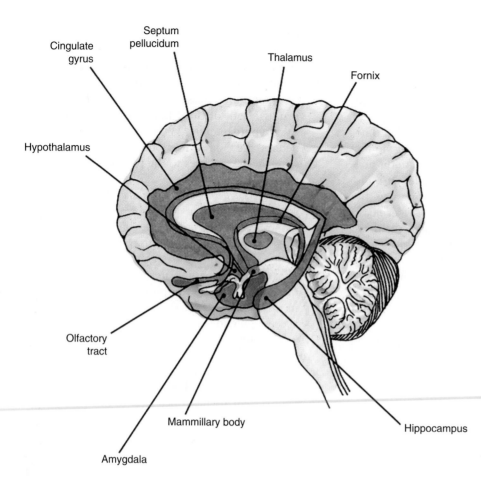

FIGURE 4–3 Structures of the limbic system (Adapted from Scanlon, V.C., & Sanders, T: *Essentials of anatomy and physiology*, ed. 5. F.A. Davis, Philadelphia, 2006.)

3. **Regulation of Appetite.** Appetite is regulated through response to blood nutrient levels.

4. **Regulation of Temperature.** The hypothalamus senses internal temperature changes in the blood that flows through the brain. It receives information through sensory input from the skin about external temperature changes. The hypothalamus then uses this information to promote certain types of responses (e.g., sweating or shivering) that help to maintain body temperature within the normal range (Scanlon & Sanders, 2006).

Limbic System. The part of the brain known as the limbic system consists of portions of the cerebrum and the diencephalon. The major components include the medially placed cortical and subcortical structures and the fiber tracts connecting them with one another and with the hypothalamus. The system is composed of the amygdala, mammillary body, olfactory tract, hypothalamus, cingulate gyrus, septum pellucidum, thalamus, hippocampus, and neuronal connecting pathways, such as the fornix and others. This system has been called "the emotional brain" and is associated with feelings of fear and anxiety; anger, rage, and aggression; love, joy, and hope; and with sexuality and social behavior.

Mesencephalon

Structures of major importance in the mesencephalon, or midbrain, include nuclei and fiber tracts. The mesencephalon extends from the pons to the hypothalamus and is responsible for integration of various reflexes, including visual reflexes (e.g., automatically turning away from a dangerous object when it comes into view), auditory reflexes (e.g., automatically turning toward a sound that is heard), and righting reflexes (e.g., automatically keeping the head upright and maintaining balance) (Scanlon & Sanders, 2006). The mesencephalon is identified in Figure 4–2.

Pons

The pons is a bulbous structure that lies between the midbrain and the medulla (Fig. 4–2). It is composed of large bundles of fibers and forms a major connection between the cerebellum and the brainstem. It also contains the central connections of cranial nerves V through VIII and centers for respiration and skeletal muscle tone.

Medulla

The medulla is the connecting structure between the spinal cord and the pons and all of the ascending and descending fiber tracts pass through it. The vital centers are contained in the medulla, and it is responsible for regulation of heart rate, blood pressure, and respiration. Also in the medulla are reflex centers for swallowing, sneezing, coughing, and vomiting (Scanlon & Sanders, 2006). It also contains nuclei for cranial nerves IX through XII. The medulla, pons, and midbrain form the structure known as the brainstem. These structures are identified in Figure 4–2.

Cerebellum

The cerebellum is separated from the brainstem by the fourth ventricle but has connections to the brainstem through bundles of fiber tracts. It is situated just below the occipital lobes of the cerebrum (Figs. 4–1 and 4–2). The functions of the cerebellum are concerned with involuntary movement, such as muscular tone and coordination and the maintenance of posture and equilibrium.

Nerve Tissue

The tissue of the central nervous system (CNS) consists of nerve cells called neurons that generate and transmit electrochemical impulses. The structure of a neuron is composed of a cell body, an axon, and dendrites. The **cell body** contains the nucleus and is essential for the continued life of the neuron. The **dendrites** are processes that transmit impulses toward the cell body, and the **axon** transmits impulses away from the cell body. The axons and dendrites are covered by layers of cells called *neuroglia* that form a coating, or "sheath," of myelin. *Myelin* is a phospholipid that provides insulation against short-circuiting of the neurons during their electrical activity and increases the velocity of the impulse. The white matter of the brain and spinal cord is so called because of the whitish appearance of the myelin sheath over the axons and dendrites. The gray matter is composed of cell bodies that contain no myelin.

The three classes of neurons include afferent (sensory), efferent (motor), and interneurons. The *afferent neurons* carry impulses from receptors in the internal and external periphery to the CNS, where they are then interpreted into various sensations. The *efferent neurons* carry impulses from the CNS to *effectors* in the periphery, such as muscles (that respond by contracting) and glands (that respond by secreting). A schematic of afferent and efferent neurons is presented in Figure 4–4.

Interneurons exist entirely within the CNS, and 99 percent of all nerve cells belong to this group. They may carry only sensory or motor impulses, or they may serve as integrators in the pathways between afferent and efferent neurons. They account in large part for thinking, feelings, learning, language, and memory. The directional pathways of afferent, efferent, and interneurons are presented in Figure 4–5.

Synapses

Information is transmitted through the body from one neuron to another. Some messages may be processed through only a few neurons, while others may require thousands of neuronal connections. The neurons that transmit the impulses do not actually touch each other. The junction between two neurons is called a **synapse**. The small space between the axon terminals of one neuron and the cell body or dendrites of another is called the *synaptic cleft*. Neurons conducting impulses toward the synapse are called *presynaptic neurons* and those conducting impulses away are called *postsynaptic neurons*.

A chemical, called a **neurotransmitter**, is stored in the axon terminals of the presynaptic neuron. An electrical impulse through the neuron causes the release of this neurotransmitter into the synaptic cleft. The neurotransmitter then diffuses across the synaptic cleft and combines with **receptor sites** that are situated on the cell membrane of the postsynaptic neuron. The result of the combination of neurotransmitter-receptor site is the determination of whether or not another electrical impulse is generated. If one is generated, the result is called an *excitatory response* and the electrical impulse moves on to the next synapse, where the same process recurs. If another electrical impulse is not generated by the neurotransmitter-receptor site combination, the result is called an *inhibitory response*, and synaptic transmission is terminated.

The cell body or dendrite of the postsynaptic neuron also contains a chemical *inactivator* that is specific to the neurotransmitter that has been released by the presynaptic neuron. When the synaptic transmission has been completed, the chemical inactivator quickly inactivates the neurotransmitter to prevent unwanted, continuous impulses, until a new impulse from the presynaptic neuron releases more neurotransmitter. A schematic representation of a synapse is presented in Figure 4–6.

Autonomic Nervous System

The autonomic nervous system (ANS) is actually considered part of the peripheral nervous system. Its regulation is integrated by the hypothalamus, however, and therefore the emotions exert a great deal of influence over its functioning. For this reason, the ANS has been implicated in the etiology of a number of psychophysiological disorders.

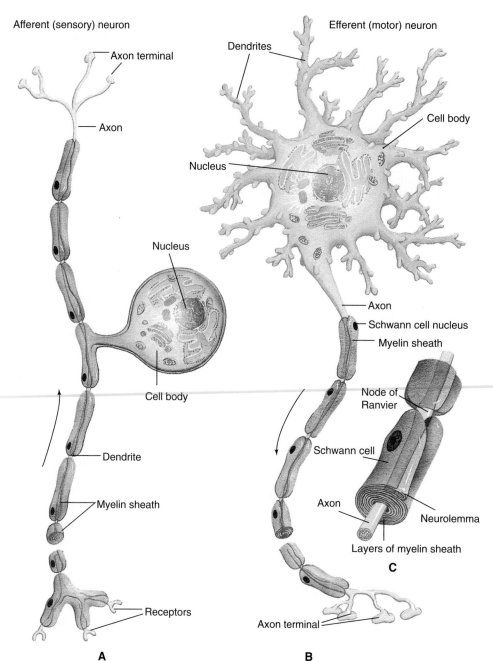

Afferent (sensory) neuron

Efferent (motor) neuron

FIGURE 4–4 Neuron structure. *(A)* A typical sensory neuron. *(B)* A typical motor neuron. The arrows indicate the direction of impulse transmission. *(C)* Details of the myelin sheath and neurolemma formed by Schwann cells. (From Scanlon, V.C., & Sanders, T: *Essentials of anatomy and physiology*, ed. 5. F.A. Davis, Philadelphia, 2006.)

The ANS has two divisions: the sympathetic and the parasympathetic. The sympathetic division is dominant in stressful situations and prepares the body for the "fight or flight" response that was discussed in Chapter 1. The neuronal cell bodies of the sympathetic division originate in the thoracolumbar region of the spinal cord. Their axons extend to the chains of sympathetic ganglia where they synapse with other neurons that subsequently innervate the visceral effectors. This results in an increase in heart rate and respirations and a decrease in digestive secretions and peristalsis. Blood is shunted to the vital organs and to skeletal muscles to ensure adequate oxygenation.

The neuronal cell bodies of the parasympathetic division originate in the brainstem and the sacral segments of the spinal cord, and extend to the parasympathetic ganglia where the synapse takes place either very close to or actually in the visceral organ being innervated. In this way, a very localized response is possible. The parasympathetic division dominates when an individual is in a relaxed, nonstressful condition. The heart and respirations are maintained at a normal rate and secretions and peristalsis increase for normal digestion. Elimination functions are promoted. A schematic representation of the autonomic nervous system is presented in Figure 4–7.

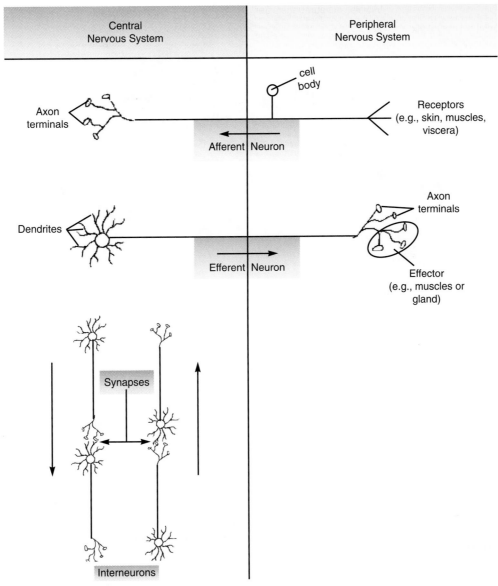

FIGURE 4–5   Directional pathways of neurons

Neurotransmitters

Neurotransmitters were described during the explanation of synaptic activity. They are being discussed separately and in detail because of the essential function they play in the role of human emotion and behavior and because they are the target for mechanism of action of many of the psychotropic medications.

Neurotransmitters are chemicals that convey information across synaptic clefts to neighboring target cells. They are stored in small vesicles in the axon terminals of neurons. When the action potential, or electrical impulse, reaches this point, the neurotransmitters are released from the vesicles. They cross the synaptic cleft and bind with receptor sites on the cell body or dendrites of the adjacent neuron to allow the impulse to continue its course or to prevent the impulse from continuing. After the neurotransmitter has performed its function in the synapse, it either returns to the vesicles to be stored and used again, or it is inactivated and dissolved by enzymes. The process of being stored for reuse is called *reuptake*, a function that holds significance for understanding the mechanism of action of certain psychotropic medications.

Many neurotransmitters exist in the central and peripheral nervous systems, but only a limited number have implications for psychiatry. Major categories include cholinergics, monoamines, amino acids, and neuropeptides. Each of these is discussed separately and summarized in Table 4–2.

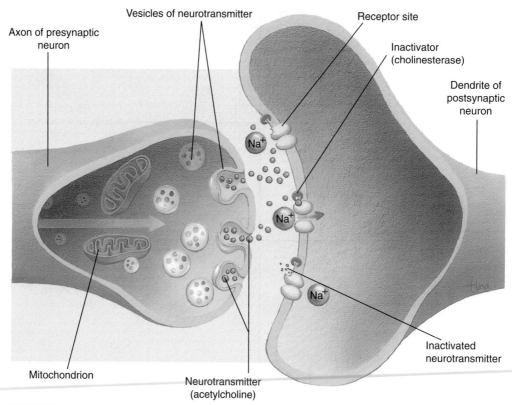

FIGURE 4–6 Impulse transmission at a synapse. The arrow indicates the direction of electrical impulses. (From Scanlon, V.C., & Sanders, T: *Essentials of anatomy and physiology*, ed. 5. F.A. Davis, Philadelphia, 2006.)

Cholinergics

Acetylcholine. Acetylcholine was the first chemical to be identified and proven as a neurotransmitter. It is a major effector chemical in the ANS, producing activity at all sympathetic and parasympathetic presynaptic nerve terminals and all parasympathetic postsynaptic nerve terminals. It is highly significant in the neurotransmission that occurs at the junctions of nerve and muscles. Acetylcholinesterase is the enzyme that destroys acetylcholine or inhibits its activity.

In the CNS, acetylcholine neurons innervate the cerebral cortex, hippocampus, and limbic structures. The pathways are especially dense through the area of the basal ganglia in the brain.

Functions of acetylcholine are manifold and include sleep, arousal, pain perception, the modulation and coordination of movement, and memory acquisition and retention (Murphy & Deutsch, 1991). Cholinergic mechanisms may have some role in certain disorders of motor behavior and memory, such as Parkinson's disease, Huntington's disease, and Alzheimer's disease.

Monoamines

Norepinephrine. Norepinephrine is the neurotransmitter that produces activity at the sympathetic postsynaptic

nerve terminals in the ANS resulting in the "fight or flight" responses in the effector organs. In the CNS, norepinephrine pathways originate in the pons and medulla and innervate the thalamus, dorsal hypothalamus, limbic system, hippocampus, cerebellum, and cerebral cortex. When norepinephrine is not returned for storage in the vesicles of the axon terminals, it is metabolized and inactivated by the enzymes monoamine oxidase (MAO) and catechol-*O*-methyl-transferase (COMT).

The functions of norepinephrine include the regulation of mood, cognition, perception, locomotion, cardiovascular functioning, and sleep and arousal (Murphy & Deutsch, 1991). The activity of norepinephrine also has been implicated in certain mood disorders such as depression and mania, in anxiety states, and in schizophrenia (Sadock & Sadock, 2007).

Dopamine. Dopamine pathways arise from the midbrain and hypothalamus and terminate in the frontal cortex, limbic system, basal ganglia, and thalamus. Dopamine neurons in the hypothalamus innervate the posterior pituitary and those from the posterior hypothalamus project to the spinal cord. As with norepinephrine, the inactivating enzymes for dopamine are MAO and COMT.

Dopamine functions include regulation of movements and coordination, emotions, voluntary decision-making ability, and because of its influence on the pituitary gland,

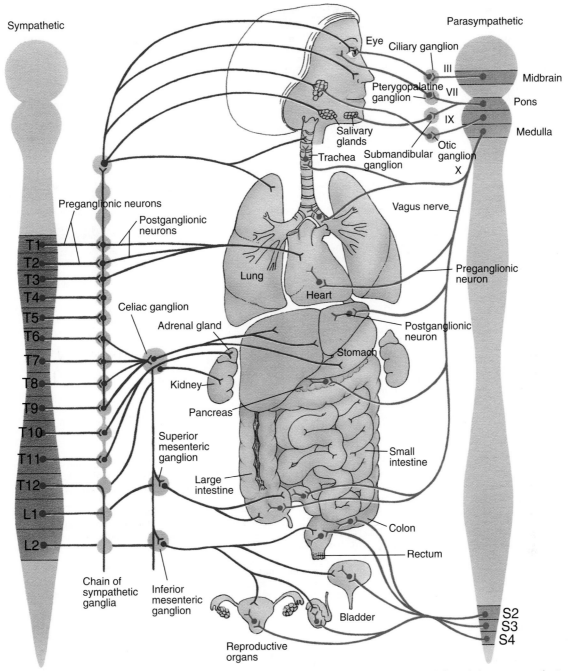

FIGURE 4–7 The autonomic nervous system. The sympathetic division is shown on the left, and the parasympathetic division is shown on the right (both divisions are bilateral). (From Scanlon, V.C., & Sanders, T: *Essentials of anatomy and physiology*, ed. 5. F.A. Davis, Philadelphia, 2006.)

it inhibits the release of prolactin (Sadock & Sadock, 2007). Increased levels of dopamine are associated with mania (Dubovsky, Davies, & Dubovsky, 2003) and schizophrenia (Ho, Black, & Andreasen, 2003).

Serotonin. Serotonin pathways originate from cell bodies located in the pons and medulla and project to areas including the hypothalamus, thalamus, limbic system, cerebral cortex, cerebellum, and spinal cord. Serotonin

that is not returned to be stored in the axon terminal vesicles is catabolized by the enzyme monoamine oxidase.

Serotonin may play a role in sleep and arousal, libido, appetite, mood, aggression, and pain perception. The serotoninergic system has been implicated in the etiology of certain psychopathological conditions including anxiety states, mood disorders, and schizophrenia (Sadock & Sadock, 2007).

TABLE 4–2 Neurotransmitters in the Central Nervous System

Neurotransmitter	Location/Function	Possible Implications for Mental Illness
I. Cholinergics		
A. Acetylcholine	ANS: Sympathetic and parasympathetic presynaptic nerve terminals; parasympathetic postsynaptic nerve terminals	Increased levels: Depression
		Decreased levels: Alzheimer's disease Huntington's disease, Parkinson's disease
	CNS: Cerebral cortex, hippocampus, limbic structures, and basal ganglia Functions: Sleep, arousal, pain perception, movement, memory	
II. Monoamines		
A. Norepinephrine	ANS: Sympathetic postsynaptic nerve terminals	Decreased levels: Depression
	CNS: Thalamus, hypothalamus, limbic system, hippocampus, cerebellum, cerebral cortex Functions: Mood, cognition, perception, locomotion, cardiovascular functioning, and sleep and arousal	Increased levels: Mania, anxiety states, schizophrenia
B. Dopamine	Frontal cortex, limbic system, basal ganglia, thalamus, posterior pituitary, and spinal cord Functions: Movement and coordination, emotions, voluntary judgment, release of prolactin	Decreased levels: Parkinson's disease and depression Increased levels: Mania and schizophrenia
C. Serotonin	Hypothalamus, thalamus, limbic system, cerebral cortex, cerebellum, spinal cord Functions: Sleep and arousal, libido, appetite, mood, aggression, pain perception, coordination, judgment	Decreased levels: Depression Increased levels: Anxiety states
D. Histamine	Hypothalamus Functions: Wakefulness; pain sensation and inflammatory response	Decreased levels: Depression
III. Amino Acids		
A. Gamma-amino-butyric acid (GABA)	Hypothalamus, hippocampus, cortex, cerebellum, basal ganglia, spinal cord, retina Functions: Slowdown of body activity	Decreased levels: Huntington's disease, anxiety disorders, schizophrenia, and various forms of epilepsy
B. Glycine	Spinal cord and brain stem Functions: Recurrent inhibition of motor neurons	Toxic levels: "glycine encephalopathy," decreased levels are correlated with spastic motor movements
C. Glutamate and Aspartate	Pyramidal cells of the cortex, cerebellum, and the primary sensory afferent systems; hippocampus, thalamus, hypothalamus, spinal cord Functions: Relay of sensory information and in the regulation of various motor and spinal reflexes	Increased levels: Huntington's disease, temporal lobe epilepsy, spinal cerebellar degeneration
IV. Neuropeptides		
A. Endorphins and Enkephalins	Hypothalamus, thalamus, limbic structures, midbrain, and brain stem; enkephalins are also found in the gastrointestinal tract Functions: Modulation of pain and reduced peristalsis (enkephalins)	Modulation of dopamine activity by opioid peptides may indicate some link to the symptoms of schizophrenia
B. Substance P	Hypothalamus, limbic structures, midbrain, brain stem, thalamus, basal ganglia, and spinal cord; also found in gastrointestinal tract and salivary glands Function: Regulation of pain	Decreased levels: Huntington's disease and Alzheimer's disease Increased levels: Depression
C. Somatostatin	Cerebral cortex, hippocampus, thalamus, basal ganglia, brain stem, and spinal cord Function: Depending on part of the brain being affected, stimulates release of dopamine, serotonin, norepinephrine, and acetylcholine, and inhibits release of norepinephrine, histamine, and glutamate. Also acts as a neuromodulator for serotonin in the hypothalamus.	Decreased levels: Alzheimer's disease Increased levels: Huntington's disease

Histamine. The role of histamine in mediating allergic and inflammatory reactions has been well documented. Its role in the CNS as a neurotransmitter has only recently been confirmed, and the availability of information is limited. The highest concentrations of histamine are found within various regions of the hypothalamus. Histaminic neurons in the posterior hypothalamus are associated with sustaining wakefulness (Gilman & Newman, 2003). The enzyme that catabolizes histamine is MAO. Although the exact processes mediated by histamine with the central nervous system are uncertain, some data suggest that histamine may play a role in depressive illness.

Amino Acids

Inhibitory Amino Acids

Gamma-Aminobutyric Acid. Gamma-aminobutyric acid (GABA) has a widespread distribution in the CNS, with high concentrations in the hypothalamus, hippocampus, cortex, cerebellum, and basal ganglia of the brain, in the gray matter of the dorsal horn of the spinal cord, and in the retina. Most GABA is associated with short inhibitory interneurons, although some long-axon pathways within the brain also have been identified. GABA is catabolized by the enzyme GABA transaminase.

Inhibitory neurotransmitters, such as GABA, prevent postsynaptic excitation, interrupting the progression of the electrical impulse at the synaptic junction. This function is significant when slowdown of body activity is advantageous. Enhancement of the GABA system is the mechanism of action by which the benzodiazepines produce their calming effect.

Alterations in the GABA system have been implicated in the etiology of anxiety disorders, movement disorders (e.g., Huntington's disease), and various forms of epilepsy.

Glycine. The highest concentrations of glycine in the CNS are found in the spinal cord and brainstem. Little is known about the possible enzymatic metabolism of glycine.

Glycine appears to be the neurotransmitter of recurrent inhibition of motor neurons within the spinal cord, and is possibly involved in the regulation of spinal and brainstem reflexes. It has been implicated in the pathogenesis of certain types of spastic disorders and in "glycine encephalopathy," which is known to occur with toxic accumulation of the neurotransmitter in the brain and cerebrospinal fluid (Murphy & Deutsch, 1991).

Excitatory Amino Acids

Glutamate and Aspartate. Glutamate and aspartate appear to be primary excitatory neurotransmitters in the pyramidal cells of the cortex, the cerebellum, and the primary sensory afferent systems. They are also found in the hippocamus, thalamus, hypothalamus, and spinal cord. Glutamate and aspartate are inactivated by uptake into the tissues and through assimilation in various metabolic pathways.

Glutamate and aspartate function in the relay of sensory information and in the regulation of various motor and spinal reflexes. Alteration in these systems has been implicated in the etiology of certain neurodegenerative disorders, such as Huntington's disease, temporal lobe epilepsy, and spinal cerebellar degeneration.

Neuropeptides

Numerous neuropeptides have been identified and studied. They are classified by the area of the body in which they are located or by their pharmacological or functional properties. Although their role as neurotransmitters has not been clearly established, it is known that they often coexist with the classic neurotransmitters within a neuron; however, the functional significance of this coexistence still requires further study. Hormonal neuropeptides are discussed in the section of this chapter on psychoendocrinology.

Opioid Peptides. Opioid peptides, which include the endorphins and enkephalins, have been widely studied. Opioid peptides are found in various concentrations in the hypothalamus, thalamus, limbic structures, midbrain, and brainstem. Enkephalins are also found in the gastrointestinal (GI) tract. Opioid peptides are thought to have a role in pain modulation, with their natural morphine-like properties. They are released in response to painful stimuli, and may be responsible for producing the analgesic effect following acupuncture. Opioid peptides alter the release of dopamine and affect the spontaneous activity of the dopaminergic neurons. These findings may have some implication for opioid peptide-dopamine interaction in the etiology of schizophrenia.

Substance P. Substance P was the first neuropeptide to be discovered. It is present in high concentrations in the hypothalamus, limbic structures, midbrain, and brainstem, and is also found in the thalamus, basal ganglia, and spinal cord. Substance P has been found to be highly concentrated in sensory fibers, and for this reason is thought to play a role in sensory transmission, and particularly in the regulation of pain. Substance P abnormalities have been associated with Huntington's disease, dementia of the Alzheimer's type, and mood disorders (Sadock & Sadock, 2007).

Somatostatin. Somatostatin (also called growth hormone-inhibiting hormone) is found in the cerebral cortex, hippocampus, thalamus, basal ganglia, brainstem, and spinal cord, and has multiple effects on the CNS. In its function as a neurotransmitter, somatostatin exerts both stimulatory and inhibitory effects. Depending on the part of the brain being affected, it has been shown to stimulate dopamine, serotonin, norepinephrine, and acetylcholine, and inhibit norepinephrine, histamine, and glutamate. It also acts as a neuromodulator for serotonin in the hypothalamus, thereby regulating its release (i.e., determining whether it is stimulated or inhibited). It is possible that somatostatin may serve this function for other neurotransmitters as well. High concentrations of somatostatin have been reported in brain specimens of clients with Huntington's disease, and low concentrations in those with Alzheimer's disease.

CORE CONCEPT

Neuroendocrinology
Study of the interaction between the nervous system and the endocrine system, and the effects of various hormones on cognitive, emotional, and behavioral functioning.

NEUROENDOCRINOLOGY

Human endocrine functioning has a strong foundation in the CNS, under the direction of the hypothalamus, which has direct control over the pituitary gland. The pituitary gland has two major lobes—the anterior lobe (also called the *adenohypophysis*) and the posterior lobe (also called the *neurohypophysis*). The pituitary gland is only about the size of a pea, but despite its size and because of the powerful control it exerts over endocrine functioning in humans, it is sometimes called the "master gland." (Figure 4–8 shows the hormones of the pituitary gland and their target organs.) Many of the hormones subject to hypothalamus-pituitary regulation may have implications for behavioral functioning. Discussion of these hormones is summarized in Table 4–3.

Pituitary Gland

The Posterior Pituitary (Neurohypophysis)

The hypothalamus has direct control over the posterior pituitary through efferent neural pathways. Two hormones are found in the posterior pituitary: vasopressin (antidiuretic hormone) and oxytocin. They are actually produced by the hypothalamus and stored in the posterior pituitary. Their release is mediated by neural impulses from the hypothalamus (Fig. 4–9).

Antidiuretic Hormone. The main function of antidiuretic hormone (ADH) is to conserve body water and maintain normal blood pressure. The release of ADH is stimulated by pain, emotional stress, dehydration, increased plasma concentration, and decreases in blood volume. An alteration in the secretion of this hormone may be a factor in the polydipsia observed in about 10 to 15 percent of hospitalized psychiatric patients. Other factors correlated with this behavior include adverse effects of psychotropic medications and features of the behavioral disorder itself. ADH also may play a role in learning and memory, in alteration of the pain response, and in the modification of sleep patterns.

Oxytocin. Oxytocin stimulates contraction of the uterus at the end of pregnancy and stimulates release of milk from the mammary glands (Scanlon & Sanders, 2006). It is also released in response to stress and during sexual arousal. Its role in behavioral functioning is unclear, although it is possible that oxytocin may act in certain situations to stimulate the release of adrenocorticotropic hormone (ACTH), thereby playing a key role in the overall hormonal response to stress.

The Anterior Pituitary (Adenohypophysis)

The hypothalamus produces *releasing hormones* that pass through capillaries and veins of the hypophyseal portal system to capillaries in the anterior pituitary, where they stimulate secretion of specialized hormones. This pathway is presented in Figure 4–9. The hormones of the anterior pituitary gland regulate multiple body functions and include growth hormone, thyroid-stimulating hormone, ACTH, prolactin, gonadotropin-stimulating hormone, and melanocyte-stimulating hormone. Most of these hormones are regulated by a *negative feedback mechanism*. Once the hormone has exerted its effects, the information is "fed back" to the anterior pituitary, which inhibits the release, and ultimately decreases the effects, of the stimulating hormones.

Growth Hormone. The release of growth hormone (GH), also called somatotropin, is stimulated by growth hormone-releasing hormone (GHRH) from the hypothalamus. Its release is inhibited by growth hormone-inhibiting hormone (GHIH), or somatostatin, also from the hypothalamus. It is responsible for growth in children, as well as continued protein synthesis throughout life. During periods of fasting, it stimulates the release of fat from the adipose tissue to be used for increased energy. The release of GHIH is stimulated in response to periods of hyperglycemia. GHRH is stimulated in response to hypoglycemia and to stressful situations. During prolonged stress, GH has a direct effect on protein, carbohydrate, and lipid metabolism, resulting in increased serum glucose and free fatty acids to be used for increased energy. There has been some indication of a possible correlation between abnormal secretion of growth hormone and anorexia nervosa.

Thyroid-Stimulating Hormone. Thyrotropin-releasing hormone (TRH) from the hypothalamus stimulates the release of thyroid-stimulating hormone (TSH), or thyrotropin, from the anterior pituitary. TSH stimulates the thyroid gland to secrete triiodothyronine (T_3) and

fundamental level—that of gene expression and interactions between molecules and cells—all the way up to the highest levels of cognition, memory, emotion, and language. The challenge requires integration of concepts from many different disciplines. A fuller understanding of development is not only important in its own right, but it is expected to pave the way for our ultimate understanding of mental health and mental illness and how different factors shape their expression at different stages of the life span. (pp. 61–62)

To ensure a smooth transition from a psychosocial focus to one of biopsychosocial emphasis, nurses must have a clear understanding of the following:

- *Neuroanatomy and neurophysiology*: the structure and functioning of the various parts of the brain and their correlation to human behavior and psychopathology.
- *Neuronal processes*: the various functions of the nerve cells, including the role of neurotransmitters, receptors, synaptic activity, and informational pathways.
- *Neuroendocrinology*: the interaction of the endocrine and nervous systems, and the role that the endocrine glands and their respective hormones play in behavioral functioning.
- *Circadian rhythms*: regulation of biochemical functioning over periods of rhythmic cycles and their influence in predicting certain behaviors.
- *Genetic influences*: hereditary factors that predispose individuals to certain psychiatric disorders.
- *Psychoimmunology*: the influence of stress on the immune system and its role in the susceptibility to illness.
- *Psychopharmacology*: the increasing use of psychotropics in the treatment of mental illness, demanding greater knowledge of psychopharmacological principles and nursing interventions necessary for safe and effective management.
- *Diagnostic technology*: the importance of keeping informed about the latest in technological procedures for diagnosing alterations in brain structure and function.

Why are these concepts important to the practice of psychiatric-mental health nursing? The interrelationship between psychosocial adaptation and physical functioning has been established. Integrating biological and behavioral concepts into psychiatric nursing practice is essential for nurses to meet the complex needs of mentally ill clients. Psychobiological perspectives must be incorporated into nursing practice, education, and research to attain the evidence-based outcomes necessary for the delivery of competent care.

SUMMARY AND KEY POINTS

- It is important for nurses to understand the interaction between biological and behavioral factors in the development and management of mental illness.
- Psychobiology is the study of the biological foundations of cognitive, emotional, and behavioral processes.
- The limbic system has been called "the emotional brain." It is associated with feelings of fear and anxiety; anger, rage, and aggression; love, joy, and hope; and with sexuality and social behavior.
- The three classes of neurons include afferent (sensory), efferent (motor), and interneurons. The junction between two neurons is called a synapse.
- Neurotransmitters are chemicals that convey information across synaptic clefts to neighboring target cells. Many neurotransmitters have implications in the etiology of emotional disorders and in the pharmacological treatment of those disorders.
- Major categories of neurotransmitters include cholinergics, monoamines, amino acids, and neuropeptides.
- The endocrine system plays an important role in human behavior through the hypothalamic-pituitary axis.
- Hormones and their circadian rhythm of regulation significantly influence a number of physiological and psychological life cycle phenomena, such as moods, sleep and arousal, stress response, appetite, libido, and fertility.
- Research continues to validate the role of genetics in psychiatric illness.
- Familial, twin, and adoption studies suggest that genetics may be implicated in the etiology of schizophrenia, bipolar disorder, depression, panic disorder, anorexia nervosa, alcoholism, and obsessive–compulsive disorder.
- Psychoimmunology examines the impact of psychological factors on the immune system.
- Evidence exists to support a link between psychosocial stressors and suppression of the immune response.
- Technologies such as magnetic resonance imagery (MRI), computed tomographic (CT) scan, positron emission tomography (PET), and electroencephalography (EEG) are used as diagnostic tools for detecting alterations in psychobiological functioning.
- Integrating knowledge of the expanding biological focus into psychiatric nursing is essential if nurses are to meet the changing needs of today's psychiatric clients.

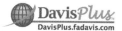 **DavisPlus**   **For additional clinical tools and study**
DavisPlus.fadavis.com   **aids, visit DavisPlus.**

REVIEW QUESTIONS

Self-Examination/Learning Exercise

Match the following parts of the brain to their functions described in the right-hand column:

_____ 1. Frontal lobe   a. Sometimes called the "emotional brain"; associated with multiple feelings and behaviors

_____ 2. Parietal lobe   b. Concerned with visual reception and interpretation

_____ 3. Temporal lobe   c. Voluntary body movement; thinking and judgment; expression of feeling

_____ 4. Occipital lobe   d. Integrates all sensory input (except smell) on way to cortex

_____ 5. Thalamus   e. Part of the cortex that deals with sensory perception and interpretation

_____ 6. Hypothalamus   f. Hearing, short-term memory, and sense of smell

_____ 7. Limbic system   g. Control over pituitary gland and autonomic nervous system; regulates appetite and temperature.

Select the answer that is most appropriate for each of the following questions.

8. At a synapse, the determination of further impulse transmission is accomplished by means of
   a. Potassium ions
   b. Interneurons
   c. Neurotransmitters
   d. The myelin sheath

9. A decrease in which of the following neurotransmitters has been implicated in depression?
   a. GABA, acetylcholine, and aspartate
   b. Norepinephrine, serotonin, and dopamine
   c. Somatostatin, substance P, and glycine
   d. Glutamate, histamine, and opioid peptides

10. Which of the following hormones has been implicated in the etiology of seasonal affective disorder (SAD)?
   a. Increased levels of melatonin
   b. Decreased levels of oxytocin
   c. Decreased levels of prolactin
   d. Increased levels of thyrotropin

11. In which of the following psychiatric disorders do genetic tendencies appear to exist?
   a. Schizophrenia
   b. Dissociative disorder
   c. Conversion disorder
   d. Narcissistic personality disorder

12. With which of the following diagnostic imaging technologies can neurotransmitter-receptor interaction be visualized?
   a. Magnetic resonance imaging (MRI)
   b. Positron emission tomography (PET)
   c. Electroencephalography (EEG)
   d. Computerized EEG mapping

13. During stressful situations, stimulation of the hypothalamic–pituitary–adrenal axis results in suppression of the immune system because of the effect of
   a. Antidiuretic hormone from the posterior pituitary
   b. Increased secretion of gonadotropins from the gonads
   c. Decreased release of growth hormone from the anterior pituitary
   d. Increased glucocorticoid release from the adrenal cortex

records, and to decide with whom their medical information may be shared. The actual document belongs to the facility or the therapist, but the information contained therein belongs to the client.

This federal privacy rule pertains to data that is called *protected health information* (PHI) and applies to most individuals and institutions involved in health care. Notice of privacy policies must be provided to clients upon entry into the health care system. PHI are individually identifiable health information indicators and "relate to past, present, or future physical or mental health or condition of the individual, or the past, present, or future payment for the provision of health care to an individual; and (1) that identifies the individual; or (2) with respect to which there is a reasonable basis to believe the information can be used to identify the individual" (U.S. Department of Health and Human Services, 2003). These specific identifiers are listed in Box 5–4.

Pertinent medical information may be released without consent in a life-threatening situation. If information is released in an emergency, the following information must be recorded in the client's record: date of disclosure, person to whom information was disclosed, reason for disclosure, reason written consent could not be obtained, and the specific information disclosed.

Box 5 – 4   Protected Health Information (PIH): Individually Identifiable Indicators

1. Names
2. Postal address information, (except State), including street address, city, county, precinct, and zip code
3. All elements of dates (except year) directly related to an individual, including birth date, admission date, discharge date, date of death; and all ages over 89 and all elements of dates (including year) indicative of such age, except that such ages and elements may be aggregated into a single category of age 90 or older
4. Telephone numbers
5. Fax numbers
6. Electronic mail addresses
7. Social security numbers
8. Medical record numbers
9. Health plan beneficiary numbers
10. Account numbers
11. Certificate/license numbers
12. Vehicle identifiers and serial numbers, including license plate numbers
13. Device identifiers and serial numbers
14. Web Universal Resource Locators (URLs)
15. Internet Protocol (IP) address numbers
16. Biometric identifiers, including finger and voice prints
17. Full face photographic images and any comparable images
18. Any other unique identifying number, characteristic, or code

SOURCE: U.S. Department of Health and Human Services.

Most states have statutes that pertain to the doctrine of **privileged communication**. Although the codes differ markedly from state to state, most grant certain professionals privileges under which they may refuse to reveal information about, and communications with, clients. In most states, the doctrine of privileged communication applies to psychiatrists and attorneys; in some instances, psychologists, clergy, and nurses are also included.

In certain instances, nurses may be called on to testify in cases in which the medical record is used as evidence. In most states, the right to privacy of these records is exempted in civil or criminal proceedings. Therefore, it is important that nurses document with these possibilities in mind. Strict record keeping using statements that are objective and nonjudgmental, having care plans that are specific in their prescriptive interventions, and keeping documentation that describes those interventions and their subsequent evaluation all serve the best interests of the client, the nurse, and the institution in case questions regarding care should arise. Documentation very often weighs heavily in malpractice case decisions.

The right to confidentiality is a basic one, and especially so in psychiatry. Although societal attitudes are improving, individuals have experienced discrimination in the past for no other reason than for having a history of emotional illness. Nurses working in psychiatry must guard the privacy of their clients with great diligence.

Informed Consent

According to law, all individuals have the right to decide whether to accept or reject treatment (Guido, 2006). A health care provider can be charged with assault and battery for providing life-sustaining treatment to a client when the client has not agreed to it. The rationale for the doctrine of **informed consent** is the preservation and protection of individual autonomy in determining what will and will not happen to the person's body (Guido, 2006).

Informed consent is a client's permission granted to a physician to perform a therapeutic procedure, before which information about the procedure has been presented to the client with adequate time given for consideration about the pros and cons. The client should receive information such as what treatment alternatives are available; why the physician believes this treatment is most appropriate; the possible outcomes, risks, and adverse effects; the possible outcome should the client select another treatment alternative; and the possible outcome should the client choose to have no treatment. An example of a treatment in the psychiatric area that requires informed consent is electroconvulsive therapy.

There are some conditions under which treatment may be performed without obtaining informed consent.

A client's refusal to accept treatment may be challenged under the following circumstances: (Aiken, 2004; Guido, 2006; Levy & Rubenstein, 1996; Mackay, 2001):

1. When a client is mentally incompetent to make a decision and treatment is necessary to preserve life or avoid serious harm.
2. When refusing treatment endangers the life or health of another.
3. During an emergency, in which a client is in no condition to exercise judgment.
4. When the client is a child (consent is obtained from parent or surrogate).
5. In the case of therapeutic privilege. In therapeutic privilege, information about a treatment may be withheld if the physician can show that full disclosure would
   a. Hinder or complicate necessary treatment
   b. Cause severe psychological harm
   c. Be so upsetting as to render a rational decision by the client impossible

Although most clients in psychiatric/mental health facilities are competent and capable of giving informed consent, those with severe psychiatric illness do not possess the cognitive ability to do so. If an individual has been legally determined to be mentally incompetent, consent is obtained from the legal guardian. Difficulty arises when no legal determination has been made, but the individual's current mental state prohibits informed decision making (e.g., the person who is psychotic, unconscious, or inebriated). In these instances, informed consent is usually obtained from the individual's nearest relative, or if none exist and time permits, the physician may ask the court to appoint a conservator or guardian. When time does not permit court intervention, permission may be sought from the hospital administrator.

A client or guardian always has the right to withdraw consent after it has been given. When this occurs, the physician should inform (or reinform) the client about the consequences of refusing treatment. If treatment has already been initiated, the physician should terminate treatment in a way least likely to cause injury to the client and inform the client or guardian of the risks associated with interrupted treatment (Guido, 2006).

The nurse's role in obtaining informed consent is usually defined by agency policy. A nurse may sign the consent form as witness for the client's signature. However, legal liability for informed consent lies with the physician. The nurse acts as client advocate to ensure that the following three major elements of informed consent have been addressed:

1. **Knowledge.** The client has received adequate information on which to base his or her decision.
2. **Competency.** The individual's cognition is not impaired to an extent that would interfere with decision

making or, if so, that the individual has a legal representative.
3. **Free Will.** The individual has given consent voluntarily without pressure or coercion from others.

Restraints and Seclusion

An individual's privacy and personal security are protected by the U.S. Constitution and supported by the Mental Health Systems Act of 1980, out of which was conceived a Bill of Rights for psychiatric patients. These include "the right to freedom from restraint or seclusion except in an emergency situation."

In psychiatry, the term *restraints* generally refers to a set of leather straps that are used to restrain the extremities of an individual whose behavior is out of control and who poses an inherent risk to the physical safety and psychological well-being of the individual and staff. Restraints are never to be used as punishment or for the convenience of staff. Other measures to decrease agitation, such as "talking down" (verbal intervention) and chemical restraints (tranquilizing medication) are usually tried first. If these interventions are ineffective, mechanical restraints may be instituted (although some controversy exists as to whether chemical restraints are indeed less restrictive than mechanical restraints). *Seclusion* is another type of physical restraint in which the client is confined alone in a room from which he or she is unable to leave. The room is usually minimally furnished with items to promote the client's comfort and safety.

The Joint Commission on Accreditation of Healthcare Organizations (JCAHO) has released a set of revisions to its previous restraint and seclusion standards. The intent of these revisions is to reduce the use of this intervention as well as to provide greater assurance of safety and protection to individuals placed in restraints or seclusion for reasons related to psychiatric disorders or substance abuse (Medscape, 2000). In addition to others, these provisions provide the following guidelines:

1. In the event of an emergency, restraints or seclusion may be initiated without a physician's order.
2. As soon as possible, but no longer than one hour after the initiation of restraints or seclusion, a qualified staff member must notify the physician about the individual's physical and psychological condition and obtain a verbal or written order for the restraints or seclusion.
3. Orders for restraints or seclusion must be reissued by a physician every 4 hours for adults age 18 and older, 2 hours for children and adolescents ages 9 to 17, and every hour for children younger than 9 years.
4. An in-person evaluation of the individual must be made by the physician within 4 hours of the initiation of restraints or seclusion of an adult age 18 or older and within 2 hours for children and adolescents ages 17 and younger.

5. Minimum time frames for an in-person re-evaluation by a physician include 8 hours for individuals ages 18 years and older, and 4 hours for individuals ages 17 and younger.
6. If an individual is no longer in restraints or seclusion when an original verbal order expires, the physician must conduct an in-person evaluation within 24 hours of initiation of the intervention.

Clients in restraints or seclusion must be observed and assessed every 10 to 15 minutes with regard to circulation, respiration, nutrition, hydration, and elimination. Such attention should be documented in the client's record.

False imprisonment is the deliberate and unauthorized confinement of a person within fixed limits by the use of verbal or physical means (Ellis & Hartley, 2004). Healthcare workers may be charged with false imprisonment for restraining or secluding—against the wishes of the client—anyone having been admitted to the hospital voluntarily. Should a voluntarily admitted client decompensate to a point that restraint or seclusion for protection of self or others is necessary, court intervention to determine competency and involuntary commitment is required to preserve the client's rights to privacy and freedom.

Commitment Issues
Voluntary Admissions

Each year, more than one million persons are admitted to healthcare facilities for psychiatric treatment, of which approximately two thirds are considered voluntary. To be admitted voluntarily, an individual makes direct application to the institution for services and may stay as long as treatment is deemed necessary. He or she may sign out of the hospital at any time, unless following a mental status examination the health care professional determines that the client may be harmful to self or others and recommends that the admission status be changed from voluntary to involuntary. Although these types of admissions are considered voluntary, it is important to ensure that the individual comprehends the meaning of his or her actions, has not been coerced in any manner, and is willing to proceed with admission.

Involuntary Commitment

Because involuntary hospitalization results in substantial restrictions of the rights of an individual, the admission process is subject to the guarantee of the Fourteenth Amendment to the U.S. Constitution that provides citizens protection against loss of liberty and ensures due process rights (Weiss-Kaffie & Purtell, 2001). Involuntary

commitments are made for various reasons. Most states commonly cite the following criteria:

1. In an emergency situation (for the client who is dangerous to self or others).
2. For observation and treatment of mentally ill persons.
3. When an individual is unable to take care of basic personal needs (the "gravely disabled").

Under the Fourth Amendment, individuals are protected from unlawful searches and seizures without probable cause. Therefore, the individual seeking the involuntary commitment must show probable cause why the client should be hospitalized against his or her wishes; that is, the person must show that there is cause to believe that the person would be dangerous to self or others, is mentally ill and in need of treatment, or is gravely disabled.

Emergency Commitments. Emergency commitments are sought when an individual manifests behavior that is clearly and imminently dangerous to self or others. These admissions are usually instigated by relatives or friends of the individual, police officers, the court, or health care professionals. Emergency commitments are time-limited, and a court hearing for the individual is scheduled, usually within 72 hours. At that time the court may decide that the client may be discharged; or, if deemed necessary, and voluntary admission is refused by the client, an additional period of involuntary commitment may be ordered. In most instances, another hearing is scheduled for a specified time (usually in 7 to 21 days).

The Mentally Ill Person in Need of Treatment. A second type of involuntary commitment is for the observation and treatment of mentally ill persons in need of treatment. Most states have established definitions of what constitutes "mentally ill" for purposes of state involuntary admission statutes. Some examples include individuals who, because of severe mental illness, are:

● Unable to make informed decisions concerning treatment
● Likely to cause harm to self or others
● Unable to fulfill basic personal needs necessary for health and safety

In determining whether commitment is required, the court looks for substantial evidence of abnormal conduct—evidence that cannot be explained as the result of a physical cause. There must be "clear and convincing evidence" as well as "probable cause" to substantiate the need for involuntary commitment to ensure that an individual's rights under the Constitution are protected. The U.S. Supreme Court in *O'Connor v. Donaldson* held that the existence of mental illness alone does not justify involuntary hospitalization. State standards require a specific impact or consequence to flow from the mental illness that involves danger or an inability to care for one's own needs. These clients are entitled to court hearings with representation, at which time determination of commitment and length of stay are considered. Legislative statutes governing involuntary commitments vary from state to state.

Involuntary Outpatient Commitment. Involuntary outpatient commitment (IOC) is a court-ordered mechanism used to compel a person with mental illness to submit to treatment on an outpatient basis. A number of eligibility criteria for commitment to outpatient treatment have been cited (Appelbaum, 2001; Maloy, 1996; Torrey & Zdanowicz, 2001). Some of these include:

1. A history of repeated decompensation requiring involuntary hospitalization
2. Likelihood that without treatment the individual will deteriorate to the point of requiring inpatient commitment
3. Presence of severe and persistent mental illness (e.g., schizophrenia or bipolar disorder) and limited awareness of the illness or need for treatment
4. The presence of severe and persistent mental illness contributing to a risk of becoming homeless, incarcerated, or violent, or of committing suicide
5. The existence of an individualized treatment plan likely to be effective and a service provider who has agreed to provide the treatment

Most states have already enacted IOC legislation or currently have resolutions that speak to this topic on their agendas. Most commonly, clients who are committed into the IOC programs are those with severe and persistent mental illness, such as schizophrenia. The rationale behind the legislation is to reduce the numbers of readmissions and lengths of hospital stays of these clients. Concern lies in the possibility of violating the individual rights of psychiatric clients without significant improvement in treatment outcomes. One study at Bellevue hospital in New York found no difference in treatment outcomes between court ordered outpatient treatment and voluntary outpatient treatment (Steadman et al., 2001). Other studies have shown positive outcomes, including a decrease in hospital readmissions, with IOC (Ridgely, Borum, & Petrila, 2001; Swartz et al., 2001). Continuing research is required to determine if IOC will improve treatment compliance and enhance quality of life in the community for individuals with severe and persistent mental illness.

The Gravely Disabled Client. A number of states have statutes that specifically define the "gravely disabled" client. For those that do not use this label, the description of the individual who, because of mental illness, is unable to take care of basic personal needs is very similar.

Gravely disabled is generally defined as a condition in which an individual, as a result of mental illness, is in danger of serious physical harm resulting from inability to provide for basic needs such as food, clothing, shelter, medical care, and personal safety. Inability to care for oneself cannot be established by showing that an individual lacks the resources to provide the necessities of life. Rather, it is the inability to make use of available resources.

Should it be determined that an individual is gravely disabled, a guardian, conservator, or committee will be appointed by the court to ensure the management of the person and his or her estate. To legally restore competency then requires another court hearing to reverse the previous ruling. The individual whose competency is being determined has the right to be represented by an attorney.

Nursing Liability

Mental health practitioners—psychiatrists, psychologists, psychiatric nurses, and social workers—have a duty to provide appropriate care based on the standards of their professions and the standards set by law. The standards of care for psychiatric/mental health nursing are presented in Chapter 9.

Malpractice and Negligence

The terms **malpractice** and **negligence** are often used interchangeably. Negligence has been defined as:

> The failure to exercise the standard of care that a reasonably prudent person would have exercised in a similar situation; any conduct that falls below the legal standard established to protect others against unreasonable risk of harm, except for conduct that is intentionally, wantonly, or willfully disregardful of others' rights. (Garner, 1999)

Any person may be negligent. In contrast, malpractice is a specialized form of negligence applicable only to professionals.

Black's Law Dictionary defines malpractice as: "An instance of negligence or incompetence on the part of a professional. To succeed in a malpractice claim, a plaintiff must also prove proximate cause and damages" (Garner, 1999). In the absence of any state statutes, common law is the basis of liability for injuries to clients caused by acts of malpractice and negligence of individual practitioners. In other words, most decisions of negligence in the professional setting are based on legal precedent (decisions that have previously been made about similar cases) rather than any specific action taken by the legislature.

To summarize, when the breach of duty is characterized as malpractice, the action is weighed against the professional standard. When it is brought forth as negligence, action is contrasted with what a reasonably prudent professional would have done in the same or similar circumstances.

Marchand (2001) cites the following basic elements of a nursing malpractice lawsuit:

1. The existence of a duty, owed by the nurse to a patient, to conform to a recognized standard of care

2. A failure to conform to the required nursing standard of care
3. Actual injury
4. A reasonably close causal connection between the nurse's conduct and the patient's injury

For the client to prevail in a malpractice claim, each of these elements must be proved. Juries' decisions are generally based on the testimony of expert witnesses, because members of the jury are laypeople and cannot be expected to know what nursing interventions should have been carried out. Without the testimony of expert witnesses, a favorable verdict usually goes to the defendant nurse.

Types of Lawsuits that Occur in Psychiatric Nursing

Most malpractice suits against nurses are civil actions; that is, they are considered breach of conduct actions on the part of the professional, for which compensation is being sought. The nurse in the psychiatric setting should be aware of the types of behaviors that may result in charges of malpractice.

Basic to the psychiatric client's hospitalization is his or her right to confidentiality and privacy. A nurse may be charged with *breach of confidentiality* for revealing aspects about a client's case, or even for revealing that an individual has been hospitalized, if that person can show that making this information known resulted in harm.

When shared information is detrimental to the client's reputation, the person sharing the information may be liable for **defamation of character**. When the information is in writing, the action is called **libel**. Oral defamation is called **slander**. Defamation of character involves communication that is malicious and false (Ellis & Hartley, 2004). Occasionally, libel arises out of critical, judgmental statements written in the client's medical record. Nurses need to be very objective in their charting, backing up all statements with factual evidence.

Invasion of privacy is a charge that may result when a client is searched without probable cause. Many institutions conduct body searches on mental clients as a routine intervention. In these cases, there should be a physician's order and written rationale showing probable cause for the intervention. Many institutions are reexamining their policies regarding this procedure.

Assault is an act that results in a person's genuine fear and apprehension that he or she will be touched without consent. **Battery** is the unconsented touching of another person. These charges can result when a treatment is administered to a client against his or her wishes and outside of an emergency situation. Harm or injury need not have occurred for these charges to be legitimate.

For confining a client against his or her wishes, and outside of an emergency situation, the nurse may be charged with false imprisonment. Examples of actions that may invoke these charges include locking an individual in a room; taking a client's clothes for purposes of detainment against his or her will; and retaining in mechanical restraints a competent voluntary client who demands to be released.

Avoiding Liability

Hall and Hall (2001) suggest the following proactive nursing actions in an effort to avoid nursing malpractice:

1. Responding to the patient
2. Educating the patient
3. Complying with the standard of care
4. Supervising care
5. Adhering to the nursing process
6. Documentation
7. Follow-up

In addition, it is a positive practice to develop and maintain a good interpersonal relationship with the client and his or her family. Some clients appear to be more "suit prone" than others. Suit-prone clients are often very critical, complaining, uncooperative, and even hostile. A natural response by the staff to these clients is to become defensive or withdrawn. Either of these behaviors increases the likelihood of a lawsuit should an unfavorable event occur (Ellis & Hartley, 2004). No matter how high the degree of technical competence and skill of the nurse, his or her insensitivity to a client's complaints and failure to meet the client's emotional needs often influence whether or not a lawsuit is generated. A great deal depends on the psychosocial skills of the health care professional.

CLINICAL PEARLS

- Always put the client's rights and welfare first.
- Develop and maintain a good interpersonal relationship with each client and his or her family.

SUMMARY AND KEY POINTS

- **Ethics** is the science that deals with the rightness and wrongness of actions.
- **Bioethics** is the term applied to these principles when they refer to concepts within the scope of medicine, nursing, and allied health.
- **Moral behavior** is defined as conduct that results from serious critical thinking about how individuals ought to treat others.

- **Values** are ideals or concepts that give meaning to the individual's life.
- A **right** is defined as, "a valid, legally recognized claim or entitlement, encompassing both freedom from government interference or discriminatory treatment and an entitlement to a benefit or service."
- The ethical theory of Utilitarianism is based on the premise that what is right and good is that which produces the most happiness for the most people.
- The ethical theory of Kantianism suggests that actions are bound by a sense of duty, and that ethical decisions are made out of respect for moral law.
- The code of Christian ethics is to treat others as moral equals and to recognize the equality of other persons by permitting them to act as we do when they occupy a position similar to ours.
- The moral precept of the Natural Law theory is "do good and avoid evil." Good is viewed as that which is inscribed by God into the nature of things. Evil acts are never condoned, even if they are intended to advance the noblest of ends.
- Ethical egoism espouses that what is right and good is what is best for the individual making the decision.
- Ethical principles include autonomy, beneficence, nonmaleficence, veracity, and justice.
- An ethical dilemma is a situation that requires an individual to make a choice between two equally unfavorable alternatives.

- Examples of ethical issues in psychiatric/mental health nursing include the right to refuse medication and the right to the least-restrictive treatment alternative.
- Statutory laws are those that have been enacted by legislative bodies, and common laws are derived from decisions made in previous cases. Both types of laws have civil and criminal components.
- Civil law protects the private and property rights of individuals and businesses, and criminal law provides protection from conduct deemed injurious to the public welfare.
- Legal issues in psychiatric/mental health nursing center around confidentiality and the right to privacy, informed consent, restraints and seclusion, and commitment issues.
- Nurses are accountable for their own actions in relation to these issues, and violation can result in malpractice lawsuits against the physician, the hospital, and the nurse.
- Developing and maintaining a good interpersonal relationship with the client and his or her family appears to be a positive factor when the question of malpractice is being considered.

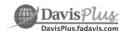 **DavisPlus**
DavisPlus.fadavis.com   For additional clinical tools and study aids, visit DavisPlus.

REVIEW QUESTIONS

Self-Examination/Learning Exercise

Match the following decision-making examples with the appropriate ethical theory:

_____ 1. Carol decides to go against family wishes and tell the client of his terminal status because that is what she would want if she were the client.

_____ 2. Carol decides to respect family wishes and not tell the client of his terminal status because that would bring the most happiness to the most people.

_____ 3. Carol decides not to tell the client about his terminal status because it would be too uncomfortable for her to do so.

_____ 4. Carol decides to tell the client of his terminal status because her reasoning tells her that to do otherwise would be an evil act.

_____ 5. Carol decides to tell the client of his terminal status because she believes it is her duty to do so.

a. Utilitarianism

b. Kantianism

c. Christian ethics

d. Natural law theories

e. Ethical egoism

Match the following nursing actions with the possible legal action with which the nurse may be charged:

_____ 6. The nurse assists the physician with electroconvulsive therapy on his client who has refused to give consent.

_____ 7. When the local newspaper calls to inquire why the mayor has been admitted to the hospital, the nurse replies, "He's here because he is an alcoholic."

_____ 8. A competent, voluntary client has stated he wants to leave the hospital. The nurse hides his clothes in an effort to keep him from leaving.

_____ 9. Jack recently lost his wife and is very depressed. He is running for reelection to the Senate and asks the staff to keep his hospitalization confidential. The nurse is excited about having a Senator on the unit and tells her boyfriend about the admission, which soon becomes common knowledge. Jack loses the election.

_____ 10. Joe is very restless and is pacing a lot. The nurse says to Joe, "If you don't sit down in the chair and be still, I'm going to put you in restraints!"

a. Breach of confidentiality

b. Defamation of character

c. Assault

d. Battery

e. False imprisonment

REFERENCES

Aiken, T.D. (2004). *Legal, ethical, and political issues in nursing* (2nd ed.). Philadelphia: F.A. Davis.

American Hospital Association (AHA). (1992). *A Patient's Bill of Rights*. Chicago: American Hospital Association.

American Nurses' Association (ANA). (2001). *Code of ethics for nurses with interpretive statements*. Washington, DC: ANA.

Appelbaum, P.S. (2001, March). Thinking carefully about outpatient commitment. *Psychiatric Services, 52*(3), 347–350.

Catalano, J.T. (2006). *Nursing now! Today's issues, tomorrow's trends* (4th ed.). Philadelphia: F.A. Davis.

Ellis, J.R., & Hartley, C.L. (2004). *Nursing in today's world: Challenges, issues, and trends* (8th ed.). Philadelphia: Lippincott Williams & Wilkins.

Fedorka, P., & Resnick, L.K. (2001). Defining nursing practice. In M.E. O'Keefe (Ed.), *Nursing practice and the law: Avoiding malpractice and other legal rights*. Philadelphia: F.A. Davis, pp. 97–117.

Garner, B.A. (Ed.). (1999). *Black's law dictionary*. St. Paul, MN: West Group.

Guido, G.W. (2006). *Legal and ethical issues in nursing* (4th ed.). Upper Saddle River, NJ: Prentice-Hall.

Hall, J.K. & Hall, D. (2001). Negligence specific to nursing. In M.E. O'Keefe (Ed.). *Nursing practice and the law: Avoiding malpractice and other legal risks*. Philadelphia: F.A. Davis, pp. 132–149.

Levy, R.M., & Rubenstein, L.S. (1996). *The rights of people with mental disabilities*. Carbondale, IL: Southern Illinois University Press.

Mackay, T.R. (2001). Informed consent. In M.E. O'Keefe (Ed.), *Nursing practice and the law: Avoiding malpractice and other legal risks*. Philadelphia: F.A. Davis, pp. 199–213.

Maloy, K.A. (1996). Does involuntary outpatient commitment work? In B.D. Sales & S.A. Shah (Eds.), *Mental health and law: Research, policy and services*. Durham, NC: Carolina Academic Press, pp. 41–74.

Marchand, L. (2001). Legal terminology. In M.E. O'Keefe (Ed.), *Nursing practice and the law: Avoiding malpractice and other legal risks*. Philadelphia: F.A. Davis, pp. 23–41.

Medscape Wire (2000). *Joint Commission releases revised restraints standards for behavioral healthcare*. Retrieved June 17, 2008 from http://www.medscape.com/ viewarticle/411832

Mental Health Systems Act. P.L. 96-398, Title V, Sect. 501.94 Stat. 1598, Oct 7, 1980.

Pappas, A. (2006). Ethical issues. In J. Zerwekh & J.C. Claborn (Eds.), *Nursing today: Transition and trends* (5th ed.). New York: Elsevier, pp. 425–453.

Peplau, H.E. (1991). *Interpersonal relations in nursing: A conceptual frame of reference for psychodynamic nursing*. New York: Springer.

Ridgely, M.S., Borum, R., & Petrila, J. (2001). *The effectiveness of involuntary outpatient treatment: Empirical evidence and the experience of eight states*. Santa Monica, CA: Rand Publications.

Sadock, B.J., & Sadock, V.A. (2007). *Synopsis of psychiatry: Behavioral sciences/clinical psychiatry* (10th ed.). Philadelphia: Lippincott Williams & Wilkins.

Schwarz, M., Swanson, J., Hiday, V., Wagner, H.R., Burns, B., & Borum, R. (2001). A randomized controlled trial of outpatient commitment in North Carolina. *Psychiatric Services, 52*(3), 325–329.

Steadman, H., Gounis, K., Dennis, D., Hopper, K., Roche, B., Swartz, M., & Robbins, P. (2001). Assessing the New York City involuntary outpatient commitment pilot program. *Psychiatric Services, 52*(3), 330–336.

Torrey, E.F. (2001). Outpatient commitment: What, Why, and for Whom. *Psychiatric Services, 52*(3), 337–341.

Weiss-Kaffie, C.J., & Purtell, N.E. (2001). Psychiatric nursing. In M.E. O'Keefe (Ed.), *Nursing practice and the law: Avoiding malpractice and other legal risks*. Philadelphia: F.A. Davis, pp. 352–371.

Cultural and Spiritual Concepts Relevant to Psychiatric/Mental Health Nursing

CHAPTER OUTLINE

OBJECTIVES

CULTURAL CONCEPTS

HOW DO CULTURES DIFFER?

APPLICATION OF THE NURSING
PROCESS

SPIRITUAL CONCEPTS

ASSESSMENT OF SPIRITUAL AND
RELIGIOUS NEEDS

SUMMARY AND KEY POINTS

REVIEW QUESTIONS

KEY TERMS

curandera
curandero
culture-bound
    syndromes
density
distance

folk medicine
shaman
stereotyping
territoriality
yin and yang

CORE CONCEPTS

culture
ethnicity
religion
spirituality

OBJECTIVES

After reading this chapter, the student will be able to:

1. Define and differentiate between *culture* and *ethnicity*.
2. Identify cultural differences based on six characteristic phenomena.
3. Describe cultural variances, based on the six phenomena, for
    a. Northern European Americans.
    b. African Americans.
    c. Native Americans.
    d. Asian/Pacific Islander Americans.
    e. Latino Americans.
    f. Western European Americans.

g. Arab Americans
    h. Jewish Americans
4. Apply the nursing process in the care of individuals from various cultural groups.
5. Define and differentiate between *spirituality* and *religion*.
6. Identify clients' spiritual and religious needs.
7. Apply the six steps of the nursing process to individuals with spiritual and religious needs.

CORE CONCEPTS

Culture describes a particular society's entire way of living, encompassing shared patterns of belief, feeling, and knowledge that guide people's conduct and are passed down from generation to generation. **Ethnicity** is a somewhat narrower term, and relates to people who identify with each other because of a shared heritage (Griffith, Gonzalez, & Blue, 2003).

CULTURAL CONCEPTS

What is culture? How does it differ from ethnicity? Why are these questions important? The answers lie in the changing face of America. Immigration is not new in the United States. Indeed, most U.S. citizens are either immigrants or descendants of immigrants. The pattern continues because of the many individuals who want to take advantage of the technological growth and upward mobility that exists in this country. A breakdown of cultural groups in the United States is presented in Figure 6–1.

Griffin (2002) states:

Most researchers agree that the United States, long a destination of immigrants, continues to grow more culturally diverse. According to the U.S. Census Bureau, the number of foreign-born residents in the country jumped from roughly 19.8 million to a little more than 28 million between 1990 and 2000. What's more, experts predict that Caucasians, who now represent about 70 percent of the U.S. population, will account for barely more than 50 percent by the year 2050. (p. 14)

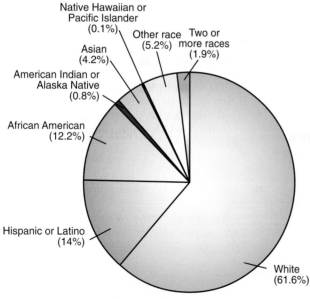

FIGURE 6–1 Breakdown of cultural groups in the United States. (Source: U.S. Census Bureau, 2006.)

Why is this important? Cultural influences affect human behavior, its interpretation, and the response to it. Therefore, it is essential for nurses to understand the effects of these cultural influences if they are to work effectively with the diverse U.S. population. Caution must be taken, however, not to assume that all individuals who share a cultural or ethnic group are identical, or exhibit behaviors perceived as characteristic of the group. This constitutes **stereotyping**, and must be avoided. Many variations and subcultures occur within a culture. The differences may be related to status, ethnic background, residence, religion, education, or other factors (Purnell & Paulanka, 2003). Every individual must be appreciated for his or her uniqueness.

This chapter explores the ways in which various cultures differ. The nursing process is applied to the delivery of psychiatric–mental health nursing care for individuals from the following cultural groups: Northern European Americans, African Americans, Native Americans, Asian/Pacific Islander Americans, Latino Americans, Western European Americans, Arab Americans, and Jewish Americans.

HOW DO CULTURES DIFFER?

It is difficult to generalize about any one specific group in a country that is known for its heterogeneity. Within our American "melting pot" any or all characteristics could apply to individuals within any or all of the cultural groups represented. As these differences continue to be integrated, one American culture will eventually emerge. This is already in evidence in certain regions of the country today, particularly in the urban coastal areas. However, some differences still exist, and it is important for nurses to be aware of certain cultural influences that may affect individuals' behaviors and beliefs, particularly as they apply to health care.

Giger and Davidhizar (2004) suggest six cultural phenomena that vary with application and use but yet are evidenced among all cultural groups: (1) communication, (2) space, (3) social organization, (4) time, (5) environmental control, and (6) biological variations.

Communication

All verbal and nonverbal behavior in connection with another individual is communication. Therapeutic communication has always been considered an essential part of the nursing process and represents a critical element in the curricula of most schools of nursing. Communication has its roots in culture. Cultural mores, norms, ideas, and customs provide the basis for our way of thinking. Cultural values are learned and differ from society to society. Individuals communicate through language (the spoken and written word), paralanguage (the voice quality, intonation, rhythm, and speed of the spoken word), and gestures (touch, facial expression, eye movements, body posture, and physical appearance). The nurse who is planning care must have an understanding of the client's needs and expectations as they are being communicated. As a third party, an interpreter often complicates matters, but one may be necessary when the client does not speak the same language as the nurse. Interpreting is a very complex process, however, that requires a keen sensitivity to cultural nuances, and not just the translating of words into another language. Tips for facilitating the communication process when employing an interpreter are presented in Box 6–1.

Space

Spatial determinants relate to the place where the communication occurs and encompass the concepts of **territoriality**, **density**, and **distance**. Territoriality refers to the innate tendency to own space. The need for territoriality

Box 6 – 1   Using an Interpreter

When using an interpreter, keep the following points in mind:

- Address the client directly rather than speaking to the interpreter. Maintain eye contact with the client to ensure the client's involvement.
- Do not interrupt the client and the interpreter. At times their interaction may take longer because of the need to clarify, and descriptions may require more time because of dialect differences or the interpreter's awareness that the client needs more preparation before being asked a particular question.
- Ask the interpreter to give you verbatim translations so that you can assess what the client is thinking and understanding.
- Avoid using medical jargon that the interpreter or client may not understand.
- Avoid talking or commenting to the interpreter at length; the client may feel left out and distrustful.
- Be aware that asking intimate or emotionally laden questions may be difficult for both the client and the interpreter. Lead up to these questions slowly. Always ask permission to discuss these topics first, and prepare the interpreter for the content of the interview.
- When possible, allow the client and the interpreter to meet each other ahead of time to establish some rapport. If possible, try to use the same interpreter for succeeding interviews with the client.
- If possible, request an interpreter of the same gender as the client and of similar age. To make good use of the interpreter's time, decide beforehand which questions you will ask. Meet with the interpreter briefly before going to see the client so that you can let the interpreter know what you are planning to ask. During the session, face the client and direct your questions to the client, not the interpreter.

SOURCE: Gorman, L.M., Raines, M.L., & Sultan, D.F. (2002). *Psychosocial Nursing for General Patient Care* (2nd ed.). Philadelphia: F.A. Davis. With permission.

is met only if the individual has control of a space, can establish rules for that space, and is able to defend the space against invasion or misuse by others (Giger & Davidhizar, 2004). Density, which refers to the number of people within a given environmental space, can influence interpersonal interaction. Distance is the means by which various cultures use space to communicate. Hall (1966) identified three primary dimensions of space in interpersonal interactions in Western culture: the intimate zone (0 to 18 inches), the personal zone (18 inches to 3 feet), and the social zone (3 to 6 feet).

Social Organization

Cultural behavior is socially acquired through a process called *acculturation*, which involves acquiring knowledge and internalizing values (Giger & Davidhizar, 2004). Children are acculturated by observing adults within their social organizations. Social organizations include families, religious groups, and ethnic groups.

Time

An awareness of the concept of time is a gradual learning process. Some cultures place great importance on values that are measured by clock time. Punctuality and efficiency are highly valued in the United States, whereas some cultures are actually scornful of clock time. For example, some peasants in Algeria label the clock as the "devil's mill" and have no notion of scheduled appointment times or meal times (Giger & Davidhizar, 2004). They are totally indifferent to the passage of clock time and despise haste in all human endeavors. Other cultural implications regarding time have to do with perception of time orientation. Whether individuals are present-oriented or future-oriented influences many aspects of their lives.

Environmental Control

The variable of environmental control has to do with the degree to which individuals perceive that they have control over their environment. Cultural beliefs and practices influence how an individual responds to his or her environment during periods of wellness and illness. To provide culturally appropriate care, the nurse should not only respect the individual's unique beliefs, but should also have an understanding of how these beliefs can be used to promote optimal health in the client's environment.

Biological Variations

Biological differences exist among people in various racial groups. Giger and Davidhizar (2004) state:

The strongest argument for including concepts on biological variations in nursing education and subsequently nursing practice is that scientific facts about biological variations can aid the nurse in giving culturally appropriate health care. (p. 136)

These differences include body structure (both size and shape), skin color, physiological responses to medication, electrocardiographic patterns, susceptibility to disease, and nutritional preferences and deficiencies.

APPLICATION OF THE NURSING PROCESS

Background Assessment Data

A format for cultural assessment that may be used to gather information related to culture and ethnicity that is important for planning client care is provided in Box 6–2.

Box 6 – 2 Cultural Assessment Tool

Client's name _____ Ethnic origin_____
Address _____
Birthdate _____
Name of significant other_____ Relationship_____
Primary language spoken_____ Second language spoken_____
How does client usually communicate with people who speak a different language?_____
Is an interpreter required?_____ Available?_____
Highest level of education achieved:_____
Occupation:_____
Presenting problem:_____
Has this problem ever occurred before?_____
    If so, in what manner was it handled previously?_____
What is the client's usual manner of coping with stress?_____
Who is (are) the client's main support system(s)?_____
Describe the family living arrangements:_____
Who is the major decision maker in the family?_____
Describe client's/family members' roles within the family._____
_____
Describe religious beliefs and practices:_____
    Are there any religious requirements or restrictions that place limitations on the client's care?_____
    If so, describe:_____
Who in the family takes responsibility for health concerns?_____
Describe any special health beliefs and practices:_____
_____
From whom does family usually seek medical assistance in time of need?_____
Describe client's usual emotional/behavioral response to:
    Anxiety: _____
    Anger: _____
    Loss/change/failure:_____
    Pain:_____
    Fear:_____
Describe any topics that are particularly sensitive or that the client is unwilling to discuss (because of
    cultural taboos):_____
Describe any activities in which the client is unwilling to participate (because of cultural customs or
    taboos):_____
What are the client's personal feelings regarding touch?_____
What are the client's personal feelings regarding eye contact?_____
What is the client's personal orientation to time? (past, present, future)_____
Describe any particular illnesses to which the client may be bioculturally susceptible (e.g., hypertension and
    sickle cell anemia in African Americans):_____
Describe any nutritional deficiencies to which the client may be bioculturally susceptible (e.g., lactose
    intolerance in Native and Asian Americans)_____
Describe the client's favorite foods:_____
Are there any foods the client requests or refuses because of cultural beliefs related to this illness (e.g., "hot" and "cold" foods for
    Latino Americans and Asian Americans)? If so, please describe: _____
Describe the client's perception of the problem and expectations of health
    care:_____

Northern European Americans

Northern European Americans have their origins in England; Ireland; Wales; Finland; Sweden; Norway; and the Baltic states of Estonia, Latvia, and Lithuania. Their language has its roots in the language of the first English settlers to the United States, with the influence of immigrants from around the world. The descendants of these immigrants now make up what is considered the dominant cultural group in the United States today. Specific dialects and rate of speech are common to various regions of the country. Northern European Americans value territory. Personal space is about 18 inches to 3 feet.

With the advent of technology and widespread mobility, less emphasis has been placed on the cohesiveness of the family. Data on marriage, divorce, and remarriage in the United States show that 43 percent of first marriages end in separation or divorce within 15 years (Centers for Disease Control [CDC], 2001). The value that was once placed on religion also seems to be diminishing in the American culture. With the exception of a few months following the terrorist attacks of September 11, 2001, when attendance increased, a steady decline in church attendance was reported from 1991 to 2004 (Barna Research Online, 2004). Punctuality and efficiency are highly valued in the culture that promoted the work ethic, and most within this cultural group tend to be future oriented (Murray & Zentner, 2001).

Northern European Americans, particularly those who achieve middle-class socioeconomic status, value preventive medicine and primary health care. This value follows along with the socioeconomic group's educational level, successful achievement, and financial capability to maintain a healthy lifestyle. Most recognize the importance of regular physical exercise. Northern European Americans have medium body structure and fair skin, the latter of which is thought to be an evolutionary result of living in cold, cloudy Northern Europe (Giger & Davidhizar, 2004).

Beef and certain seafoods, such as lobster, are regarded as high-status foods among many people in this culture (Giger & Davidhizar, 2004). Changing food habits, however, may bring both good news and bad news. The good news is that people are learning to eat healthier by decreasing the amount of fat and increasing the nutrients in their diets. The bad news is that Americans still enjoy fast food, and it conforms to their fast-paced lifestyles.

African Americans

The language dialect of many African Americans is different from what is considered standard English. The origin of the black dialect is not clearly understood but is thought to be a combination of various African languages and the languages of other cultural groups (e.g., Dutch, French, English, and Spanish) present in the United States at the time of its settlement. Personal space tends to be smaller than that of the dominant culture.

Patterns of discrimination date back to the days of slavery, and evidence of segregation still exists, usually in the form of predominantly black neighborhoods, churches, and schools, still visible in some U.S. cities. Some African Americans find it too difficult to try to assimilate into the mainstream culture and choose to remain within their own social organization.

In 2005, 31 percent of African American households were headed by a woman (U.S. Census Bureau, 2006). Social support systems may be large and include sisters, brothers, aunts, uncles, cousins, boyfriends, girlfriends, neighbors, and friends. Many African Americans have a strong religious orientation, with the vast majority practicing some form of Protestantism (Harris, 2004).

African Americans who have assimilated into the dominant culture are likely to be well educated, professional, and future-oriented. Some who have not become assimilated may believe that planning for the future is hopeless, given their previous experiences and encounters with racism and discrimination (Cherry & Giger, 2004). They may be unemployed or have low-paying jobs, with little expectation of improvement. They are unlikely to value time or punctuality to the same degree as the dominant cultural group, which often causes them to be labeled as irresponsible.

Some African Americans, particularly those from the rural South, may reach adulthood never having seen a physician. They receive their medical care from the local folk practitioner known as "granny," or "the old lady," or a "spiritualist." Incorporated into the system of **folk medicine** is the belief that health is a gift from God, whereas illness is a punishment from God or a retribution for sin and evil. Historically, African Americans have turned to folk medicine either because they could not afford the cost of mainstream medical treatment or because of insensitive treatment by caregivers in the health care delivery system.

The height of African Americans varies little from that of their Northern European American counterparts. Skin color varies from white to very dark brown or black, which offered the ancestors of African Americans protection from the sun and tropical heat.

Hypertension occurs more frequently, and sickle cell anemia occurs predominantly, in African Americans. Hypertension carries a strong hereditary risk factor, whereas sickle cell anemia is genetically derived. Alcoholism is a serious problem among members of the black community, leading to a high incidence of alcohol-related illness and death (Cherry & Giger, 2004).

The diet of most African Americans differs little from that of the mainstream culture. However, some African Americans follow their heritage and still enjoy what has come to be known as "soul" food, which includes poke salad, collard greens, beans, corn, fried chicken, black-eyed peas, grits, okra, and cornbread. These foods are now considered typical Southern fare and are regularly consumed and enjoyed by most individuals who live in the Southern region of the United States.

Native Americans

The Bureau of Indian Affairs (BIA) recognizes 563 Indian tribes and Alaska Native groups in the U.S. today (Wikipedia, 2007). Some 250 tribal languages are spoken and many are written (Office of Tribal Justice, 2007). Fewer than half of these still live on reservations, but most return home often to participate in family and tribal life and sometimes to retire. Touch is an aspect of communication that is not the same among Native Americans as in the dominant American culture. Some Native Americans view the traditional handshake as somewhat aggressive. Instead, if a hand is offered to another, it may be accepted with a light touch or just a passing of hands (Still & Hodgins, 2003). Some Native Americans will not touch a dead person (Hanley, 2004).

Native Americans may appear silent and reserved. They may be uncomfortable expressing emotions because the culture encourages keeping private thoughts to oneself.

The concept of space is very concrete to Native Americans. Living space is often crowded with members of both nuclear and extended families. A large network of kin is very important to Native Americans. However, a need for extended space exists, as demonstrated by a distance of many miles between individual homes or camps.

The primary social organizations of Native Americans are the family and the tribe. From infancy, Native American children are taught the importance of these units. Traditions are passed down by the elderly, and children are taught to respect tradition and to honor wisdom.

Native Americans are very present-time oriented. Time sequences, in order of importance, are present, past, and future, with little emphasis on the future (Still & Hodgins, 2003). Not only are Native Americans not ruled by the clock, some do not even own clocks. The concept of time is very casual, and tasks are accomplished, not with the notion of a particular time in mind, but merely in a present-oriented time frame.

Religion and health practices are intertwined in the Native American culture. The medicine man (or woman) is called the **shaman**, who may use a variety of methods in his or her practice. Some depend on "crystal gazing" to diagnose illness, some sing and perform elaborate healing ceremonies, and some use herbs and other plants or roots to concoct remedies with healing properties. The Native American healers and U.S. Indian Health Service have worked together with mutual respect for many years. Hanley (2004) relates that a medicine man or woman may confer with a physician regarding the care of a client

in the hospital. Clients may sometimes receive hospital passes to participate in a healing ceremony held outside the hospital. Research studies have continued to show the importance of each of these health care systems in the overall wellness of Native American people.

Native Americans are typically of average height with reddish-tinted skin that may be light to medium brown. Their cheekbones are usually high and their noses have high bridges, probably an evolutionary result of living in very dry climates.

The risks of illness and premature death from alcoholism, diabetes, tuberculosis, heart disease, accidents, homicide, suicide, pneumonia, and influenza are greater for Native Americans than for the U.S. population as a whole (Indian Health Service [IHS], 2001). Alcoholism is a significant problem among Native Americans (National Institute on Alcohol Abuse and Alcoholism [NIAAA], 2004). It is thought to be a symptom of depression in many cases and to contribute to a number of other serious problems such as automobile accidents, homicides, spouse and child abuse, and suicides.

Nutritional deficiencies are not uncommon among tribal Native Americans. Fruits and green vegetables are often scarce in many of the federally defined Indian geographical regions. Meat and corn products are identified as preferred foods. Fiber intake is relatively low, while fat intake is often of the saturated variety. A large number of Native Americans living on or near reservations recognized by the federal or state government receive commodity foods supplied by the U.S. Department of Agriculture's food distribution program (U.S. Department of Agriculture, 2004).

Asian/Pacific Islander Americans

Asian Americans comprise approximately 4 percent of the U.S. population. The Asian American culture includes peoples (and their descendants) from Japan, China, Vietnam, the Philippines, Thailand, Cambodia, Korea, Laos, India, and the Pacific Islands. Although this discussion relates to these peoples as a single culture, it is important to keep in mind that a multiplicity of differences regarding attitudes, beliefs, values, religious practices, and language exist among these subcultures.

Many Asian Americans, particularly Japanese, are third- and even fourth-generation Americans. These individuals are likely to be acculturated to the U.S. culture. Ng (2001) describes three patterns common to Asian Americans in their attempt to adjust to the American culture:

1. The Traditionalists. These individuals tend to be the older generation Asians who hold on to the traditional values and practices of their native culture. They have strong internalized Asian values. Primary allegiance is to the biological family.

2. The Marginal People. These individuals reject the traditional values and totally embrace Western culture. Often they are members of the younger generations.

3. Asian Americans. These individuals incorporate traditional values and beliefs with Western values and beliefs. They become integrated into the American culture, while maintaining a connection with their ancestral culture.

The languages and dialects of Asian Americans are very diverse. In general, they do share a similar belief in harmonious interaction. To raise one's voice is likely to be interpreted as a sign of loss of control. The English language is very difficult to master, and even bilingual Asian Americans may encounter communication problems because of the differences in meaning assigned to nonverbal cues, such as facial gestures, verbal intonation and speed, and body movements. In Asian cultures, touching during communication has historically been considered unacceptable. However, with the advent of Western acculturation, younger generations of Asian Americans accept touching as more appropriate than did their ancestors. Eye contact is often avoided as it connotes rudeness and lack of respect in some Asian cultures. Acceptable personal and social spaces are larger than in the dominant American culture. Some Asian Americans have a great deal of difficulty expressing emotions. Because of their reserved public demeanor, Asian Americans may be perceived as shy, cold, or uninterested.

The family is the ultimate social organization in the Asian American culture, and loyalty to family is emphasized above all else. Children are expected to obey and honor their parents. Misbehavior is perceived as bringing dishonor to the entire family. Filial piety (one's social obligation or duty to one's parents) is held in high regard. Failure to fulfill these obligations can create a great deal of guilt and shame in an individual. A chronological hierarchy exists, with the elderly maintaining positions of authority. Several generations, or even extended families, may share a single household.

Although education is highly valued among Asian Americans, many remain undereducated. Religious beliefs and practices are very diverse and exhibit influences of Taoism, Buddhism, Confucianism, Islam, Hinduism, and Christianity (Giger & Davidhizar, 2004).

Many Asian Americans are both past- and present-oriented. Emphasis is placed on the wishes of one's ancestors, while adjusting to demands of the present. Little value is given to prompt adherence to schedules or rigid standards of activities.

Restoring the balance of **yin and yang** is the fundamental concept of Asian health practices (Spector, 2004). Yin and yang represent opposite forces of energy, such as negative/positive, dark/light, cold/hot, hard/soft, and feminine/masculine. When there is a disruption in the balance of these forces of energy, illness can occur. In medicine, the opposites are expressed as "hot" and "cold," and health is the result of a balance between hot and cold elements (Wang, 2003). Food, medicines, and herbs are classified according to their hot and cold properties and are used to restore balance between yin and yang (cold and hot), thereby restoring health.

Asian Americans are generally small of frame and build. Obesity is very uncommon in this culture. Skin color ranges from white to medium brown, with yellow tones. Other physical characteristics include almond-shaped eyes with a slight droop to eyelids and sparse body hair, particularly in men, in whom chest hair is often absent. Hair on the head is commonly coarse, thick, straight, and black.

Rice, vegetables, and fish are the main staple foods of Asian Americans. Milk is seldom consumed because a large majority of Asian Americans experience lactose intolerance. With Western acculturation, their diet is changing, and unfortunately, with more meat being consumed, the percentage of fat in the diet is increasing.

Many Asian Americans believe that psychiatric illness is merely behavior that is out of control and view it as a great shame to the individual and the family. They often attempt to manage the ill person on their own until they can no longer handle the situation. It is not uncommon for Asian Americans to somaticize. Expressing mental distress through various physical ailments may be viewed as more acceptable than expressing true emotions (Ishida & Inouye, 2004).

The incidence of alcohol dependence is low among Asians. This may be a result of a possible genetic intolerance of the substance. Some Asians develop unpleasant symptoms, such as flushing, headaches, and palpitations, on drinking alcohol. Research indicates that this is due to an isoenzyme variant that quickly converts alcohol to acetaldehyde and the absence of an isoenzyme that is needed to oxidize acetaldehyde. The result is a rapid accumulation of acetaldehyde that produces the unpleasant symptoms (Wall et al., 1997).

Latino Americans

Latino Americans are the fastest growing group of people in the United States, comprising approximately 14 percent of the population (U.S. Census Bureau, 2006). They represent the largest ethnic minority group.

Latino Americans trace their ancestry to countries such as Spain, Mexico, Puerto Rico, Cuba, and other countries of Central and South America. The common language is Spanish, spoken with a number of dialects by the various peoples. Touch is a common form of communication among Latinos; however, they are very modest and are likely to withdraw from any infringement on their modesty (Murray & Zentner, 2001). Latinos tend to be very tactful and diplomatic and will often appear agreeable on the surface out of courtesy for the person with whom they are communicating. It is only after the fact, when agreements may remain unfulfilled, that the true context of the interaction becomes clear.

Latino Americans are very group-oriented. It is important for them to interact with large groups of relatives, where a great deal of touching and embracing occurs. The family is the primary social organization and includes nuclear family members as well as numerous extended family members. The nuclear family is male dominated, and the father possesses ultimate authority.

Latino Americans tend to be present-oriented. The concept of being punctual and giving attention to activities that relate to concern about the future are perceived as less important than present-oriented activities that cannot be retrieved beyond the present time.

Roman Catholicism is the predominant religion among Latino Americans. Most Latinos identify with the Roman Catholic Church, even if they do not attend services. Religious beliefs and practices are likely to be strong influences in their lives. Especially in times of crisis, such as in cases of illness and hospitalization, Latino Americans rely on priest and family to carry out important religious rituals, such as promise making, offering candles, visiting shrines, and offering prayers (Spector, 2004).

Folk beliefs regarding health are a combination of elements incorporating views of Roman Catholicism and Indian and Spanish ancestries. The folk healer is called a **curandero** (male) or **curandera** (female). Among traditional Latino Americans, the *curandero* is believed to have a gift from God for healing the sick and is often the first contact made when illness is encountered. Treatments used include massage, diet, rest, suggestions, practical advice, indigenous herbs, prayers, magic, and supernatural rituals (Gonzalez & Kuipers, 2004). Many Latino Americans still subscribe to the "hot and cold theory" of disease. This concept is similar to the Asian perception of yin and yang discussed earlier in this chapter. Diseases and the foods and medicines used to treat them are classified as "hot" or "cold," and the intention is to restore the body to a balanced state.

Latino Americans are usually shorter than the average member of the dominant American culture. Skin color can vary from light tan to dark brown. Research indicates that there is less mental illness among Latino Americans than in the general population. This may have to do with the strong cohesiveness of the family and the support that is given during times of stress. Because Latino Americans have clearly defined rules of conduct, fewer role conflicts occur within the family.

Western European Americans

Western European Americans have their origins in France, Italy, and Greece. Each of these cultures possesses its own unique language, in which a number of dialects are noticeable. Western Europeans are known to be very warm and affectionate people and tend to be physically expressive, using a great deal of body language, including hugging and kissing.

Like Latino Americans, Western European Americans are very family-oriented. They interact in large groups, and it is not uncommon for several generations to live together or in close proximity of each other. A strong allegiance to the cultural heritage exists, and it is not uncommon, particularly among Italians, to find settlements of immigrants clustering together.

Roles within the family are clearly defined, with the man as the head of the household. Western European women view their role principally as mother and homemaker, and children are prized and cherished. The elderly are held in positions of respect and often are cared for in the home rather than placed in nursing homes.

Roman Catholicism is the predominant religion for the French and Italians, Greek Orthodox for the Greeks. A number of religious traditions are observed surrounding rites of passage. Masses and rituals are observed for births, first communions, confirmations, marriages, anniversaries, and deaths.

Western Europeans tend to be present-oriented with a somewhat fatalistic view of the future. A priority is placed on the here and now, and whatever will happen in the future is perceived as God's will.

Most Western European Americans follow health beliefs and practices of the dominant American culture, but some folk beliefs and superstitions still endure. Spector (2004, p. 285) reports the following superstitions and practices of Italians as they relate to health and illness:

1. Congenital abnormalities can be attributed to the unsatisfied desire for a particular food during pregnancy.
2. If a woman is not given food that she craves or smells, the fetus will move inside, and a miscarriage can result.
3. If a pregnant woman bends or turns or moves in a certain way, the fetus may not develop normally.
4. A woman must not reach during pregnancy because reaching can harm the fetus.
5. Sitting in a draft can cause a cold that can lead to pneumonia.

This author recalls her own Italian immigrant grandmother warming large collard greens in oil and placing them on swollen parotid glands during a bout with the mumps. The greens most likely did nothing for the mumps, but they (along with the tender loving care) felt wonderful!

Western Europeans are typically of average stature. Skin color ranges from fair to medium brown. Hair and eyes are commonly dark, but some Italians have blue eyes and blond hair. Food is very important in the Western European American culture. Italian, Greek, and French cuisine is world famous, and food is used in a social manner, as well as for nutritional purposes. Wine is consumed by all (even the children, who are given a mixture of water and wine) and is the beverage of choice with meals. However, among Greek Americans, drunkenness engenders social disgrace on the individual and the family (Tripp-Reimer & Sorofman, 1998).

Arab Americans*

Arab Americans trace their ancestry and traditions to the nomadic desert tribes of the Arabian Peninsula. The Arab countries include Algeria, Bahrain, Comoros, Djibouti, Egypt, Iraq, Jordan, Kuwait, Lebanon, Libya, Mauritania, Morocco, Oman, Palestine, Qatar, Saudi Arabia, Somalia, Sudan, Syria, Tunisia, United Arab Emirates, and Yemen. First-wave immigrants, primarily Christians, came to the United States between 1887 and 1913 seeking economic opportunity. First-wave immigrants and their descendants typically resided in urban centers of the Northeast. Second-wave immigrants entered the United States after World War II. Most are refugees from nations beset by war and political instability. This group includes a large number of professionals and individuals seeking educational degrees who have subsequently remained in the United States. Most are Muslims and favor professional occupations. Many second-wave Arab Americans have settled in Texas and Ohio.

Arabic is the official language of the Arab world. Although English is a common second language, language and communication can pose formidable problems in health care settings. Communication is highly contextual, where unspoken expectations are more important than the actual spoken words. Conversants stand close together, maintain steady eye contact, and touch (only between members of the same sex) the other's hand or shoulder.

Speech is loud and expressive and is characterized by repetition and gesturing, particularly when involved in serious discussions. Observers witnessing impassioned communication may incorrectly assume that Arabs are argumentative, confrontational, or aggressive. Privacy is valued, and many resist disclosure of personal information to strangers, especially when it relates to familial disease conditions. Among friends and relatives, Arabs express feelings freely. Devout Muslim men may not shake hands with women. When an Arab man is introduced to an Arab woman, the man waits for the woman to extend her hand.

Punctuality is not taken seriously except for business or professional meetings. Social events and appointments tend not to have a fixed beginning or end time.

Gender roles are clearly defined. The man is the head of the household and women are subordinate to men. Men are breadwinners, protectors, and decision-makers. Women are responsible for the care and education of children and for the maintenance of a successful marriage by tending to their husbands' needs.

The family is the primary social organization, and children are loved and indulged. The father is the disciplinarian and the mother is an ally and mediator. Loyalty to one's family takes precedence over personal needs. Sons are responsible for supporting elderly parents.

Women, especially devout Muslims, value modesty, which is expressed through their attire. Many Muslim women view the *hijab*, "covering the body except for one's face and hands," as offering them protection in situations in which men and women mix.

Most Arabs have dark or olive-colored skin, but some have blonde or auburn hair, blue eyes, and fair complexions. Infectious diseases such as tuberculosis, malaria, trachoma, typhus, hepatitis, typhoid fever, dysentery, and parasitic infestations are common among newer immigrants. Sickle cell anemia and the thalassemias are common in the eastern Mediterranean. Sedentary lifestyle and high fat intake among Arab Americans place them at higher risk for cardiovascular diseases. The rates of breast cancer screening, mammography, and cervical Pap smears are low because of modesty.

Arab cooking shares many general characteristics. Typical spices and herbs include cinnamon, allspice, cloves, ginger, cumin, mint, parsley, bay leaves, garlic, and onions. Bread accompanies every meal and is viewed as a gift from God. Lamb and chicken are the most popular meats. Muslims are prohibited from eating pork and pork products. Food is eaten with the right hand because it is regarded as clean. Eating and drinking at the same time is viewed as unhealthy. Eating properly, consuming nutritious foods, and fasting are believed to cure disease. Gastrointestinal complaints are the most frequent reason for seeking health care. Lactose intolerance is common.

Most Arabs are Muslims. Islam is the religion of most Arab countries, and in Islam there is no separation of church and state; a certain amount of religious participation is obligatory. Many Muslims believe in combining spiritual healing, performing daily prayers, and reading or listening to the Qur'an with conventional medical treatment. A devout client may request that his or her chair or bed be turned to face in the direction of Mecca and that a basin of water be provided for ritual washing or ablution before prayer. Sometimes illness is perceived as punishment for one's sins.

Mental illness is a major social stigma. Psychiatric symptoms may be denied or attributed to "bad nerves" or evil spirits. When individuals suffering from mental distress seek medical care, they are likely to present with a variety of vague complaints such as abdominal pain, lassitude, anorexia, and shortness of breath. Clients often

---

*This section on Arab Americans is taken from Purnell, L.D. & Paulanka, B.J. *Guide to Culturally Competent Health Care.* (2005). © F.A. Davis. Used with permission.

expect and may insist on somatic treatment, at least "vitamins and tonics." When mental illness is accepted as a diagnosis, treatment with medications, rather than counseling, is preferred.

Jewish Americans

To be Jewish is to belong to a specific group of people and a specific religion. The term *Jewish* does not refer to a race. The Jewish people came to the United States predominantly from Spain, Portugal, Germany, and Eastern Europe (Schwartz, 2004). There are more than 5 million Jewish Americans living in the United States, and they are located primarily in the larger urban areas.

Four main Jewish religious groups exist today: Orthodox, Reform, Conservative, and Reconstructionist. Orthodox Jews adhere to strict interpretation and application of Jewish laws and ethics. They believe that the laws outlined in the Torah (the five books of Moses) are divine, eternal, and unalterable. Reform Judaism is the largest Jewish religious group in the United States. The Reform group believes in the autonomy of the individual in interpreting the Jewish code of law, and a more liberal interpretation is followed. Conservative Jews also accept a less strict interpretation. They believe that the code of laws comes from God, but accept flexibility and adaptation of those laws to absorb aspects of the culture, while remaining true to Judaism's values. The Reconstructionists have modern views that generally override traditional Jewish laws. They do not believe that Jews are God's chosen people, they reject the notion of divine intervention, and there is general acceptance of interfaith marriage.

The primary language of Jewish Americans is English. Hebrew, the official language of Israel and the Torah, is used for prayers and is taught in Jewish religious education. Early Jewish immigrants spoke a Judeo-German dialect called Yiddish, and some of those words have become part of American English (e.g., *klutz, kosher, tush*).

Although traditional Jewish law is clearly male-oriented, with acculturation little difference is seen today with regard to gender roles. Formal education is a highly respected value among the Jewish people. A larger percentage of Jewish Americans hold advanced degrees and are employed as professionals (e.g., science, medicine, law, education) than that of the total U.S. white population.

While most Jewish people live for today and plan for and worry about tomorrow, they are raised with stories of their past, especially of the Holocaust. They are warned to "never forget," lest history be repeated. Therefore, their time orientation is simultaneously to the past, the present, and the future (Purnell & Paulanka, 2005).

Children are considered blessings and valued treasures, treated with respect, and deeply loved. They play an active role in most holiday celebrations and services. Respecting and honoring one's parents is one of the Ten Commandments. Children are expected to be forever grateful to their parents for giving them the gift of life (Purnell & Paulanka, 2005). The rite of passage into adulthood occurs during a religious ceremony called a *bar* or *bat mitzvah* (son or daughter of the commandment) and is usually commemorated by a family celebration.

Jewish people differ greatly in physical appearance, depending on the area of the world from which they migrated. Ancestors of Mediterranean region and Eastern European immigrants may have fair skin and blonde hair or darker skin and brunette hair, Asian descendants share oriental features, and Ethiopian Jews (*Falashas*) are Black (Schwartz, 2004).

Because of the respect afforded physicians and the emphasis on keeping the body and mind healthy, Jewish Americans are health conscious. In general, they practice preventive health care, with routine physical, dental, and vision screening. Circumcision for male infants is both a medical procedure and a religious rite and is performed on the eighth day of life. The procedure is a family festivity. It is usually performed at home, and many relatives are invited.

A number of genetic diseases are more common in the Jewish population, including Tay–Sachs disease, Gaucher's disease, and familial dysautonomia. Other conditions that occur with increased incidence in the Jewish population include inflammatory bowel disease (ulcerative colitis and Crohn's disease), colorectal cancer, and breast and ovarian cancer. Jewish people have a higher rate of side effects from the antipsychotic clozapine. About 20 percent develop agranulocytosis, which has been attributed to a specific gene that was recently identified (Purnell & Paulanka, 2005).

Alcohol, especially wine, is an essential part of religious holidays and festive occasions. It is viewed as appropriate and acceptable as long as it is used in moderation. For Jewish people who follow the dietary laws, a tremendous amount of attention is given to the slaughter of livestock and preparation and consumption of food. Religious laws dictate which foods are permissible. The term *kosher* means "fit to eat," and following these guidelines is thought to be a commandment of God. Meat may be eaten only if the permitted animal has been slaughtered, cooked, and served following kosher guidelines. Pigs are considered unclean, and pork and pork products are forbidden. Dairy products and meat may not be mixed together in cooking, serving, or eating.

Judaism opposes discrimination against people with physical, mental, and developmental conditions. The maintenance of one's mental health is considered just as important as the maintenance of one's physical health. Mental incapacity has always been recognized as grounds for exemption from all obligations under Jewish law (Purnell & Paulanka, 2005).

A summary of information related to the six cultural phenomena as they apply to the cultural groups discussed here is presented in Table 6–1.

and cold" theory of disease are very important to the well-being of some Asians and Latinos, respectively. Try to ensure that a balance of these foods are included in the diet as an important reinforcement for traditional medical care.

7. Be aware of favorite foods of individuals from different cultures. The health care setting may seem strange and somewhat isolated, and for some individuals it is comforting to have anything around them that is familiar. They may even refuse to eat foods that are unfamiliar to them. If it does not interfere with his or her care, allow family members to provide favorite foods for the client.

8. The nurse working in psychiatry must realize that psychiatric illness is stigmatized in some cultures. Individuals who believe that expressing emotions is unacceptable (e.g., Asian Americans and Native Americans) will present unique problems when they are clients in a psychiatric setting. Nurses must have patience and work slowly to establish trust in order to provide these individuals with the assistance they require.

Evaluation

Evaluation of nursing actions is directed at achievement of the established outcomes. Part of the evaluation process is continuous reassessment to ensure that the selected actions are appropriate and the goals and outcomes are realistic. Including the family and extended support systems in the evaluation process is essential if cultural implications of nursing care are to be measured. Modifications to the plan of care are made as the need is determined.

CORE CONCEPT

Spirituality
The human quality that gives meaning and sense of purpose to an individual's existence. Spirituality exists within each individual regardless of belief system and serves as a force for interconnectedness between the self and others, the environment, and a higher power.

SPIRITUAL CONCEPTS

Spirituality is difficult to describe. It cannot be seen, and it undoubtedly means something different to all people. Perhaps this is partly the reason it has been somewhat ignored in the nursing literature. This aspect is changing, however, with the following transformations occurring in nursing: The inclusion of nursing responsibility for spiritual care cited by the International Council of Nurses in their Code of Ethics; by the American

Holistic Nurses Association in their Standards for Holistic Nursing Practice; and through the development of a nursing diagnostic category, Spiritual Distress, by NANDA International (Wright, 2005). In addition, contemporary research has produced evidence that spirituality and religion can make a positive difference in health and illness.

Smucker (2001) states:

Spirituality is the recognition or experience of a dimension of life that is invisible, and both within us and yet beyond our material world, providing a sense of connectedness and interrelatedness with the universe. (p. 5)

Smucker (2001) identifies the following factors as types of spiritual needs associated with human beings:

1. Meaning and purpose in life
2. Faith or trust in someone or something beyond ourselves
3. Hope
4. Love
5. Forgiveness

Spiritual Needs

Meaning and Purpose in Life

Humans by nature appreciate order and structure in their lives. Having a purpose in life gives one a sense of control and the feeling that life is worth living. Smucker (2001) states, "Meaning provides us with a basic understanding of life and our place in it" (p. 6). Walsh (1999) describes "seven perennial practices" that he believes provide meaning and purpose to life. He suggests that these practices promote enlightenment and transformation and encourage spiritual growth. He identifies the seven perennial practices as follows:

1. **Transform your motivation:** Reduce craving and find your soul's desire.
2. **Cultivate emotional wisdom:** Heal your heart and learn to love.
3. **Live ethically:** Feel good by doing good.
4. **Concentrate and calm your mind:** Accept the challenge of mastering attention.
5. **Awaken your spiritual vision:** See clearly and recognize the sacred in all things.
6. **Cultivate spiritual intelligence:** Develop wisdom and understand life.
7. **Express spirit in action:** Embrace generosity and the joy of service. (p. 14)

In the final analysis, each individual must determine his or her own perception of what is important and what gives meaning to life. Throughout one's existence, the meaning of life will undoubtedly be challenged many times. A solid spiritual foundation may help an individual confront the challenges that result from life's experiences.

Faith

Faith is often thought of as the acceptance of a belief in the absence of physical or empirical evidence. Smucker (2001) states,

> For all people, faith is an important concept. From childhood on, our psychological health depends on having faith or trust in something or someone to help meet our needs. (p. 7)

Having faith requires that individuals rise above that which they can only experience through the five senses. Indeed, faith transcends the appearance of the physical world. An increasing amount of medical and scientific research is showing that what individuals believe exists can have as powerful an impact as what actually exists. Karren and associates (2002) state:

> Personal belief gives us an unseen power that enables us to do the impossible, to perform miracles—even to heal ourselves. It has been found that patients who exhibit faith become less concerned about their symptoms, have less-severe symptoms, and have less-frequent symptoms with longer periods of relief between them than patients who lack faith. (p. 485)

Evidence suggests that faith, combined with conventional treatment and an optimistic attitude, can be a very powerful element in the healing process.

Hope

Hope has been defined as a special kind of positive expectation (Karren et al., 2002). With hope, individuals look at a situation, and no matter how negative, find something positive on which to focus. Hope functions as an energizing force. In addition, research indicates that hope may promote healing, facilitate coping, and enhance quality of life (Nekolaichuk, Jevne, & Maguire, 1999).

Kübler-Ross (1969), in her classic study of dying patients, stressed the importance of hope. She suggested that, even though these patients could not hope for a cure, they could hope for additional time to live, to be with loved ones, for freedom from pain, or for a peaceful death with dignity. She found hope to be a satisfaction unto itself, whether or not it was fulfilled. She stated, "If a patient stops expressing hope, it is usually a sign of imminent death" (p. 140).

Karren and associates (2002) state:

> Researchers in the field of psychoneuroimmunology have found that what happens in the brain—the thoughts and emotions we experience, the attitudes with which we face the world—can have a definite effect on the body. An attitude like hope is not just a mental state; it causes specific electrochemical changes in the body that influence not only the strength of the immune system but can even influence the workings of the individual organs in the body. (p. 518)

The medical literature abounds with countless examples of individuals with terminal conditions who suddenly improve when they find something to live for. Conversely, there are also many accounts of patients whose conditions deteriorate when they lose hope.

Love

Love may be identified as a projection of one's own good feelings onto others. To love others, one must first experience love of self, and then be able and willing to project that warmth and affectionate concern for others (Karren et al., 2002).

Smucker (2001) states:

> Love, in its purest unconditional form, is probably life's most powerful force and our greatest spiritual need. Not only is it important to receive love, but equally important to give love to others. Thinking about and caring for the needs of others keeps us from being too absorbed with ourselves and our needs to the exclusion of others. We all have experienced the good feelings that come from caring for and loving others. (p. 10)

Love may be a very important key in the healing process. Karren and associates (2002) state:

> People who become more loving and less fearful, who replace negative thoughts with the emotion of love, are often able to achieve physical healing. Most of us are familiar with the emotional effects of love, the way love makes us feel inside. But...true love—a love that is patient, trusting, protecting, optimistic, and kind—has actual physical effects on the body, too. (p. 479)

Some researchers suggest that love has a positive effect on the immune system. This has been shown to be true in adults and children, and also in animals (Fox & Fox, 1988; Ornish, 1998). The giving and receiving of love may also result in higher levels of endorphins, thereby contributing to a sense of euphoria and helping to reduce pain.

In one long-term study, Werner and Smith (1992) studied children who were reared in impoverished environments. Their homes were troubled by discord, desertion, or divorce, or marred by parental alcoholism or mental illness. The subjects were studied at birth, childhood, adolescence, and adulthood. Two out of three of these high-risk children had developed serious learning and/or behavioral problems by age 10, or had a record of delinquencies, mental health problems, or pregnancies by age 18. One-fourth of them had developed "very serious" physical and psychosocial problems. By the time they reached adulthood, more than three-fourths of them suffered from profound psychological and behavioral problems and even more were in poor physical health. But of particular interest to the researchers were the 15 to 20 percent who remained resilient and well despite their impoverished and difficult existence. The children who remained resilient and well had experienced a warm and loving relationship with another person during their first year of life, whereas those who developed serious psychological and physical problems had not. This research indicates that the earlier people have the benefit of a strong, loving relationship, the better they seem able to resist the effects of a deleterious lifestyle.

Forgiveness

Karren and associates (2002) state, "Essential to a spiritual nature is forgiveness—the ability to release from the mind all the past hurts and failures, all sense of guilt and loss." Feelings of bitterness and resentment take a physical toll on an individual by generating stress hormones, which maintained for long periods can have a detrimental effect on a person's health. Forgiveness enables a person to cast off resentment and begin the pathway to healing.

Forgiveness is not easy. Individuals often have great difficulty when called upon to forgive others, and even greater difficulty in attempting to forgive themselves. Many people carry throughout their lives a sense of guilt for having committed a mistake for which they do not believe they have been forgiven, or for which they have not forgiven themselves.

To forgive is not necessarily to condone or excuse one's own or someone else's inappropriate behavior. Karren and associates (2002) suggest that forgiveness is

> . . . a decision to see beyond the limits of another's personality; to be willing to accept responsibility for your own perceptions; to shift your perceptions repeatedly; and to gradually transform yourself from being a helpless victim of your circumstances to being a powerful and loving co-creator of your reality. (p. 451)

Holding on to grievances causes pain, suffering, and conflict. Forgiveness (of self and others) is a gift to oneself. It offers freedom and peace of mind.

It is important for nurses to be able to assess the spiritual needs of their clients. Nurses need not serve the role of professional counselor or spiritual guide, but because of the closeness of their relationship with clients, nurses may be the part of the health care team to whom clients may reveal the most intimate details of their lives. Smucker (2001) states:

> Just as answering a patient's question honestly and with accurate information and responding to his needs in a timely and sensitive manner communicates caring, so also does high-quality professional nursing care reach beyond the physical body or the illness to that part of the person where identity, self-worth, and spirit lie. In this sense, good nursing care is also good spiritual care. (pp. 11–12)

 CORE CONCEPT

Religion
A set of beliefs, values, rites, and rituals adopted by a group of people. The practices are usually grounded in the teachings of a spiritual leader.

Religion

Religion is one way in which an individual's spirituality may be expressed. There are more than 6500 religions in the world (Bronson, 2005). Some individuals seek out various religions in an attempt to find answers to fundamental questions that they have about life, and indeed, about their very existence. Others, although they may regard themselves as spiritual, choose not to affiliate with an organized religious group. In either situation, however, it is inevitable that questions related to life and the human condition arise during the progression of spiritual maturation.

Brodd (2003) suggests that all religious traditions manifest seven dimensions: experiential, mythic, doctrinal, ethical, ritual, social, and material. He explains that these seven dimensions are intertwined and complementary and, depending on the particular religion, certain dimensions are emphasized more than others. For example, Zen Buddhism has a strong experiential dimension, but says little about doctrines. Roman Catholicism is strong in both ritual and doctrine. The social dimension is a significant aspect of religion, as it provides a sense of community, of belonging to a group, such as a parish or a congregation, which is empowering for some individuals.

Affiliation with a religious group has been shown to be a health-enhancing endeavor (Karren et al., 2002). A number of studies have been conducted that indicate a correlation between religious faith/church attendance and increased chance of survival following serious illness, less depression and other mental illness, longer life, and overall better physical and mental health. In an extensive review of the literature, Maryland psychologist John Gartner (1998) found that individuals with a religious commitment had lower suicide rates, lower drug use and abuse, less juvenile delinquency, lower divorce rates, and improved mental illness outcomes.

It is not known how religious participation protects health and promotes well-being. Some churches actively promote healthy lifestyles and discourage behavior that would be harmful to health or interfere with treatment of disease. But some researchers believe that the strong social support network found in churches may be the most important force in boosting the health and well-being of their members. More so than merely an affiliation, however, it is regular church attendance and participation that appear to be the key factors.

ASSESSMENT OF SPIRITUAL AND RELIGIOUS NEEDS

It is important for nurses to consider spiritual and religious needs when planning care for their clients. The Joint Commission on Accreditation of Healthcare Organizations (JCAHO) requires that nurses address the psychosocial, spiritual, and cultural variables that influence the perception of illness. Dossey (1998) has developed a spiritual assessment tool (Box 6–3) about which she states:

BOX 6 – 3   Spiritual Assessment Tool

The following reflective questions may assist you in assessing, evaluating, and increasing awareness of spirituality in yourself and others.

Meaning and Purpose

These questions assess a person's ability to seek meaning and fulfillment in life, manifest hope, and accept ambiguity and uncertainty.

- What gives your life meaning?
- Do you have a sense of purpose in life?
- Does your illness interfere with your life goals?
- Why do you want to get well?
- How hopeful are you about obtaining a better degree of health?
- Do you feel that you have a responsibility in maintaining your health?
- Will you be able to make changes in your life to maintain your health?
- Are you motivated to get well?
- What is the most important or powerful thing in your life?

Inner Strengths

These questions assess a person's ability to manifest joy and recognize strengths, choices, goals, and faith.

- What brings you joy and peace in your life?
- What can you do to feel alive and full of spirit?
- What traits do you like about yourself?
- What are your personal strengths?
- What choices are available to you to enhance your healing?
- What life goals have you set for yourself?
- Do you think that stress in any way caused your illness?
- How aware were you of your body before you became sick?
- What do you believe in?
- Is faith important in your life?
- How has your illness influenced your faith?
- Does faith play a role in recognizing your health?

Interconnections

These questions assess a person's positive self-concept, self-esteem, and sense of self; sense of belonging in the world with others; capacity to pursue personal interests; and ability to demonstrate love of self and self-forgiveness.

- How do you feel about yourself right now?
- How do you feel when you have a true sense of yourself?
- Do you pursue things of personal interest?
- What do you do to show love for yourself?

- Can you forgive yourself?
- What do you do to heal your spirit?

These questions assess a person's ability to connect in life-giving ways with family, friends, and social groups and to engage in the forgiveness of others.

- Who are the significant people in your life?
- Do you have friends or family in town who are available to help you?
- Who are the people to whom you are closest?
- Do you belong to any groups?
- Can you ask people for help when you need it?
- Can you share your feelings with others?
- What are some of the most loving things that others have done for you?
- What are the loving things that you do for other people?
- Are you able to forgive others?

These questions assess a person's capacity for finding meaning in worship or religious activities, and a connectedness with a divinity.

- Is worship important to you?
- What do you consider the most significant act of worship in your life?
- Do you participate in any religious activities?
- Do you believe in God or a higher power?
- Do you think that prayer is powerful?
- Have you ever tried to empty your mind of all thoughts to see what the experience might be?
- Do you use relaxation or imagery skills?
- Do you meditate?
- Do you pray?
- What is your prayer?
- How are your prayers answered?
- Do you have a sense of belonging in this world?

These questions assess a person's ability to experience a sense of connection with life and nature, an awareness of the effects of the environment on life and well-being, and a capacity or concern for the health of the environment.

- Do you ever feel a connection with the world or universe?
- How does your environment have an impact on your state of well-being?
- What are your environmental stressors at work and at home?
- What strategies reduce your environmental stressors?
- Do you have any concerns for the state of your immediate environment?
- Are you involved with environmental issues such as recycling environmental resources at home, work, or in your community?
- Are you concerned about the survival of the planet?

SOURCES: Dossey, B.M. (1998). Holistic modalities and healing moments, *American Journal of Nursing, 98*(6), 44–47. With permission. Burkhardt, M.A. (1989). Spirituality: An analysis of the concept. *Holist Nurs Pract, 3*(3), 69-77; Dossey, B.M. et al. (Eds.) (1995). *Holistic nursing: A handbook for practice* (2nd ed.). Gaithersburg, MD: Aspen.

The Spiritual Assessment Tool provides reflective questions for assessing, evaluating, and increasing awareness of spirituality in patients and their significant others. The tool's reflective questions can facilitate healing because they stimulate spontaneous, independent, meaningful initiatives to improve the patient's capacity for recovery and healing.

Diagnoses/Outcome Identification/Evaluation

Nursing diagnoses that may be used when addressing spiritual and religious needs of clients include:

● Risk for Spiritual Distress
● Spiritual Distress
● Readiness for Enhanced Spiritual Well-being
● Risk for Impaired Religiosity
● Impaired Religiosity
● Readiness for Enhanced Religiosity

The following outcomes may be used as guidelines for care and to evaluate effectiveness of the nursing interventions.

The client will:

1. Identify meaning and purpose in life that reinforce hope, peace, and contentment.
2. Verbalize acceptance of self as worthwhile human being.
3. Accept and incorporate change into life in a healthy manner.
4. Express understanding of relationship between difficulties in current life situation and interruption in previous religious beliefs and activities.
5. Discuss beliefs and values about spiritual and religious issues.
6. Express desire and ability to participate in beliefs and activities of desired religion.

Planning/Implementation

NANDA International (2007) information related to the diagnoses Risk for Spiritual Distress and Risk for Impaired Religiosity is provided in the subsections that follow.

Risk for Spiritual Distress

Definition. At risk for an impaired ability to experience and integrate meaning and purpose in life through a person's connectedness with self, other persons, art, music, literature, nature, and/or a power greater than oneself.

Risk Factors

Physical. Physical/chronic illness; substance abuse/excessive drinking.
  Psychosocial. Low self-esteem; depression; anxiety; stress; poor relationships; separate from support systems; blocks to experiencing love; inability to forgive; loss; racial/cultural conflict; change in religious rituals; change in spiritual practices.
  Developmental. Life change; developmental life changes.
  Environmental. Environmental changes; natural disasters.

Risk for Impaired Religiosity

Definition. At risk for an impaired ability to exercise reliance on religious beliefs and/or participate in rituals of a particular faith tradition.

Risk Factors

Physical. Illness/hospitalization; pain.
  Psychological. Ineffective support/coping/caregiving; depression; lack of security.
  Sociocultural. Lack of social interaction; cultural barrier to practicing religion; social isolation.
  Spiritual. Suffering.
  Environmental. Lack of transportation; environmental barriers to practicing religion.
  Developmental. Life transitions.
  A plan of care addressing client's spiritual/religious needs is provided in Table 6–3. Selected nursing diagnoses are presented, along with appropriate nursing interventions and rationales for each.

Evaluation

Evaluation of nursing actions is directed at achievement of the established outcomes. Part of the evaluation process is continuous reassessment to ensure that the selected actions are appropriate and the goals and outcomes are realistic. Including the family and extended support systems in the evaluation process is essential if spiritual and religious implications of nursing care are to be measured. Modifications to the plan of care are made as the need is determined.

Table 6-3 Care Plan for the Client with Spiritual and Religious Needs*

NURSING DIAGNOSIS: RISK FOR SPIRITUAL DISTRESS

RELATED TO: Life changes; environmental changes; stress; anxiety; depression

EVIDENCED BY: Questioning meaning of life and own existence; inner conflict about personal beliefs and values

Outcome Criteria	Nursing Interventions	Rationale
Client will identify meaning and purpose in life that reinforce hope, peace, contentment, and self-satisfaction.	1. Assess current situation.	1–8. Thorough assessment is necessary to develop an accurate care plan for the client.
	2. Listen to client's expressions of anger, concern, self-blame.	
	3. Note reason for living and whether it is directly related to situation.	
	4. Determine client's religious/spiritual orientation, current involvement, presence of conflicts, especially in current circumstances.	
	5. Assess sense of self-concept, worth, ability to enter into loving relationships.	
	6. Observe behavior indicative of poor relationships with others.	
	7. Determine support systems available to and used by client and significant others.	
	8. Assess substance use/abuse.	
	9. Establish an environment that promotes free expression of feelings and concerns.	9. Trust is the basis of a therapeutic nurse-client relationship.
	10. Have client identify and prioritize current/immediate needs.	10. Helps client focus on what needs to be done and identify manageable steps to take.
	11. Discuss philosophical issues related to impact of current situation on spiritual beliefs and values.	11. Helps client to understand that certain life experiences can cause individuals to question personal values and that this response is not uncommon.
	12. Use therapeutic communication skills of reflection and active listening.	12. Helps client find own solutions to concerns.
	13. Review coping skills used and their effectiveness in current situation.	13. Identifies strengths to incorporate into plan and techniques that need revision.
	14. Provide a role model (e.g., nurse, individual experiencing similar situation)	14. Sharing of experiences and hope assists client to deal with reality.
	15. Suggest use of journaling.	15. Journaling can assist in clarifying beliefs and values and in recognizing and resolving feelings about current life situation.
	16. Discuss client's interest in the arts, music, literature.	16. Provides insight into meaning of these issues and how they are integrated into an individual's life.
	17. Role-play new coping techniques. Discuss possibilities of taking classes, becoming involved in discussion groups, cultural activities of their choice.	17. These activities will help to enhance integration of new skills and necessary changes in client's lifestyle
	18. Refer client to appropriate resources for help.	18. Client may require additional assistance with an individual who specializes in these types of concerns.

Continued on following page

Table 6–3 *(Continued)*

NURSING DIAGNOSIS: RISK FOR IMPAIRED RELIGIOSITY

RELATED TO: Suffering; depression; illness; life transitions

EVIDENCED BY: Concerns about relationship with deity; unable to participate in usual religious practices; anger toward God

Outcome Criteria	Nursing Interventions	Rationale
Client will express achievement of support and personal satisfaction from spiritual/religious practices.	1. Assess current situation (e.g., illness, hospitalization, prognosis of death, presence of support systems, financial concerns)	1. This information identifies problems client is dealing with in the moment that is affecting desire to be involved with religious activities.
	2. Listen nonjudgmentally to client's expressions of anger and possible belief that illness/condition may be a result of lack of faith.	2. Individuals often blame themselves for what has happened and reject previous religious beliefs and/or God.
	3. Determine client's usual religious/spiritual beliefs, current involvement in specific church activities.	3. This is important background for establishing a database.
	4. Note quality of relationships with significant others and friends.	4. Individual may withdraw from others in relation to the stress of illness, pain, and suffering.
	5. Assess substance use/abuse.	5. Individuals often turn to use of various substances in distress and this can affect the ability to deal with problems in a positive manner.
	6. Develop nurse–client relationship in which individual can express feelings and concerns freely.	6. Trust is the basis for a therapeutic nurse–client relationship.
	7. Use therapeutic communications skills of active listening, reflection, and I-messages.	7. Helps client to find own solutions to problems and concerns and promotes sense of control.
	8. Be accepting and nonjudgmental when client expresses anger and bitterness toward God. Stay with the client.	8. The nurse's presence and nonjudgmental attitude increase the client's feelings of self-worth and promote trust in the relationship.
	9. Encourage client to discuss previous religious practices and how these practices provided support in the past.	9. A nonjudgmental discussion of previous sources of support may help the client work through current rejection of them as potential sources of support.
	10. Allow the client to take the lead in initiating participation in religious activities, such as prayer.	10. Client may be vulnerable in current situation and needs to be allowed to decide own resumption of these actions.
	11. Contact spiritual leader of client's choice, if he or she requests.	11. These individuals serve to provide relief from spiritual distress and often can do so when other support persons cannot.

*The interventions for this care plan were adapted from Doenges, Moorhouse, and Murr (2006).

SUMMARY AND KEY POINTS

- Culture encompasses shared patterns of belief, feeling, and knowledge that guide people's conduct and are passed down from generation to generation.
- Ethnic groups are bound together by a shared heritage.
- Cultural groups differ in terms of communication, space, social organization, time, environmental control, and biological variations.
- Northern European Americans are the descendants of the first immigrants to the United States and make up the current dominant cultural group. They value punctuality, a responsible work ethic, and a healthy lifestyle.

- African Americans trace their roots in the United States to the days of slavery. Most have large support systems and a strong religious orientation. Many have assimilated into and have many of the same characteristics as the dominant culture. Some African Americans from the rural South may receive health care from a folk practitioner.
- Many Native Americans still live on reservations. They speak many different languages and dialects. They often appear silent and reserved and many are uncomfortable with touch and expressing emotions. Health care may be delivered by a medicine man or woman called a *shaman*.
- Asian American languages are very diverse. Touching during communication has historically been considered unacceptable. Individuals may have difficulty expressing emotions and appear cold and aloof. Family loyalty is emphasized. Psychiatric illness is viewed as behavior that is out of control and brings shame on the family.
- The common language of Latino Americans is Spanish. Large family groups are important, and touch is a common form of communication. The predominant religion is Roman Catholicism and the church is often a source of strength in times of crisis. Health care may be delivered by a folk healer called a *curandero*, who uses various forms of treatment to restore the body to a balanced state.
- Western European Americans have their origins in Italy, France, and Greece. They are warm and expressive and use touch as a common form of communication. The dominant religion is Roman Catholicism for the Italians and French and Greek Orthodoxy for the Greeks. Most Western European Americans follow the health practices of the dominant culture, but some folk beliefs and superstitions endure.
- Arab Americans trace their ancestry and traditions to the nomadic desert tribes of the Arabian Peninsula.

Arabic is the official language of the Arab world and the dominant religion is Islam. Mental illness is considered a social stigma, and symptoms are often somaticized.

- The Jewish people came to the United States predominantly from Spain, Portugal, Germany, and Eastern Europe. Four main Jewish religious groups exist today: Orthodox, Reform, Conservative, and Reconstructionist. The primary language is English. A high value is placed on education. Jewish Americans are very health conscious and practice preventive health care. The maintenance of one's mental health is considered just as important as the maintenance of one's physical health.
- Culture-bound syndromes are clusters of physical and behavioral symptoms that are considered as illnesses or "afflictions" by specific cultures and recognized as such by the *DSM-IV-TR*.
- Spirituality is the human quality that gives meaning and sense of purpose to an individual's existence.
- Individuals possess a number of spiritual needs that include meaning and purpose in life, faith or trust in someone or something beyond themselves, hope, love, and forgiveness.
- Religion is a set of beliefs, values, rites, and rituals adopted by a group of people.
- It is one way in which an individual's spirituality may be expressed.
- Affiliation with a religious group has been shown to be a health-enhancing endeavor.
- Nurses must consider cultural, spiritual, and religious needs when planning care for their clients.

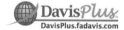 **For additional clinical tools and study aids, visit DavisPlus.**

REVIEW QUESTIONS

Self-Examination/Learning Exercise

Select the answer that is most appropriate for each of the following questions.

1. Miss Lee is an Asian American on the psychiatric unit. She tells the nurse, "I must have the hot ginger root for my headache. It is the only thing that will help." What meaning does the nurse attach to this statement by Miss Lee?

   a. She is being obstinate and wants control over her care.
   b. She believes that ginger root has magical qualities.
   c. She subscribes to the restoration of health through the balance of yin and yang.
   d. Asian Americans refuse to take traditional medicine for pain.

2. Miss Lee (the same client from the previous question) says she is afraid that no one from her family will visit her. On what belief does Miss Lee base her statement?

   a. Many Asian Americans do not believe in hospitals.
   b. Many Asian Americans do not have close family support systems.
   c. Many Asian Americans believe the body will heal itself if left alone.
   d. Many Asian Americans view psychiatric problems as bringing shame to the family.

3. Joe, a Native American, appears at the community health clinic with an oozing stasis ulcer on his lower right leg. It is obviously infected, and he tells the nurse that the shaman has been treating it with herbs. The nurse determines that Joe needs emergency care, but Joe states he will not go to the emergency department (ED) unless the shaman is allowed to help treat him. How should the nurse handle this situation?

   a. Contact the shaman and have him meet them at the ED to consult with the attending physician.
   b. Tell Joe that the shaman is not allowed in the ED.
   c. Explain to Joe that the shaman is at fault for his leg being in the condition it is in now.
   d. Have the shaman try to talk Joe into going to the ED without him.

4. When the shaman arrives at the hospital, Joe's physician extends his hand for a handshake. The shaman lightly touches the physician's hand, then quickly moves away. How should the physician interpret this gesture?

   a. The shaman is snubbing the physician.
   b. The shaman is angry that he was called away from his supper.
   c. The shaman does not believe in traditional medicine.
   d. The shaman does not feel comfortable with touch.

5. Sarah is an African American woman who receives a visit from the psychiatric home health nurse. A referral for a mental health assessment was made by the public health nurse, who noticed that Sarah was becoming exceedingly withdrawn. When the psychiatric nurse arrives, Sarah says to her, "No one can help me. I was an evil person in my youth, and now I must pay." How might the nurse assess this statement?

   a. Sarah is having delusions of persecution.
   b. Some African Americans believe illness is God's punishment for their sins.
   c. Sarah is depressed and just wants to be left alone.
   d. African Americans do not believe in psychiatric help.

6. Sarah says to the nurse, "Granny told me to eat a lot of poke greens and I would feel better." How should the nurse interpret this statement?

   a. Sarah's grandmother believes in the healing power of poke greens.
   b. Sarah believes everything her grandmother tells her.
   c. Sarah has been receiving health care from a "folk practitioner."
   d. Sarah is trying to determine if the nurse agrees with her grandmother.

7. Frank is a Latino American who has an appointment at the community health center for 1:00 p.m. The nurse is angry when Frank shows up at 3:30 p.m., stating, "I was visiting with my brother." How must the nurse interpret this behavior?

   a. Frank is being passive–aggressive by showing up late.
   b. This is Frank's way of defying authority.
   c. Frank is a member of a cultural group that is present-oriented.
   d. Frank is a member of a cultural group that rejects traditional medicine.

8. The nurse must give Frank (the client from the previous question) a physical examination. She tells him to remove his clothing and put on an examination gown. Frank refuses. How should the nurse interpret this behavior?

   a. Frank does not believe in taking orders from a woman.
   b. Frank is modest and embarrassed to remove his clothes.
   c. Frank does not understand why he must remove his clothes.
   d. Frank does not think he needs a physical examination.

9. Maria is an Italian American who is in the hospital after having suffered a miscarriage at 5 months' gestation. Her room is filled with relatives who have brought a variety of foods and gifts for Maria. They are all talking, seemingly at the same time, and some, including Maria, are crying. They repeatedly touch and hug Maria and each other. How should the nurse handle this situation?

   a. Explain to the family that Maria needs her rest and they must all leave.
   b. Allow the family to remain and continue their activity as described, as long as they do not disturb other clients.
   c. Explain that Maria will not get over her loss if they keep bringing it up and causing her to cry so much.
   d. Call the family priest to come and take charge of this family situation.

10. Maria's mother says to the nurse, "If only Maria had told me she wanted the biscotti. I would have made them for her." What is the meaning behind Maria's mother's statement?

    a. Some Italian Americans believe a miscarriage can occur if a woman does not eat a food she craves.
    b. Some Italian Americans think biscotti can prevent miscarriage.
    c. Maria's mother is taking the blame for Maria's miscarriage.
    d. Maria's mother believes the physician should have told Maria to eat biscotti.

11. Joe, who has come to the mental health clinic with symptoms of depression, says to the nurse, "My father is dying. I have always hated my father. He physically abused me when I was a child. We haven't spoken for many years. He wants to see me now, but I don't know if I want to see him." With which spiritual need is Joe struggling?

    a. Forgiveness
    b. Faith
    c. Hope
    d. Meaning and purpose in life

12. Joe (from the previous question) says to the nurse, "I'm so angry! Why did God have to give me a father like this? I feel cheated of a father! I've always been a good person. I deserved better. I hate God!!" From this subjective data, which nursing diagnosis might the nurse apply to Joe?

    a. Readiness for enhanced religiosity
    b. Risk for impaired religiosity
    c. Readiness for enhanced spiritual well-being
    d. Spiritual distress

REFERENCES

American Psychiatric Association (APA). (2000). *Diagnostic and statistical manual of mental disorders* (4th ed.). *Text revision.* Washington, DC: American Psychiatric Association.

Barna Research Online. (2004). Church attendance. Retrieved October 8, 2004 from http://www.barna.org/

Brodd, J. (2003). *World religions: A voyage of discovery* (2nd ed.). Winona, MN: Saint Mary's Press.

Bronson, M. (2005). *Why are there so many religions?* Retrieved September 28, 2005 from http://www.biblehelp.org/relig.htm

Centers for Disease Control (CDC). (2001). *First marriage dissolution, divorce, and remarriage in the United States.* Atlanta: CDC Office of Enterprise Communication.

Cherry, B., & Giger, J.N. (2004). African-Americans. In J.N. Giger & R.E. Davidhizar (Eds.), *Transcultural nursing: Assessment and intervention* (4th ed.). St. Louis: C.V. Mosby.

Doenges, M.E., Moorhouse, M.F., & Murr, A.C. (2006). *Nurse's pocket guide: Diagnoses, interventions, and rationales* (10th ed.). Philadelphia: F.A. Davis.

Dossey, B.M. (1998). Holistic modalities and healing moments. *American Journal of Nursing, 98*(6), 44–47.

Fox, A., & Fox, B. (1988). *Wake up! You're alive.* Deerfield Beach, FL: Health Communications, Inc.

Gartner, J. (1998). Religious commitment, mental health, and prosocial behavior: A review of the empirical literature. In E. Shafranske (Ed.), *Religion and the clinical practice of psychology.* Washington, DC: American Psychological Association.

Giger, J.N., & Davidhizar, R.E. (2004). *Transcultural nursing: Assessment and intervention* (4th ed.). St. Louis: C.V. Mosby.

Gonzalez, T., & Kuipers, J. (2004). Mexican Americans. In J.N. Giger & R.E. Davidhizar (Eds.), *Transcultural nursing: Assessment and intervention* (4th ed.). St. Louis: C.V. Mosby.

Griffin, H.C. (2002, December 12). Embracing diversity. *NurseWeek* [Special Edition], 14–15.

Griffith, E.E.H., Gonzalez, C.A., & Blue, H.C. (2003). Introduction to cultural psychiatry. In R.E. Hales & S.C. Yudofsky (Eds.), *Textbook of clinical psychiatry* (4th ed.). Washington, DC: American Psychiatric Publishing.

Hanley, C.E. (2004). Navajos. In J.N. Giger & R.E. Davidhizar (Eds.), *Transcultural nursing: Assessment and intervention* (4th ed.). St. Louis: C.V. Mosby.

Harris, L.M. (2004). *African Americans.* Microsoft Encarta Online Encyclopedia. Retrieved October 13, 2004 from http://encarta.msn.com

Indian Health Service (IHS). (2001). *Important strides in Indian health.* Retrieved November 1, 2001 from http://www.ihs.gov/MedicalPrograms/Nursing/nursing-strides.asp.

Ishida, D., & Inouye, J. (2004). Japanese Americans. In J.N. Giger & R.E. Davidhizar (Eds.), *Transcultural nursing: Assessment and intervention* (4th ed.). St. Louis: C.V. Mosby.

Karren, K.J., Hafen, B.Q., Smith, N.L., & Frandsen, K.J. (2002). *Mind/body health: The effects of attitudes, emotions, and relationships.* (2nd ed.). San Francisco: Benjamin Cummings.

Murray, R.B., & Zentner, J.P. (2001). *Health promotion strategies through the life span* (7th ed.). Upper Saddle River, NJ: Prentice-Hall.

NANDA International. (2007). *Nursing diagnoses: Definitions & classification 2007–2008.* Philadelphia: NANDA International.

National Institute on Alcohol Abuse and Alcoholism (NIAAA). (2004). *Alcohol abuse increases, dependence declines across decade: Young adult minorities emerge as high-risk subgroups.* News Release, June 10, 2004. Washington, DC: NIAAA.

Nekolaichuk, C.L., Jevne, R.F., & Maguire, T.O. (1999). Structuring the meaning of hope in health and illness. *Social Science and Medicine, 48*(5), 591–605.

Ng, M. (2001). *The Asian-American struggle for identity and battle with racism.* Retrieved November 2, 2001 from http://www.stern.nyu.edu/~myn1/racism.htm

Office of Tribal Justice. (2007). *FAQs About Native Americans.* Retrieved January 11, 2007 from http://www.usdoj.gov/otj/nafaqs.htm

Ornish, D. (1998). *Love and survival: Eight pathways to intimacy and health.* New York: HarperPerennial.

Purnell, L.D., & Paulanka, B.J. (2003). *Transcultural health care: A culturally competent approach* (2nd ed.). Philadelphia: F.A. Davis.

Purnell, L.D., & Paulanka, B.J. (2005). *Guide to culturally competent health care.* Philadelphia: F.A. Davis.

Schwartz, E.A. (2004). Jewish Americans. In J.N. Giger & R.E. Davidhizar (Eds.). *Transcultural nursing: Assessment & intervention* (4th ed.). St. Louis: Mosby.

Smucker, C.J. (2001). Overview of Nursing the Spirit. In D.L. Wilt & C.J. Smucker (Eds.), *Nursing the spirit: The art and science of applying spiritual care.* Washington, DC: American Nurses Publishing.

Spector, R.E. (2004). *Cultural diversity in health and illness* (6th ed.). Upper Saddle River, NJ: Pearson Prentice-Hall.

Still, O., & Hodgins, D. (2003). Navajo Indians. In L.D. Purnell & B.J. Paulanka, (Eds.), *Transcultural health care: A culturally competent approach* (2nd ed.). Philadelphia: F.A. Davis.

Tripp-Reimer, T., & Sorofman, B. (1998). Greek-Americans. In L.D. Purnell & B.J. Paulanka, (Eds.), *Transcultural health care: A culturally competent approach.* Philadelphia: F.A. Davis.

U.S. Census Bureau. (2006). *2005 American Community Survey.* Retrieved November 3, 2006 from http://factfinder.census.gov/servlet/DatasetMainPageServlet?_program=ACS&_submenuId=&_lang=en&_ts=

U.S. Department of Agriculture. (2004). *Food, nutrition, and consumer services.* Retrieved October 24, 2004 from http://www.aphis.usda.gov/anawg/Bluebook/guidefive.html

Wall, T.L., Peterson, C.M., Peterson, K.P., Johnson, M.L., Thomasson, H.R., Cole, M., & Ehlers, C.L. (1997). Alcohol metabolism in Asian-American men with genetic polymorphisms of aldehyde dehydrogenase. *Annals of Internal Medicine, 127,* 376–379.

Walsh, R. (1999). *Essential spirituality.* New York: John Wiley & Sons.

Wang, Y. (2003). People of Chinese heritage. In L.D. Purnell & B.J. Paulanka (Eds.), *Transcultural health care: A culturally competent approach* (2nd ed.). Philadelphia: F.A. Davis.

Werner, E.E., & Smith, R.S. (1992). *Overcoming the odds: High risk children from birth to adulthood.* Ithaca, NY: Cornell University Press.

Wikipedia. (2007). *Native Americans in the United States.* Retrieved January 11, 2007 from http://en.wikipedia.org/wiki/Native_Americans_in_the_United_States

Wright, L.M. (2005). *Spirituality, suffering, and illness.* Philadelphia: F.A. Davis.

CLASSICAL REFERENCES

Hall, E.T. (1966). *The hidden dimension.* Garden City, NY: Doubleday.

Kübler-Ross, E. (1969). *On death and dying.* New York: Macmillan.

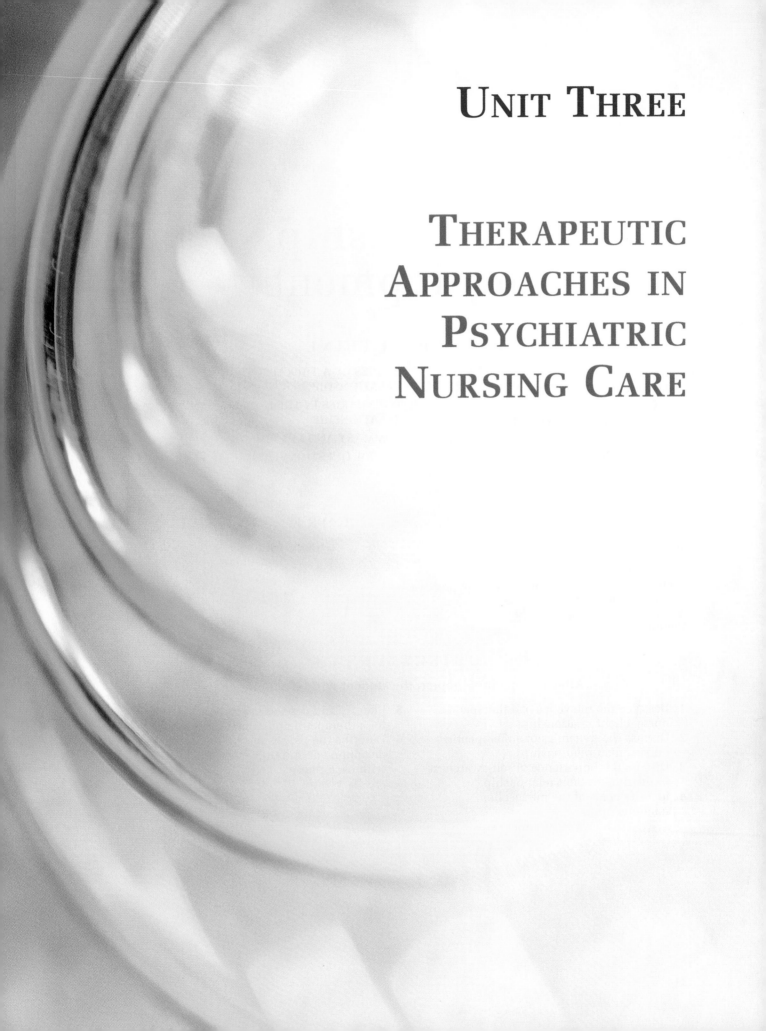

UNIT THREE

THERAPEUTIC APPROACHES IN PSYCHIATRIC NURSING CARE

7

C H A P T E R

Relationship Development

C H A P T E R   O U T L I N E

K E Y   T E R M S

attitude
belief
concrete thinking
confidentiality
countertransference
empathy
genuineness

rapport
sympathy
transference
unconditional positive
    regard
values

C O R E   C O N C E P T

therapeutic
    relationship

O B J E C T I V E S

After reading this chapter, the student will be able to:

1. Describe the relevance of a therapeutic nurse–client relationship.
2. Discuss the dynamics of a therapeutic nurse–client relationship.
3. Discuss the importance of self-awareness in the nurse–client relationship.
4. Identify goals of the nurse–client relationship.

5. Identify and discuss essential conditions for a therapeutic relationship to occur.
6. Describe the phases of relationship development and the tasks associated with each phase.

The nurse–client relationship is the foundation upon which psychiatric nursing is established. It is a relationship in which both participants must recognize each other as unique and important human beings. It is also a relationship in which mutual learning occurs. Peplau (1991) states:

> Shall a nurse do things *for* a patient or can participant relationships be emphasized so that a nurse comes to do things *with* a patient as her share of an agenda of work to be accomplished in reaching a goal—health. It is likely that the nursing process is educative and therapeutic when nurse and patient can come to know and to respect each other, as persons who are alike, and yet, different, as persons who share in the solution of problems. (p. 9.)

This chapter examines the role of the psychiatric nurse and the use of self as the therapeutic tool in the nursing of clients with emotional illness. Phases of the therapeutic relationship are explored and conditions essential to the development of a therapeutic relationship are discussed. The importance of values clarification in the development of self-awareness is emphasized.

CORE CONCEPT

Therapeutic Relationship
An interaction between two people (usually a caregiver and a care receiver) in which input from both participants contributes to a climate of healing, growth promotion, and/or illness prevention.

ROLE OF THE PSYCHIATRIC NURSE

What is a nurse? Undoubtedly, this question would elicit as many different answers as the number of people to whom it was presented. Nursing as a *concept* has probably existed since the beginning of the civilized world, with the provision of "care" to the ill or infirm by anyone in the environment who took the time to administer to those in need. However, the emergence of nursing as a *profession* only began in the late 1800s with the graduation of Linda Richards from the New England Hospital for Women and Children in Boston upon achievement of the diploma in nursing. Since that time, the nurse's role has evolved from that of custodial caregiver and physician's handmaiden to recognition as a unique, independent member of the professional healthcare team.

Peplau (1991) has identified several subroles within the role of the nurse:

1. **The Stranger.** A nurse is at first a stranger to the client. The client is also a stranger to the nurse. Peplau (1991) states:

> Respect and positive interest accorded a stranger is at first nonpersonal and includes the same ordinary

courtesies that are accorded to a new guest who has been brought into any situation. This principle implies: (1) accepting the patient as he is; (2) treating the patient as an emotionally able stranger and relating to him on this basis until evidence shows him to be otherwise. (p. 44)

2. **The Resource Person.** According to Peplau, "a resource person provides specific answers to questions usually formulated with relation to a larger problem" (p. 47). In the role of resource person, the nurse explains, in language that the client can understand, information related to the client's health care.

3. **The Teacher.** In this subrole, the nurse identifies learning needs and provides information required by the client or family to improve the health situation.

4. **The Leader.** According to Peplau, "democratic leadership in nursing situations implies that the patient will be permitted to be an active participant in designing nursing plans for him" (p. 49). Autocratic leadership promotes overvaluation of the nurse and clients' substitution of the nurse's goals for their own. Laissez-faire leaders convey a lack of personal interest in the client.

5. **The Surrogate.** Outside of their awareness, clients often perceive nurses as symbols of other individuals. They may view the nurse as a mother figure, a sibling, a former teacher, or another nurse who has provided care in the past. This occurs when a client is placed in a situation that generates feelings similar to ones he or she has experienced previously. Peplau (1991) explains that the nurse–client relationship progresses along a continuum. When a client is acutely ill, he or she may incur the role of infant or child, while the nurse is perceived as the mother surrogate. Peplau (1991) states, "Each nurse has the responsibility for exercising her professional skill in aiding the relationship to move forward on the continuum, so that person to person relations compatible with chronological age levels can develop" (p. 55).

6. **The Counselor.** The nurse uses "interpersonal techniques" to assist clients to learn to adapt to difficulties or changes in life experiences. Peplau states, "Counseling in nursing has to do with helping the patient to remember and to understand fully what is happening to him in the present situation, so that the experience can be integrated with, rather than dissociated from, other experiences in life" (p. 64).

Peplau (1962) believed that the emphasis in psychiatric nursing is on the counseling subrole. How then does this emphasis influence the role of the nurse in the psychiatric setting? Many sources define the *nurse therapist* as having graduate preparation in psychiatric/mental health nursing. He or she has developed skills thro intensive supervised educational experiences to r helpful individual, group, or family therapy.

Peplau suggests that it is essential for the *staff nurse working in psychiatry* to have a general knowledge of basic counseling techniques. A therapeutic or "helping" relationship is established through use of these interpersonal techniques and is based on a knowledge of theories of personality development and human behavior.

Sullivan (1953) believed that emotional problems stem from difficulties with interpersonal relationships. Interpersonal theorists, such as Peplau and Sullivan, emphasize the importance of relationship development in the provision of emotional care. Through establishment of a satisfactory nurse–client relationship, individuals learn to generalize the ability to achieve satisfactory interpersonal relationships to other aspects of their lives.

DYNAMICS OF A THERAPEUTIC NURSE–CLIENT RELATIONSHIP

Travelbee (1971), who expanded on Peplau's theory of interpersonal relations in nursing, has stated that it is only when each individual in the interaction perceives the other as a unique human being that a relationship is possible. She refers not to a nurse–client relationship, but rather to a human-to-human relationship, which she describes as a "mutually significant experience." That is, both the nurse and the recipient of care have needs met when each views the other as a unique human being, not as "an illness," as "a room number," or as "all nurses" in general.

Therapeutic relationships are goal oriented. Ideally, the nurse and client decide together what the goal of the relationship will be. Most often, the goal is directed at learning and growth promotion, in an effort to bring about some type of change in the client's life. In general, the goal of a therapeutic relationship may be based on a problem-solving model.

Example:

Goal
The client will demonstrate more adaptive coping strategies for dealing with (specific life situation).

Interventions

1. Identify what is troubling the client at the present time.
2. Encourage the client to discuss changes he or she would like to make.
3. Discuss with the client which changes are possible and which are not possible.
4. Have the client explore feelings about aspects that cannot be changed and alternative ways of coping more adaptively.
5. Discuss alternative strategies for creating changes the client desires to make.

6. Weigh the benefits and consequences of each alternative.
7. Assist the client to select an alternative.
8. Encourage the client to implement the change.
9. Provide positive feedback for the client's attempts to create change.
10. Assist the client to evaluate outcomes of the change and make modifications as required.

Therapeutic Use of Self

Travelbee (1971) described the instrument for delivery of the process of interpersonal nursing as the *therapeutic use of self*, which she defined as "the ability to use one's personality consciously and in full awareness in an attempt to establish relatedness and to structure nursing interventions."

Use of the self in a therapeutic manner requires that the nurse have a great deal of self-awareness and self-understanding; that he or she has arrived at a philosophical belief about life, death, and the overall human condition. The nurse must understand that the ability and extent to which one can effectively help others in time of need is strongly influenced by this internal value system—a combination of intellect and emotions.

Gaining Self-Awareness

Values Clarification

Knowing and understanding oneself enhances the ability to form satisfactory interpersonal relationships. Self-awareness requires that an individual recognize and accept what he or she values and learn to accept the uniqueness and differences in others. This concept is important in everyday life and in the nursing profession in general; but it is *essential* in psychiatric nursing.

An individual's value system is established very early in life and has its foundations in the value system held by the primary caregivers. It is culturally oriented; it may change many times over the course of a lifetime; and it consists of beliefs, attitudes, and values. Values clarification is one process by which an individual may gain self-awareness.

Beliefs. A **belief** is an idea that one holds to be true, and it can take any of several forms:

1. *Rational beliefs.* Ideas for which objective evidence exists to substantiate its truth.

Example:

Alcoholism is a disease.

2. *Irrational beliefs.* Ideas that an individual holds as true despite the existence of objective contradictory evidence. Delusions can be a form of irrational beliefs.

Example:

Once an alcoholic has been through detox and rehab, he or she can drink socially if desired.

3. *Faith (sometimes called "blind beliefs").* An ideal that an individual holds as true for which no objective evidence exists.

Example:

Belief in a higher power can help an alcoholic stop drinking.

4. *Stereotype.* A socially shared belief that describes a concept in an oversimplified or undifferentiated matter.

Example:

All alcoholics are skid-row bums.

Attitudes. An **attitude** is a frame of reference around which an individual organizes knowledge about his or her world. An attitude also has an emotional component. It can be a prejudgment and may be selective and biased. Attitudes fulfill the need to find meaning in life and to provide clarity and consistency for the individual. The prevailing stigma attached to mental illness is an example of a negative attitude. An associated belief might be that "all people with mental illness are dangerous."

Values. **Values** are abstract standards, positive or negative, that represent an individual's ideal mode of conduct and ideal goals. Some examples of ideal mode of conduct include seeking truth and beauty; being clean and orderly; and behaving with sincerity, justice, reason, compassion, humility, respect, honor, and loyalty. Examples of ideal goals are security, happiness, freedom, equality, ecstasy, fame, and power.

Values differ from attitudes and beliefs in that they are action oriented or action producing. One may hold many attitudes and beliefs without behaving in a way that shows they hold those attitudes and beliefs. For example, a nurse may believe that all clients have the right to be told the truth about their diagnosis; however, he or she may not always act on the belief and tell all clients the complete truth about their condition. Only when the belief is acted on does it become a value.

Attitudes and beliefs flow out of one's set of values. An individual may have thousands of beliefs and hundreds of attitudes, but his or her values probably only number in the dozens. Values may be viewed as a kind of core concept or basic standards that determine one's attitudes and beliefs, and ultimately, one's behavior. Raths, Merril, and Simon (1966) identified a seven-step process of valuing that can be used to help clarify personal values. This process is presented in Table 7–1. The process can be used by applying these seven steps to an attitude or belief that one holds. When an attitude or belief has met each of the seven criteria, it can be considered a value.

The Johari Window

The self arises out of self-appraisal and the appraisal of others and represents each individual's unique pattern of values, attitudes, beliefs, behaviors, emotions, and needs. Self-awareness is the recognition of these aspects and understanding about their impact on the self and others. The Johari Window is a representation of the self and a tool that can be used to increase self-awareness (Luft, 1970). The Johari Window is presented in Figure 7–1 and is divided into four quadrants.

The Open or Public Self

The upper left quadrant of the window represents the part of the self that is public; that is, aspects of the self about which both the individual and others are aware.

TABLE 7–1	The Process of Values Clarification		
Level of Operations	**Category**	**Criteria**	**Explanation**
Cognitive	Choosing	1. Freely 2. From alternatives. 3. After careful consideration of the consequences	"This value is mine. No one forced me to choose it. I understand and accept the consequences of holding this value."
Emotional	Prizing	4. Satisfied; pleased with the choice 5. Making public affirmation of the choice, if necessary	"I am proud that I hold this value, and I am willing to tell others about it."
Behavioral	Acting	6. Taking action to demonstrate the value behaviorally 7. Demonstrating this pattern of behavior consistently and repeatedly	The value is reflected in the individual's behavior for as long as he or she holds it.

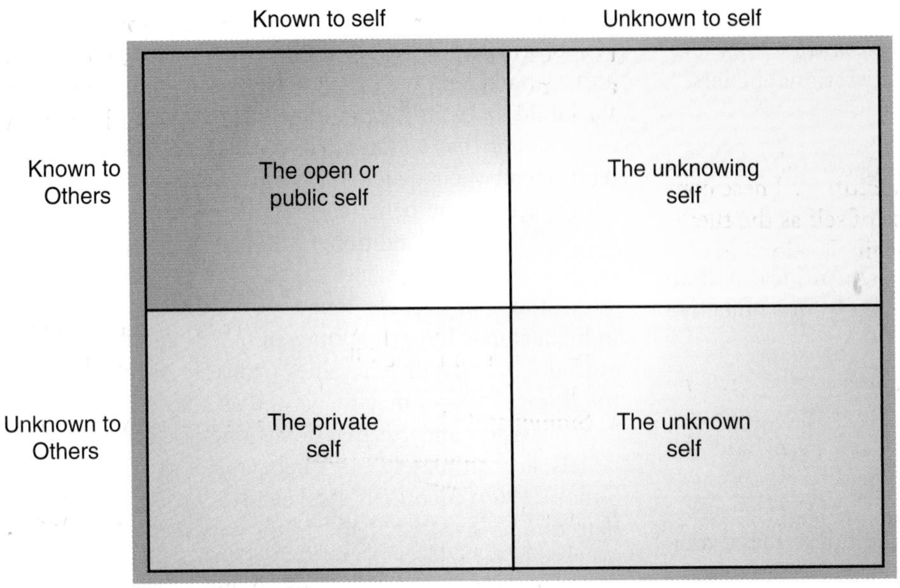

FIGURE 7–1 The Johari Window. (From Luft, J: *Group Processes: An Introduction to Group Dynamics.* National Press Books, Palo Alto, CA, 1970.)

Example:

Susan, a nurse who is the adult child of an alcoholic has strong feelings about helping alcoholics to achieve sobriety. She volunteers her time to be a support person on call to help recovering alcoholics. She is aware of her feelings and her desire to help others. Members of the Alcoholics Anonymous group in which she volunteers her time are also aware of Susan's feelings and they feel comfortable calling her when they need help refraining from drinking.

The Unknowing Self

The upper right (blind) quadrant of the window represents the part of the self that is known to others but remains hidden from the awareness of the individual.

Example:

When Susan takes care of patients in detox, she does so without emotion, tending to the technical aspects of the task in a way that the clients perceive as cold and judgmental. She is unaware that she comes across to the clients in this way.

The Private Self

The lower left quadrant of the window represents the part of the self that is known to the individual, but which the individual deliberately and consciously conceals from others.

Example:

Susan would prefer not to take care of the clients in detox because doing so provokes painful memories from her childhood. However, because she does not want the other staff members to know about these feelings, she volunteers to take care of the detox clients whenever they are assigned to her unit.

The Unknown Self

The lower right quadrant of the window represents the part of the self that is unknown to both the individual and to others.

Example:

Susan felt very powerless as a child growing up with an alcoholic father. She seldom knew in what condition she would find her father or what his behavior would be. She learned over the years to find small ways to maintain control over her life situation, and left home as soon as she graduated from high school. The need to stay in control has always been very important to Susan, and she is unaware that working with recovering alcoholics helps to fulfill this need in her. The people she is helping are also unaware that Susan is satisfying an unfulfilled personal need as she provides them with assistance.

The goal of increasing self-awareness by using the Johari Window is to increase the size of the quadrant that represents the open or public self. The individual who is open to self and others has the ability to be spontaneous and to share emotions and experiences with others. This individual also has a greater understanding of personal behavior and of others' responses to him or her. Increased self-awareness allows an individual to interact with others comfortably, to accept the differences in others, and to observe each person's right to respect and dignity.

CONDITIONS ESSENTIAL TO DEVELOPMENT OF A THERAPEUTIC RELATIONSHIP

Several characteristics that enhance the achievement of a therapeutic relationship have been identified. These concepts are highly significant to the use of self as the therapeutic tool in interpersonal relationship development.

✓ Rapport

Getting acquainted and establishing **rapport** is the primary task in relationship development. Rapport implies special feelings on the part of both the client and the nurse based on acceptance, warmth, friendliness, common interest, a sense of trust, and a nonjudgmental attitude. Establishing rapport may be accomplished by discussing non-health-related topics. Travelbee (1971) states:

> [To establish rapport] is to create a sense of harmony based on knowledge and appreciation of each individual's uniqueness. It is the ability to be still and experience the other as a human being—to appreciate the unfolding of each personality one to the other. The ability to truly care for and about others is the core of rapport.

✓ Trust

To trust another, one must feel confidence in that person's presence, reliability, integrity, veracity, and sincere desire to provide assistance when requested. As previously discussed, trust is the initial developmental task described by Erikson. When this task has not been achieved, this component of relationship development becomes more difficult. That is not to say that trust cannot be established, but only that additional time and patience may be required on the part of the nurse.

CLINICAL PEARL

The nurse must convey an aura of trustworthiness, which requires that he or she possess a sense of self-confidence. Confidence in the self is derived out of knowledge gained through achievement of personal and professional goals, as well as the ability to integrate these roles and to function as a unified whole.

Trust cannot be presumed; it must be earned. Trustworthiness is demonstrated through nursing interventions that convey a sense of warmth and caring to the client. These interventions are initiated simply and concretely and directed toward activities that address the client's basic needs for physiological and psychological safety and security. Many psychiatric clients experience **concrete thinking**, which focuses their thought processes on specifics rather than generalities, and immediate issues rather than eventual outcomes. Examples of nursing interventions that would promote trust in an individual who is thinking concretely include the following:

- Providing a blanket when the client is cold
- Providing food when the client is hungry
- Keeping promises
- Being honest (e.g., saying "I don't know the answer to your question, but I'll try to find out") and then following through
- Simply and clearly providing reasons for certain policies, procedures, and rules
- Providing a written, structured schedule of activities
- Attending activities with the client if he or she is reluctant to go alone
- Being consistent in adhering to unit guidelines
- Taking the client's preferences, requests, and opinions into consideration when possible in decisions concerning his or her care
- Ensuring **confidentiality**; providing reassurance that what is discussed will not be repeated outside the boundaries of the healthcare team

Trust is the basis of a therapeutic relationship. The nurse working in psychiatry must perfect the skills that foster the development of trust. Trust must be established in order for the nurse–client relationship to progress beyond the superficial level of tending to the client's immediate needs.

✓ Respect

To show respect is to believe in the dignity and worth of an individual regardless of his or her unacceptable behavior. Rogers (1951) called this **unconditional positive regard**. The attitude is nonjudgmental, and the respect is unconditional in that it does not depend on the behavior of the client to meet certain standards. The nurse, in fact, may not approve of the client's lifestyle or pattern of behaving. With unconditional positive regard, however, the client is accepted and respected for no other reason than that he or she is considered to be a worthwhile and unique human being.

Many psychiatric clients have very little self-respect owing to the fact that, because of their behavior, they were frequently rejected by others in the past. Recognition that they are being accepted and respected as unique individuals on an unconditional basis can serve to elevate feelings of self-worth and self-respect. The nurse can convey an attitude of respect with the following interventions:

- Calling the client by name (and title, if the client prefers)
- Spending time with the client

- Allowing for sufficient time to answer the client's questions and concerns
- Promoting an atmosphere of privacy during therapeutic interactions with the client or when the client may be undergoing physical examination or therapy
- Always being open and honest with the client, even when the truth may be difficult to discuss
- Taking the client's ideas, preferences, and opinions into considerations when planning care
- Striving to understand the motivation behind the client's behavior, regardless of how unacceptable it may seem

Genuineness

The concept of **genuineness** refers to the nurse's ability to be open, honest, and "real" in interactions with the client. To be "real" is to be aware of what one is experiencing internally and to express this awareness in the therapeutic relationship. When one is genuine, there is *congruence* between what is felt and what is being expressed (Raskin & Rogers, 2005). The nurse who possesses the quality of genuineness responds to the client with truth and honesty, rather than with responses he or she may consider more "professional" or ones that merely reflect the "nursing role."

Genuineness may call for a degree of *self-disclosure* on the part of the nurse. This is not to say that the nurse must disclose to the client *everything* he or she is feeling or *all* personal experiences that may relate to what the client is going through. Indeed, care must be taken when using self-disclosure, to avoid reversing the roles of nurse and client.

When the nurse uses self-disclosure, a quality of "humanness" is revealed to the client, creating a role for the client to model in similar situations. The client may then feel more comfortable revealing personal information to the nurse.

Most individuals have an uncanny ability to detect other peoples' artificiality. When the nurse does not bring the quality of genuineness to the relationship, a reality base for trust cannot be established. These qualities are essential if the actualizing potential of the client is to be released and for change and growth to occur (Raskin & Rogers, 2005).

Empathy

Empathy is the ability to see beyond outward behavior and to understand the situation from the client's point of view. With empathy, the nurse can accurately perceive and comprehend the meaning and relevance of the client's thoughts and feelings. The nurse must also be able to communicate this perception to the client by attempting to translate words and behaviors into feelings.

It is not uncommon for the concept of empathy to be confused with that of **sympathy**. The major difference is that with *empathy* the nurse "accurately perceives or understands" what the client is feeling and encourages the client to explore these feelings. With *sympathy* the nurse actually "shares" what the client is feeling, and experiences a need to alleviate distress. Schuster (2000) states:

> Empathy means that you remain emotionally separate from the other person, even though you can see the patient's viewpoint clearly. This is different from sympathy. Sympathy implies taking on the other's needs and problems as if they were your own and becoming emotionally involved to the point of losing your objectivity. To empathize rather then sympathize, you must show feelings but not get caught up in feelings or overly identify with the patient's and family's concerns. (p. 102)

Empathy is considered to be one of the most important characteristics of a therapeutic relationship. Accurate empathetic perceptions on the part of the nurse assist the client to identify feelings that may have been suppressed or denied. Positive emotions are generated as the client realizes that he or she is truly understood by another. As the feelings surface and are explored, the client learns aspects about self of which he or she may have been unaware. This contributes to the process of personal identification and the promotion of positive self-concept.

With empathy, while understanding the client's thoughts and feelings, the nurse is able to maintain sufficient objectivity to allow the client to achieve problem resolution with minimal assistance. With sympathy, the nurse actually feels what the client is feeling, objectivity is lost, and the nurse may become focused on relief of personal distress rather than on helping the client resolve the problem at hand. The following is an example of an empathetic and sympathetic response to the same situation.

Situation: **B.J.** is a client on the psychiatric unit with a diagnosis of major depressive disorder. She is 5'5" tall and weighs 295 lbs. B.J. has been overweight all her life. She is single, has no close friends, and has never had an intimate relationship with another person. It is her first day on the unit, and she is refusing to come out of her room. When she appeared for lunch in the dining room following admission, she was embarrassed when several of the other clients laughed out loud and called her "fatso."

Sympathetic response: Nurse: "I can certainly identify with what you are feeling. I've been overweight most of my life, too. I just get so angry when people act like that. They are so insensitive! It's just so typical of skinny people to act that way. You have a right to want to stay away from them. We'll just see how loud they laugh when *you* get to choose what movie is shown on the unit after dinner tonight."

Empathetic response: Nurse: "You feel angry and embarrassed by what happened at lunch today." As tears fill BJ's eyes, the nurse encourages her to cry if she feels like it and to express her anger at the situation. She stays with BJ but does not dwell on her *own* feelings about what happened. Instead she focuses on BJ and what the client perceives are her most immediate needs at this time.

PHASES OF A THERAPEUTIC NURSE–CLIENT RELATIONSHIP

Psychiatric nurses use interpersonal relationship development as the primary intervention with clients in various psychiatric/mental health settings. This is congruent with Peplau's (1962) identification of *counseling* as the major subrole of nursing in psychiatry. Sullivan (1953), from whom Peplau patterned her own interpersonal theory of nursing, strongly believed that many emotional problems were closely related to difficulties with interpersonal relationships. With this concept in mind, this role of the nurse in psychiatry becomes especially meaningful and purposeful. It becomes an integral part of the total therapeutic regimen.

The therapeutic interpersonal relationship is the means by which the nursing process is implemented. Through the relationship, problems are identified and resolution is sought. Tasks of the relationship have been categorized into four phases: the preinteraction phase, the orientation (introductory) phase, the working phase, and the termination phase. Although each phase is presented as specific and distinct from the others, there may be some overlapping of tasks, particularly when the interaction is limited. The major nursing goals during each phase of the nurse–client relationship are listed in Table 7–2.

The Preinteraction Phase

The preinteraction phase involves preparation for the first encounter with the client. Tasks include the following:

1. Obtaining available information about the client from his or her chart, significant others, or other health team members. From this information, the initial assessment is begun. This initial information may also allow the nurse to become aware of personal responses to knowledge about the client.
2. Examining one's feelings, fears, and anxieties about working with a particular client. For example, the nurse may have been reared in an alcoholic family and have ambivalent feelings about caring for a client who is alcohol dependent. All individuals bring attitudes and feelings from prior experiences to the clinical setting. The nurse needs to be aware of how these preconceptions may affect his or her ability to care for individual clients.

The Orientation (Introductory) Phase

During the orientation phase, the nurse and client become acquainted. Tasks include:

1. Creating an environment for the establishment of trust and rapport.
2. Establishing a contract for intervention that details the expectations and responsibilities of both nurse and client.
3. Gathering assessment information to build a strong client data base.
4. Identifying the client's strengths and limitations.
5. Formulating nursing diagnoses.
6. Setting goals that are mutually agreeable to the nurse and client.
7. Developing a plan of action that is realistic for meeting the established goals.
8. Exploring feelings of both the client and nurse in terms of the introductory phase. Introductions are often uncomfortable, and the participants may experience some anxiety until a degree of rapport has been established.

Interactions may remain on a superficial level until anxiety subsides. Several interactions may be required to fulfill the tasks associated with this phase.

The Working Phase

The therapeutic work of the relationship is accomplished during this phase. Tasks include:

1. Maintaining the trust and rapport that was established during the orientation phase.
2. Promoting the client's insight and perception of reality.

TABLE 7–2	Phases of Relationship Development and Major Nursing Goals	
Phase	**Goals**
1. Preinteraction ✓	Explore self-perceptions
2. Orientation (introductory)	Establish trust
	Formulate contract for intervention
3. Working counter transference &	Promote client change
4. Termination transference	Evaluate goal attainment
	Ensure therapeutic closure

3. Problem solving using the model presented earlier in this chapter.
4. Overcoming resistance behaviors on the part of the client as the level of anxiety rises in response to discussion of painful issues.
5. Continuously evaluating progress toward goal attainment.

Transference and Countertransference

Transference and countertransference are common phenomena that often arise during the course of a therapeutic relationship.

Transference

Transference occurs when the client unconsciously displaces (or "transfers") to the nurse feelings formed toward a person from the past (Sadock & Sadock, 2007). These feelings toward the nurse may be triggered by something about the nurse's appearance or personality characteristics that remind the client of the person. Transference can interfere with the therapeutic interaction when the feelings being expressed include anger and hostility. Anger toward the nurse can be manifested by uncooperativeness and resistance to the therapy.

Transference can also take the form of overwhelming affection for the nurse or excessive dependency on the nurse. The nurse is overvalued and the client forms unrealistic expectations of the nurse. When the nurse is unable to fulfill those expectations or meet the excessive dependency needs, the client becomes angry and hostile.

Interventions for Transference. Hilz (2008) states,

In cases of transference, the relationship does not usually need to be terminated, except when the transference poses a serious barrier to therapy or safety. The nurse should work with the patient in sorting out the past from the present, and assist the patient into identifying the transference and reassign a new and more appropriate meaning to the current nurse-patient relationship. The goal is to guide the patient to independence by teaching them to assume responsibility for their own behaviors, feelings, and thoughts, and to assign the correct meanings to the relationships based on present circumstances instead of the past.

Countertransference

Countertransference refers to the nurse's behavioral and emotional response to the client. These responses may be related to unresolved feelings toward significant others from the nurse's past, or they may be generated in response to transference feelings on the part of the client. It is not easy to refrain from becoming angry when the client is consistently antagonistic, to feel flattered when showered with affection and attention by the client, or even to feel quite powerful when the client exhibits excessive dependency on the nurse. These feelings can interfere with the therapeutic relationship when they initiate the following types of behaviors:

● The nurse overidentifies with the client's feelings, as they remind him or her of problems from the nurse's past or present.
● The nurse and client develop a social or personal relationship.
● The nurse begins to give advice or attempts to "rescue" the client.
● The nurse encourages and promotes the client's dependence.
● The nurse's anger engenders feelings of disgust toward the client.
● The nurse feels anxious and uneasy in the presence of the client.
● The nurse is bored and apathetic in sessions with the client.
● The nurse has difficulty setting limits on the client's behavior.
● The nurse defends the client's behavior to other staff members.

The nurse may be completely unaware or only minimally aware of the counter-transference as it is occurring (Hilz, 2008).

Interventions for Countertransference. Hilz (2008) states:

A relationship usually should not be terminated in the presence of countertransference. Rather, the nurse or staff member experiencing the countertransference should be supportively assisted by other staff members to identify his or her feelings and behaviors and recognize the occurrence of the phenomenon. It may be helpful to have evaluative sessions with the nurse after his or her encounter with the patient, in which both the nurse and other staff members (who are observing the interactions) discuss and compare the exhibited behaviors in the relationship.

Termination Phase

Termination of the relationship may occur for a variety of reasons: the mutually agreed-on goals may have been reached, the client may be discharged from the hospital, or in the case of a student nurse, it may be the end of a clinical rotation. Termination can be a difficult phase for both the client and nurse. Tasks include the following:

1. Bringing a therapeutic conclusion to the relationship. This occurs when:
   a. Progress has been made toward attainment of mutually set goals.
   b. A plan for continuing care or for assistance during stressful life experiences is mutually established by the nurse and client.

c. Feelings about termination of the relationship are recognized and explored. Both the nurse and client may experience feelings of sadness and loss. The nurse should share his or her feelings with the client. Through these interactions, the client learns that it is acceptable to have these kinds of feelings at a time of separation. Through this knowledge, the client experiences growth during the process of termination.

NOTE: When the client feels sadness and loss, behaviors to delay termination may become evident. If the nurse experiences the same feelings, he or she may allow the client's behaviors to delay termination. For therapeutic closure, the nurse must establish the reality of the separation and resist being manipulated into repeated delays by the client.

BOUNDARIES IN THE NURSE–CLIENT RELATIONSHIP

A boundary indicates a border or a limit. It determines the extent of acceptable limits. Many types of boundaries exist. Examples include the following:

● **Material boundaries.** These are physical property that can be seen, such as fences that border land.
● **Social boundaries.** These are established within a culture and define how individuals are expected to behave in social situations
● **Personal boundaries.** These are boundaries that individuals define for themselves. These include physical distance boundaries, or just how close individuals will allow others to invade their physical space; and emotional boundaries, or how much individuals choose to disclose of their most private and intimate selves to others.
● **Professional boundaries.** These boundaries limit and outline expectations for appropriate professional relationships with clients. They separate therapeutic behavior from any other behavior which, well intentioned or not, could lessen the benefit of care to clients (College and Association of Registered Nurses of Alberta [CARNA], 2005).

Concerns related to professional boundaries commonly refer to the following types of issues:

● **Self-disclosure.** Self-disclosure on the part of the nurse may be appropriate when it is judged that the information may therapeutically benefit the client. It should never be undertaken for the purpose of meeting the nurse's needs.
● **Gift-giving.** Individuals who are receiving care often feel indebted toward healthcare providers. And, indeed, gift giving may be part of the therapeutic process for people who receive care (CARNA, 2005).

Cultural belief and values may also enter into the decision of whether to accept a gift from a client. In some cultures, failure to do so would be interpreted as an insult. Accepting financial gifts is never appropriate, but in some instances nurses may be permitted to suggest instead a donation to a charity of the client's choice. If acceptance of a small gift of gratitude is deemed appropriate, the nurse may choose to share it with other staff members who have been involved in the client's care. In all instances, nurses should exercise professional judgment when deciding whether to accept a gift from a client. Attention should be given to what the gift-giving means to the client, as well as to institutional policy, the ANA *Code of Ethics for Nurses*, and the ANA *Scope and Standards of Practice*.

● **Touch.** Nursing by its very nature involves touching clients. Touching is required to perform the many therapeutic procedures involved in the physical care of clients. Caring touch is the touching of clients when there is no physical need (Registered Nurses Association of British Columbia [RNABC], 2003). Caring touch often provides comfort or encouragement and, when it is used appropriately, it can have a therapeutic effect on the client. However, certain vulnerable clients may misinterpret the meaning of touch. Certain cultures, such as Native Americans and Asian Americans, are often uncomfortable with touch. The nurse must be sensitive to these cultural nuances and aware when touch is crossing a personal boundary. In addition, clients who are experiencing high levels of anxiety or suspicious or psychotic behaviors may interpret touch as aggressive. These are times when touch should be avoided or considered with extreme caution.
● **Friendship or romantic association.** When a nurse is acquainted with a client, the relationship must move from one of a personal nature to professional. If the nurse is unable to accomplish this separation, he or she should withdraw from the nurse–client relationship. Likewise, nurses must guard against personal relationships developing as a result of the nurse–client relationship. Romantic, sexual, or similar personal relationships are never appropriate between nurse and client.

Certain warning signs exist that indicate that professional boundaries of the nurse–client relationship may be in jeopardy. Some of these include the following (Coltrane & Pugh, 1978):

● Favoring one client's care over another's
● Keeping secrets with a client
● Changing dress style for working with a particular client
● Swapping client assignments to care for a particular client
● Giving special attention or treatment to one client over others

- Spending free time with a client
- Frequently thinking about the client when away from work
- Sharing personal information or work concerns with the client
- Receiving of gifts or continued contact/communication with the client after discharge

Boundary crossings can threaten the integrity of the nurse–client relationship. Nurses must gain self-awareness and insight to be able to recognize when professional integrity is being compromised. Peternelj-Taylor and Yonge (2003) state:

> The nursing profession needs nurses who have the ability to make decisions about boundaries based on the best interests of the clients in their care. This requires nurses to reflect on their knowledge and experiences, on how they think and how they feel, and not simply to buy blindly into a framework that says, "do this," "don't do that." (p. 65)

SUMMARY AND KEY POINTS

- Nurses who work in the psychiatric/mental health field use special skills, or "interpersonal techniques," to assist clients in adapting to difficulties or changes in life experiences.
- Therapeutic nurse–client relationships are goal oriented, and the problem-solving model is used to try to bring about some type of change in the client's life.
- The instrument for delivery of the process of interpersonal nursing is the therapeutic use of self, which requires that the nurse possess a strong sense of self-awareness and self-understanding.
- Hildegard Peplau identified six subroles within the role of nurse: stranger, resource person, teacher, leader, surrogate, and counselor.
- Characteristics that enhance the achievement of a therapeutic relationship include rapport, trust, respect, genuineness, and empathy.
- Phases of a therapeutic nurse–client relationship include the preinteraction phase, the orientation (introductory) phase, the working phase, and the termination phase.
- Transference occurs when the client unconsciously displaces (or "transfers") to the nurse feelings formed toward a person from the past.
- Countertransference refers to the nurse's behavioral and emotional response to the client. These responses may be related to unresolved feelings toward significant others from the nurse's past, or they may be generated in response to transference feelings on the part of the client.
- Types of boundaries include material, social, personal, and professional.
- Concerns associated with professional boundaries include self-disclosure, gift-giving, touch, and developing a friendship or romantic association.
- Boundary crossings can threaten the integrity of the nurse–client relationship.

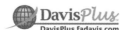 **DavisPlus** For additional clinical tools and study aids, visit DavisPlus. DavisPlus.fadavis.com

REVIEW QUESTIONS

Self-Examination/Learning Exercise

Test your knowledge of therapeutic nurse–client relationships by answering the following questions:

1. Name the six subroles of nursing identified by Peplau. *Stranger, Resource Person, teacher, leader Surrogate, Counselor*
2. Which subrole is emphasized in psychiatric nursing? *The Counselor*
3. Why is relationship development so important in the provision of emotional care? *It is through establishment of a satisfactory relationship that individuals learn to generalize the ability to achieve satisfactory interpersonal relationships to other*
4. In general, what is the goal of a therapeutic relationship? What method is recommended for intervention? *most often the goal is directed at learning & growth promotion, aspects of their lives*
5. What is the instrument for delivery of the process of interpersonal nursing? *therapeutic use of self*
6. Several characteristics that enhance the achievement of a therapeutic relationship have been identified. Match the therapeutic concept with the corresponding definition.

___ *d* 1. Rapport   a. The feeling of confidence in another person's presence, reliability, integrity, and desire to provide assistance.

___ *a* 2. Trust   b. Congruence between what is felt and what is being expressed.

___ *e* 3. Respect   c. The ability to see beyond outward behavior and to understand the situation from the client's point of view.

___ *b* 4. Genuineness   d. Special feelings between two people based on acceptance, warmth, friendliness, and shared common interest.

___ *c* 5. Empathy   e. Unconditional acceptance of an individual as a worthwhile and unique human being.

7. Match the actions listed on the right to the appropriate phase of nurse–client relationship development on the left.

___ *c* 1. Preinteraction Phase   a. Kim tells Nurse Jones she wants to learn more adaptive ways to handle her anger. Together, they set some goals.

___ *a* 2. Orientation (Introductory) Phase   b. The goals of therapy have been met, but Kim cries and says she has to keep coming to therapy in order to be able to handle her anger appropriately.

___ *d* 3. Working Phase   c. Nurse Jones reads Kim's previous medical records. She explores her feelings about working with a woman who has abused her child.

___ *b* 4. Termination Phase   d. Nurse Jones helps Kim practice various techniques to control her angry outbursts. She gives Kim positive feedback for attempting to improve maladaptive behaviors.

8. Nurse Mary has been providing care for Tom during his hospital stay. On Tom's day of discharge, his wife brings a bouquet of flowers and box of chocolates to his room. He presents these gifts to Nurse Mary saying, "Thank you for taking care of me." What is a correct response by the nurse?
   a. "I don't accept gifts from patients."
   b. "Thank you so much! It is so nice to be appreciated."
   c. "Thank you. I will share these with the rest of the staff."
   d. "Hospital policy forbids me to accept gifts from patients."
9. Nancy says to the nurse, "I worked as a secretary to put my husband through college, and as soon as he graduated, he left me. I hate him! I hate all men!" Which is an empathetic response by the nurse?
   a. "You are very angry now. This is a normal response to your loss."
   b. "I know what you mean. Men can be very insensitive."

  c. "I understand completely. My husband divorced me, too."
  d. "You are depressed now, but you will feel better in time."

10. Which of the following behaviors suggests a possible breach of professional boundaries?

  a. The nurse repeatedly requests to be assigned to a specific client.
  b. The nurse shares the details of her divorce with the client.
  c. The nurse makes arrangements to meet the client outside of the therapeutic environment.
  d. C only.
  e. A, B, and C

REFERENCES

College and Association of Registered Nurses of Alberta (CARNA). (2005). *Professional boundaries for registered nurses: Guidelines for the nurse–client relationship.* Edmonton, AB: CARNA.

Hilz, L.M. (2008). Transference and countertransference. *Kathi's mental health review.* Retrieved June 21, 2008 from http://www.toddlertime.com/mh/terms/countertransference-transference-3.htm

Peplau, H.E. (1991). *Interpersonal relations in nursing.* New York: Springer.

Peternelj-Taylor, C.A., & Yonge, O. (2003). Exploring boundaries in the nurse–client relationship: Professional roles and responsibilities. *Perspectives in Psychiatric Care, 39*(2), 55–66.

Raskin, N.J., & Rogers, C.R. (2005). Person-centered therapy. In R.J. Corsini & D. Wedding (Eds.), *Current psychotherapies* (7th ed.). Belmont, CA: Wadsworth.

Registered Nurses' Association of British Columbia (RNABC). (2003). *Nurse–client Relationships.* Vancouver, BC: RNABC.

Sadock, B.J., & Sadock, V. A. (2007). *Synopsis of psychiatry: Behavioral sciences/clinical psychiatry* (10th ed.). Philadelphia: Lippincott Williams & Wilkins.

Schuster, P.M. (2000). *Communication: The key to the therapeutic relationship.* Philadelphia: F.A. Davis.

CLASSICAL REFERENCES

Coltrane, F., & Pugh, C. (1978). Danger signals in staff/patient relationships. *Journal of Psychiatric Nursing & Mental Health Services, 16*(6), 34–36.

Luft, J. (1970). *Group processes: An introduction to group dynamics.* Palo Alto, CA: National Press Books.

Peplau, H.E. (1962). Interpersonal techniques: The crux of psychiatric nursing. *American Journal of Nursing, 62*(6), 50–54.

Raths, L., Merril, H., & Simon, S. (1966). *Values and teaching.* Columbus, OH: Merrill.

Rogers, C.R. (1951). *Client-centered therapy.* Boston: Houghton Mifflin.

Sullivan, H.S. (1953). *The interpersonal theory of psychiatry.* New York: W.W. Norton.

Travelbee, J. (1971). *Interpersonal aspects of nursing* (2nd ed.). Philadelphia: F.A. Davis.

Example:

Prompt response   "I saw you hit the wall with your fist just now when you hung up the phone after talking to your mother."

Delayed response   "You need to learn some more appropriate ways of dealing with your anger. Last week after group I saw you pounding your fist against the wall."

SUMMARY AND KEY POINTS

● Interpersonal communication is a transaction between the sender and the receiver.
● In all interpersonal transactions, both the sender and receiver bring certain preexisting conditions to the exchange that influences both the intended message and the way in which it is interpreted.
● Examples of these preexisting conditions include one's value system, internalized attitudes and beliefs, culture or religion, social status, gender, background knowledge and experience, age or developmental level, and the type of environment in which the communication takes place.
● Nonverbal expression is a primary communication system in which meaning is assigned to various gestures and patterns of behavior.
● Some components of nonverbal communication include physical appearance and dress, body movement and posture, touch, facial expressions, eye behavior, and vocal cues or paralanguage.
● Meaning of the nonverbal components of communication is culturally determined.
● Therapeutic communication includes verbal and nonverbal techniques that focus on the care receiver's needs and advance the promotion of healing and change.
● Nurses must also be aware of and avoid a number of techniques that are considered to be barriers to effective communication.
● Active listening is described as being attentive to what the client is saying, through both verbal and nonverbal cues. Skills associated with active listening include sitting squarely facing the client, observing an open posture, leaning forward toward the client, establishing eye contact, and being relaxed.
● Process recordings are written reports of verbal interactions with clients. They are used as learning tools for professional development.
● Feedback is a method of communication for helping the client consider a modification of behavior.
● The nurse must be aware of the therapeutic or nontherapeutic value of the communication techniques used with the client because they are the "tools" of psychosocial intervention.

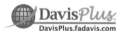 **DavisPlus**   For additional clinical tools and
DavisPlus.fadavis.com   study aids, visit DavisPlus.

REVIEW QUESTIONS

Self-Examination/Learning Exercise

Test your knowledge about the concept of communication by answering the following questions:

1. Describe the transactional model of communication.

2. List eight types of preexisting conditions that can influence the outcome of the communication process.

3. Define *territoriality*. How does it affect communication?

4. Define *density*. How does it affect communication?

5. Identify four types of spatial distance and give an example of each.

6. Identify six components of nonverbal communication that convey special messages and give an example of each.

7. Describe five facilitative skills for active, or attentive, listening that can be identified by the acronym SOLER.

Identify the correct answer in each of the following questions. Provide explanation where requested. Identify the technique used (both therapeutic and nontherapeutic) in all choices given.

8. A client states: "I refuse to shower in this room. I must be very cautious. The FBI has placed a camera in here to monitor my every move." Which of the following is the therapeutic response? What is this technique called?

   a. "That's not true."
   b. "I have a hard time believing that is true."

9. Nancy, a depressed client who has been unkept and untidy for weeks, today comes to group therapy wearing a clean dress, makeup, and having washed and combed her hair. Which of the following responses by the nurse is most appropriate? Give the rationale.

   a. "Nancy, I see you have put on a clean dress and combed your hair."
   b. "Nancy, you look wonderful today!"

10. Dorothy was involved in an automobile accident while under the influence of alcohol. She swerved her car into a tree and narrowly missed hitting a child on a bicycle. She is in the hospital with multiple abrasions and contusions. She is talking about the accident with the nurse. Which of the following statements by the nurse is most appropriate? Identify the therapeutic or nontherapeutic technique in each.

    a. "Now that you know what can happen when you drink and drive, I'm sure you won't let it happen again. I'm sure everything will be okay."
    b. "That was a terrible thing you did. You could have killed that child!"
    c. "Now I guess you'll have to buy a new car. Can you afford that?"
    d. "What made you do such a thing?"
    e. "Tell me how you are feeling about what happened."

11. Judy has been under doctor's care for several weeks undergoing careful dosage tapering for withdrawal from Valium. She has used Valium "to settle my nerves" for the past 15 years. She is getting close to the time of discharge from treatment. She states to the nurse, "I don't know if I will be able to make it without Valium. I'm already starting to feel nervous. I have so many personal problems." Which is the most appropriate response by the nurse? Identify the technique in each.

    a. "Why do you think you have to have drugs to deal with your problems?"
    b. "You'll just have to pull yourself together. Everybody has problems, and everybody doesn't use drugs to deal with them. They just do the best that they can."

c. "I don't want to talk about that now. Look at that sunshine. It's beautiful outside. You and I are going to take a walk!"

d. "Starting today you and I are going to think about some alternative ways for you to deal with those problems—things that you can do to decrease your anxiety without resorting to drugs."

12. Mrs. S. asks the nurse, "Do you think I should tell my husband about my affair with my boss?" Give one therapeutic response and one nontherapeutic response, give your rationale, and identify the technique used in each response.

13. Carol, an adolescent, just returned from group therapy and is crying. She says to the nurse, "All the other kids laughed at me! I try to fit in, but I always seem to say the wrong thing. I've never had a close friend. I guess I never will." Which is the most appropriate response by the nurse? Identify each technique used.

a. "You're feeling pretty down on yourself right now."
b. "Why do you feel this way about yourself?"
c. "What makes you think you will never have any friends?"
d. "The next they laugh at you, you should just get up and leave the room!"
e. "I'm sure they didn't mean to hurt your feelings."
f. "Keep your chin up and hang in there. Your time will come."

REFERENCES

Archer, D. (2006). *Exploring nonverbal communication.* Retrieved June 21, 2008 from http://nonverbal.ucsc.edu/index.html

Givens, D.B. (2006a). The nonverbal dictionary. Center for Nonverbal Studies. Retrieved June 21, 2008 from http://members.aol.com/nonverbal2/diction1.htm

Givens, D.B. (2006b). The nonverbal dictionary. Center for Nonverbal Studies. Retrieved June 21, 2008 from http://members.aol.com/nonverbal3/facialx.htm

Givens, D.B. (2006c). The nonverbal dictionary. Center for Nonverbal Studies. Retrieved June 21, 2008 from http://members.aol.com/nonverbal3/eyecon.htm

Hughey, J.D. (1990). *Speech communication.* Stillwater, OK: Oklahoma State University.

Oak, C. (2004, November 8). Enhancing communication skills. *Insurance Journal Online.* Retrieved June 21, 2008 from http://www.insurancejournal.com

Schuster, P.M. (2000). *Communication: The key to the therapeutic relationship.* Philadelphia: F.A. Davis.

Yates, D. (2006). Communication models. Seton Hall University. Department of Communication. Retrieved June 21, 2008 from http://pirate.shu.edu/~yatesdan/Tutorial.htm

CLASSICAL REFERENCES

Hall, E.T. (1966). *The hidden dimension.* Garden City, NY: Doubleday.

Hays, J.S., & Larson, K.H. (1963). *Interacting with patients.* New York: Macmillan.

Knapp, M.L. (1980). *Essentials of nonverbal communication.* New York: Holt, Rinehart & Winston.

Reece, M., & Whitman, R. (1962). Expressive movements, warmth, and verbal reinforcement. *Journal of Abnormal and Social Psychology, 64,* 234–236.

9
CHAPTER

The Nursing Process in Psychiatric/Mental Health Nursing

CHAPTER OUTLINE

OBJECTIVES

THE NURSING PROCESS

WHY NURSING DIAGNOSIS?

NURSING CASE MANAGEMENT

APPLYING THE NURSING PROCESS IN THE PSYCHIATRIC SETTING

CONCEPT MAPPING

DOCUMENTATION OF THE NURSING PROCESS

SUMMARY AND KEY POINTS

REVIEW QUESTIONS

KEY TERMS

case management
case manager
concept mapping
critical pathways
    of care
Focus Charting®
interdisciplinary
managed care

nursing interventions
    classification (NIC)
nursing outcomes
    classification (NOC)
nursing process
PIE charting
problem-oriented
    recording

CORE CONCEPTS

assessment
evaluation
nursing diagnosis
outcomes

OBJECTIVES

After reading this chapter, the student will be able to:

1. Define *nursing process*.
2. Identify six steps of the nursing process and describe nursing actions associated with each.
3. Describe the benefits of using nursing diagnosis.
4. Discuss the list of nursing diagnoses approved by NANDA International (NANDA-I) for clinical use and testing.
5. Define and discuss the use of case management and critical pathways of care in the clinical setting.
6. Apply the six steps of the nursing process in the care of a client within the psychiatric setting.
7. Document client care that validates use of the nursing process.

Box 9 – 1   (Continued)

2. Drug history and assessment:
   Use of prescribed drugs:

NAME	DOSAGE	PRESCRIBED FOR	RESULTS

   Use of over-the-counter drugs:

NAME	DOSAGE	USED FOR	RESULTS

   Use of street drugs or alcohol:

NAME	AMOUNT USED	HOW OFTEN USED	WHEN LAST USED	EFFECTS PRODUCED

3. Pertinent physical assessments:
   a. Respirations: normal_____ labored_____
      Rate_____ Rhythm_____
   b. Skin: warm_____ dry_____ moist_____ cool_____ clammy_____ pink_____ cyanotic_____
      poor turgor _____ edematous_____
      Evidence of: rash_____ bruising_____ needle tracts_____ hirsutism_____ loss of hair_____ other_____

   c. Musculoskeletal status: weakness_____ tremors_____
      Degree of range of motion (describe limitations)_____

      Pain (describe)_____

      Skeletal deformities (describe)_____
      Coordination (describe limitations)_____
   d. Neurological status:
      History of (check all that apply): seizures_____ (describe method of control)_____

      headaches (describe location and frequency)_____
      fainting spells_____ dizziness _____
      tingling/numbness (describe location)_____
   e. Cardiovascular: B/P_____ Pulse_____
      History of (check all that apply):
      hypertension_____ palpitations_____
      heart murmur_____ chest pain_____
      shortness of breath_____ pain in legs_____
      phlebitis_____ ankle/leg edema_____
      numbness/tingling in extremities_____
      varicose veins_____
   f. Gastrointestinal:
      Usual diet pattern:_____
      Food allergies:_____
      Dentures? Upper_____ Lower_____
      Any problems with chewing or swallowing?_____
      Any recent change in weight?_____
      Any problems with:
      indigestion/heartburn?_____
         relieved by_____
      nausea/vomiting?_____
         relieved by_____
      History of ulcers?_____
      Usual bowel pattern_____
         Constipation?_____ Diarrhea?_____
      Type of self-care assistance provided for either of the above problems_____

(continued)

Box 9 – 1 *(Continued)*

g. Genitourinary/Reproductive:
Usual voiding pattern_____
Urinary hesitancy?_____ Frequency?_____
Nocturia?_____ Pain/burning?_____
Incontinence?_____
Any genital lesions?_____
  Discharge?_____ Odor?_____
History of sexually transmitted disease?_____
  If yes, please explain:_____
  _____

Any concerns about sexuality/sexual activity?_____
_____

Method of birth control used_____
Females:
  Date of last menstrual cycle_____
  Length of cycle_____
  Problems associated with menstruation?_____
  _____

  Breasts: Pain/tenderness?_____
    Swelling?_____ Discharge?_____
    Lumps?_____ Dimpling?_____
  Practice breast self-examination?_____
    Frequency?_____
Males:
  Penile discharge?_____
  Prostate problems?_____

h. Eyes: YES   NO   EXPLAIN
  Glasses?   ____   ____   _____
  Contacts?   ____   ____   _____
  Swelling?   ____   ____   _____
  Discharge?   ____   ____   _____
  Itching?   ____   ____   _____
  Blurring?   ____   ____   _____
  Double vision?   ____   ____   _____

i. Ears   YES   NO   EXPLAIN
  Pain?   ____   ____   _____
  Drainage?   ____   ____   _____
  Difficulty hearing? ____ ____   _____
  Hearing aid?   ____   ____   _____
  Tinnitus?   ____   ____   _____

j. Medication side effects:
  What symptoms is the client experiencing that may be attributed to current medication usage?_____
  _____

k. Altered lab values and possible significance:_____
  _____
  _____

l. Activity/rest patterns:
  Exercise (amount, type, frequency)_____
  _____

  Leisure time activities:_____
  _____

  Patterns of sleep: Number of hours per night_____
    Use of sleep aids?_____
    Pattern of awakening during the night?_____
    _____
    Feel rested upon awakening?_____

m. Personal hygiene/activities of daily living:
  Patterns of self-care: independent_____
  Requires assistance with: mobility_____
    hygiene_____
    toileting_____
    feeding_____
    dressing_____
    other _____

> **Box 9 – 1** *(Continued)*
>
> Statement describing personal hygiene and general appearance_____
> _____
> _____
>
> n. Other pertinent physical assessments:_____
> _____
> _____
>
> VI. Summary of Initial Psychosocial/Physical Assessment:
> Knowledge Deficits Identified:
> Nursing Diagnoses Indicated:

TABLE 9–1 Brief Mental Status Evaluation

Area of Mental Function Evaluated	Evaluation Activity
Orientation to time	"What year is it? What month is it? What day is it? (3 points)
Orientation to place	"Where are you now?" (1 point)
Attention and immediate recall	"Repeat these words now: bell, book, & candle" (3 points)
	"Remember these words and I will ask you to repeat them in a few minutes."
Abstract thinking	"What does this mean: No use crying over spilled milk." (3 points)
Recent memory	"Say the 3 words I asked you to remember earlier." (3 points)
Naming objects	Point to eyeglasses and ask, "What is this?" Repeat with 1 other item (e.g., calendar, watch, pencil). (2 points possible)
Ability to follow simple verbal command	"Tear this piece of paper in half and put it in the trash container." (2 points)
Ability to follow simple written command	Write a command on a piece of paper (e.g., TOUCH YOUR NOSE), give the paper to the patient and say, "Do what it says on this paper". (1 point for correct action)
Ability to use language correctly	Ask the patient to write a sentence. (3 points if sentence has a subject, a verb, and has valid meaning).
Ability to concentrate	"Say the months of the year in reverse, starting with December." (1 point each for correct answers from November through August. 4 points possible.)
Understanding spatial relationships	Draw a clock; put in all the numbers; and set the hands on 3 o'clock. (clock circle = 1 pt; numbers in correct sequence = 1 pt; numbers placed on clock correctly = 1 pt; two hands on the clock = 1 pt; hands set at correct time=1 pt. (5 points possible)

SOURCES: *The Merck Manual of Health & Aging* (2004); Folstein, Folstein, & McHugh (1975); Kaufman & Zun (1995); Kokman et al. (1991); and Pfeiffer (1975).
Scoring: 30–21 = normal; 20–11 = mild cognitive impairment; 10–0 = severe cognitive impairment (scores are not absolute and must be considered within the comprehensive diagnostic assessment)

CORE CONCEPT

Nursing Diagnosis
Nursing diagnoses are clinical judgments about individual, family, or community responses to actual or potential health problems/life processes. A nursing diagnosis provides the basis for selection of nursing interventions to achieve outcomes for which the nurse is accountable. (NANDA, 2007)

Standard 2. Diagnosis

The Psychiatric-Mental Health Registered Nurse analyzes the assessment data to determine diagnoses or problems, including level of risk.

In the second step, data gathered during the assessment are analyzed. Diagnoses and potential problem statements are formulated and prioritized. Diagnoses conform to accepted classification systems, such as the NANDA International Nursing Diagnosis Classification (see Appendix D); International Classification of Diseases (WHO, 1993); and *DSM-IV-TR* (APA, 2000; see Appendix C.)

CORE CONCEPT

Outcomes
Measurable, expected, patient-focused goals that translate into observable behaviors (ANA, 2004).

Standard 3. Outcomes Identification

The Psychiatric-Mental Health Registered Nurse identifies expected outcomes for a plan individualized to the patient or to the situation.

Expected outcomes are derived from the diagnosis. They must be measurable and include a time estimate for attainment. They must be realistic for the client's capabilities, and are most effective when formulated cooperatively by the interdisciplinary team members, the client, and significant others.

Nursing Outcomes Classification

The **nursing outcomes classification (NOC)** is a comprehensive, standardized classification of patient/client outcomes developed to evaluate the effects of nursing interventions (Johnson, Maas, & Moorhead, 2004). The outcomes have been linked to NANDA diagnoses and to the **Nursing Interventions Classification (NIC)**. NANDA, NIC, and NOC represent all domains of nursing and can be used together or separately (Johnson et al, 2006).

Each NOC outcome has a label name, a definition, a list of indicators to evaluate client status in relation to the outcome, and a five-point Likert scale to measure client status (Johnson et al, 2006). The 330 NOC outcomes include 311 individual, 10 family, and 9 community level outcomes (Johnson, Maas, & Moorhead, 2004).

Standard 4. Planning

The Psychiatric-Mental Health Registered Nurse develops a plan that prescribes strategies and alternatives to attain expected outcomes.

The care plan is individualized to the client's mental health problems, condition, or needs and is developed in collaboration with the client, significant others, and interdisciplinary team members, if possible. For each diagnosis identified, the most appropriate interventions, based on current psychiatric/mental health nursing practice and research, are selected. Client education and necessary referrals are included. Priorities for delivery of nursing care are determined.

Nursing Interventions Classification

The Nursing Interventions Classification (NIC) is a comprehensive, standardized language describing treatments that nurses perform in all settings and in all specialties. NIC includes both physiological and psychosocial interventions, as well as those for illness treatment, illness prevention, and health promotion (Dochterman & Bulechek, 2004). NIC interventions are comprehensive, based on research, and reflect current clinical practice. They were developed inductively based on existing practice.

NIC contains 542 interventions each with a definition and a detailed set of activities that describe what a nurse does to implement the intervention. The use of a standardized language is thought to enhance continuity of care and facilitate communication among nurses and between nurses and other providers.

Standard 5. Implementation

The Psychiatric-Mental Health Registered Nurse implements the identified plan.

Interventions selected during the planning stage are executed, taking into consideration the nurse's level of practice, education, and certification. The care plan serves as a blueprint for delivery of safe, ethical, and appropriate interventions. Documentation of interventions also occurs at this step in the nursing process.

Several specific interventions are included among the standards of psychiatric/mental health clinical nursing practice (ANA, 2000):

Standard 5A. Coordination of Care

The psychiatric-mental health registered nurse coordinates care delivery.

Standard 5B. Health Teaching and Health Promotion

The psychiatric-mental health registered nurse employs strategies to promote health and a safe environment.

Standard 5C. Milieu Therapy

The psychiatric-mental health registered nurse provides, structures, and maintains a safe and therapeutic environment in collaboration with patients, families, and other healthcare clinicians.

Standard 5D. Pharmacological, Biological, and Integrative Therapies

The psychiatric-mental health registered nurse incorporates knowledge of pharmacological, biological, and complementary interventions with applied clinical skills to restore the patient's health and prevent further disability.

Standard 5E. Prescriptive Authority and Treatment

The psychiatric-mental health advanced practice registered nurse uses prescriptive authority, procedures, referrals, treatments, and therapies in accordance with state and federal laws and regulations.

Standard 5F. Psychotherapy

The psychiatric-mental health advanced practice registered nurse conducts individual, couples, group, and family psychotherapy using evidence-based psychotherapeutic frameworks and nurse–patient therapeutic relationships.

Standard 5G. Consultation

The psychiatric-mental health advanced practice registered nurse provides consultation to influence the identified plan, enhance the abilities of other clinicians to provide services for patients, and effect change.

Evaluation
The process of determining both the client's progress toward the attainment of expected outcomes and the effectiveness of nursing care.

Standard 6. Evaluation

The Psychiatric-Mental Health Registered Nurse evaluates progress toward attainment of expected outcomes.

During the evaluation step, the nurse measures the success of the interventions in meeting the outcome criteria. The client's response to treatment is documented, validating use of the nursing process in the delivery of care. The diagnoses, outcomes, and plan of care are reviewed and revised as need is determined by the evaluation.

WHY NURSING DIAGNOSIS?

The concept of nursing diagnosis is not new. For centuries, nurses have identified specific client responses for which nursing interventions were used in an effort to improve quality of life. Historically, however, the autonomy of practice to which nurses were entitled by virtue of their licensure was lacking in the provision of nursing care. Nurses assisted physicians as required, and performed a group of specific tasks that were considered within their scope of responsibility.

The term *diagnosis* in relation to nursing first began to appear in the literature in the early 1950s. The formalized organization of the concept, however, was initiated only in 1973 with the convening of the First Task Force to Name and Classify Nursing Diagnoses. The Task Force of the National Conference Group on the Classification of Nursing Diagnoses was developed during this conference (NANDA International, 2006a). These individuals were charged with the task of identifying and classifying nursing diagnoses.

Also in the 1970s, the ANA began to write standards of practice around the steps of the nursing process, of which nursing diagnosis is an inherent part. This format encompassed both the general and specialty standards outlined by the ANA. The standards of psychiatric-mental health nursing practice are summarized in Box 9–2.

From this progression a statement of policy was published in 1980 and included a definition of nursing. The ANA defined nursing as "the diagnosis and treatment of human responses to actual or potential health problems" (ANA, 2003). This definition has been expanded to describe more appropriately nursing's commitment to society and to the profession itself. The ANA (2003) defines nursing as follows:

Nursing is the protection, promotion, and optimization of health and abilities, prevention of illness and injury, alleviation of suffering through the diagnosis and treatment of human response, and advocacy in the care of individuals, families, communities, and populations. (p. 6)

Nursing diagnosis is an inherent component of both the original and expanded definitions.

Decisions regarding professional negligence are made based on the standards of practice defined by the ANA and the individual state nursing practice acts. A number of states have incorporated the steps of the nursing process, including nursing diagnosis, into the scope of nursing practice described in their nursing practice acts. When this is the case, it is the legal duty of the nurse to show that nursing process and nursing diagnosis were accurately implemented in the delivery of nursing care.

NANDA International evolved from the original task force that was convened in 1973 to name and classify nursing diagnoses. The major purpose of NANDA International is to "increase the visibility of nursing's contribution to patient care by continuing to develop, refine, and classify phenomena of concern to nurses" (NANDA International, 2006b). A list of nursing diagnoses approved by NANDA-I for use and testing is presented in Appendix D. This list is by no means exhaustive or all-inclusive. For purposes of this text, however, the existing list will be used in an effort to maintain a common language within nursing and to encourage clinical testing of what is available.

The use of nursing diagnosis affords a degree of autonomy that historically has been lacking in the practice of nursing. Nursing diagnosis describes the client's condition, facilitating the prescription of interventions and establishment of parameters for outcome criteria based on what is uniquely nursing. The ultimate benefit is to the client, who receives effective and consistent nursing care based on knowledge of the problems that he or she is experiencing and of the most effective nursing interventions to resolve them.

NURSING CASE MANAGEMENT

The concept of **case management** evolved with the advent of diagnosis-related groups (DRGs) and shorter hospital stays. Case management is an innovative model of care delivery that can result in improved client care. Within this model, clients are assigned a manager who negotiates with multiple providers to obtain diverse services. This type of healthcare delivery process serves to decrease fragmentation of care while striving to contain cost of services.

Case management in the acute care setting strives to organize client care through an episode of illness so that specific clinical and financial outcomes are achieved within an allotted time frame. Commonly, the allotted

---

BOX 9–2   Standards of Psychiatric-Mental Health Clinical Nursing Practice

Standard 1. Assessment

The psychiatric-mental health registered nurse collects comprehensive health data that is pertinent to the patient's health or situation.

Standard 2. Diagnosis

The psychiatric-mental health registered nurse analyzes the assessment data to determine diagnoses or problems, including level of risk.

Standard 3. Outcomes Identification

The psychiatric-mental health registered nurse identifies expected outcomes for a plan individualized to the patient or to the situation.

Standard 4. Planning

The psychiatric-mental health registered nurse develops a plan that prescribes strategies and alternatives to attain expected outcomes.

Standard 5. Implementation

The psychiatric-mental health registered nurse implements the identified plan.

Standard 5A. Coordination of Care

The psychiatric-mental health registered nurse coordinates care delivery.

Standard 5B. Health Teaching and Health Promotion

The psychiatric-mental health registered nurse employs strategies to promote health and a safe environment.

Standard 5C. Milieu Therapy — environment conducive to learn

The psychiatric-mental health registered nurse provides, structures, and maintains a safe and therapeutic environment in collaboration with patients, families, and other healthcare clinicians.

Standard 5D. Pharmacological, Biological, and Integrative Therapies

The psychiatric-mental health registered nurse incorporates knowledge of pharmacological, biological, and complementary interventions with applied clinical skills to restore the patient's health and prevent further disability.

Standard 5E. Prescriptive Authority and Treatment

The psychiatric-mental health advanced practice registered nurse uses prescriptive authority, procedures, referrals, treatments, and therapies in accordance with state and federal laws and regulations.

Standard 5F. Psychotherapy

The psychiatric-mental health advanced practice registered nurse conducts individual, couples, group, and family psychotherapy using evidence-based psychotherapeutic frameworks and nurse-patient therapeutic relationships.

Standard 5G. Consultation

The psychiatric-mental health advanced practice registered nurse provides consultation to influence the identified plan, enhance the abilities of other clinicians to provide services for patients, and effect change.

Standard 6. Evaluation

The psychiatric-mental health registered nurse evaluates progress toward attainment of expected outcomes.

SOURCE: *Psychiatric-Mental Health Nursing: Scope and Standards of Practice.* ANA, APNA, & ISPN (2007). With permission.

---

time frame is determined by the established protocols for length of stay as defined by the DRGs.

Case management has been shown to be an effective method of treatment for individuals with a chronic mental illness. This type of care strives to improve functioning by assisting the individual to solve problems, improve work and socialization skills, promote leisure-time activities, and enhance overall independence.

Ideally, case management incorporates concepts of care at the primary, secondary, and tertiary levels of prevention. Various definitions have emerged and are clarified as follows.

Managed care refers to a strategy employed by purchasers of health services who make determinations about various types of services in order to maintain quality and control costs. In a managed care program, individuals receive health care based on need, as assessed by coordi-

nators of the providership. Managed care exists in many settings, including (but not limited to) the following:

● Insurance-based programs
● Employer-based medical providerships
● Social service programs
● The public health sector

Managed care may exist in virtually any setting in which medical providership is a part of the service; that is, in any setting in which an organization (whether private or government-based) is responsible for payment of healthcare services for a group of people. Examples of managed care are health maintenance organizations (HMOs) and preferred provider organizations (PPOs).

Case management is the method used to achieve managed care. It is the actual coordination of services required to meet the needs of a client within the fragmented healthcare system. Case management strives to help at-risk clients prevent avoidable episodes of illness. Its goal is to provide these services while attempting to control healthcare costs to the consumer and third-party payers.

Types of clients who benefit from case management include (but are not limited to) the following:

● The frail elderly
● The developmentally disabled
● The physically handicapped
● The mentally handicapped
● Individuals with long-term medically complex problems that require multifaceted, costly care (e.g., high-risk infants, those with human immunodeficiency virus [HIV] or acquired immunodeficiency syndrome [AIDS], and transplant clients)
● Individuals who are severely compromised by an acute episode of illness or an acute exacerbation of a chronic illness (e.g., schizophrenia)

The **case manager** is responsible for negotiating with multiple healthcare providers to obtain a variety of services for the client. Nurses are very well qualified to serve as case managers. The very nature of nursing, which incorporates knowledge about the biological, psychological, and sociocultural aspects related to human functioning, makes nurses highly appropriate as case managers. Several years of experience as a registered nurse is usually required for employment as a case manager. Some case management programs prefer master's-prepared clinical nurse specialists who have experience working with the specific populations for whom the case management service will be rendered.

Critical Pathways of Care

Critical pathways of care (CPCs) have emerged as the tools for provision of care in a case management system. A critical pathway is a type of abbreviated plan of care that provides outcome-based guidelines for goal achievement within a designated length of stay. A sample CPC is presented in Table 9–2. Only one nursing diagnosis is used in this sample. A CPC may have nursing diagnoses for several individual problems.

Critical pathways of care are intended to be used by the entire interdisciplinary team, which may include nurse case manager, clinical nurse specialist, social worker, psychiatrist, psychologist, dietitian, occupational therapist, recreational therapist, chaplain, and others. The team decides what categories of care are to be performed, by what date, and by whom. Each member of the team is then expected to carry out his or her functions according to the time line designated on the CPC. The nurse, as case manager, is ultimately responsible for ensuring that each of the assignments is carried out. If variations occur at any time in any of the categories of care, rationales must be documented in the progress notes.

For example, with the sample CPC presented, the nurse case manager may admit the client into the detoxification center. The nurse contacts the psychiatrist to inform him or her of the admission. The psychiatrist performs additional assessments to determine if other consults are required. The psychiatrist also writes the orders for the initial diagnostic work-up and medication regimen. Within 24 hours, the interdisciplinary team meets to decide on other categories of care, to complete the CPC, and to make individual care assignments from the CPC. This particular sample CPC relies heavily on nursing care of the client through the critical withdrawal period. However, other problems for the same client, such as imbalanced nutrition, impaired physical mobility, or spiritual distress, may involve other members of the team to a greater degree. Each member of the team stays in contact with the nurse case manager regarding individual assignments. Ideally, team meetings are held daily or every other day to review progress and modify the plan as required.

CPCs can be standardized, as they are intended to be used with uncomplicated cases. A CPC can be viewed as protocol for various clients with problems for which a designated outcome can be predicted.

APPLYING THE NURSING PROCESS IN THE PSYCHIATRIC SETTING

Based on the definition of mental health set forth in Chapter 2, the role of the nurse in psychiatry focuses on helping the client successfully adapt to stressors within the environment. Goals are directed toward changes in thoughts, feelings, and behaviors that are age appropriate and congruent with local and cultural norms.

Therapy within the psychiatric setting is very often team, or **interdisciplinary**, oriented. Therefore, it is important to delineate nursing's involvement in the treatment regimen. Nurses are indeed valuable members of the team. Having progressed beyond the role of custodial caregiver in the psychiatric setting, nurses now provide services that are defined within the scope of nursing practice. Nursing diagnosis is helping to define these nursing boundaries, providing the degree of autonomy and professionalism that has for so long been unrealized.

For example, a newly admitted client with the medical diagnosis of schizophrenia may be demonstrating the following behaviors:

● Inability to trust others
● Verbalizing hearing voices
● Refusing to interact with staff and peers
● Expressing a fear of failure
● Poor personal hygiene

TABLE 9–2	Sample Critical Pathway of Care for Client in Alcohol Withdrawal

Estimated Length of Stay: 7 Days—Variations from Designated Pathway Should Be Documented in Progress Notes

Nursing Diagnoses and Categories of Care	Time Dimension	Goals and/or Actions	Time Dimension	Goals and/or Actions	Time Dimension	Discharge Outcome
Risk for injury related to CNS agitation					Day 7	Client shows no evidence of injury obtained during ETOH withdrawal
Referrals	Day 1	Psychiatrist Assess need for: Neurologist Cardiologist Internist			Day 7	Discharge with follow-up appointments as required.
Diagnostic Studies	Day 1	Blood alcohol level Drug screen (urine and blood) Chemistry Profile Urinalysis Chest x-ray ECG	Day 4	Repeat of selected diagnostic studies as necessary.		
Additional assessments	Day 1 Day 1–5 Ongoing Ongoing	VS q4h I&O Restraints p.r.n. Assess withdrawal symptoms: tremors, nausea/ vomiting, tachycardia, sweating, high blood pressure, seizures, insomnia, hallucinations	Day 2–3 Day 6 Day 4	VS q8h if stable DC I&O Marked decrease in objective withdrawal symptoms	Day 4–7 Day 7	VS b.i.d.; remain stable Discharge; absence of objective withdrawal symptoms
Medications	Day 1 Day 2 Day 1–6 Day 1–7	*Librium 200 mg in divided doses Librium 160 mg in divided doses Librium p.r.n. Maalox ac & hs *NOTE: Some physicians may elect to use Serax or Tegretol in the detoxification process	Day 3 Day 4	Librium 120 mg in divided doses Librium 80 mg in divided doses	Day 5 Day 6 Day 7	Librium 40 mg DC Librium Discharge; no withdrawal symptoms
Client education			Day 5	Discuss goals of AA and need for outpatient therapy	Day 7	Discharge with information regarding AA attendance or outpatient treatment

From these assessments, the treatment team may determine that the client has the following problems:

● Paranoid delusions
● Auditory hallucinations
● Social withdrawal
● Developmental regression

Team goals would be directed toward the following:

● Reducing suspiciousness
● Terminating auditory hallucinations
● Increasing feelings of self-worth

TABLE 9–5	**Validation of the Nursing Process with APIE Method**	
APIE Charting	**What Is Recorded**	**Nursing Process**
A (Assessment)	Subjective and objective data about the client that are gathered at the beginning of each shift	Assessment
P (Problem)	Name (or number) of nursing diagnosis being addressed from written problem list, and identified outcome for that problem. **NOTE:** If outcome appears on written care plan, it need not be repeated in daily documentation unless a change occurs.	Diagnosis and outcome identification
I (Intervention)	Nursing actions performed, directed at problem resolution	Plan and implementation
E (Evaluation)	Appraisal of client responses to determine effectiveness of nursing interventions	Evaluation

Explanation of any deviation from the norm is included in the progress notes.

P = Problem: A problem list, or list of nursing diagnoses, is an important part of the APIE method of charting. The name or number of the problem being addressed is documented in this section.

I = Intervention: Nursing actions are performed, directed at resolution of the problem.

E = Evaluation: Outcomes of the implemented interventions are documented, including an evaluation of client responses to determine the effectiveness of nursing interventions and the presence or absence of progress toward resolution of a problem.

Table 9–5 shows how APIE charting corresponds to the steps of the nursing process. Following is an example of a three-column documentation in the APIE format.

Date/Time	Problem	Progress Notes
6/22/08 1000	Social Isolation	**A:** States he does not want to sit with or talk to others; they "frighten" him; stays in room alone unless strongly encouraged to come out; no group involvement; at times listens to group conversations from a distance but does not interact; some hypervigilance and scanning noted **P:** Social isolation related to inability to trust, panic level of anxiety, and delusional thinking **I:** Initiated trusting relationship by spending time alone with client; discussed his feelings regarding interactions with others; accompanied client to group activities; provided positive feedback for voluntarily participating in assertiveness training **E:** Cooperative with therapy; still uncomfortable in the presence of a group of people; accepted positive feedback from nurse.

Electronic Documentation

Most healthcare facilities have implemented—or are in the process of implementing—some type of electronic health records (EHR) or electronic documentation system. EHRs have been shown to improve both the quality of client care and the efficiency of the healthcare system (Hopper & Ames, 2004). In 2003, the U.S. Department of Health and Human Services commissioned the Institute of Medicine (IOM) to study the capabilities of an EHR system. The IOM identified a set of eight core functions that EHR systems should perform in the delivery of safer, higher quality, and more efficient health care. These eight core capabilities include the following (Tang, 2003):

- **Health Information and Data**. EHRs would provide more rapid access to important patient information (e.g., allergies, lab test results, a medication list, demographic information, and clinical narratives), thereby improving care providers' ability to make sound clinical decisions in a timely manner.
- **Results Management.** Computerized results of all types (e.g., laboratory test results, radiology procedure result reports) can be accessed more easily by the provider at the time and place they are needed.
- **Order Entry/Order Management.** Computer-based order entries improve workflow processes by eliminating lost orders and ambiguities caused by illegible handwriting, generating related orders automatically, monitoring for duplicate orders, and improving the speed with which orders are executed.
- **Decision Support.** Computerized decision support systems enhance clinical performance for many aspects of health care. Using reminders and prompts, improvement in regular screenings and other preventive practices can be accomplished. Other aspects of healthcare support include identifying possible drug interactions and facilitating diagnosis and treatment.
- **Electronic Communication and Connectivity.** Improved communication among care associates, such as medicine, nursing, laboratory, pharmacy, and radiology, can enhance client safety and quality of care. Efficient communication among providers improves

TABLE 9–6	Advantages and Disadvantages of Paper Records and EHRs

Paper*	EHR
Advantages	**Advantages**
● People know how to use it.	● Can be accessed by multiple providers from remote sites.
● It is fast for current practice.	● Facilitates communication between disciplines.
● It is portable.	● Provides reminders about completing information.
● It is nonbreakable.	● Provides warnings about incompatibilities of medications or variances from normal standards.
● It accepts multiple data types, such as graphs, photographs, drawings, and text.	● Reduces redundancy of information.
● Legal issues and costs are understood.	● Requires less storage space and more difficult to lose.
	● Easier to research for audits, quality assurance, and epidemiological surveillance.
Disadvantages	● Provides immediate retrieval of information (e.g., test results).
● It can be lost.	● Provides links to multiple databases of healthcare knowledge, thus providing diagnostic support.
● It is often illegible and incomplete.	● Decreases charting time.
● It has no remote access.	● Reduces errors due to illegible handwriting.
● It can be accessed by only one person at a time.	● Facilitates billing and claims procedures.
● It is often disorganized.	
● Information is duplicated.	**Disadvantages**
● It is hard to store.	● Excessive expense to initiate the system.
● It is difficult to research, and continuous quality improvement is laborious.	● Substantial learning curve involved for new users; training and re-training required.
● Same client has separate records at each facility (physician office, hospital, home care).	● Stringent requirements to maintain security and confidentiality.
● Records are shared only through hard copy.	● Technical difficulties are possible.
	● Legal and ethical issues involving privacy and access to client information.
	● Requires consistent use of standardized terminology to support information sharing across wide networks.

*From Young, K.M. (2006). Nursing Informatics. In J.T. Catalano (Ed.), *Nursing Now! Today's issues, tomorrow's trends* (4th ed.). Philadelphia: F.A. Davis. With permission.

continuity of care, allows for more timely interventions, and reduces the risk of adverse events.

● **Patient Support.** Computer-based interactive client education, self-testing, and self-monitoring have been shown to improve control of chronic illnesses.

● **Administrative Processes.** Electronic scheduling systems (e.g., for hospital admissions and outpatient procedures) increase the efficiency of healthcare organizations and provide more timely service to patients.

● **Reporting and Population Health Management.** Healthcare organizations are required to report healthcare data to government and private sectors for patient safety and public health. Uniform electronic data standards facilitate this process at the provider level, reduce the associated costs, and increase the speed and accuracy of the data reported.

Table 9–6 lists some of the advantages and disadvantages of paper records and EHRs.

SUMMARY AND KEY POINTS

● The nursing process provides a methodology by which nurses may deliver care using a systematic, scientific approach.

● The focus of nursing process is goal directed and based on a decision-making or problem-solving model, consisting of six steps: assessment, diagnosis, outcome identification, planning, implementation, and evaluation.

● Assessment is a systematic, dynamic process by which the nurse, through interaction with the client, significant others, and healthcare providers, collects and analyzes data about the client.

● Nursing diagnoses are clinical judgments about individual, family, or community responses to actual or potential health problems/life processes.

● Outcomes are measurable, expected, patient-focused goals that translate into observable behaviors.

● Evaluation is the process of determining both the client's progress toward the attainment of expected outcomes and the effectiveness of nursing care.

● The psychiatric nurse uses the nursing process to assist clients to adapt successfully to stressors within the environment.

● The nurse serves as a valuable member of the interdisciplinary treatment team, working both independently and cooperatively with other team members.

● Case management is an innovative model of care delivery that serves to provide quality client care while controlling healthcare costs. Critical pathways of care (CPCs) serve as the tools for provision of care in a case management system.

● Nurses may serve as case managers, who are responsible for negotiating with multiple healthcare providers to obtain a variety of services for the client.

● Concept mapping is a diagrammatic teaching and learning strategy that allows students and faculty to visualize interrelationships between medical diagnoses, nursing diagnoses, assessment data, and treatments. The concept map care plan is an innovative approach to planning and organizing nursing care.

● Nurses must document that the nursing process has been used in the delivery of care. Three methods of documentation that reflect use of the nursing process include POR, Focus Charting, and the PIE method.

● Many healthcare facilities have implemented the use of electronic health records (EHR) or electronic documentation systems. EHRs have been shown to improve both the quality of client care and the efficiency of the healthcare system.

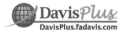 **DavisPlus**
DavisPlus.fadavis.com   **For additional clinical tools and study aids, visit DavisPlus.**

REVIEW QUESTIONS

Self-Examination/Learning Exercise

Test your knowledge of the nursing process by supplying the information requested.

1. Name the six steps of the nursing process.
2. Identify the step of the nursing process to which each of the following nursing actions applies:
   a. Obtains a short-term contract from the client to seek out staff if feeling suicidal.
   b. Identifies nursing diagnosis: Risk for suicide.
   c. Determines if nursing interventions have been appropriate to achieve desired results.
   d. Client's family reports recent suicide attempt.
   e. Prioritizes the necessity for maintaining a safe environment for the client.
   f. Establishes goal of care: Client will not harm self during hospitalization.
3. S.T. is a 15-year-old girl who has just been admitted to the adolescent psychiatric unit with a diagnosis of anorexia nervosa. She is 5'5" tall and weighs 82 lb. She was elected to the cheerleading squad for the fall but states that she is not as good as the others on the squad. The treatment team has identified the following problems: refusal to eat, occasional purging, refusing to interact with staff and peers, and fear of failure.

   Formulate three nursing diagnoses and identify outcomes for each that nursing could use as a part of the treatment team to contribute both independently and cooperatively to the team treatment plan.
4. Review various methods of documentation that reflect delivery of nursing care via the nursing process. Practice making entries for the case described in question 3 using the various methods presented in the text.

REFERENCES

American Nurses' Association (ANA). (2003). *Nursing's social policy statement* (2nd ed). Washington, DC: Author.

American Nurses' Association (ANA). (2004). *Nursing: Scope and standards of practice*. Washington, DC: Author.

American Nurses' Association (ANA), American Psychiatric Nurses Association (APNA), & International Society of Psychiatric-Mental Health Nurses (ISPN). (2007). *Psychiatric-mental health nursing: Scope and standards of practice*. Silver Spring, MD: ANA.

American Psychiatric Association (APA). (2000). *Diagnosis and statistical manual of mental disorders* (4th ed.) Text revision. Washington, DC: American Psychiatric Association.

Dochterman, J.M., & Bulechek, G. (2004). Nursing interventions classification overview. Retrieved June 21, 2008 from http://www.nursing.uiowa.edu/excellence/nursing_knowledge/clinical_effectiveness/nicoverview.htm

Doenges, M.E., Moorhouse, M.F., & Murr, A.C. (2005). *Nursing diagnosis manual: Planning, individualizing, and documenting client care*. Philadelphia: F.A. Davis.

Folstein, M.F., Folstein, S.E., & McHugh, P.R. (1975). Mini-mental state: A practical method for grading the cognitive state of patients for the clinician. *Journal of Psychiatric Research, 12*(3), 189–198.

Hopper, K., & Ames, K.J. (2004). *Health policy analysis: Standardized EMRs*. Durham, NC: Duke University.

Johnson, M., Bulechek, G., Dochterman, J.M., Maas, M., & Moorhead, S., Swanson, E., & Butcher, H. (2006). *NANDA, NOC, and NIC linkages: Nursing diagnoses, outcomes, & interventions* (2nd ed.). New York: Elsevier.

Johnson, M., Maas, M., & Moorhead, S. (2004). Nursing outcomes classification overview. Retrieved June 21, 2008 from

http://www.nursing.uiowa.edu/excellence/nursing_knowledge/clinical_effectiveness/nocoverview.htm

Kaufman, D.M., & Zun, L. (1995). A quantifiable, brief mental status examination for emergency patients. *Journal of Emergency Medicine, 13*(4), 440–456.

Kokman, E., Smith, G.E., Petersen, R.C., Tangalos, E., & Ivnik, R.C. (1991). The short test of mental status: Correlations with standardized psychometric testing. *Archives of Neurology, 48*(7), 725–728.

Lampe, S.S. (1985). Focus charting: Streamlining documentation. *Nursing Management, 16*(7), 43–46.

Merck Manual of Health & Aging, The. (2004). Whitehouse Station, NJ: Merck Research Laboratories.

NANDA International. (2007). *Nursing diagnoses: Definitions and classification, 2007–2008*. Philadelphia: NANDA International.

NANDA International. (2006a). *History and historical highlights 1973 through 1998*. Retrieved June 21, 2008 from http://www.nanda.org/html/history1.html

NANDA International. (2006b). *About NANDA International*. Retrieved June 21, 2008 from http://www.nanda.org/html/about.html

Pfeiffer, E. (1975). A short portable mental status questionnaire for the assessment of organic brain deficit in elderly patients. *Journal of the American Geriatric Society, 23*(10), 433–441.

Schuster, P.M. (2002). *Concept mapping: A critical-thinking approach to care planning*. Philadelphia: F.A. Davis.

Tang, P. (2003). *Key capabilities of an electronic health record system*. Institute of Medicine Committee on Data Standards for Patient Safety. Board on Health Care Services. Washington, DC: National Academies Press.

World Health Organization (WHO). (1993). *International classification of diseases* (10th ed.). Geneva: World Health Organization.

Therapeutic Groups

CHAPTER OUTLINE

KEY TERMS

altruism
autocratic
catharsis
democratic
laissez-faire
psychodrama
universality

CORE CONCEPTS

group
group therapy

OBJECTIVES

After reading this chapter, the student will be able to:

1. Define a *group*.
2. Discuss eight functions of a group.
3. Identify various types of groups.
4. Describe physical conditions that influence groups.
5. Discuss "curative factors" that occur in groups.
6. Describe the phases of group development.
7. Identify various leadership styles in groups.
8. Identify various roles that members assume within a group.
9. Discuss psychodrama as a specialized form of group therapy.
10. Describe the role of the nurse in group therapy.

Human beings are complex creatures who share their activities of daily living with various *groups* of people. Sampson and Marthas (1990) state:

We are *biological* organisms possessing qualities shared with all living systems and with others of our species. We are *psychological* beings with distinctly human capabilities for thought, feeling, and action. We are also *social* beings, who function as part of the complex webs that link us with other people. (p. 3)

Healthcare professionals not only share their personal lives with groups of people but also encounter multiple group situations in their professional operations. Team conferences, committee meetings, grand rounds, and inservice sessions are but a few. In psychiatry, work with clients and families often takes the form of groups. With group work, not only does the nurse have the opportunity to reach out to a greater number of people at one time, but those individuals also assist each other by bringing to the group and sharing their feelings, opinions, ideas, and behaviors. Clients learn from each other in a group setting.

This chapter explores various types and methods of therapeutic groups that can be used with psychiatric clients, and the role of the nurse in group intervention.

CORE CONCEPT

Group

A *group* is a collection of individuals whose association is founded on shared commonalities of interest, values, norms, or purpose. Membership in a group is generally by chance (born into the group), by choice (voluntary affiliation), or by circumstance (the result of life-cycle events over which an individual may or may not have control).

FUNCTIONS OF A GROUP

Sampson and Marthas (1990) outlined eight functions that groups serve for their members. They contend that groups may serve more than one function and usually serve different functions for different members of the group. The eight functions are as follows:

1. **Socialization.** The cultural group into which we are born begins the process of teaching social norms. This is continued throughout our lives by members of other groups with which we become affiliated.
2. **Support.** One's fellow group members are available in time of need. Individuals derive a feeling of security from group involvement.
3. **Task completion.** Group members provide assistance in endeavors that are beyond the capacity of one individual alone or when results can be achieved more effectively as a team.
4. **Camaraderie.** Members of a group provide the joy and pleasure that individuals seek from interactions with significant others.
5. **Informational.** Learning takes place within groups. Explanations regarding world events occur in groups. Knowledge is gained when individual members learn how others in the group have resolved situations similar to those with which they are currently struggling.
6. **Normative.** This function relates to the ways in which groups enforce the established norms.
7. **Empowerment.** Groups help to bring about improvement in existing conditions by providing support to individual members who seek to bring about change. Groups have power that individuals alone do not.
8. **Governance.** An example of the governing function is that of rules being made by committees within a larger organization.

TYPES OF GROUPS

The functions of a group vary depending on the reason the group was formed. Clark (1994) identifies three types of groups in which nurses most often participate: task, teaching, and supportive/therapeutic groups.

Task Groups

The function of a task group is to accomplish a specific outcome or task. The focus is on solving problems and making decisions to achieve this outcome. Often a deadline is placed on completion of the task, and such importance is placed on a satisfactory outcome that conflict in the group may be smoothed over or ignored in order to focus on the priority at hand.

Teaching Groups

Teaching, or educational, groups exist to convey knowledge and information to a number of individuals. Nurses can be involved in teaching groups of many varieties, such as medication education, childbirth education, breast self-examination, and effective parenting classes. These groups usually have a set time frame or a set number of meetings. Members learn from each other as well as from the designated instructor. The objective of teaching groups is verbalization or demonstration by the learner of the material presented by the end of the designated period.

Supportive/Therapeutic Groups

The primary concern of support groups is to prevent future upsets by teaching participants effective ways of dealing with emotional stress arising from situational or developmental crises.

CORE CONCEPT

Group Therapy

A form of psychosocial treatment in which a number of clients meet together with a therapist for purposes of sharing, gaining personal insight, and improving interpersonal coping strategies.

For the purposes of this text, it is important to differentiate between "therapeutic groups" and "group therapy." Leaders of group therapy generally have advanced degrees in psychology, social work, nursing, or medicine. They often have additional training or experience under the supervision of an accomplished

REVIEW QUESTIONS

Self-Examination/Learning Exercise

Test your knowledge of group process by supplying the information requested.

1. Define a *group*.

2. Identify the type of group and leadership style in each of the following situations:

   a. N.J. is the nurse leader of a childbirth preparation group. Each week she shows various films and sets out various reading materials. She expects the participants to utilize their time on a topic of their choice or practice skills they have observed on the films. Two couples have dropped out of the group, stating, "This is a big waste of time."
   Type of group _____
   Style of leadership _____

   b. M.K. is a psychiatric nurse who has been selected to lead a group for women who desire to lose weight. The criterion for membership is that they must be at least 20 lb. overweight. All have tried to lose weight on their own many times in the past without success. At their first meeting, M.K. provides suggestions as the members determine what their goals will be and how they plan to go about achieving those goals. They decided how often they wanted to meet, and what they planned to do at each meeting.
   Type of group _____
   Style of leadership _____

   c. J.J. is a staff nurse on a surgical unit. He has been selected as leader of a newly established group of staff nurses organized to determine ways to decrease the number of medication errors occurring on the unit. J.J. has definite ideas about how to bring this about. He has also applied for the position of Head Nurse on the unit and believes that if he is successful in leading the group toward achievement of its goals, he can also facilitate his chances for promotion. At each meeting he addresses the group in an effort to convince the members to adopt his ideas.
   Type of group _____
   Style of leadership _____

Match the situation on the right to the curative factor or benefit it describes on the left.

_____ 3. Instillation of hope

_____ 4. Universality

_____ 5. Imparting of information

_____ 6. Altruism

_____ 7. Corrective recapitulation of the primary family group

_____ 8. Development of socializing techniques

_____ 9. Imitative behavior

a. Sam admires the way Jack stands up for what he believes. He decides to practice this himself.

b. Nancy sees that Jane has been a widow for 5 years now, and has adjusted well.
She thinks maybe she can too.

c. Susan has come to realize that she has the power to shape the direction of her life.

d. John is able to have a discussion with another person for the first time in his life.

e. Linda now understands that her mother really did love her, although she was not able to show it.

f. Alice has come to feel as though the other group members are like a family to her. She looks forward to the meetings each week.

g. Tony talks in the group about the abuse he experienced as a child. He has never told anyone about this before.

_____ 10. Interpersonal learning

_____ 11. Group cohesiveness

_____ 12. Catharsis

_____ 13. Existential factors

h. Sandra felt good about herself when she left group tonight. She had provided both physical and emotional support to Judy who shared for the first time about being raped.

i. Judy appreciated Sandra's support as she expressed her feelings related to the rape. She had come to believe that no one else felt as she did.

j. Paul knew that people did not want to be his friend because of his violent temper. In the group, he has learned to control his temper and form satisfactory interpersonal relationships with others.

k. Henry learned about the effects of alcohol on the body when a nurse from the chemical dependency unit spoke to the group.

Match the individual on the right to the role he or she is playing within the group.

_____ 14. Aggressor

_____ 15. Blocker

_____ 16. Dominator

_____ 17. Help seeker

_____ 18. Monopolizer

_____ 19. Mute or silent member

_____ 20. Recognition seeker

_____ 21. Seducer

a. Nancy talks incessantly in group. When someone else tries to make a comment, she refuses to allow him or her to speak.

b. On the first day the group meets, Valerie shares the intimate details of her incestuous relationship with her father.

c. Colleen listens with interest to everything the other members say, but she does not say anything herself in group.

d. Violet is obsessed with her physical appearance. Although she is beautiful, she has little self-confidence and needs continuous positive feedback. She states, "Maybe if I became a blond my boyfriend would love me more."

e. Larry states to Violet, "Listen, dummy, you need more than blond hair to keep the guy around. A bit more in the brains department would help!"

f. At the beginning of the group meeting, Dan says, "All right now, I have a date tonight. I want this meeting over on time! I'll keep track of the time and let everyone know when their time is up. When I say you're done, you're done, understand?"

g. Joyce says, "I won my first beauty contest when I was 6 months old. Can you imagine? And I've been winning them ever since. I was prom queen when I was 16, Miss Rose Petal when I was 19, Miss Silver City at 21. Next I go to the state contest. It's just all so exciting!"

h. Joe, an RN on the care-planning committee says, "What a stupid suggestion. Nursing Diagnosis!?!? I won't even discuss the matter. We have been doing our care plans this way for 20 years. I refuse to even consider changing."

theory is viewed as the foundation for this model. Communication is the actual transmission of information among individuals. All behavior sends a message, so all behavior in the presence of two or more individuals is communication. In this model, families considered to be functional are open systems where clear and precise messages, congruent with the situation, are sent and received. Healthy communication patterns promote nurturance and individual self-worth. Dysfunctional families are viewed as partially closed systems in which communication is vague, and messages are often inconsistent and incongruent with the situation. Destructive patterns of communication tend to inhibit healthful nurturing and decrease individual feelings of self-worth.

Major Concepts

Double-Bind Communication. Double-bind communication occurs when a statement is made and succeeded by a contradictory statement. It also occurs when a statement is made accompanied by nonverbal expression that is inconsistent with the verbal communication. These incompatible communications can interfere with ego development in an individual and promote mistrust of all communications. Double-bind communication often results in a "damned if I do and damned if I don't" situation.

> **Example:**
>
> A mother freely gives and receives hugs and kisses from her 6-year-old son some of the time, while at other times she pushes him away saying, "Big boys don't act like that." The little boy receives a conflicting message and is presented with an impossible dilemma: "To please my mother I must not show her that I love her, but if I do not show her that I love her, I'm afraid I will lose her."

Pseudomutuality and Pseudohostility. A healthy functioning individual is able to relate to other people while still maintaining a sense of separate identity. In a dysfunctional family, patterns of interaction may be reflected in the remoteness or closeness of relationships. These relationships may reflect erratic interaction (i.e., sometimes remote and sometimes close), or inappropriate interaction (i.e., excessive closeness or remoteness). **Pseudomutuality** and **pseudohostility** are seen as collective defenses against reality of the underlying meaning of the relationships in a dysfunctional family system. Pseudomutuality is characterized by a facade of mutual regard. Emotional investment is directed at maintaining outward representation of reciprocal fulfillment rather than in the relationship itself. The style of relating is fixed and rigid, and pseudomutuality allows family members to deny underlying fears of separation and hostility.

> **Example:**
>
> Janet, age 16, is the only child of State Senator J. and his wife. Janet was recently involved in a joyriding experience with a group of teenagers her parents call "the wrong crowd." In family therapy, Mrs. J. says, "We have always been a close family. I can't imagine why she is doing these things." Senator J. states, "I don't know another colleague who has a family that is as close as mine." Janet responds, "Yes, we are close. I just don't see my parents very much. Dad has been in politics since I was a baby, and Mom is always with him. I wish I could spend more time with them. But we are a close family."

Pseudohostility is also a fixed and rigid style of relating, but the facade being maintained is that of a state of chronic conflict and alienation among family members. This relationship pattern allows family members to deny underlying fears of tenderness and intimacy.

> **Example:**
>
> Jack, 14, and his sister Jill, 15, will have nothing to do with each other. When they are together they can agree on nothing, and the barrage of "putdowns" is constant. This behavior reflects pseudohostility used by individuals who are afraid to reveal feelings of intimacy.

Schism and Skew

Schism and Skew. Lidz, Cornelison, Fleck, and Terry (1957) observed two patterns within families that relate to a dysfunctional marital dyad. A **marital schism** is defined as "a state of severe chronic disequilibrium and discord, with recurrent threats of separation." Each partner undermines the other, mutual trust is absent, and a competition exists for closeness with the children. Often a partner establishes an alliance with his or her parent against the spouse. Children lack appropriate role models.

Marital skew describes a relationship in which there is lack of equal partnership. One partner dominates the relationship and the other partner. The marriage remains intact as long as the passive partner allows the domination to continue. Children also lack role models when a marital skew exists.

Goal and Techniques of Therapy

The goal of strategic family therapy is to create change in destructive behavior and communication patterns among family members. The identified family *problem* is the unit of therapy, and all family members need not be counseled together. In fact, strategic therapists may prefer to see subgroups or individuals separately in an effort to achieve problem resolution. Therapy is oriented in the present and the therapist assumes full responsibility for devising an effective strategy for family change. Therapeutic techniques include the following:

● **Paradoxical Intervention.** A paradox can be called a contradiction in therapy, or "prescribing the symptom." With **paradoxical intervention**, the therapist requests that the family continue to engage in the behavior that they are trying to change. Alternatively, specific directions may be given for continuing the defeating behavior. For example, a couple that regularly engages in insulting shouting matches is instructed to have one of these encounters on Tuesdays and Thursdays from 8:30 to 9:00 P.M. Boyer and Jeffrey (1994) explain:

A family using its maladaptive behavior to control or punish other people loses control of the situation when it finds itself continuing the behavior under a therapist's direction and being praised for following instructions. If the family disobeys the therapist's instruction, the price it pays is sacrificing the old behavior pattern and experiencing more satisfying ways of interacting with one another. A family that maintains it has no control over its behavior, or whose members contend that others must change before they can themselves, suddenly finds itself unable to defend such statements. (p. 125)

● **Reframing.** Goldenberg and Goldenberg (2005) describe reframing as "relabeling problematic behavior by putting it into a new, more positive perspective that emphasizes its good intention." Therefore, with reframing, the *behavior* may not actually change, but the *consequences* of the behavior may change, owing to a change in the meaning attached to the behavior. This technique is sometimes referred to as *positive reframing*.

| Example: |

Tom has a construction job and makes a comfortable living for his wife, Sue, and their two children. Tom and Sue have been arguing a lot and came to the therapist for counseling. Sue says Tom frequently drinks too much and is often late getting home from work. Tom counters, "I never used to drink on my way home from work, but Sue started complaining to me the minute I walked in the door about being so dirty and about tracking dirt and mud on 'her nice, clean floors.' It was the last straw when she made me undress before I came in the house and leave my dirty clothes and shoes in the garage. I thought a man's home was his castle. Well, I sure don't feel like a king. I need a few stiff drinks to face her nagging!"

The therapist used reframing to attempt change by helping Sue to view the situation in a more positive light. He suggested to Sue that she try to change her thinking by focusing on how much her husband must love her and her children to work as hard has he does. He asked her to focus on the dirty clothes and shoes as symbols of his love

for them and to respond to his "dirty" arrivals home with greater affection. This positive reframing set the tone for healing and for increased intimacy within the marital relationship.

The Evolution of Family Therapy

Goldenberg and Goldenberg (2004) describe Bowen's family theory and the structural and strategic models as "basic models of family therapy." They state:

While noteworthy differences continue to exist in the theoretical assumptions each school of thought makes about the nature and origin of psychological dysfunction, in what precisely they look for in understanding family patterns, and in their strategies for therapeutic intervention, in practice the trend today is toward electicism and integration in family therapy. (p. 125)

Nichols and Schwartz (2004) suggest that contemporary family therapists "borrow from each other's arsenal of techniques." The basic models described here have provided a foundation for the progression and growth of the discipline of family therapy. Examples of newer models include the following:

● **Narrative Therapy:** An approach to treatment that emphasizes the role of the stories people construct about their experience (Nichols & Schwartz, 2004, p. 442).
● **Feminist Family Therapy:** A form of collaborative, egalitarian, nonsexist intervention, applicable to both men and women, addressing family gender roles, patriarchal attitudes, and social and economic inequalities in male-female relationships (Goldenberg & Goldenberg, 2004, p. 508).
● **Social Constructionist Therapy:** Concerned with the assumptions or premises different family members hold about the problem. Efforts are focused on engaging families in conversations to solicit everyone's views, and not in imposing on families what is considered objectivity, truth, or "established knowledge" (Goldenberg & Goldenberg, 2004, p. 327).
● **Psychoeducational Family Therapy:** Therapy that emphasizes educating family members to help them understand and cope with a seriously disturbed family member (Nichols & Schwartz, 2004, p. 443).

The goal of most family therapy models is to provide the opportunity for change based on family members' perceptions of available options. The basic differences among models arise in how they go about achieving this goal. Goldenberg and Goldenberg (2004) state:

Regardless of procedures, all attempt to create a therapeutic environment conducive to self-examination, to reduce discomfort and conflict, to mobilize family resilience and empowerment, and to help the family members improve their overall functioning. (p. 463)

THE NURSING PROCESS—A CASE STUDY

Assessment

Wright and Leahey (2005) have developed the Calgary Family Assessment Model (CFAM), a multidimensional model originally adapted from a framework developed by Tomm and Sanders (1983). The CFAM consists of three major categories: structural, developmental, and functional. Wright and Leahey (2005) state:

> Each category contains several subcategories. It is important for each nurse to decide which subcategories are relevant and appropriate to explore and assess with each family at each point in time. That is, not all subcategories need to be assessed at a first meeting with a family, and some subcategories need never be assessed. If the nurse uses too many

subcategories, he or she may become overwhelmed by all the data. If the nurse and the family discuss too few subcategories, each may have a distorted view of the family's strengths or problems and the family situation. (p. 57)

A diagram of the CFAM is presented in Figure 11–3. The three major categories are listed, along with the subcategories for assessment under each. This diagram is used to assess the Marino family in the following case study.

Structural Assessment

A graphic representation of the Marino family structure is presented in the genogram in Figure 11–4.

Internal Structure. This is a family that consists of a husband, wife, and their biological son and daughter who

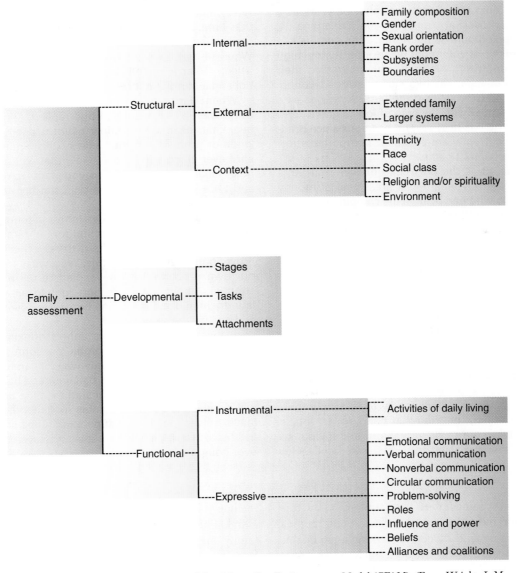

FIGURE 11–3 Branching diagram of the Calgary Family Assessment Model (CFAM). (From Wright, L.M., & Leahey, M. [2005]. *Nurses and families: A guide to family assessment and intervention* (4th ed.). Philadelphia: F.A. Davis.)

CASE STUDY

THE MARINO FAMILY

John and Nancy Marino have been married for 19 years. They have a 17-year-old son, Peter, and a 15-year-old daughter, Anna. Anna was recently hospitalized for taking an overdose of fluoxetine, her mother's prescription antidepressant. The family is attending family therapy sessions while Anna is in the hospital. Anna states, "I just couldn't take the fighting anymore! Our house is an awful place to be. Everyone hates each other, and everyone is unhappy. Dad drinks too much and Mom is always sick! Peter stays away as much as he can and I don't blame him. I would too if I had someplace to stay. I just thought I'd be better off dead."

John Marino, age 44, is the oldest of five children. His father, Paulo, age 66, is a first-generation Italian American whose parents emigrated from Italy in the early 1900s. Paulo retired last year after 32 years as a cutter in a meatpacking plant. His wife, Carla, age 64, has never worked outside the home. John and his siblings all worked at minimum-wage jobs during high school, and John and his two brothers worked their way through college. His two sisters married young, and both are housewives and mothers. John was able to go to law school with the help of loans, grants, and scholarships. He has held several positions since graduation and is currently employed as a corporate attorney for a large aircraft company.

Nancy, age 43, is the only child of Sam and Ethyl Jones. Sam, age 67, inherited a great deal of money from his family who had been in the shipping business. He is currently the Chief Executive Officer of this business. Ethyl, also 67, was an aspiring concert pianist when she met Sam. She chose to give up her career for marriage and family, although Nancy believes her mother always resented doing so. Nancy was reared in an affluent lifestyle. She attended private boarding schools as she was growing up and chose an exclusive college in the East to pursue her interest in art. She studied in Paris during her junior year. Nancy states that she was never emotionally close to her parents. They traveled a great deal, and she spent much of her time under the supervision of a nanny.

Nancy's parents were opposed to her marrying John. They perceived John's family to be below their social status. Nancy, on the other hand, loved John's family. She felt them to be very warm and loving, so unlike what she was used to in her own family. Her family is Protestant and also disapproved of her marrying in the Roman Catholic Church.

Family Dynamics

As their marriage progressed, Nancy's health became very fragile. She had continued her artistic pursuits but seemed to achieve little satisfaction from it. She tried to keep in touch with her parents but often felt spurned by them. They traveled a great deal and often did not even inform her of their whereabouts. They were not present at the birth of her children. She experiences many aches and pains and spends many days in bed. She sees several physicians, who have prescribed various pain medications, antianxiety agents, and antidepressants but can find nothing organically wrong. Five years ago she learned that John had been having an affair with his secretary. He promised to break it off and fired the secretary, but Nancy has had difficulty trusting him since that time. She brings up his infidelity whenever they have an argument, which is more and more often lately. When he is home, John drinks, usually until he falls asleep. Peter frequently comes home smelling of alcohol and a number of times has been clearly intoxicated.

When Nancy called her parents to tell them that Anna was in the hospital, Ethyl replied, "I'm sorry to hear that, dear. We certainly never had any of those kinds of problems on our side of the family. But I'm sure everything will be okay now that you are getting help. Please give our love to your family. Your father and I are leaving for Europe on Saturday and will be gone for 6 weeks."

Although more supportive, John's parents view this situation as somewhat shameful for the family. John's dad responded, "We had hard times when you were growing up, but never like this. We always took care of our own problems. We never had to tell a bunch of strangers about them. It's not right to air your dirty laundry in public. Bring Anna home. Give her your love and she will be okay."

In therapy, Nancy blames John's drinking and his admitted affair for all their problems. John states that he drinks because it is the only way he can tolerate his wife's complaining about his behavior and her many illnesses. Peter is very quiet most of the time but says he will be glad when he graduates in 4 months and can leave "this looney bunch of people." Anna cries as she listens to her family in therapy and says, "Nothing's ever going to change."

live together in the same home. They conform to the traditional gender roles. John is the eldest child from a rather large family, and Nancy has no siblings. In this family, their son, Peter, is the first-born and his sister, Anna, is 2 years younger. Neither spousal, sibling, nor spousal-sibling subsystems appear to be close in this family, and some are clearly conflictual. Problematic subsystems include John-Nancy, John-Nancy-children, and Nancy-Ethyl. The subsystem boundaries are quite rigid, and the family members appear to be emotionally disengaged from one another.

External Structure. This family has ties to extended family, although the availability of support is questionable. Nancy's parents offered little emotional support to

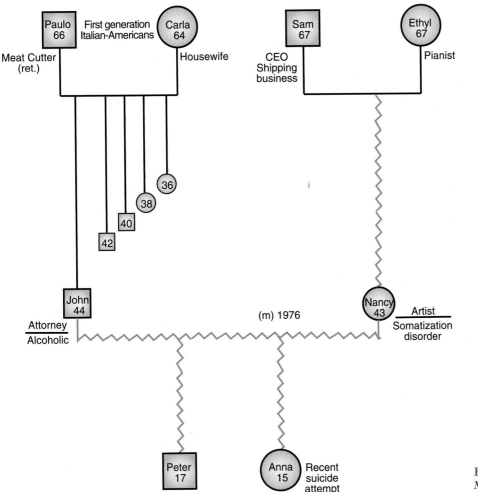

FIGURE 11-4 Genogram of the Marino family.

her as a developing child. They never approved of her marriage to John and still remain distant and cold. John's family consists of a father, mother, two brothers, and two sisters. They are warm and supportive most of the time, but cultural influences interfere with their understanding of this current situation. At this time, the Marino family is probably receiving the most support from healthcare professionals who have intervened during Anna's hospitalization.

Context. John is a second-generation Italian American. His family of origin is large, warm, and supportive. However, John's parents believe that family problems should be dealt with in the family, and disapprove of bringing "strangers" in to hear what they consider to be private information. They believe that Anna's physical condition should be stabilized, and then she should be discharged to deal with family problems at home.

John and Nancy were reared in different social classes. In John's family, money was not available to seek out professional help for every problem that arose. Italian cultural beliefs promote the provision of help within the nuclear and extended family network. If outside counseling is sought, it is often with the family priest. John and Nancy did not seek this type of counseling because they no longer attend church regularly.

In Nancy's family, money was available to obtain the very best professional help at the first sign of trouble. However, Nancy's parents refused to acknowledge, both then and now, that any difficulty ever existed in their family situation.

The Marino family lives comfortably on John's salary as a corporate attorney. They have health insurance and access to any referrals that are deemed necessary. They are well educated but have been attempting to deny the dysfunctional dynamics that exist in their family.

Developmental Assessment

The Marino family is in stage IV of Carter and McGoldrick's family life cycle: the family with adolescents. In stage IV, parents are expected to respond to adolescents' requests for increasing independence, while being available to continue to fulfill dependency needs. They may also be required to provide additional support to aging grandparents. This may be a time when parents may also begin to reexamine their own marital and career issues.

The Marino family is not fulfilling the dependency needs of its adolescents; in fact, they may be establishing premature independence. The parents are absorbed in their own personal problems to the exclusion of their children. Peter responds to this neglect by staying away as much as possible, drinking with his friends, and planning to leave home at the first opportunity. Anna's attempted suicide is a cry for help. She has needs that are unfulfilled by her parents, and this crisis situation may be required for them to recognize that a problem exists. This may be the time when they begin to reexamine their unresolved marital issues. Extended family are still self-supporting and do not require assistance from John and Nancy at this time.

Functional Assessment

Instrumental Functioning. This family has managed to adjust to the maladaptive functioning in an effort to meet physical activities of daily living. They subsist on fast food, or sometimes Nancy or Anna will prepare a meal. Seldom do they sit down at table to eat together. Nancy must take pain medication or sedatives to sleep. John usually drinks himself to sleep. Anna and Peter take care of their own needs independently. Often they do not even see their parents in the evenings. Each manages to do fairly well in school. Peter says, "I don't intend to ruin my chances of getting out of this hell hole as soon as I can!"

Expressive Functioning. John and Nancy Marino argue a great deal about many topics. This family seldom shows affection to one another. Nancy and Anna express sadness with tears, whereas John and Peter have a tendency to withdraw or turn to alcohol when experiencing unhappiness. Nancy somaticizes her internal pain, and numbs this pain with medication. Anna internalized her emotional pain until it became unbearable. A notable lack of constructive communication is evident.

This family is unable to solve its problems effectively. In fact, it is unlikely that it has even identified its problems, which undoubtedly have been in existence for a long while. These problems have only recently been revealed in light of Anna's suicide attempt.

Diagnosis

The following nursing diagnoses were identified for the Marino family:

● **Interrupted family processes** related to unsuccessful achievement of family developmental tasks and dysfunctional coping strategies evidenced by inability of family members to relate to each other in an adaptive manner; adolescents' unmet dependency needs; inability of family members to express a wide range of feelings and to send and receive clear messages.

● **Disabled family coping** related to highly ambivalent family relationships and lack of support evidenced by inability to problem-solve; each member copes in response to dysfunctional family processes with destructive behavior (John drinks, Nancy somaticizes, Peter drinks and withdraws; and Anna attempts suicide).

Outcome Identification

The following criteria were identified as measurement of outcomes in counseling of the Marino family:

● Family members will demonstrate effective communication patterns.
● Family members will express feelings openly and honestly.
● Family members will establish more adaptive coping strategies.
● Family members will be able to identify destructive patterns of functioning and problem-solve them effectively.
● Boundaries between spousal subsystems and spousal-children subsystems will become more clearly defined.
● Family members will establish stronger bonds with extended family.

Planning/Implementation

The Marino family will undoubtedly require many months of outpatient therapy. It is even likely that each member will need individual psychotherapy in addition to the family therapy. Once Anna has been stabilized physiologically and is discharged from the hospital, family/individual therapy will begin.

Several strategies for family therapy have been discussed in this chapter. As mentioned previously, family therapy has a strong theoretical framework and is performed by individuals with specialized education in family theory and process. Some advanced practice nurses possess the credentials required to perform family therapy. It is important, however, for all nurses to have some knowledge about working with families, to be able to assess family interaction, and to recognize when problems exist.

Some interventions with the Marino family might include the following:

1. Create a therapeutic environment that fosters trust, and in which the family members can feel safe and comfortable. The nurse can promote this type of environment by being empathetic, listening actively (see Chapter 8), accepting feelings and attitudes, and being nonjudgmental.
2. Promote effective communication by
   a. Seeking clarification when vague and generalized statements are made (e.g., Anna states, "I just want

my family to be like my friends' families." Nurse: "Anna, would you please explain to the group exactly what you mean by that?").

b. Setting clear limits (e.g., "Peter, it is okay to state when you are angry about something that has been said. It is not okay to throw the chair against the wall.").

c. Being consistent and fair (e.g., "I encourage each of you to contribute to the group process and to respect one another's opportunity to contribute equally.").

d. Addressing each individual clearly and directly and encouraging family members to do the same (e.g., "Nancy, I think it would be more appropriate if you directed that statement to John instead of to me.").

3. Identify patterns of interaction that interfere with successful problem resolution. For example, John asks Nancy many "Why?" questions that keep her on the defensive. He criticizes her for "always being sick." Nancy responds by frequently reminding John of his infidelity. Peter and Anna interrupt each other and their parents when the level of conflict reaches a certain point. Provide examples of more appropriate ways to communicate that can improve interpersonal relations and lead to more effective patterns of interaction.

4. Help the Marino family to identify problems that may necessitate change. Encourage each member to discuss a family process that he or she would like to change. As a group, promote discussion of what must take place for change to occur and allow each member to explore whether he or she could realistically cooperate with the necessary requirements for change.

5. As the problem-solving process progresses, encourage all family members to express honest feelings. Address each one directly, "John (Nancy, Peter, Anna), how do you feel about what the others are suggesting?" Ensure that all participants understand that each member may express honest feelings (e.g., anger, sadness, fear, anxiety, guilt, disgust, helplessness) without criticism, judgment, or fear of personal reprisal.

6. Avoid becoming triangled in the family emotional system. Remain neutral and objective. Do not take sides in family disagreements; instead, provide alternative explanations and suggestions (e.g., "Perhaps we can look at that situation in a different light. . .").

7. Reframe vague problem descriptions into ones for which resolution is more realistic. For example, rather than defining the problem as "We don't love each other any more," the problem could be defined as, "We do not spend time together in family activities any more." This definition evolves from the family members' description of what they mean by the more general problem description.

8. Discuss present coping strategies. Encourage each family member to describe how he or she copes with

stress and with the adversity within the family. Explore each member's possible contribution to the family's problems. Encourage family members to discuss possible solutions among themselves.

9. Identify community resources that may assist individual family members and provide support for establishing more adaptive coping mechanisms. For example, Alcoholics Anonymous for John; Al Anon for Nancy; and Al Ateen for Peter and Anna. Other groups that may be of assistance to this family include Emotions Anonymous, Parent's Support Group, Families Helping Families, Marriage Enrichment, Parents of Teenagers, and We Saved Our Marriage (WESOM). Local self-help networks often provide a directory of resources within specific communities.

10. Discuss with the family the possible need for psychotherapy for individual members. Provide names of therapists who would perform assessments to determine individual needs. Encourage follow-through with appointments.

11. Assist family members in planning leisure time activities together. This could include time to play together, exercise together, or engage in a shared project.

Evaluation

Evaluation is the final step in the nursing process. In this step, progress toward attainment of outcomes is measured.

1. Do family members demonstrate effective patterns of communication?
2. Can family members express feelings openly and honestly without fear of reprisal?
3. Can family members accept their own personal contribution to the family's problems?
4. Can individual members identify maladaptive coping methods and express a desire to improve?
5. Do family members work together to solve problems?
6. Can family members identify resources in the community from which they can seek assistance and support?
7. Do family members express a desire to form stronger bonds with the extended family?
8. Are family members willing to seek individual psychotherapy?
9. Are family members pursuing shared activities?

SUMMARY AND KEY POINTS

● Nurses must have sufficient knowledge of family functioning to assess family interaction and recognize when problems exist.
● Carter and McGoldrick (2005) identified six stages that describe the family life cycle. They include the following:
  ● The single young adult
  ● The newly married couple

- The family with young children
- The family with adolescents
- The family launching grown children
- The family in later life
- Tasks of families experiencing divorce and remarriage, and those that vary according to cultural norms were also presented.
- Families are assessed as functional or dysfunctional based on the following six elements: communication, self-concept reinforcement, family members' expectations, handling differences, family interactional patterns, and family climate.
- Bowen viewed the family as a system that was composed of various subsystems. His theoretical approach to family therapy includes eight major concepts: differentiation of self, triangles, nuclear family emotional process, family projection process, multigenerational transmission process, sibling position profiles, emotional cutoff, and societal regression.

- In the structural model of family therapy, the family is viewed as a social system within which the individual lives and to which the individual must adapt.
- In the strategic model of family therapy, communication is viewed as the foundation of functioning. Functional families are open systems where clear and precise messages are sent and received. Dysfunctional families are viewed as partially closed systems in which communication is vague, and messages are often inconsistent and incongruent with the situation.
- Many family therapists today follow an eclectic approach and incorporate concepts from several models into their practices.
- The nursing process is used as a framework for assessing, diagnosing, planning, implementing, and evaluating care to families who require assistance to maintain or regain adaptive functioning.

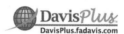

DavisPlus
DavisPlus.fadavis.com   For additional clinical tools and study aids, visit DavisPlus.

REVIEW QUESTIONS

Self-Examination/Learning Exercise

Match the tasks in the column on the left to the family life cycle stages listed on the right.

_____ 1. Renegotiation of the marital system as a dyad

_____ 2. Differentiation of self in relation to family of origin.

_____ 3. Dealing with loss of spouse, siblings, and peers.

_____ 4. Adjusting marital system to make space for children

_____ 5. Formation of the marital system.

_____ 6. Refocus on midlife marital and career issues.

a. The Single Young Adult

b. The Newly Married Couple

c. The Family With Young Children

d. The Family with Adolescents

e. The Family Launching Grown Children

f. The Family in Later Life

Select the answer that is most appropriate in each of the following questions.

7. The nurse-therapist is counseling the Smith family: Mr. and Mrs. Smith, 10-year-old Rob, and 8-year-old Lisa. When Mr. and Mrs. Smith start to argue, Rob hits Lisa and Lisa starts to cry. The Smiths then turn their attention to comforting Lisa and scolding Rob, complaining that he is "out of control and we don't know what to do about his behavior." These dynamics are an example of

   a. Double-bind messages.
   b. Triangulation.
   c. Pseudohostility.
   d. Multigenerational transmission.

8. Using Bowen's systems approach to therapy with the Smith's, the therapist would:

   a. Try to change family principles that may be promoting dysfunctional behavior patterns.
   b. Strive to create change in destructive behavior through improvement in communication and interaction patterns.
   c. Encourage increase in the differentiation of individual family members.
   d. Promote change in dysfunctional behavior by encouraging the formation of more diffuse boundaries between family members.

9. Using the structural approach to therapy with the Smith's, the therapist would:

   a. Try to change family principles that may be promoting dysfunctional behavior patterns.
   b. Strive to create change in destructive behavior through improvement in communications and interaction patterns.
   c. Encourage increase in the differentiation of individual family members.
   d. Promote change in dysfunctional behavior by encouraging the formation of more diffuse boundaries between family members.

10. Using the strategic approach to therapy with the Smith's, the therapist would:

   a. Try to change family principles that may be promoting dysfunctional behavior patterns.
   b. Strive to create change in destructive behavior through improvement in communication and interaction patterns.
   c. Encourage increase in the differentiation of individual family members.
   d. Promote change in dysfunctional behavior by encouraging the formation of more diffuse boundaries between family members.

REFERENCES

Bleifeld, B. (2006). Jewish families. *Building a Jewish Home.* Retrieved June 22, 2008 from http://www.chsweb.org/mc/building02. html

Boyer, P.A., & Jeffrey, R.J. (1994). *A guide for the family therapist.* Northvale, NJ: Jason Aronson.

Bramlett, M.D., & Mosher, W.D. (2002). Cohabitation, marriage, divorce, and remarriage in the United States. National Center for Health Statistics. *Vital and Health Statistics, 23*(22).

Carter, B., & McGoldrick, M. (2005). Overview: The expanded family life cycle: Individual, family, and social perspectives. In B. Carter & M. McGoldrick (Eds.), *The expanded family life cycle: Individual, family, and social perspectives* (3rd ed.). Boston: Allyn & Bacon.

Compendium of the Catechism of the Catholic Church. (2006). Washington, DC: United States Conference of Catholic Bishops.

Earp, J.B. K. (2004). Korean Americans. In J.N. Giger and R.E. Davidhizar (Eds.), *Transcultural nursing: Assessment and Intervention* (4th ed.). St. Louis: Mosby.

Georgetown Family Center. (2004a). Bowen theory: Differentiation of self. Retrieved June 22, 2008 from http://www.georgetownfamilycenter. org/ pages/conceptds.html

Georgetown Family Center. (2004b). Bowen theory: Societal emotional process. Retrieved June 22, 2008 from http:// www. georgetownfamilycenter.org/pages/conceptsep. html

Goldenberg, I., & Goldenberg. H. (2004). *Family therapy: An overview* (6th ed.). Belmont, CA: Wadsworth.

Goldenberg, I., & Goldenberg, H. (2005). Family therapy. In R.J. Corsini & D. Wedding (Eds.), *Current psychotherapies* (7th ed.). Belmont, CA: Wadsworth.

Kreider, R.M., & Fields, J.M. (2002). Number, timing, and duration of marriages and divorces. *Current population reports, P70–80.* Washington, DC: U.S. Census Bureau.

Kreider, R.M., & Fields, J.M. (2005). Living arrangements of children. *Current Population reports, P70–104.* Washington, DC: U.S. Census Bureau.

Leman, K. (2004). The birth order book: Why you are the way you are. Grand Rapids, MI: Baker Books.

Moriarty, H.J., & Brennan, S.M. (2005). Family mental health nursing. In S.M.H. Hanson, V. Gedaly-Duff, & J.R. Kaakinen (Eds.), *Family health care nursing: Theory, practice, and research* (3rd ed.). Philadelphia: F.A. Davis.

Nichols, M.P. & Schwartz, R.C. (2004). *Family therapy: Concepts and methods* (6th ed.). Boston, MA: Allyn and Bacon.

Parents Without Partners. (2006). *Facts about single parent families.* Retrieved June 22, 2008 from http://www.parentswithoutpartners. org/Support1.htm

Puri, S. (2004). Sex selection alive and well in South Asian immigrant communities in the U.S. *Pacific News Service.* Retrieved June 22, 2008 from http://news.newamericanmedia.org

Purnell, L.D. & Paulanka, B.J. (2003). Purnell's model for cultural competence. In L.D. Purnell & B.J. Paulanka (Eds.), *Transcultural health care: A culturally competent approach* (2nd ed.). Philadelphia: F.A. Davis.

Tomm, K., & Sanders, G. (1983). Family assessment in a problem oriented record. In J.C. Hansen, & B.F. Keeney (Eds.), *Diagnosis and assessment in family therapy.* London: Aspen Systems.

Wright, L.M., and Leahey, M. (2005). *Nurses and families: A guide to family assessment and intervention* (4th ed.). Philadelphia: F.A. Davis.

Wright, L.M., Watson, W.L., & Bell, J.M. (1996). *Beliefs: The heart of healing in families and illness.* New York: Basic Books.

CLASSICAL REFERENCES

Bowen, M. (1971). The use of family theory in clinical practice. In J. Haley (Ed.), *Changing families.* New York: Grune & Stratton.

Bowen, M. (1976). Theory in the practice of psychotherapy. In P. Guerin (Ed.), *Family therapy: Theory and practice.* New York: Gardner Press.

Bowen, M. (1978). *Family therapy in clinical practice.* New York: Jason Aronson.

Lidz, T., Cornelison, A., Fleck, S., & Terry, D. (1957). The intra-familial environment of schizophrenic patients: II. Marital schism and marital skew. *American Journal of Psychiatry, 114,* 241–248.

Minuchin, S. (1974). *Families and family therapy.* Cambridge, MA: Harvard University Press.

Milieu Therapy—The Therapeutic Community

CHAPTER OUTLINE

KEY TERMS

milieu
therapeutic community

CORE CONCEPT

milieu therapy

OBJECTIVES

After reading this chapter, the student will be able to:

1. Define *milieu therapy*.
2. Explain the goal of therapeutic community/milieu therapy.
3. Identify seven basic assumptions of a therapeutic community.
4. Discuss conditions that characterize a therapeutic community.

5. Identify the various therapies that may be included within the program of the therapeutic community and the health-care workers that make up the interdisciplinary treatment team.
6. Describe the role of the nurse on the interdisciplinary treatment team.

Standard 5c of the Psychiatric-Mental Health Nursing: Scope and Standards of Practice (ANA, 2007) states that, "The psychiatric-mental health nurse provides, structures, and maintains a safe and therapeutic environment in collaboration with patients, families, and other health care clinicians" (p. 39).

This chapter defines and explains the goal of milieu therapy. The conditions necessary for a therapeutic environment are discussed, and the roles of the various healthcare workers within the interdisciplinary team are

delineated. An interpretation of the nurse's role in milieu therapy is included.

MILIEU, DEFINED

The word *milieu* is French for "middle." The English translation of the word is "surroundings, or environment." In psychiatry, therapy involving the milieu, or environment, may be called milieu therapy, **therapeutic**

community, or therapeutic environment. The goal of milieu therapy is to manipulate the environment so that all aspects of the client's hospital experience are considered therapeutic. Within this therapeutic community setting the client is expected to learn adaptive coping, interaction, and relationship skills that can be generalized to other aspects of his or her life.

Milieu Therapy
A scientific structuring of the environment in order to effect behavioral changes and to improve the psychological health and functioning of the individual (Skinner, 1979).

CURRENT STATUS OF THE THERAPEUTIC COMMUNITY

Milieu therapy came into its own during the 1960s through early 1980s. During this period, psychiatric inpatient treatment provided sufficient time to implement programs of therapy that were aimed at social rehabilitation. Nursing's focus of establishing interpersonal relationships with clients fit well within this concept of therapy. Patients were encouraged to be active participants in their therapy, and individual autonomy was emphasized.

The current focus of inpatient psychiatric care has changed. Hall (1995) states:

Care in inpatient psychiatric facilities can now be characterized as short and biologically based. By the time patients have stabilized enough to benefit from the socialization that would take place in a milieu as treatment program, they [often] have been discharged. (p. 51)

Although strategies for milieu therapy are still used, they have been modified to conform to the short-term approach to care or to outpatient treatment programs. Some programs (e.g., those for children and adolescents, clients with substance addictions, and geriatric clients) have successfully adapted the concepts of milieu treatment to their specialty needs (Bowler, 1991; DeSocio, Bowllan, & Staschak, 1997; Whall, 1991).

Echternacht (2001) suggests that more emphasis should be placed on unstructured components of milieu therapy. She describes the unstructured components as a multitude of complex interactions between clients, staff, and visitors that occur around the clock. Echternacht calls these interactions "fluid group work." They involve spontaneous opportunities within the milieu environment for the psychiatric nurse to provide "on-the-spot therapeutic interventions designed to enhance socialization competency

and interpersonal relationship awareness. Emphasis is on social skills and activities in the context of interpersonal interactions" (p. 40). With fluid group work, the nurse applies psychotherapeutic knowledge and skills to brief clinical encounters that occur spontaneously in the therapeutic milieu setting. Echternacht (2001) believes that by using these techniques, nurses can "reclaim their milieu therapy functions in the midst of a changing health care environment" (p. 40).

Many of the original concepts of milieu therapy are presented in this chapter. It is important to remember that a number of modifications to these concepts have been applied in practice for use in a variety of settings.

BASIC ASSUMPTIONS

Skinner (1979) outlined seven basic assumptions on which a therapeutic community is based:

1. **The Health in Each Individual Is to Be Realized and Encouraged to Grow.** All individuals are considered to have strengths as well as limitations. These healthy aspects of the individual are identified and serve as a foundation for growth in the personality and in the ability to function more adaptively and productively in all aspects of life.
2. **Every Interaction Is an Opportunity for Therapeutic Intervention.** Within this structured setting, it is virtually impossible to avoid interpersonal interaction. The ideal situation exists for clients to improve communication and relationship development skills. Learning occurs from immediate feedback of personal perceptions.
3. **The Client Owns His or Her Own Environment.** Clients make decisions and solve problems related to government of the unit. In this way, personal needs for autonomy as well as needs that pertain to the group as a whole are fulfilled.
4. **Each Client Owns His or Her Behavior.** Each individual within the therapeutic community is expected to take responsibility for his or her own behavior.
5. **Peer Pressure Is a Useful and a Powerful Tool.** Behavioral group norms are established through peer pressure. Feedback is direct and frequent, so that behaving in a manner acceptable to the other members of the community becomes essential.
6. **Inappropriate Behaviors Are Dealt with as They Occur.** Individuals examine the significance of their behavior, look at how it affects other people, and discuss more appropriate ways of behaving in certain situations.
7. **Restrictions and Punishment Are to Be Avoided.** Destructive behaviors can usually be controlled with group discussion. However, if an individual requires external controls, temporary isolation is preferred over lengthy restriction or other harsh punishment.

CONDITIONS THAT PROMOTE A THERAPEUTIC COMMUNITY

In a **therapeutic community** setting, everything that happens to the client, or within the client's environment, is considered to be part of the treatment program. The community setting is the foundation for the program of treatment. Community factors—such as social interactions, the physical structure of the treatment setting, and schedule of activities—may generate negative responses from some clients. These stressful experiences are used as examples to help the client learn how to manage stress more adaptively in real-life situations.

Under what conditions, then, is a hospital environment considered therapeutic? A number of criteria have been identified:

1. **Basic Physiological Needs Are Fulfilled.** As Maslow (1968) has suggested, individuals do not move to higher levels of functioning until the basic biological needs for food, water, air, sleep, exercise, elimination, shelter, and sexual expression have been met.

2. **The Physical Facilities Are Conducive to Achievement of the Goals of Therapy.** Space is provided so that each client has sufficient privacy, as well as physical space, for therapeutic interaction with others. Furnishings are arranged to present a homelike atmosphere—usually in spaces that accommodate communal living, dining, and activity areas—for facilitation of interpersonal interaction and communication.

3. **A Democratic Form of Self-Government Exists.** In the therapeutic community, clients participate in the decision making and problem solving that affect the management of the treatment setting. This is accomplished through regularly scheduled community meetings. These meetings are attended by staff and clients, and all individuals have equal input into the discussions. At these meetings, the norms and rules and behavioral limits of the treatment setting are set forth. This reinforces the democratic posture of the treatment setting, because these are expectations that affect all clients on an equal basis. An example might be the rule that no client may enter a room being occupied by a client of the opposite sex. Consequences of violating the rules are explained. Other issues that may be discussed at the community meetings include those with which certain clients have some disagreements. A decision is then made by the entire group in a democratic manner. For example, several clients in an inpatient unit may disagree with the hours that have been designated for watching television on a weekend night. They may elect to bring up this issue at a community meeting and suggest an extension in television-viewing time. After discussion by the group, a vote will be taken, and clients and staff agree to abide by the expressed preference of the majority. Some therapeutic communities elect officers (usually a president and a secretary) who serve for a specified time. The president calls the meeting to order, conducts the business of discussing old and new issues, and asks for volunteers (or makes appointments, alternately, so that all clients have a turn) to accomplish the daily tasks associated with community living; for example, cleaning the tables after each meal and watering plants in the treatment facility. New assignments are made at each meeting. The secretary reads the minutes of the previous meeting and takes minutes of the current meeting. Minutes are important in the event that clients have a disagreement about issues that were discussed at various meetings. Minutes provide written evidence of decisions made by the group. In treatment settings where clients have short attention spans or disorganized thinking, meetings are brief. Business is generally limited to introductions and expectations of the here and now. Discussions also may include comments about a recent occurrence in the group or something that has been bothering a member and about which he or she has some questions. These meetings are usually conducted by staff, although all clients have equal input into the discussions.

All clients are expected to attend the meetings. Exceptions are made for times when aspects of therapy interfere (e.g., scheduled testing, X-ray examinations, electroencephalograms). An explanation is made to clients present so that false perceptions of danger are not generated by another person's absence. All staff members are expected to attend the meetings, unless client care precludes their attendance.

4. **Responsibilities Are Assigned According to Client Capabilities.** Increasing self-esteem is an ultimate goal of the therapeutic community. Therefore, a client should not be set up for failure by being assigned a responsibility that is beyond his or her level of ability. By assigning clients responsibilities that promote achievement, self-esteem is enhanced. Consideration must also be given to times during which the client will show some regression in the treatment regimen. Adjustments in assignments should be made in a way that preserves self-esteem and provides for progression to greater degrees of responsibility as the client returns to previous level of functioning.

5. **A Structured Program of Social and Work-Related Activities Is Scheduled as Part of the Treatment Program.** Each client's therapeutic program consists of group activities in which interpersonal interaction and communication with other individuals are emphasized. Time is also devoted to personal problems. Various group activities may be selected for clients with specific needs (e.g., an exercise group for a person who expresses anger inappropriately, an assertiveness group for a person who is passive-aggressive, or a

stress-management group for a person who is anxious). A structured schedule of activities is the major focus of a therapeutic community. Through these activities, change in the client's personality and behavior can be achieved. New coping strategies are learned and social skills are developed. In the group situation, the client is able to practice what he or she has learned to prepare for transition to the general community.

6. **Community and Family Are Included in the Program of Therapy in an Effort to Facilitate Discharge from Treatment.** An attempt is made to include family members, as well as certain aspects of the community that affect the client, in the treatment program. It is important to keep as many links to the client's life outside of therapy as possible. Family members are invited to participate in specific therapy groups and, in some instances, to share meals with the client in the communal dining room. Connection with community life may be maintained through client group activities, such as shopping, picnicking, attending movies, bowling, and visiting the zoo. Inpatient clients may be awarded passes to visit family or may participate in work-related activities, the length of time being determined by the activity and the client's condition. These connections with family and community facilitate the discharge process and may help to prevent the client from becoming too dependent on the therapy.

THE PROGRAM OF THERAPEUTIC COMMUNITY

Care for clients in the therapeutic community is directed by an interdisciplinary treatment (IDT) team. An initial assessment is made by the admitting psychiatrist, nurse, or other designated admitting agent who establishes a priority of care. The IDT team determines a comprehensive treatment plan and goals of therapy and assigns intervention responsibilities. All members sign the treatment plan and meet regularly to update the plan as needed. Depending on the size of the treatment facility and scope of the therapy program, members representing a variety of disciplines may participate in the promotion of a therapeutic community. For example, an IDT team may include a psychiatrist, clinical psychologist, psychiatric clinical nurse specialist, psychiatric nurse, mental health technician, psychiatric social worker, occupational therapist, recreational therapist, art therapist, music therapist, psychodramatist, dietitian, and chaplain. Table 12–1 provides an explanation of responsibilities and educational preparation required for these members of the IDT team.

TABLE 12–1	The Interdisciplinary Treatment Team in Psychiatry	
Team Member	**Responsibilities**	**Credentials**
Psychiatrist	Serves as the leader of the team. Responsible for diagnosis and treatment of mental disorders. Performs psychotherapy; prescribes medication and other somatic therapies.	Medical degree with residency in psychiatry and license to practice medicine.
Clinical psychologist	Conducts individual, group, and family therapy. Administers, interprets, and evaluates psychological tests that assist in the diagnostic process.	Doctorate in clinical psychology with 2- to 3-year internship supervised by a licensed clinical psychologist. State license is required to practice.
Psychiatric clinical nurse specialist	Conducts individual, group, and family therapy. Presents educational programs for nursing staff. Provides consultation services to nurses who require assistance in the planning and implementation of care for individual clients.	Registered nurse with minimum of a master's degree in psychiatric nursing. Some institutions require certification by national credentialing association
Psychiatric nurse	Provides ongoing assessment of client condition, both mentally and physically. Manages the therapeutic milieu on a 24-hour basis. Administers medications. Assists clients with all therapeutic activities as required. Focus is on one-to-one relationship development.	Registered nurse with hospital diploma, associate degree, or baccalaureate degree. Some psychiatric nurses have national certification.
Mental health technician (also called psychiatric aide or assistant or psychiatric technician)	Functions under the supervision of the psychiatric nurse. Provides assistance to clients in the fulfillment of their activities of daily living. Assists activity therapists as required in conducting their groups. May also participate in one-to-one relationship development.	Varies from state to state. Requirements include high school education, with additional vocational education or on-the-job training. Some hospitals hire individuals with baccalaureate degree in psychology in this capacity. Some states require a licensure examination to practice.
Psychiatric social worker	Conducts individual, group, and family therapy. Is concerned with client's social needs, such as placement, financial support, and community requirements. Conducts in-depth psychosocial history on which the needs assessment is based. Works with client and family to ensure that requirements for discharge are fulfilled and needs can be met by appropriate community resources.	Minimum of a master's degree in social work. Some states require additional supervision and subsequent licensure by examination.

Team Member	Responsibilities	Credentials
Occupational therapist	Works with clients to help develop (or redevelop) independence in performance of activities of daily living. Focus is on rehabilitation and vocational training in which clients learn to be productive, thereby enhancing self-esteem. Creative activities and therapeutic relationship skills are used.	Baccalaureate or master's degree in occupational therapy.
Recreational therapist	Uses recreational activities to promote clients to redirect their thinking or to rechannel destructive energy in an appropriate manner. Clients learn skills that can be used during leisure time and during times of stress following discharge from treatment. Examples include bowling, volleyball, exercises, and jogging. Some programs include activities such as picnics, swimming, and even group attendance at the state fair when it is in session.	Baccalaureate or master's degree in recreational therapy.
Music therapist	Encourages clients in self-expression through music. Clients listen to music, play instruments, sing, dance, and compose songs that help them get in touch with feelings and emotions that they may not be able to experience in any other way.	Graduate degree with specialty in music therapy.
Art therapist	Uses the client's creative abilities to encourage expression of emotions and feelings through artwork. Helps clients to analyze their own work in an effort to recognize and resolve underlying conflict.	Graduate degree with specialty in art therapy.
Psychodramatist	Directs clients in the creation of a "drama" that portrays real-life situations. Individuals select problems they wish to enact, and other clients play the roles of significant others in the situations. Some clients are able to "act out" problems that they are unable to work through in a more traditional manner. All members benefit through intensive discussion that follows.	Graduate degree in psychology, social work, nursing, or medicine with additional training in group therapy and specialty preparation to become a psychodramatist.
Dietitian	Plans nutritious meals for all clients. Works on consulting basis for clients with specific eating disorders, such as anorexia nervosa, bulimia nervosa, obesity, & pica.	Baccalaureate or master's degree with specialty in dietetics.
Chaplain	Assesses, identifies, and attends to the spiritual needs of clients and their family members. Provides spiritual support and comfort as requested by client or family. May provide counseling if educational background includes this type of preparation.	College degree with advanced education in theology, seminary, or rabbinical studies.

THE ROLE OF THE NURSE

Milieu therapy can take place in a variety of inpatient and outpatient settings. In the hospital, nurses are generally the only members of the IDT team who spend time with the clients on a 24-hour basis, and they assume responsibility for management of the therapeutic milieu. In all settings, the nursing process is used for the delivery of nursing care. Ongoing assessment, diagnosis, outcome identification, planning, implementation, and evaluation of the environment are necessary for the successful management of a therapeutic milieu. Nurses are involved in all day-to-day activities that pertain to client care. Suggestions and opinions of nursing staff are given serious consideration in the planning of care for individual clients. Information from the initial nursing assessment is used to create the IDT plan. Nurses have input into therapy goals and participate in the regular updates and modification of treatment plans.

In some treatment facilities, a separate nursing care plan is required in addition to the IDT plan. When this is the case, the nursing care plan must reflect diagnoses that are specific to nursing and include problems and interventions from the IDT plan that have been assigned specifically to the discipline of nursing.

In the therapeutic milieu, nurses are responsible for ensuring that clients' physiological needs are met. Clients must be encouraged to perform as independently as possible in fulfilling activities of daily living. However, the nurse must make ongoing assessments to provide assistance for those who require it. Assessing physical status is an important nursing responsibility that must not be overlooked in a psychiatric setting that emphasizes holistic care.

Reality orientation for clients who have disorganized thinking or who are disoriented or confused is important in the therapeutic milieu. Clocks with large hands and numbers, calendars that give the day and date in large print, and orientation boards that discuss daily activities and news happenings can help keep clients oriented to reality. Nurses should ensure that clients have written schedules of activities to which they are assigned and that they arrive at those activities on schedule. Some clients may require an identification sign on their door to remind them which room is theirs. On short-term units, nurses who are dealing with psychotic clients usually rely on a basic activity or topic that helps keep people oriented. For example, showing pictures of the hospital where they are housed, introducing people who were admitted during the night, and providing name badges with their first name.

Nurses are responsible for the management of medication administration on inpatient psychiatric units. In some treatment programs, clients are expected to accept the responsibility and request their medication at the appropriate time. Although ultimate responsibility lies with the nurse, he or she must encourage clients to be self-reliant. Nurses must work with the clients to determine methods that result in achievement and provide positive feedback for successes.

A major focus of nursing in the therapeutic milieu is the one-to-one relationship, which grows out of a developing trust between client and nurse. Many clients with psychiatric disorders have never achieved the ability to trust. If this can be accomplished in a relationship with the nurse, the trust may be generalized to other relationships in the client's life. Developing trust means keeping promises that have been made. It means total acceptance of the individual as a person, separate from behavior that is unacceptable. It means responding to the client with concrete behaviors that are understandable to him or her (e.g., "If you are frightened, I will stay with you"; "If you are cold, I will bring you a blanket"; "If you are thirsty, I will bring you a drink of water"). Within an atmosphere of trust, the client is encouraged to express feelings and emotions and to discuss unresolved issues that are creating problems in his or her life.

The nurse is responsible for setting limits on unacceptable behavior in the therapeutic milieu. This requires stating to the client in understandable terminology what behaviors are not acceptable and what the consequences will be should the limits be violated. These limits must be established, written, and carried out by all staff. Consistency in carrying out the consequences of violation of the established limits is essential if the learning is to be reinforced.

The role of client teacher is important in the psychiatric area, as it is in all areas of nursing. Nurses must be able to assess learning readiness in individual clients. Do they want to learn? What is their level of anxiety? What is their level of ability to understand the information being presented? Topics for client education in psychiatry include information about medical diagnoses, side effects of medications, the importance of continuing to take medications, and stress management, among others.

Some topics must be individualized for specific clients, whereas others may be taught in group situations. Box 12–1 outlines various topics of nursing concern for client education in psychiatry.

Echternacht (2001) states:

Milieu therapy interventions are recognized as one of the basic-level functions of psychiatric mental health nurses as addressed [in the Psychiatric-Mental Health Nursing: Scope and Standard of Practice (ANA, 2007)]. Milieu therapy has been described as an excellent framework for operationalizing [Hildegard] Peplau's interpretation and extension of Harry Stack Sullivan's Interpersonal Theory for use in nursing practice. (p. 39)

Now is the time to rekindle interest in the therapeutic milieu concept and to reclaim nursing's traditional milieu intervention functions. Nurses need to identify the number of registered nurses necessary to carry out structured and unstructured milieu functions consistent with their Standards of Practice. (p. 43)

BOX 1 2 – 1 The Therapeutic Milieu—Topics for Client Education

1. Ways to increase self-esteem
2. Ways to deal with anger appropriately
3. Stress-management techniques
4. How to recognize signs of increasing anxiety and intervene to stop progression
5. Normal stages of grieving and behaviors associated with each stage
6. Assertiveness techniques
7. Relaxation techniques
   a. Progressive relaxation
   b. Tense and relax
   c. Deep breathing
   d. Autogenics
8. Medications (specify)
   a. Reason for taking
   b. Harmless side effects
   c. Side effects to report to physician
   d. Importance of taking regularly
   e. Importance of not stopping abruptly
9. Effects of (substance) on the body
   a. Alcohol
   b. Other depressants
   c. Stimulants
   d. Hallucinogens
   e. Narcotics
   f. Cannabinols
10. Problem-solving skills
11. Thought-stopping/thought-switching techniques
12. Sex education
    a. Structure and function of reproductive system
    b. Contraceptives
    c. Sexually transmitted diseases
13. The essentials of good nutrition
14. (For parents/guardians)
    a. Signs and symptoms of substance abuse
    b. Effective parenting techniques

SUMMARY AND KEY POINTS

- In psychiatry, milieu therapy (or a therapeutic community) constitutes a manipulation of the environment in an effort to create behavioral changes and to improve the psychological health and functioning of the individual.
- The goal of therapeutic community is for the client to learn adaptive coping, interaction, and relationship skills that can be generalized to other aspects of his or her life.
- The community environment itself serves as the primary tool of therapy.
- According to Skinner (1979), a therapeutic community is based on seven basic assumptions:
  - The health in each individual is to be realized and encouraged to grow.
  - Every interaction is an opportunity for therapeutic intervention.
  - The client owns his or her own environment.
  - Each client owns his or her behavior.
  - Peer pressure is a useful and a powerful tool.
  - Inappropriate behaviors are dealt with as they occur.
  - Restrictions and punishment are to be avoided.
- Because the goals of milieu therapy relate to helping the client learn to generalize that which is learned to other aspects of his or her life, the conditions that promote a therapeutic community in the psychiatric setting are similar to the types of conditions that exist in real-life situations.
- Conditions that promote a therapeutic community include the following:
  - The fulfillment of basic physiological needs.
  - Physical facilities that are conducive to achievement of the goals of therapy.
  - The existence of a democratic form of self-government.
  - The assignment of responsibilities according to client capabilities.
  - A structured program of social and work-related activities.
  - The inclusion of community and family in the program of therapy in an effort to facilitate discharge from treatment.
- The program of therapy on the milieu unit is conducted by the IDT team.
- The team includes some, or all, of the following disciplines and may include others that are not specified here: psychiatrist, clinical psychologist, psychiatric clinical nurse specialist, psychiatric nurse, mental health technician, psychiatric social worker, occupational therapist, recreational therapists, art therapist, music therapist, psychodramatist, dietitian, and chaplain.
- Nurses play a crucial role in the management of a therapeutic milieu. They are involved in the assessment, diagnosis, outcome identification, planning, implementation, and evaluation of all treatment programs.
- Nurses have significant input into the IDT plans, which are developed for all clients. They are responsible for ensuring that clients' basic needs are fulfilled; assessing physical and psychosocial status; administering medication; helping the client develop trusting relationships; setting limits on unacceptable behaviors; educating clients; and ultimately, helping clients, within the limits of their capability, to become productive members of society.

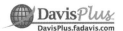 **DavisPlus** For additional clinical tools and
DavisPlus.fadavis.com study aids, visit DavisPlus.

REVIEW QUESTIONS

Self-Examination/Learning Exercise

Test your knowledge of milieu therapy by supplying the information requested.

1. Define *milieu therapy*.

2. What is the goal of milieu therapy/therapeutic community?

Select the best response in each of the following questions:

3. In prioritizing care within the therapeutic environment, which of the following nursing interventions would receive the highest priority?
   a. Ensuring that the physical facilities are conducive to achievement of the goals of therapy.
   b. Scheduling a community meeting for 8:30 each morning.
   c. Attending to the nutritional and comfort needs of all clients.
   d. Establishing contacts with community resources.

4. In the community meeting, which of the following actions is most important for reinforcing the democratic posture of the therapy setting?
   a. Allowing each person a specific and equal amount of time to talk.
   b. Reviewing group rules and behavioral limits that apply to all clients.
   c. Reading the minutes from yesterday's meeting.
   d. Waiting until all clients are present before initiating the meeting.

5. One of the goals of therapeutic community is for clients to become more independent and accept self-responsibility. Which of the following approaches by staff best encourages fulfillment of this goal?
   a. Including client input and decisions into the treatment plan.
   b. Insisting that each client take a turn as "president" of the community meeting.
   c. Making decisions for the client regarding plans for treatment.
   d. Requiring that the client be bathed, dressed and attend breakfast on time each morning.

6. Client teaching is an important nursing function in milieu therapy. Which of the following statements by the client indicates the need for knowledge and a readiness to learn?
   a. "Get away from me with that medicine! I'm not sick!"
   b. "I don't need psychiatric treatment. It's my migraine headaches that I need help with."
   c. "I've taken Valium every day of my life for the last 20 years. I'll stop when I'm good and ready!"
   d. "The doctor says I have bipolar disorder. What does that really mean?"

Match the following activities with the responsible therapist from the IDT team.

_____ 7. Psychiatrist   a. Helps clients plan, shop for, and cook a meal.

_____ 8. Clinical psychologist   b. Locates halfway house and arranges living conditions for client being discharged from the hospital.

_____ 9. Psychiatric social worker   c. Helps clients get to know themselves better by having them describe what they feel when they hear a certain song.

_____ 10. Psychiatric clinical nurse specialist   d. Helps clients to recognize their own beliefs so that they may draw comfort from those beliefs in time of spiritual need.

_____ 11. Psychiatric nurse   e. Accompanies clients on community trip to the zoo.

_____ 12. Mental health technician   f. Diagnoses mental disorders, conducts psychotherapy, and prescribes somatic therapies.

_____13. Occupational therapist

g. Manages the therapeutic milieu on a 24-hour basis.

_____14. Recreational therapist

h. Conducts group and family therapies and administers and evaluates psychological tests that assist in the diagnostic process.

_____15. Music therapist

i. Conducts group therapies and provides consultation and education to staff nurses.

_____16. Art therapist

j. Assists staff nurses in the management of the milieu.

_____17. Psychodramatist

k. Encourages clients to express painful emotions by drawing pictures on paper.

_____18. Dietitian

l. Assesses needs, establishes, monitors, and evaluates a nutritional program for a client with anorexia nervosa.

_____19. Chaplain

m. Directs a group of clients in acting out a situation that is otherwise too painful for a client to discuss openly.

REFERENCES

American Nurses' Association (2007). *Psychiatric-mental health nursing: Scope and standards of practice.* Silver Spring, MD: American Nurses' Association.

Bowler, J.B. (1991). Transformation into a healing healthcare environment: Recovering the possibilities of psychiatric/mental health nursing. *Perspectives in Psychiatric Care, 27*(2), 21–25.

DeSocio, J., Bowllan, N., & Staschak, S. (1997). Lessons learned in creating a safe and therapeutic milieu for children, adolescents, and families: Developmental considerations. *Journal of Child and Adolescent Psychiatric Nursing, 10*(4), 18–26.

Echternacht, M.R. (2001). Fluid group: Concept and clinical application in the therapeutic milieu. *Journal of the American Psychiatric Nurses Association, 7*(2), 39–44.

Hall, B.A. (1995). Use of milieu therapy: The context and environment as therapeutic practice for psychiatric-mental health nurses. In C.A. Anderson (Ed.), *Psychiatric nursing 1974 to 1994: A report on the state of the art.* St. Louis: Mosby-Year Book.

Whall, A.L. (1991). Using the environment to improve the mental health of the elderly. *Journal of Gerontological Nursing, 17*(7), 39.

CLASSICAL REFERENCES

Maslow, A. (1968). *Towards a psychology of being* (2nd ed.). New York: D. Van Nostrand.

Skinner, K. (1979, August). The therapeutic milieu: Making it work. *Journal of Psychiatric Nursing and Mental Health Services,* 38–44.

Crisis Intervention

CHAPTER OUTLINE

KEY TERMS

crisis intervention   disaster

CORE CONCEPT

crisis

OBJECTIVES

After reading this chapter, the student will be able to:

1. Define *crisis*.
2. Describe four phases in the development of a crisis.
3. Identify types of crises that occur in people's lives.
4. Discuss the goal of crisis intervention.
5. Describe the steps in crisis intervention.
6. Identify the role of the nurse in crisis intervention.
7. Apply the nursing process to care of victims of disasters.

Stressful situations are a part of everyday life. Any stressful situation can precipitate a crisis. Crises result in a disequilibrium from which many individuals require assistance to recover. Crisis intervention requires problem-solving skills that are often diminished by the level of anxiety accompanying disequilibrium. Assistance with problem solving

CORE CONCEPT

Crisis

A sudden event in one's life that disturbs homeostasis, during which usual coping mechanisms cannot resolve the problem (Lagerquist, 2006).

during the crisis period preserves self-esteem and promotes growth with resolution.

In recent years, individuals in the United States have been faced with a number of catastrophic events, including natural disasters such as tornados, earthquakes, hurricanes, and floods. Also, manmade disasters, such as the Oklahoma City bombing and the attacks on the World Trade Center and the Pentagon, have created psychological stress of astronomical proportions in populations around the world.

This chapter examines the phases in the development of a crisis and the types of crises that occur in people's lives. The methodology of crisis intervention, including the role of the nurse, is explored. A discussion of disaster nursing is also presented.

CHARACTERISTICS OF A CRISIS

A number of characteristics have been identified that can be viewed as assumptions upon which the concept of crisis is based (Aguilera, 1998; Caplan, 1964; Winston, 2008). They include the following:

1. Crisis occurs in all individuals at one time or another and is not necessarily equated with psychopathology.
2. Crises are precipitated by specific identifiable events.
3. Crises are personal by nature. What may be considered a crisis situation by one individual may not be so for another.
4. Crises are acute, not chronic, and will be resolved in one way or another within a brief period.
5. A crisis situation contains the potential for psychological growth or deterioration.

Individuals who are in crisis feel helpless to change. They do not believe they have the resources to deal with the precipitating stressor. Levels of anxiety rise to the point that the individual becomes nonfunctional, thoughts become obsessional, and all behavior is aimed at relief of the anxiety being experienced. The feeling is overwhelming and may affect the individual physically as well as psychologically.

Bateman and Peternelj-Taylor (1998) state:

> Outside Western culture, a crisis is often viewed as a time for movement and growth. The Chinese symbol for crisis consists of the characters for *danger* and *opportunity* [Figure 13–1]. When a crisis is viewed as an opportunity for growth, those involved are much more capable of resolving related issues and more able to move toward positive changes. When the crisis experience is overwhelming because of its scope and nature or when there has not been adequate preparation for the necessary changes, the dangers seem paramount and overshadow any potential growth. The results are maladaptive coping and dysfunctional behavior. (pp. 144–145)

PHASES IN THE DEVELOPMENT OF A CRISIS

The development of a crisis situation follows a relatively predictable course. Caplan (1964) outlined four specific phases through which individuals progress in response to

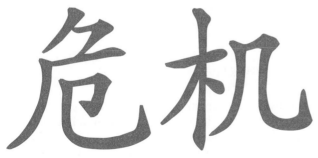

FIGURE 13–1 Chinese symbol for crisis.

a precipitating stressor and that culminate in the state of acute crisis.

Phase 1. *The individual is exposed to a precipitating stressor.* Anxiety increases; previous problem-solving techniques are employed.

Phase 2. *When previous problem-solving techniques do not relieve the stressor, anxiety increases further.* The individual begins to feel a great deal of discomfort at this point. Coping techniques that have worked in the past are attempted, only to create feelings of helplessness when they are not successful. Feelings of confusion and disorganization prevail.

Phase 3. *All possible resources, both internal and external, are called on to resolve the problem and relieve the discomfort.* The individual may try to view the problem from a different perspective, or even to overlook certain aspects of it. New problem-solving techniques may be used, and, if effectual, resolution may occur at this phase, with the individual returning to a higher, a lower, or the previous level of premorbid functioning.

Phase 4. *If resolution does not occur in previous phases, Caplan states that "the tension mounts beyond a further threshold or its burden increases over time to a breaking point. Major disorganization of the individual with drastic results often occurs."* Anxiety may reach panic levels. Cognitive functions are disordered, emotions are labile, and behavior may reflect the presence of psychotic thinking.

These phases are congruent with the transactional model of stress/adaptation outlined in Chapter 1. The relationship between the two perspectives is presented in Figure 13–2. Similarly, Aguilera (1998) spoke of "balancing factors" that affect the way in which an individual perceives and responds to a precipitating stressor. A schematic of these balancing factors is illustrated in Figure 13–3.

The paradigm set forth by Aguilera suggests that whether or not an individual experiences a crisis in response to a stressful situation depends upon the following three factors:

1. **The individual's perception of the event.** If the event is perceived realistically, the individual is more likely to draw upon adequate resources to restore equilibrium. If the perception of the event is distorted, attempts at problem solving are likely to be ineffective, and restoration of equilibrium goes unresolved.
2. **The availability of situational supports.** Aguilera states, "Situational supports are those persons who are available in the environment and who can be depended on to help solve the problem" (p. 37). Without adequate situational supports during a stressful situation, an individual is most likely to feel overwhelmed and alone.
3. **The availability of adequate coping mechanisms.** When a stressful situation occurs, individuals draw upon behavioral strategies that have been successful

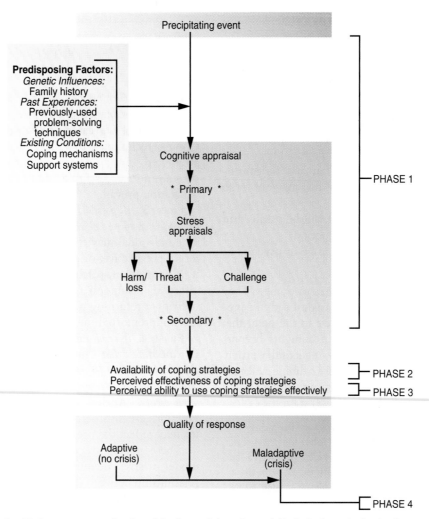

FIGURE 13–2 Relationship between transactional models of stress/adaptation and Caplan's phases in the development of a crisis.

for them in the past. If these coping strategies work, a crisis may be diverted. If not, disequilibrium may continue and tension and anxiety increase.

As previously set forth, it is assumed that crises are acute, not chronic, situations that will be resolved in one way or another within a brief period. Winston (2008) states, "Crises tend to be time limited, generally lasting no more than a few months; the duration depends on the stressor and on the individual's perception of and response to the stressor" (p. 1270). Crises can become growth opportunities when individuals learn new methods of coping that can be preserved and used when similar stressors recur.

TYPES OF CRISES

Baldwin (1978) identified six classes of emotional crises, which progress by degree of severity. As the measure of psychopathology increases, the source of the stressor changes from external to internal. The type of crisis determines the method of intervention selected.

Class 1: Dispositional Crises

Definition: An acute response to an external situational stressor.

Example:

Nancy and Ted have been married for 3 years and have a 1-year-old daughter. Ted has been having difficulty with his boss at work. Twice during the past 6 months he has exploded in anger at home and become abusive with Nancy. Last night he became angry that dinner was not ready when he expected. He grabbed the baby from Nancy and tossed her, screaming, into her crib. He hit and punched Nancy until she feared for her life. This morning when he left for work, she took the baby and went to the emergency department of the city hospital, not having anywhere else to go.

Intervention: Nancy's physical wounds were cared for in the emergency department. The mental health counselor provided support and guidance in terms of presenting alternatives to her. Needs and issues were clarified, and referrals for agency assistance were made.

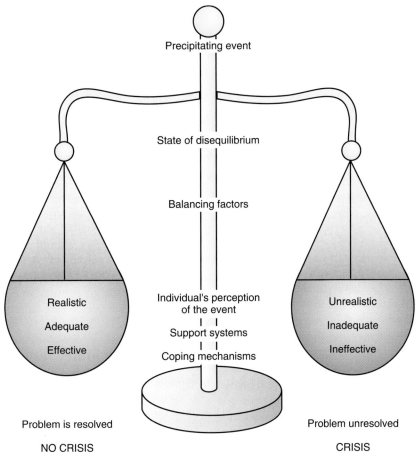

FIGURE 13–3   Effects of balancing factors in a stressful event.

Class 2: Crises of Anticipated Life Transitions

Definition: Normal life-cycle transitions that may be anticipated but over which the individual may feel a lack of control.

Example:

College student J.T. is placed on probationary status because of low grades this semester. His wife had a baby and had to quit her job. He increased his working hours from part time to full time to compensate, and therefore had little time for studies. He presents himself to the student-health nurse practitioner complaining of numerous vague physical complaints.

Intervention: Physical examination should be performed (physical symptoms could be caused by depression) and ventilation of feelings encouraged. Reassurance and support should be provided as needed. The client should be referred to services that can provide financial and other types of needed assistance. Problematic areas should be identified and approaches to change discussed.

Class 3: Crises Resulting from Traumatic Stress

Definition: Crises precipitated by unexpected external stresses over which the individual has little or no control and from which he or she feels emotionally overwhelmed and defeated.

Example:

Sally is a waitress whose shift ends at midnight. Two weeks ago, while walking to her car in the deserted parking lot, she was abducted by two men with guns, taken to an abandoned building, and raped and beaten. Since that time, her physical wounds have nearly healed. However, Sally cannot be alone, is constantly fearful, relives the experience in flashbacks and dreams, and is unable to eat, sleep, or work at her job in the restaurant. Her friend offers to accompany her to the mental health clinic.

Intervention: The nurse should encourage Sally to talk about the experience and to express her feelings associated with it. The nurse should offer reassurance and support; discuss stages of grief and how rape causes a loss of self-worth, triggering the grief response; identify support systems that can help Sally to resume her normal activities; and explore new methods of coping with emotions arising from a situation with which she has had no previous experience.

Class 4: Maturational/Developmental Crises

Definition: Crises that occur in response to situations that trigger emotions related to unresolved conflicts in one's life. These crises are of internal origin and reflect underlying developmental issues that involve dependency, value conflicts, sexual identity, control, and capacity for emotional intimacy.

Example:

Bob is 40 years old. He has just been passed over for a job promotion for the third time. He has moved many times within the large company for which he works, usually after angering and alienating himself from the supervisor. His father was domineering and became abusive when Bob did not comply with his every command. Over the years, Bob's behavioral response became one of passive-aggressiveness—first with his father, then with his supervisors. This third rejection has created feelings of depression and intense anxiety in Bob. At his wife's insistence, he has sought help at the mental health clinic.

Intervention: The primary intervention is to help the individual identify the unresolved developmental issue that is creating the conflict. Support and guidance are offered during the initial crisis period, then assistance is given to help the individual work through the underlying conflict in an effort to change response patterns that are creating problems in his current life situation.

Class 5: Crises Reflecting Psychopathology

Definition: Emotional crises in which preexisting psychopathology has been instrumental in precipitating the crisis or in which psychopathology significantly impairs or complicates adaptive resolution. Examples of psychopathology that may precipitate crises include borderline personality, severe neuroses, characterological disorders, or schizophrenia.

Example:

Sonja, age 29, was diagnosed with borderline personality at age 18. She has been in therapy on a weekly basis for 10 years, with several hospitalizations for suicide attempts during that time. She has had the same therapist for the past 6 years. This therapist told Sonja today that

she is to be married in 1 month and will be moving across the country with her new husband. Sonja is distraught and experiencing intense feelings of abandonment. She is found wandering in and out of traffic on a busy expressway, oblivious to her surroundings. Police bring her to the emergency department of the hospital.

Intervention: The initial intervention is to help bring down the level of anxiety in Sonja that has created feelings of unreality in her. She requires that someone stay with her and reassure her of her safety and security. After the feelings of panic anxiety have subsided, she should be encouraged to verbalize her feelings of abandonment. Regressive behaviors should be discouraged. Positive reinforcement should be given for independent activities and accomplishments. The primary therapist will need to pursue this issue of termination with Sonja at length. Referral to a long-term care facility may be required.

Class 6: Psychiatric Emergencies

Definition: Crisis situations in which general functioning has been severely impaired and the individual rendered incompetent or unable to assume personal responsibility. Examples include acutely suicidal individuals, drug overdoses, reactions to hallucinogenic drugs, acute psychoses, uncontrollable anger, and alcohol intoxication.

Example:

Jennifer, age 16, had been dating Joe, the star high school football player, for 6 months. After the game on Friday night, Jennifer and Joe went to Jackie's house, where a number of high school students had gathered for an after-game party. No adults were present. About midnight, Joe told Jennifer that he did not want to date her anymore. Jennifer became hysterical, and Jackie was frightened by her behavior. She took Jennifer to her parent's bedroom and gave her a Valium from a bottle in her mother's medicine cabinet. She left Jennifer lying on her parent's bed and returned to the party downstairs. About an hour later, she returned to her parent's bedroom and found that Jennifer had removed the bottle of Valium from the cabinet and swallowed all of the tablets. Jennifer was unconscious and Jackie could not awaken her. An ambulance was called and Jennifer was transported to the local hospital.

Intervention: The crisis team monitored vital signs, ensured maintenance of adequate airway, initiated gastric lavage, and administered activated charcoal to minimize absorption. Jennifer's parents were notified and rushed to the hospital.

The situation was explained to them, and they were encouraged to stay by her side. When the physical crisis was resolved, Jennifer was transferred to the psychiatric unit. In therapy, she was encouraged to ventilate her feelings regarding the rejection and subsequent overdose. Family therapy sessions were conducted in an effort to clarify interpersonal issues and to identify areas for change. On an individual level, Jennifer's therapist worked with her to establish more adaptive methods of coping with stressful situations.

CRISIS INTERVENTION

Individuals experiencing crises have an urgent need for assistance. In **crisis intervention** the therapist, or other intervener, becomes a part of the individual's life situation. Because of the individual's emotional state, he or she is unable to problem solve, so requires guidance and support from another to help mobilize the resources needed to resolve the crisis.

Lengthy psychological interpretations are obviously not appropriate for crisis intervention. It is a time for doing what is needed to help the individual get relief and for calling into action all the people and other resources required to do so.

Aguilera (1998) states:

The goal of crisis intervention is the resolution of an immediate crisis. Its focus is on the supportive, with the restoration of the individual to his precrisis level of functioning or possibly to a higher level of functioning. The therapist's role is direct, supportive, and that of an active participant. (p. 24)

Crisis intervention takes place in both inpatient and outpatient settings. The basic methodology relies heavily on orderly problem-solving techniques and structured activities that are focused on change. Through adaptive change, crises are resolved and growth occurs. Because of the time limitation of crisis intervention, the individual must experience some degree of relief almost from the first interaction. Crisis intervention, then, is not aimed at major personality change or reconstruction (as may be the case in long-term psychotherapy), but rather at using a given crisis situation, at the very least, to restore functioning and, at most, to enhance personal growth.

PHASES OF CRISIS INTERVENTION: THE ROLE OF THE NURSE

Nurses respond to crisis situations on a daily basis. Crises can occur on every unit in the general hospital, in the home setting, the community healthcare setting, schools, offices, and in private practice. Indeed, nurses may be called on to function as crisis helpers in virtually any setting committed to the practice of nursing.

Roberts and Ottens (2005) provide a seven-stage model of crisis intervention. This model is summarized in Table 13–1. Aguilera (1998) describes four specific phases in the technique of crisis intervention that are clearly comparable to the steps of the nursing process. These phases are discussed in the following paragraphs.

Phase 1. Assessment

In this phase, the crisis helper gathers information regarding the precipitating stressor and the resulting crisis that prompted the individual to seek professional help. A nurse in crisis intervention might perform some of the following assessments:

1. Ask the individual to describe the event that precipitated this crisis.
2. Determine when it occurred.
3. Assess the individual's physical and mental status.
4. Determine if the individual has experienced this stressor before. If so, what method of coping was used? Have these methods been tried this time?
5. If previous coping methods were tried, what was the result?
6. If new coping methods were tried, what was the result?
7. Assess suicide or homicide potential, plan, and means.
8. Assess the adequacy of support systems.
9. Determine level of precrisis functioning. Assess the usual coping methods, available support systems, and ability to problem solve.
10. Assess the individual's perception of personal strengths and limitations.
11. Assess the individual's use of substances.

Information from the comprehensive assessment is then analyzed, and appropriate nursing diagnoses reflecting the immediacy of the crisis situation are identified. Some nursing diagnoses that may be relevant include

1. Ineffective coping
2. Anxiety (severe to panic)
3. Disturbed thought processes
4. Risk for self- or other-directed violence
5. Rape-trauma syndrome
6. Post-trauma syndrome
7. Fear

Phase 2. Planning of Therapeutic Intervention

In the planning phase of the nursing process, the nurse selects the appropriate nursing actions for the identified nursing diagnoses. In planning the interventions, the type of crisis, as well as the individual's strengths and available resources for support, are taken into consideration. Goals

TABLE 13–1	Roberts' Seven-Stage Crisis Intervention Model
Stage	**Interventions**
Stage I. Psychosocial and Lethality Assessment	● Conduct a rapid but thorough biopsychosocial assessment
Stage II. Rapidly Establish Rapport	● The counselor uses genuineness, respect, and unconditional acceptance to establish rapport with the client. ● Skills such as good eye contact, a nonjudgmental attitude, flexibility, and maintaining a positive mental attitude are important.
Stage III. Identify the Major Problems or Crisis Precipitants	● Identify the precipitating event that has led the client to seek help at the present time. ● Identify other situations that led up to the precipitating event. ● Prioritize major problems with which the client needs help. ● Discuss client's current style of coping, and offer assistance in areas where modification would be helpful in resolving the present crisis and preventing future crises.
Stage IV. Deal with Feelings and Emotions	● Encourage client to vent feelings. Provide validation. ● Use therapeutic communication techniques to help client explain his or her story about the current crisis situation. ● Eventually, and cautiously, begin to challenge maladaptive beliefs and behaviors, and help client adopt more rational and adaptive options.
Stage V. Generate and Explore Alternatives	● Collaboratively explore options with client. ● Identify coping strategies that have been successful for the client in the past ● Help client problem-solve strategies for confronting current crisis adaptively.
Stage VI. Implement an Action Plan	● There is a shift at this stage from crisis to resolution. ● Develop a concrete plan of action to deal directly with the current crisis. ● Having a concrete plan restores the client's equilibrium and psychological balance. ● Work through the meaning of the event that precipitated the crisis. How could it have been prevented? What responses may have aggravated the situation?
Stage VII. Follow-Up	● Plan a follow-up visit with the client to evaluate the postcrisis status of the client. ● Beneficial scheduling of follow-up visits include 1-month and 1-year anniversaries of the crisis event.

SOURCE: Adapted from Roberts and Ottens (2005).

are established for crisis resolution and a return to, or increase in, the precrisis level of functioning.

Phase 3. Intervention

During phase 3, the actions that were identified in phase 2 are implemented. The following interventions are the focus of nursing in crisis intervention:

1. Use a reality-oriented approach. The focus of the problem is on the here and now.
2. Remain with the individual who is experiencing panic anxiety.
3. Establish a rapid working relationship by showing unconditional acceptance, by active listening, and by attending to immediate needs.
4. Discourage lengthy explanations or rationalizations of the situation; promote an atmosphere for verbalization of true feelings.
5. Set firm limits on aggressive, destructive behaviors. At high levels of anxiety, behavior is likely to be impulsive and regressive. Establish at the outset what is acceptable and what is not, and maintain consistency.
6. Clarify the problem that the individual is facing. The nurse does this by describing his or her perception of the problem and comparing it with the individual's perception of the problem.

7. Help the individual determine what he or she believes precipitated the crisis.
8. Acknowledge feelings of anger, guilt, helplessness, and powerlessness, while taking care not to provide positive feedback for these feelings.
9. Guide the individual through a problem-solving process by which he or she may move in the direction of positive life change:
   a. Help the individual confront the source of the problem that is creating the crisis response.
   b. Encourage the individual to discuss changes he or she would like to make. Jointly determine whether or not desired changes are realistic.
   c. Encourage exploration of feelings about aspects that cannot be changed, and explore alternative ways of coping more adaptively in these situations.

CLINICAL PEARL

Coping mechanisms are highly individual and the choice ultimately must be made by the client. The nurse may offer suggestions and provide guidance to help the client identify coping mechanisms that are realistic for him or her, and that can promote positive outcomes in a crisis situation.

d. Discuss alternative strategies for creating changes that are realistically possible.

e. Weigh benefits and consequences of each alternative.

f. Assist the individual to select alternative coping strategies that will help alleviate future crisis situations.

10. Identify external support systems and new social networks from whom the individual may seek assistance in times of stress.

Phase 4. Evaluation of Crisis Resolution and Anticipatory Planning

To evaluate the outcome of crisis intervention, a reassessment is made to determine if the stated objective was achieved:

1. Have positive behavioral changes occurred?
2. Has the individual developed more adaptive coping strategies? Have they been effective?
3. Has the individual grown from the experience by gaining insight into his or her responses to crisis situations?
4. Does the individual believe that he or she could respond with healthy adaptation in future stressful situations to prevent crisis development?
5. Can the individual describe a plan of action for dealing with stressors similar to the one that precipitated this crisis?

During the evaluation period, the nurse and client summarize what has occurred during the intervention. They review what the individual has learned and "anticipate" how he or she will respond in the future. A determination is made regarding follow-up therapy; if needed, the nurse provides referral information.

DISASTER NURSING

Although there are many definitions of **disaster**, a common feature is that the event overwhelms local resources and threatens the function and safety of the community (Norwood, Ursano, & Fullerton, 2006). A violent disaster, whether natural or man-made, may leave devastation of property or life. Such tragedies also leave victims with a damaged sense of safety and well-being, and varying degrees of emotional trauma (Oklahoma State Department of Health [OSDH], 2001). Children, who lack life experiences and coping skills, are particularly vulnerable. Their sense of order and security has been seriously disrupted, and they are unable to understand that the disruption is time-limited and that their world will eventually return to normal.

APPLICATION OF THE NURSING PROCESS TO DISASTER NURSING

Background Assessment Data

Individuals respond to traumatic events in many ways. Grieving is a natural response following any loss, and it may be more extreme if the disaster is directly experienced or witnessed (OSDH, 2001). The emotional effects of loss and disruption may show up immediately or may appear weeks or months later.

Psychological and behavioral responses common in adults following trauma and disaster include: anger; disbelief; sadness; anxiety; fear; irritability; arousal; numbing; sleep disturbance; and increases in alcohol, caffeine, and tobacco use (Norwood, Ursano, & Fullerton, 2006). Preschool children commonly experience separation anxiety, regressive behaviors, nightmares, and hyperactive or withdrawn behaviors. Older children may have difficulty concentrating, somatic complaints, sleep disturbances, and concerns about safety. Adolescents' responses are often similar to those of adults.

Norwood, Ursano, and Fullerton (2006) state:

> Traumatic bereavement is recognized as posing special challenges to survivors. While the death of loved ones is always painful, and unexpected and violent death can be more difficult to assimilate. Family members may develop intrusive images of the death based on information gleaned from authorities or the media. Witnessing or learning of violence to a loved one also increases vulnerability to psychiatric disorders. The knowledge that one has been exposed to toxins is a potent traumatic stressor . . . and the focus of much concern in the medical community preparing for responses to terrorist attacks using biological, chemical, or nuclear agents. (p. 3)

Nursing Diagnoses/Outcome Identification

Information from the assessment is analyzed, and appropriate nursing diagnoses reflecting the immediacy of the situation are identified. Some nursing diagnoses that may be relevant include:

● Risk for injury (trauma, suffocation, poisoning)
● Risk for infection
● Anxiety (panic)
● Fear
● Spiritual distress
● Risk for posttrauma syndrome
● Ineffective community coping

The following criteria may be used for measurement of outcomes in the care of the client having experienced a traumatic event. Timelines are individually determined.

The client:

1. Experiences minimal/no injury to self.
2. Demonstrates behaviors necessary to protect self from further injury.

3. Identifies interventions to prevent/reduce risk of infection.
4. Is free of infection.
5. Maintains anxiety at manageable level.
6. Expresses beliefs and values about spiritual issues.
7. Demonstrates ability to deal with emotional reactions in an individually appropriate manner.
8. Demonstrates an increase in activities to improve community functioning.

Planning/Implementation

Table 13–2 provides a plan of care for the client who has experienced a traumatic event. Selected nursing diagnoses are presented, along with outcome criteria, appropriate nursing interventions, and rationales for each.

Evaluation

In the final step of the nursing process, a reassessment is conducted to determine if the nursing actions have been successful in achieving the objectives of care. Evaluation of the nursing actions for the client who has experienced a traumatic event may be facilitated by gathering information utilizing the following types of questions:

1. Has the client escaped serious injury, or have injuries been resolved?
2. Have infections been prevented or resolved?
3. Is the client able to maintain anxiety at a manageable level?
4. Does he or she demonstrate appropriate problem-solving skills?
5. Is the client able to discuss his or her beliefs about spiritual issues?
6. Does the client demonstrate the ability to deal with emotional reactions in an individually appropriate manner?
7. Does he or she verbalize a subsiding of the physical manifestations (e.g., pain, nightmares, flashbacks, fatigue) associated with the traumatic event?
8. Has there been recognition of factors affecting the community's ability to meet its own demands or needs?
9. Has there been a demonstration of increased activities to improve community functioning?
10. Has a plan been established and put in place to deal with future contingencies?

Table 13–2	Care Plan for the Client Who Has Experienced a Traumatic Event

NURSING DIAGNOSIS: ANXIETY (PANIC)/FEAR

RELATED TO: Real or perceived threat to physical well-being; threat of death; situational crisis; exposure to toxins; unmet needs

EVIDENCED BY: Persistent feelings of apprehension and uneasiness; sense of impending doom; impaired functioning; verbal expressions of having no control or influence over situation, outcome, or self-care; sympathetic stimulation; extraneous physical movements

Outcome Criteria	Nursing Interventions	Rationale
Client will maintain anxiety at manageable level.	1. Determine degree of anxiety/fear present, associated behaviors (e.g., laughter, crying, calm or agitation, excited/hysterical behavior, expressions of disbelief and/or self-blame), and reality of perceived threat.	1. Clearly understanding client's perception is pivotal to providing appropriate assistance in overcoming the fear. Individual may be agitated or totally overwhelmed. Panic state increases risk for client's own safety as well as the safety of others in the environment.
	2. Note degree of disorganization.	2. Client may be unable to handle ADLs or work requirements and need more intensive intervention.
	3. Create as quiet an area as possible. Maintain a calm confident manner. Speak in even tone using short simple sentences.	3. Decreases sense of confusion or overstimulation; enhances sense of safety. Helps client focus on what is said and reduces transmission of anxiety.
	4. Develop trusting relationship with the client.	4. Trust is the basis of a therapeutic nurse-client relationship and enables them to work effectively together.
	5. Identify whether incident has reactivated preexisting or coexisting situations (physical or psychological).	5. Concerns and psychological issues will be recycled every time trauma is reexperienced and affect how the client views the current situation.

Outcome Criteria	✓ Nursing Interventions	Rationale
	6. Determine presence of physical symptoms (e.g., numbness, headache, tightness in chest, nausea, and pounding heart)	6. Physical problems need to be differentiated from anxiety symptoms so appropriate treatment can be given.
	7. Identify psychological responses (e.g., anger, shock, acute anxiety, panic, confusion, denial). Record emotional changes.	7. Although these are normal responses at the time of the trauma, they will recycle again and again until they are dealt with adequately.
	8. Discuss with client the perception of what is causing the anxiety.	8. Increases the ability to connect symptoms to subjective feeling of anxiety, providing opportunity to gain insight/control and make desired changes.
	9. Assist client to correct any distortions being experienced. Share perceptions with client.	9. Perceptions based on reality will help to decrease fearfulness. How the nurse views the situation may help client to see it differently.
	10. Explore with client or significant other the manner in which client has previously coped with anxiety-producing events.	10. May help client regain sense of control and recognize significance of trauma.
	11. Engage client in learning new coping behaviors (e.g., progressive muscle relaxation, thought-stopping)	11. Replacing maladaptive behaviors can enhance ability to manage and deal with stress. Interrupting obsessive thinking allows client to use energy to address underlying anxiety, whereas continued rumination about the incident can retard recovery.
	12. Encourage use of techniques to manage stress and vent emotions such as anger and hostility.	12. Reduces the likelihood of eruptions that can result in abusive behavior.
	13. Give positive feedback when client demonstrates better ways to manage anxiety and is able to calmly and realistically appraise the situation.	13. Provides acknowledgment and reinforcement, encouraging use of new coping strategies. Enhances ability to deal with fearful feelings and gain control over situation, promoting future successes.
	14. Administer medications as indicated: Antianxiety: diazepam, alprazolam, oxazepam; or Antidepressants: fluoxetine, paroxetine, bupropion.	14. Provides temporary relief of anxiety symptoms, enhancing ability to cope with situation. To lift mood and help suppress intrusive thoughts and explosive anger.

NURSING DIAGNOSIS: SPIRITUAL DISTRESS

RELATED TO: Physical or psychological stress; energy-consuming anxiety; loss(es), intense suffering; separation from religious or cultural ties; challenged belief and value system

EVIDENCED BY: Expressions of concern about disaster and the meaning of life and death or belief systems; inner conflict about current loss of normality and effects of the disaster; anger directed at deity; engaging in self-blame; seeking spiritual assistance

Outcome Criteria	✓ Nursing Interventions	Rationale
Client expresses beliefs and values about spiritual issues.	1. Determine client's religious/spiritual orientation, current involvement, and presence of conflicts.	1. Provides baseline for planning care and accessing appropriate resources.
	2. Establish environment that promotes free expression of feelings and concerns. Provide calm, peaceful setting when possible.	2. Promotes awareness and identification of feelings so they can be dealt with.

Continued on following page

Table 13-2	(Continued)

NURSING DIAGNOSIS: SPIRITUAL DISTRESS

RELATED TO: Physical or psychological stress; energy-consuming anxiety; loss(es), intense suffering; separation from religious or cultural ties; challenged belief and value system

EVIDENCED BY: Expressions of concern about disaster and the meaning of life and death or belief systems; inner conflict about current loss of normality and effects of the disaster; anger directed at deity; engaging in self-blame; seeking spiritual assistance

Outcome Criteria	Nursing Interventions	Rationale
	3. Listen to client's and significant others' expressions of anger, concern, alienation from God, belief that situation is a punishment for wrongdoing, etc.	3. It is helpful to understand the client's and significant others' points of view and how they are questioning their faith in the face of tragedy.
	4. Note sense of futility, feelings of hopelessness and helplessness, lack of motivation to help self.	4. These thoughts and feelings can result in the client feeling paralyzed and unable to move forward to resolve the situation.
	5. Listen to expressions of inability to find meaning in life and reason for living. Evaluate for suicidal ideation.	5. May indicate need for further intervention to prevent suicide attempt.
	6. Determine support systems available to client.	6. Presence or lack of support systems can affect client's recovery.
	7. Ask how you can be most helpful. Convey acceptance of client's spiritual beliefs and concerns.	7. Promotes trust and comfort, encouraging client to be open about sensitive matters.
	8. Make time for nonjudgmental discussion of philosophic issues and questions about spiritual impact of current situation.	8. Helps client to begin to look at basis for spiritual confusion. *Note:* There is a potential for care provider's belief system to interfere with client finding own way. Therefore, it is most beneficial to remain neutral and not espouse own beliefs.
	9. Discuss difference between grief and guilt and help client to identify and deal with each, assuming responsibility for own actions, expressing awareness of the consequences of acting out of false guilt.	9. Blaming self for what has happened impedes dealing with the grief process and needs to be discussed and dealt with.
	10. Use therapeutic communication skills of reflection and active-listening.	10. Helps client find own solutions to concerns.
	11. Encourage client to experience meditation, prayer, and forgiveness. Provide information that anger with God is a normal part of the grieving process.	11. This can help to heal past and present pain.
	12. Assist client to develop goals for dealing with life situation.	12. Enhances commitment to goal, optimizing outcomes and promoting sense of hope.
	13. Identify and refer to resources that can be helpful, e.g., pastoral/parish nurse or religious counselor, crisis counselor, psychotherapy, Alcoholics/Narcotics Anonymous.	13. Specific assistance may be helpful to recovery (e.g., relationship problems, substance abuse, suicidal ideation).
	14. Encourage participation in support groups.	14. Discussing concerns and questions with others can help client resolve feelings.

NURSING DIAGNOSIS: RISK FOR POSTTRAUMA SYNDROME

RELATED TO: Events outside the range of usual human experience; serious threat or injury to self or loved ones; witnessing horrors or tragic events; exaggerated sense of responsibility; survivor's guilt or role in the event; inadequate social support

Outcome Criteria	Nursing Interventions	Rationale
Client demonstrates ability to deal with emotional reactions in an individually appropriate manner.	1. Determine involvement in event (e.g., survivor, significant other, rescue/aid worker, healthcare provider, family member).	1. All those concerned with a traumatic event are at risk for emotional trauma and have needs related to their involvement in the event. *Note:* Close involvement with victims affects individual responses and may prolong emotional suffering.
	2. Evaluate current factors associated with the event, such as displacement from home due to illness/injury, natural disaster, or terrorist attack. Identify how client's past experiences may affect current situation.	2. Affects client's reaction to current event and is basis for planning care and identifying appropriate support systems and resources.
	3. Listen for comments of taking on responsibility (e.g., "I should have been more careful or gone back to get her.")	3. Statements such as these are indicators of "survivor's guilt" and blaming self for actions.
	4. Identify client's current coping mechanisms.	4. Noting positive or negative coping skills provides direction for care.
	5. Determine availability and usefulness of client's support systems, family, social contacts, and community resources.	5. Family and others close to the client may also be at risk and require assistance to cope with the trauma.
	6. Provide information about signs and symptoms of post-trauma response, especially if individual is involved in a high-risk occupation.	6. Awareness of these factors helps individual identify need for assistance when signs and symptoms occur.
	7. Identify and discuss client's strengths as well as vulnerabilities.	7. Provides information to build on for coping with traumatic experience.
	8. Evaluate individual's perceptions of events and personal significance (e.g., rescue worker trained to provide lifesaving assistance but recovering only dead bodies).	8. Events that trigger feelings of despair and hopelessness may be more difficult to deal with, and require long-term interventions.
	9. Provide emotional and physical presence by sitting with client/significant other and offering solace.	9. Strengthens coping abilities
	10. Encourage expression of feelings. Note whether feelings expressed appear congruent with events experienced.	10. It is important to talk about the incident repeatedly. Incongruencies may indicate deeper conflict and can impede resolution.
	11. Note presence of nightmares, reliving the incident, loss of appetite, irritability, numbness and crying, and family or relationship disruption.	11. These responses are normal in the early post-incident time frame. If prolonged and persistent, they may indicate need for more intensive therapy.
	12. Provide a calm, safe environment.	12. Helps client deal with the disruption in their life.
	13. Encourage and assist client in learning stress-management techniques.	13. Promotes relaxation and helps individual exercise control over self and what has happened.
	14. Recommend participation in debriefing sessions that may be provided following major disaster events.	14. Dealing with the stresses promptly may facilitate recovery from the event or prevent exacerbation.

Continued on following page

Table 13–2 *(Continued)*

NURSING DIAGNOSIS: RISK FOR POSTTRAUMA SYNDROME

RELATED TO: Events outside the range of usual human experience; serious threat or injury to self or loved ones; witnessing horrors or tragic events; exaggerated sense of responsibility; survivor's guilt or role in the event; inadequate social support

Outcome Criteria	Nursing Interventions	Rationale
	15. Identify employment, community resource groups.	15. Provides opportunity for ongoing support to deal with recurrent feelings related to the trauma.
	16. Administer medications as indicated, such as antipsychotics (e.g., chlorpromazine, haloperidol, olanzapine, or quetiapine) or carbamazepine (Tegretol).	16. Low doses may be used for reduction of psychotic symptoms when loss of contact with reality occurs, usually for clients with especially disturbing flashbacks. Tegretol may be used to alleviate intrusive recollections/flashbacks, impulsivity, and violent behavior.

NURSING DIAGNOSIS: INEFFECTIVE COMMUNITY COPING

RELATED TO: Natural or man-made disasters (earthquakes, tornados, floods, reemerging infectious agents, terrorist activity); ineffective or nonexistent community systems (e.g., lack of or inadequate emergency medical system, transportation system, or disaster planning systems)

EVIDENCED BY: Deficits of community participation; community does not meet its own expectations; expressed vulnerability; community powerlessness; stressors perceived as excessive; excessive community conflicts; high illness rates

Outcome Criteria	Nursing Interventions	Rationale
Client demonstrates an increase in activities to improve community functioning.	1. Evaluate community activities that are related to meeting collective needs within the community itself and between the community and the larger society. Note immediate needs, such as health care, food, shelter, funds.	1. Provides a baseline to determine community needs in relation to current concerns or threats.
	2. Note community reports of functioning including areas of weakness or conflict.	2. Provides a view of how the community itself sees these areas.
	3. Identify effects of related factors on community activities.	3. In the face of a current threat, local or national, community resources need to be evaluated, updated, and given priority to meet the identified need.
	4. Determine availability and use of resources. Identify unmet demands or needs of the community.	4. Information necessary to identify what else is needed to meet the current situation.
	5. Determine community strengths.	5. Promotes understanding of the ways in which the community is already meeting the identified needs.
	6. Encourage community members/groups to engage in problem-solving activities.	6. Promotes a sense of working together to meet the needs.
	7. Develop a plan jointly with the members of the community to address immediate needs.	7. Deals with deficits in support of identified goals.
	8. Create plans managing interactions within the community itself and between the community and the larger society.	8. Meets collective needs when the concerns/threats are shared beyond a local community.

Outcome Criteria	Nursing Interventions	Rationale
	9. Make information accessible to the public. Provide channels for dissemination of information to the community as a whole (e.g., print media, radio/television reports and community bulletin boards, internet sites, speaker's bureau, reports to committees/councils/advisory boards).	9. Readily available accurate information can help citizens deal with the situation.
	10. Make information available in different modalities and geared to differing educational levels/cultures of the community.	10. Using languages other than English and making written materials accessible to all members of the community will promote understanding.
	11. Seek out and evaluate needs of underserved populations.	11. Homeless and those residing in lower income areas may have special requirements that need to be addressed with additional resources.

SOURCE: Doenges, Moorhouse, & Murr (2006). With permission.

SUMMARY AND KEY POINTS

- A *crisis* is defined as "a sudden event in one's life that disturbs homeostasis, during which usual coping mechanisms cannot resolve the problem." (Lagerquist, 2006).
- All individuals experience crises at one time or another. This does not necessarily indicate psychopathology.
- Crises are precipitated by specific identifiable events and are determined by an individual's personal perception of the situation.
- Crises are acute rather than chronic and generally last no more than a few weeks to a few months.
- Crises occur when an individual is exposed to a stressor and previous problem-solving techniques are ineffective. This causes the level of anxiety to rise. Panic may ensue when new techniques are tried and resolution fails to occur.
- Six types of crises have been identified. They include dispositional crises, crises of anticipated life transitions, crises resulting from traumatic stress, maturation/developmental crises, crises reflecting psychopathology, and psychiatric emergencies. The type of crisis determines the method of intervention selected.
- Crisis intervention is designed to provide rapid assistance for individuals who have an urgent need.

- The minimum therapeutic goal of crisis intervention is psychological resolution of the individual's immediate crisis and restoration to at least the level of functioning that existed before the crisis period. A maximum goal is improvement in functioning above the precrisis level.
- Nurses regularly respond to individuals in crisis in all types of settings. Nursing process is the vehicle by which nurses assist individuals in crisis with a short-term problem-solving approach to change.
- A four-phase technique of crisis intervention includes assessment/analysis, planning of therapeutic intervention, intervention, and evaluation of crisis resolution and anticipatory planning.
- Through this structured method of assistance, nurses help individuals in crisis to develop more adaptive coping strategies for dealing with stressful situations in the future.
- Nurses have many important skills that can assist individuals and communities in the wake of traumatic events. Nursing interventions presented in this chapter were developed for the nursing diagnoses of panic anxiety/fear, spiritual distress, risk for post-trauma syndrome, and ineffective community coping.

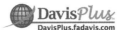 DavisPlus
DavisPlus.fadavis.com

For additional clinical tools and study aids, visit DavisPlus.

REVIEW QUESTIONS

Self-Examination/Learning Exercise

Select the best response to each of the following questions.

1. Which of the following is a correct assumption regarding the concept of crisis?
   a. Crises occur only in individuals with psychopathology.
   b. The stressful event that precipitates crisis is seldom identifiable.
   c. A crisis situation contains the potential for psychological growth or deterioration.
   d. Crises are chronic situations that recur many times during an individual's life.

2. Crises occur when an individual:
   a. Is exposed to a precipitating stressor.
   b. Perceives a stressor to be threatening.
   c. Has no support systems.
   d. Experiences a stressor and perceives coping strategies to be ineffective.

3. Amanda's mobile home was destroyed by a tornado. Amanda received only minor injuries, but is experiencing disabling anxiety in the aftermath of the event. This type of crisis is called:
   a. Crisis resulting from traumatic stress.
   b. Maturational/developmental crisis.
   c. Dispositional crisis.
   d. Crisis of anticipated life transitions.

4. The most appropriate crisis intervention with Amanda would be to:
   a. Encourage her to recognize how lucky she is to be alive.
   b. Discuss stages of grief and feelings associated with each.
   c. Identify community resources that can help Amanda.
   d. Suggest that she find a place to live that provides a storm shelter.

5. Jenny reported to the high school nurse that her mother drinks too much. She is drunk every afternoon when Jenny gets home from school. Jenny is afraid to invite friends over because of her mother's behavior. This type of crisis is called:
   a. Crisis resulting from traumatic stress.
   b. Maturational/developmental crisis.
   c. Dispositional crisis.
   d. Crisis reflecting psychopathology.

6. The most appropriate nursing intervention with Jenny would be to:
   a. Make arrangements for her to start attending Al-Ateen meetings.
   b. Help her identify the positive things in her life and recognize that her situation could be a lot worse than it is.
   c. Teach her about the effects of alcohol on the body and that it can be hereditary.
   d. Refer her to a psychiatrist for private therapy to learn to deal with her home situation.

7. Ginger, age 19 and an only child, left 3 months ago to attend a college of her choice 500 miles away from her parents. It is Ginger's first time away from home. She has difficulty making decisions and will not undertake anything new without first consulting her mother. They talk on the phone almost every day. Ginger has recently started having anxiety attacks. She consults the nurse practitioner in the student health center. This type of crisis is called:
   a. Crisis resulting from traumatic stress.
   b. Dispositional crisis.
   c. Psychiatric emergency.
   d. Maturational/developmental crisis.

8. The most appropriate nursing intervention with Ginger would be to:
   a. Suggest she move to a college closer to home.
   b. Work with Ginger on unresolved dependency issues.

CHAPTER 14 ● RELAXATION THERAPY 223

TABLE 14–1 Physiological, Cognitive, and Behavioral Manifestations of Stress

Physiological	Cognitive	Behavioral
Epinephrine and norepinephrine are released into the bloodstream. Pupils dilate. Respiration rate increases. Heart rate increases. Blood pressure increases. Digestion subsides. Blood sugar increases. Metabolism increases. Serum free fatty acids, cholesterol, and triglycerides increase.	Anxiety increases. Confusion and disorientation may be evident. The person is unable to problem solve. The person is unable to concentrate. Cognitive processes focus on achieving relief from anxiety. Learning is inhibited. Thoughts may reflect obsessions and ruminations.	Restlessness Irritability Use or misuse of defense mechanisms Disorganized routine functioning Insomnia and anorexia Compulsive or bizarre behaviors (depending on level of anxiety being experienced)

Virtually no muscle activity is observed. Eyes are closed, jaws may be slightly parted, and palms are open with fingers curled, but not clenched. Head may be slightly tilted to the side.

A summary of the physiological, cognitive, and behavioral manifestations of relaxation is presented in Table 14–2.

METHODS OF ACHIEVING RELAXATION

Deep Breathing Exercises

Deep breathing is a simple technique that is basic to most other relaxation skills. Tension is released when the lungs are allowed to breathe in as much oxygen as possible (Sobel & Ornstein, 1996). Breathing exercises have been found to be effective in reducing anxiety, depression, irritability, muscular tension, and fatigue (Davis, Eshelman, & McKay, 2008; Sobel & Ornstein, 1996). An advantage of this exercise is that it may be accomplished anywhere and at any time. A good guideline is to practice deep breathing for a few minutes three or four times a day or whenever a feeling of tenseness occurs.

Technique

1. Sit, stand, or lie in a comfortable position, ensuring that the spine is straight.
2. Place one hand on your abdomen and the other on your chest.
3. Inhale slowly and deeply through your nose. The abdomen should be expanding and pushing up on your hand. The chest should be moving only slightly.
4. When you have breathed in as much as possible, hold your breath for a few seconds before exhaling.
5. Begin exhaling slowly through the mouth, pursing your lips as if you were going to whistle. Pursing the lips helps to control how fast you exhale and keeps airways open as long as possible.
6. Feel the abdomen deflate as the lungs are emptied of air.
7. Begin the inhale-exhale cycle again. Focus on the sound and feeling of your breathing as you become more and more relaxed.
8. Continue the deep-breathing exercises for 5 to 10 minutes at a time. Once mastered, the technique may be used as often as required to relieve tension.

Progressive Relaxation

Progressive relaxation, a method of deep-muscle relaxation, was developed in 1929 by Chicago physician Edmond Jacobson. His technique is based on the premise that the body responds to anxiety-provoking thoughts and events with muscle tension. Excellent results have been observed with this method in the treatment of muscular tension, anxiety, insomnia, depression, fatigue, irritable bowel, muscle spasms, neck and back pain, high

TABLE 14–2 Physiological, Cognitive, and Behavioral Manifestations of Relaxation

Physiological	Cognitive	Behavioral
Lower levels of epinephrine and norepinephrine in the blood Respiration rate decreases (sometimes as low as 4–6 breaths per minute) Heart rate decreases (sometimes as low as 24 beats per minute) Blood pressure decreases Metabolic rate slows down Muscle tension diminishes Pupils constrict Vasodilation and increased temperature in the extremities	Change from beta consciousness to alpha consciousness Creativity and memory are enhanced Increased ability to concentrate	Distractibility to environmental stimuli is decreased Will respond to questions but does not initiate verbal interaction Calm, tranquil demeanor; no evidence of restlessness Common mannerisms include eyes closed, jaws parted, palms open, fingers curled, and head slightly tilted to the side

blood pressure, mild phobias, and stuttering (Davis, Eshelman, & McKay, 2008).

Technique

Each muscle group is tensed for 5 to 7 seconds and then relaxed for 20 to 30 seconds, during which time the individual concentrates on the difference in sensations between the two conditions. Soft, slow background music may facilitate relaxation.

1. Sit in a comfortable chair with your hands in your lap, your feet flat on the floor, and your eyes closed.
2. Begin by taking three deep, slow breaths, inhaling through the nose and releasing the air slowly through the mouth.
3. Now starting with the feet, pull the toes forward toward the knees, stiffen your calves, and hold for a count of five.
4. Now release the hold. Let go of the tension. Feel the sensation of relaxation and warmth as the tension flows out of the muscles.
5. Next, tense the muscles of the thighs and buttocks, and hold for a count of five.
6. Now release the hold. Feel the tension drain away, and be aware of the difference in sensation—perhaps a heavyness or feeling of warmth that you did not feel when the muscles were tensed. Concentrate on this feeling for a few seconds.
7. Next, tense the abdominal muscles. Hold for a count of five.
8. Now release the hold. Concentrate on the feeling of relaxation in the muscles. You may feel a warming sensation. Hold on to that feeling for 15 to 20 seconds.
9. Next, tense the muscles in the back and hold for a count of five.
10. Now release the hold. Feel the sensation of relaxation and warmth as the tension flows out of the muscles.
11. Next, tense the muscles of your hands, biceps, and forearms. Clench your hands into a tight fist. Hold for a count of five.
12. Now release the hold. Notice the sensations. You may feel tingling, warmth, or a light, airy feeling. Recognize these sensations as tension leaves the muscles.
13. Next, tense the muscles of the shoulders and neck. Shrug the shoulders tightly and hold for a count of five.
14. Now relea1se the hold. Sense the tension as it leaves the muscles and experience the feeling of relaxation.
15. Next, tense the muscles of the face. Wrinkle the forehead, frown, squint the eyes, and purse the lips. Hold for a count of five.
16. Now release the hold. Recognize a light, warm feeling flowing into the muscles.
17. Now feel the relaxation in your whole body. As the tension leaves your entire being, you feel completely relaxed.
18. Open your eyes and enjoy renewed energy.

Modified (or Passive) Progressive Relaxation

Technique

In this version of total-body relaxation, the muscles are not tensed. The individual learns to relax muscles by concentrating on the feeling of relaxation within the muscle. These instructions may be presented by one person for another or they may be self-administered. Relaxation may be facilitated by playing soft, slow background music during the activity.

1. Assume a comfortable position. Some suggestions include the following:
   a. Sitting straight up in a chair with hands in the lap or at sides and feet flat on the floor.
   b. Sitting in a reclining chair with hands in the lap or at sides and legs up on an elevated surface.
   c. Lying flat with head slightly elevated on pillow and arms at sides.
2. Close your eyes and take three deep breaths through your nose, slowly releasing the air through your mouth.
3. Allow a feeling of peacefulness to descend over you—a pleasant, enjoyable sensation of being comfortable and at ease.
4. Remain in this state for several minutes.
5. It is now time to turn your attention to various parts of your body.
6. Begin with the muscles of the head, face, throat, and shoulders. Concentrate on these muscles, paying particular attention to those in the forehead and jaws. Feel the tension leave the area. The muscles start to feel relaxed, heavy, and warm. Concentrate on this feeling for a few minutes.
7. Now let the feeling of relaxation continue to spread downward to the muscles of your biceps, forearms, and hands. Concentrate on these muscles. Feel the tension dissolve, the muscles starting to feel relaxed and heavy. A feeling of warmth spreads through these muscles all the way to the fingertips. They are feeling very warm and very heavy. Concentrate on this feeling for a few minutes.
8. The tension is continuing to dissolve now, and you are feeling very relaxed. Turn your attention to the muscles in your chest, abdomen, and lower back. Feel the tension leave these areas. Allow these muscles to become very relaxed. They start to feel very warm and very heavy. Concentrate on this feeling for a few minutes.

9. The feeling of relaxation continues to move downward now as you move to the muscles of the thighs, buttocks, calves, and feet. Feel the tension moving down and out of your body. These muscles feel very relaxed now. Your legs are feeling very heavy and very limp. A feeling of warmth spreads over the area, all the way to the toes. You can feel that all the tension has been released.

10. Your whole body feels relaxed and warm. Listen to the music for a few moments and concentrate on this relaxed, warm feeling. Take several deep, slow breaths through your nose, releasing the air through your mouth. Continue to concentrate on how relaxed and warm you feel.

11. It is now time to refocus your concentration on the present and wake up your body to resume activity. Open your eyes and stretch or massage your muscles. Wiggle your fingers and toes. Take another deep breath, arise, and enjoy the feeling of renewed energy.

Meditation

Records and phenomenological accounts of meditative practices date back more than 2000 years, but only recently have empirical studies revealed the psychophysiological benefits of regular use (Pelletier, 1992). The goal of **meditation** is to gain "mastery over attention." It brings on a special state of consciousness as attention is concentrated solely on one thought or object.

Historically, meditation has been associated with religious doctrines and disciplines by which individuals sought enlightenment with God or another higher power. However, meditation can be practiced independently from any religious philosophy and purely as a means of achieving inner harmony and increasing self-awareness.

During meditation, the respiration rate, heart rate, and blood pressure decrease. The overall metabolism declines, and the need for oxygen consumption is reduced. Alpha brain waves—those associated with brain activity during periods of relaxation—predominate (Pelletier, 1992).

Meditation has been used successfully in the prevention and treatment of various cardiovascular diseases. It has proved helpful in curtailing obsessive thinking, anxiety, depression, and hostility (Davis, Eshelman, & McKay, 2008). Meditation improves concentration and attention.

Technique

1. Select a quiet place and a comfortable position. Various sitting positions are appropriate for meditation. Examples include:
   a. Sitting in a chair with your feet flat on the floor approximately 6 inches apart, arms resting comfortably in your lap.
   b. Cross-legged on the floor or on a cushion.
   c. In the Japanese fashion with knees on floor, great toes together, pointed backward, and buttocks resting comfortably on bottom of feet.
   d. In the lotus yoga position, sitting on the floor with the legs flexed at the knees. The ankles are crossed and each foot rests on top of the opposite thigh.

2. Select an object, word, or thought on which to dwell. During meditation the individual becomes preoccupied with the selected focus. This total preoccupation serves to prevent distractions from interrupting attention. Examples of foci include:
   a. *Counting One's Breaths*. All attention is focused on breathing in and out.
   b. *Mantras*. A *mantra* is a syllable, word, or name that is repeated many times as you free your mind of thoughts. Any mantra is appropriate if it works to focus attention and prevent distracting thoughts.
   c. *Objects for Contemplation*. Select an object, such as a rock, a marble, or anything that does not hold a symbolic meaning that might cause distraction. Contemplate the object both visually and tactilely. Focus total attention on the object.
   d. *A Thought That Has Special Meaning to You*. With eyes closed, focus total attention on a specific thought or idea.

3. Practice directing attention on your selected focus for 10 to 15 minutes a day for several weeks. It is essential that the individual does not become upset if intrusive thoughts find their way into the meditation practice. They should merely be dealt with and dismissed as the individual returns to the selected focus of attention. Worrying about one's progress in the ability to meditate is a self-inhibiting behavior.

Mental Imagery

Mental imagery uses the imagination in an effort to reduce the body's response to stress. The frame of reference is very personal, based on what each individual considers to be a relaxing environment. Some might select a scene at the seashore, some might choose a mountain atmosphere, and some might choose floating through the air on a fluffy white cloud. The choices are as limitless as one's imagination. Following is an example of how one individual uses imagery for relaxation. The information is most useful when taped and played back at a time when the individual wishes to achieve relaxation.

Technique

Sit or lie down in a comfortable position. Close your eyes. Imagine that you and someone you love are walking along the seashore. No other people are in sight in any direction. The sun is shining, the sky is blue, and a gentle breeze is blowing. You select a spot to stop and rest. You lie on the sand and close your eyes. You hear the sound of the waves as they splash against the shore. The sun feels warm on your face and body. The sand feels soft and warm against your back. An occasional wave splashes you with a cool mist that dries rapidly in the warm sun. The coconut fragrance of your suntan lotion wafts gently and pleasantly in the air. You lie in this quiet place for what seems like a very long time, taking in the sounds of the waves, the warmth of the sun, and the cooling sensations of the mist and ocean breeze. It is very quiet. It is very warm. You feel very relaxed, very contented. This is your special place. You may come to this special place whenever you want to relax.

Biofeedback

Biofeedback is the use of instrumentation to become aware of processes in your body that you usually do not notice and to help bring them under voluntary control. Biofeedback machines give immediate information about an individual's own biological conditions, such as muscle tension, skin surface temperature, brain-wave activity, skin conductivity, blood pressure, and heart rate (Sadock & Sadock, 2007). Some conditions that can be treated successfully with biofeedback include spastic colon, hypertension, tension and migraine headaches, muscle spasms/pain, anxiety, phobias, stuttering, and teeth grinding.

Technique

Biological conditions are monitored by the biofeedback equipment. Sensors relate muscle spasticity, body temperature, brain-wave activity, heart rate, and blood pressure. Each of these conditions will elicit a signal from the equipment, such as a blinking light, a measure on a meter, or an audible tone. The individual practices using relaxation and voluntary control to modify the signal, in turn indicating a modification of the autonomic function it represents.

Various types of biofeedback equipment have been developed for home use. Often they are less than effective, however, because they usually measure only one autonomic function. In fact, modification of several functions may be required to achieve the benefits of total relaxation.

Biofeedback can help monitor the progress an individual is making toward learning to relax. It is often used together with other relaxation techniques such as deep breathing, progressive relaxation, and mental imagery.

Special training is required to become a biofeedback practitioner. Nurses can support and encourage individuals learning to use this method of stress management. Nurses can also teach other techniques of relaxation that enhance the results of biofeedback training.

Physical Exercise

Regular exercise is viewed by many as one of the most effective methods for relieving stress. Physical exertion provides a natural outlet for the tension produced by the body in its state of arousal for "fight or flight." Following exercise, physiological equilibrium is restored, resulting in a feeling of relaxation and revitalization. Physical inactivity increases all causes of mortality and doubles the risk of cardiovascular disease, type 2 diabetes, and obesity. It also increases the risks of colon and breast cancer, high blood pressure, lipid disorders, osteoporosis, depression, and anxiety (World Health Organization [WHO], 2006).

Aerobic exercises strengthen the cardiovascular system and increase the body's ability to use oxygen more efficiently. Aerobic exercises include brisk walking, jogging, running, cycling, swimming, and dancing, among other activities. To achieve the benefits of aerobic exercises, they must be performed regularly—for at least 30 minutes, three times per week.

Individuals can also benefit from low-intensity physical exercise. Although there is little benefit to the cardiovascular system, low-intensity exercise can help prevent obesity, relieve muscular tension, prevent muscle spasms, and increase flexibility. Examples of low-intensity exercise include slow walking, house cleaning, shopping, light gardening, calisthenics, and weight lifting.

Studies indicate that physical exercise can be effective in reducing general anxiety and depression. Vigorous exercise has been shown to increase levels of beta-endorphins and monoamines (serotonin, norepinephrine, and dopamine), all of which have been implicated in mood regulation (Craft & Perna, 2004). Depressed people are often deficient in these monoamines. Endorphins act as natural narcotics and mood elevators.

THE ROLE OF THE NURSE IN RELAXATION THERAPY

Nurses work with anxious clients in all departments of the hospital and in community and home health services. Individuals experience stress daily; it cannot be eliminated. Stress is a response to both pleasant and unpleasant events, and usually requires some readjustment on the part of the individual to adapt to it.

CLINICAL PEARL

Management of stress must be considered a lifelong function. Nurses can help individuals recognize the sources of stress in their lives and identify methods of adaptive coping.

Assessment

Stress management requires a holistic approach. Physical and psychosocial dimensions are considered in determining the individual's adaptation to stress. Following are some examples of assessment data for collection. Other assessments may need to be made, depending on specific circumstances of each individual.

1. Genetic influences
   a. Identify medical/psychiatric history of client and biological family members.
2. Past experiences
   a. Describe your living/working conditions.
   b. When did you last have a physical examination?
   c. Do you have a spiritual or religious position from which you derive support?
   d. Do you have a job? Have you experienced any recent employment changes or other difficulties on your job?
   e. What significant changes have occurred in your life in the last year?
   f. What is your usual way of coping with stress?
   g. Do you have someone to whom you can go for support when you feel stressed?
3. Client's perception of the stressor
   a. What do you feel is the major source of stress in your life right now?
4. Adaptation responses
   a. Do you ever feel anxious? Confused? Unable to concentrate? Fearful?
   b. Do you have tremors? Stutter or stammer? Sweat profusely?
   c. Do you often feel angry? Irritable? Moody?
   d. Do you ever feel depressed? Do you ever feel like harming yourself or others?
   e. Do you have difficulty communicating with others?
   f. Do you experience pain? What part of your body? When do you experience it? When does it worsen?
   g. Do you ever experience stomach upset? Constipation? Diarrhea? Nausea and vomiting?
   h. Do you ever feel your heart pounding in your chest?
   i. Do you take any drugs (prescription, over-the-counter, or street)?
   j. Do you drink alcohol? Smoke cigarettes? How much?
   k. Are you eating more/less than usual?
   l. Do you have difficulty sleeping?
   m. Do you have a significant other? Describe the relationship.
   n. Describe your relationship with other family members.
   o. Do you perceive any problems in your sexual lifestyle or behavior?

Diagnosis

Possible nursing diagnoses for individuals requiring assistance with stress management are listed here. Others may be appropriate for individuals with particular problems.

1. Risk-prone health behavior
2. Anxiety (specify level)
3. Disturbed body image
4. Coping, defensive
5. Coping, ineffective
6. Decisional conflict (specify)
7. Denial, ineffective
8. Fear
9. Grieving
10. Grieving, complicated
11. Hopelessness
12. Deficient knowledge (specify)
13. Pain (acute or chronic)
14. Parental role conflict
15. Post-trauma syndrome
16. Powerlessness
17. Rape-trauma syndrome
18. Role performance, ineffective
19. Low self-esteem
20. Sexual dysfunction
21. Sexuality pattern, ineffective
22. Sleep pattern, disturbed
23. Social interaction, impaired
24. Social isolation
25. Spiritual distress
26. Violence, risk for self-directed or other-directed

Outcome Identification/Implementation

The immediate goal for nurses working with individuals needing assistance with stress management is to help minimize current maladaptive symptoms. The long-term goal is to assist individuals toward achievement of their highest potential for wellness. Examples of outcome criteria may include:

1. Client will verbalize a reduction in pain following progressive relaxation techniques.
2. Client will be able to voluntarily control a decrease in blood pressure following 3 weeks of biofeedback training.
3. Client will be able to maintain stress at a manageable level by performing deep breathing exercises when feeling anxious.

Implementation of nursing actions has a strong focus on the role of client teacher. Relaxation therapy, as described in this chapter, is one way to help individuals manage stress. These techniques are well within the scope of nursing practice.

Evaluation

Evaluation requires that the nurse and client assess whether or not these techniques are achieving the desired outcomes. Various alternatives may be attempted and reevaluated.

Relaxation therapy provides alternatives to old, maladaptive methods of coping with stress. Lifestyle changes may be required and change does not come easily. Nurses must help individuals analyze the usefulness of these techniques in the management of stress in their daily lives.

SUMMARY AND KEY POINTS

- Stress is part of our everyday lives. It can be positive or negative, but it cannot be eliminated.
- Keeping stress at a manageable level is a lifelong process.
- Individuals under stress respond with a physiological arousal that can be dangerous over long periods.
- The stress response has been shown to be a major contributor, either directly or indirectly, to coronary heart disease, cancer, lung ailments, accidental injuries, cirrhosis of the liver, and suicide—six of the leading causes of death in the United States.
- Relaxation therapy is an effective means of reducing the stress response in some individuals.

- The degree of anxiety that an individual experiences in response to stress is related to certain predisposing factors, such as characteristics of temperament with which he or she was born, past experiences resulting in learned patterns of responding, and existing conditions, such as health status, coping strategies, and adequate support systems.
- Deep relaxation can counteract the physiological and behavioral manifestations of stress.
- Some examples of relaxation therapy include deep breathing exercises, progressive relaxation, passive progressive relaxation, meditation, mental imagery, biofeedback, and physical exercise.
- Nurses use the nursing process to assist individuals in the management of stress.
- Assessment data are collected from which nursing diagnoses are derived.
- Outcome criteria that help individuals reduce current maladaptive symptoms and ultimately achieve their highest potential for wellness are identified.
- Implementation includes instructing clients and their families in the various techniques for achieving relaxation. Behavioral changes provide objective measurements for evaluation.

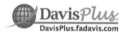 For additional clinical tools and study aids, visit DavisPlus.

DavisPlus.fadavis.com

REVIEW QUESTIONS

Self-Examination/Learning Exercise

1. **Learning exercise:** Practice some of the relaxation exercises presented in this chapter. It may be helpful to tape some of the exercises with soft music in the background. These tapes may be used with anxious clients or when you are feeling anxious yourself.

2. **Clinical activity:** Teach a relaxation exercise to a client. Practice it together. Evaluate the client's ability to achieve relaxation by performing the exercise.

3. **Case study:** Linda has just been admitted to the psychiatric unit. She was experiencing attacks of severe anxiety. Linda has worked in the typing pool of a large corporation for 10 years. She was recently promoted to private secretary for one of the executives. Some of her new duties include attending the board meetings and taking minutes, screening all calls and visitors for her boss, keeping track of his schedule, reminding him of important appointments, and making decisions for him in his absence. Linda felt comfortable in her old position, but has become increasingly fearful of making errors and incorrect decisions in her new job. Even though she is proud to have been selected for this position, she is constantly "nervous," has lost 10 pounds in 3 weeks, is having difficulty sleeping, and is having a recurrence of the severe migraine headaches she experienced as a teenager. She is often irritable with her husband and children for no apparent reason.

   a. Discuss some possible nursing diagnoses for Linda.
   b. Identify outcome criteria for Linda.
   c. Describe some relaxation techniques that may be helpful for her.

REFERENCES

Craft, L.L., & Perna, F.M. (2004). The benefits of exercise for the clinically depressed. *Primary Care Companion Journal of Clinical Psychiatry, 6*(4), 104–111.

Davis, M.D., Eshelman, E.R., & McKay, M. (2008). *The relaxation and stress reduction workbook* (6th ed.) Oakland, CA: New Harbinger Publications.

Karren, K.J., Hafen, B.Q., Smith, N.L., & Frandsen, K.J. (2006). *Mind/Body Health: The effects of attitudes, emotions, and relationships* (3rd ed.). San Francisco: Benjamin Cummings.

Miller, M.A., & Rahe, R.H. (1997). Life changes scaling for the 1990s. *Journal of Psychosomatic Research, 43*(3), 279–292.

Pelletier, K.R. (1992). *Mind as healer, mind as slayer*. New York: Dell.

Sadock, B.J., & Sadock, V.A. (2007). *Synopsis of psychiatry: Behavioral sciences/clinical psychiatry* (10th ed.). Philadelphia: Lippincott Williams & Wilkins.

Sobel, D.S., & Ornstein, R. (1996). *The healthy mind, healthy body handbook*. Los Altos, CA: DR^X.

World Health Organization (WHO). (2006). *Sedentary lifestyle: A global public health problem*. Retrieved June 24, 2008 from http://www.emro.who.int/whd2002/Readings-Section3.htm

Assertiveness Training

CHAPTER OUTLINE

KEY TERMS

aggressive
assertive
nonassertive

passive–aggressive
thought stopping

CORE CONCEPT

assertive behavior

OBJECTIVES

After reading this chapter, the student will be able to:

1. Define *assertive behavior*.
2. Discuss basic human rights.
3. Differentiate among nonassertive, assertive, aggressive, and passive–aggressive behaviors.
4. Describe techniques that promote assertive behavior.
5. Demonstrate thought-stopping techniques.
6. Discuss the role of the nurse in assertiveness training.

Alberti and Emmons (2001) ask:

Are you able to express warm, positive feelings to another person? Are you comfortable starting a conversation with strangers at a party? Do you sometimes feel ineffective in making your desires clear to others? Do you have difficulty saying "no" to persuasive people? Are you often at the bottom of the "pecking order," pushed around by others? Or maybe you're the one who pushes others around to get your way? (pp. 4, 5)

Assertive behavior promotes a feeling of personal power and self-confidence. These two components are commonly lacking in clients with emotional disorders. Becoming more assertive empowers individuals by promoting self-esteem, without diminishing the esteem of others.

This chapter describes a number of rights that are considered basic to human beings. Various kinds of behaviors are explored, including assertive, nonassertive, aggressive, and passive–aggressive. Techniques that promote assertive behavior and the nurse's role in assertiveness training are presented.

CORE CONCEPT

Assertive Behavior
Assertive behavior promotes equality in human relationships, enabling us to act in our own best interests, to stand up for ourselves without undue anxiety, to express honest feelings comfortably, to exercise personal rights without denying the rights of others (Alberti & Emmons, 2001).

ASSERTIVE COMMUNICATION

Assertive behavior helps us feel good about ourselves and increases our self-esteem. It helps us feel good about other people and increases our ability to develop satisfying relationships with others. This is accomplished out of honesty, directness, appropriateness, and respecting one's own basic rights as well as the rights of others.

Honesty is basic to assertive behavior. Assertive honesty is not an outspoken declaration of everything that is on one's mind. It is instead an accurate representation of feelings, opinions, or preferences expressed in a manner that promotes self-respect and respect for others.

Direct communication is stating what one wants to convey with clarity and candor. Hinting and "beating around the bush" are indirect forms of communication.

Communication must occur in an appropriate context to be considered assertive. The location and timing, as well as the manner (tone of voice, nonverbal gestures) in which the communication is presented, must be correct for the situation.

BASIC HUMAN RIGHTS

A number of authors have identified a variety of "assertive rights" (Davis, McKay, & Eshelman, 2008; Lloyd, 2002; Powell & Enright, 1990; Schuster, 2000; Sobel & Ornstein, 1996). Following is a composite of 10 basic assertive human rights adapted from the aggregation of sources.

1. The right to be treated with respect.
2. The right to express feelings, opinions, and beliefs.
3. The right to say "no" without feeling guilty.
4. The right to make mistakes and accept the responsibility for them.
5. The right to be listened to and taken seriously.
6. The right to change your mind.
7. The right to ask for what you want.
8. The right to put yourself first, sometimes.
9. The right to set your own priorities.
10. The right to refuse justification for your feelings or behavior.

In accepting these rights, an individual also accepts the responsibilities that accompany them. Rights and responsibilities are reciprocal entities. To experience one without the other is inherently destructive to an individual. Some responsibilities associated with basic assertive human rights are presented in Table 15–1.

RESPONSE PATTERNS

Individuals develop patterns of responding to others. Some of these patterns that have been identified include:

1. Watching other people (role modeling).
2. Being positively reinforced or punished for a certain response.
3. Inventing a response.
4. Not being able to think of a better way to respond.
5. Not developing the proper skills for a better response.
6. Consciously choosing a response style.

The nurse should be able to recognize his or her own pattern of responding, as well as that of others. Four response patterns will be discussed here: nonassertive, assertive, aggressive, and passive–aggressive.

Nonassertive Behavior

Individuals who are **nonassertive** (sometimes called *passive*) seek to please others at the expense of denying their own basic human rights. They seldom let their true feelings show and often feel hurt and anxious because they allow others to choose for them. They seldom achieve their own desired goals (Alberti & Emmons, 2001). They come across as being very apologetic and tend to be

TABLE 15–1	Assertive Rights and Responsibilities
Rights ◀━━━━━━━━━━━━━━━━━━━▶	**Responsibilities**
1. To be treated with respect ◀━━▶	To treat others in a way that recognizes their human dignity
2. To express feelings, opinions, and beliefs ◀━━▶	To accept ownership of our feelings and show respect for those that differ from our own
3. To say "no" ◀━━▶	To analyze each situation individually, recognizing all human rights as equal (others have the right to say "no," too)
4. To make mistakes ◀━━▶	To accept responsibility for own mistakes and to try to correct them
5. To be listened to ◀━━▶	To listen to others
6. To change your mind ◀━━▶	To accept the possible consequences that the change may incur; to accept the same flexibility in others
7. To ask for what you want ◀━━▶	To accept others' right to refuse your request
8. To put yourself first, sometimes ◀━━▶	To put others first, sometimes
9. To set your own priorities ◀━━▶	To consider one's limitations as well as strengths in directing independent activities; to be a dependable person
10. To refuse to justify feelings or behavior ◀━━▶	To accept ownership of own feelings/behavior; to accept others without requiring justification for their feelings/behavior

self-deprecating. They use actions instead of words and hope someone will "guess" what they want. Their voices are hesitant, weak, and expressed in a monotone. Their eyes are usually downcast. They feel uncomfortable in interpersonal interactions. All they want is to please and to be liked by others. Their behavior helps them avoid unpleasant situations and confrontations with others; however, they often harbor anger and resentment.

Assertive Behavior

Assertive individuals stand up for their own rights while protecting the rights of others. Feelings are expressed openly and honestly. They assume responsibility for their own choices and allow others to choose for themselves. They maintain self-respect and respect for others by treating everyone equally and with human dignity. They communicate tactfully, using lots of "I" statements. Their voices are warm and expressive, and eye contact is intermittent but direct. These individuals desire to communicate effectively with, and be respected by, others. They are self-confident and experience satisfactory and pleasurable relationships with others.

Aggressive Behavior

Individuals who are **aggressive** defend their own basic rights by violating the basic rights of others. Feelings are often expressed dishonestly and inappropriately. They say what is on their mind, often at the expense of others. Aggressive behavior commonly results in a *putdown* of the receiver. Rights denied, the receiver feels hurt, defensive, and humiliated (Alberti & Emmons, 2001). Aggressive individuals devalue the self-worth of others on whom they impose their choices. They express an air of superiority, and their voices are often loud, demanding, angry, or cold, without emotion. Eye contact may be "to intimidate others by staring them down." They want to increase their feeling of power by dominating or humiliating others. Aggressive behavior hinders interpersonal relationships.

Passive–Aggressive Behavior

Passive–aggressive individuals defend their own rights by expressing resistance to social and occupational demands (American Psychiatric Association [APA], 2000). Sometimes called *indirect aggression*, this behavior takes the form of passive, nonconfrontive action (Alberti & Emmons, 2001). These individuals are devious, manipulative, and sly, and they undermine others with behavior that expresses the opposite of what they are feeling. They are highly critical and sarcastic. They allow others to make choices for them, then resist by using passive behaviors, such as procrastination, dawdling, stubbornness, and

"forgetfulness." They use actions instead of words to convey their message, and the actions express covert aggression. They become sulky, irritable, or argumentative when asked to do something they do not want to do. They may protest to others about the demands but will not confront the person who is making the demands. Instead, they may deal with the demand by "forgetting" to do it. The goal is domination through retaliation. This behavior offers a feeling of control and power, although passive–aggressive individuals actually feel resentment and that they are being taken advantage of. They possess extremely low self-confidence.

A comparison of these four behavior patterns is presented in Table 15–2.

BEHAVIORAL COMPONENTS OF ASSERTIVE BEHAVIOR

Alberti and Emmons (2001) have identified several defining characteristics of assertive behavior:

1. **Eye contact.** Eye contact is considered appropriate when it is intermittent (i.e., looking directly at the person to whom one is speaking but looking away now and then). Individuals feel uncomfortable when someone stares at them continuously and intently. Intermittent eye contact conveys the message that one is interested in what is being said.
2. **Body posture.** Sitting and leaning slightly toward the other person in a conversation suggests an active interest in what is being said. Emphasis on an assertive stance can be achieved by standing with an erect posture, squarely facing the other person. A slumped posture conveys passivity or nonassertiveness.
3. **Distance/physical contact.** The distance between two individuals in an interaction or the physical contact between them has a strong cultural influence. For example, in the United States, intimate distance is considered approximately 18 inches from the body. We are very careful about whom we allow to enter this intimate space. Invasion of this space may be interpreted by some individuals as very aggressive.
4. **Gestures.** Nonverbal gestures may also be culturally related. Gesturing can add emphasis, warmth, depth, or power to the spoken word.
5. **Facial expression.** Various facial expressions convey different messages (e.g., frown, smile, surprise, anger, fear). It is difficult to "fake" these messages. In assertive communication, the facial expression is congruent with the verbal message.
6. **Voice.** The voice conveys a message by its loudness, softness, degree and placement of emphasis, and evidence of emotional tone.
7. **Fluency.** Being able to discuss a subject with ease and with obvious knowledge conveys assertiveness and self-confidence. This message is impeded by

Does the client participate in decisions that affect his or her life?

Can the client make rational decisions independently?

Has he or she become more assertive in interpersonal relations?

Is improvement observed in the physical presentation of self-esteem, such as eye contact, posture, changes in eating and sleeping, fatigue, libido, elimination patterns, self-care, and complaints of aches and pains?

SUMMARY AND KEY POINTS

- Emotional wellness requires that an individual have some degree of self-worth—a perception that he or she possesses a measure of value to self and others.
- Self-concept consists of body image, personal identity, and self-esteem.
- Body image encompasses one's appraisal of personal attributes, functioning, sexuality, wellness-illness state, and appearance.
- The personal identity component is composed of the moral–ethical self, the self-consistency, and the self-ideal.
- The moral–ethical self functions as observer, standard setter, dreamer, comparer, and most of all evaluator of who the individual says he or she is.
- Self-consistency is the component of the personal identity that strives to maintain a stable self-image.
- Self-ideal relates to an individual's perception of what he or she wants to be, do, or become.
- Self-esteem refers to the degree of regard or respect that individuals have for themselves and is a measure

of worth that they place on their abilities and judgments. It is largely influenced by the perceptions of how one is viewed by significant others.

- Predisposing factors to the development of positive self-esteem include a sense of competence, unconditional love, a sense of survival, realistic goals, a sense of responsibility, and reality orientation. Genetics and environmental conditions may also be influencing factors.
- The development of self-esteem progresses throughout the life span. Erikson's theory of personality development was used in this chapter as a framework for illustration of this progression.
- The behaviors associated with low self-esteem are numerous.
- Stimuli that trigger these behaviors were presented according to focal, contextual, or residual types.
- Boundaries, or personal limits, help individuals define the self and are part of the individuation process.
- Boundaries are physical and psychological and may be rigid, flexible, or enmeshed.
- Unhealthy boundaries are often the result of dysfunctional family systems.
- The nursing process is the vehicle for delivery of care to clients needing assistance with self-esteem disturbances.
- The three nursing diagnoses relating to self-esteem that have been accepted by NANDA International include: chronic low self-esteem, situational low self-esteem, and risk for situational low self-esteem.

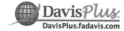 **DavisPlus.** **For additional clinical tools and**
DavisPlus.fadavis.com **study aids, visit DavisPlus.**

REVIEW QUESTIONS

Self-Examination/Learning Exercise

Situation: Karen is 23 years old. She has always been a good student and liked by her peers. She made As and Bs in high school, was captain of the cheerleading squad, and was chosen best-liked girl by her senior classmates at graduation. She entered nursing school at a nearby university and graduated with a 3.2/4.0 grade point average in 4 years.

The summer after graduation, Karen took the state board examination and did not pass. She was disappointed but was allowed to continue working at her hospital job as a graduate nurse until she was able to take the examination again. After a few months, she retook the exam and again did not pass. She was no longer able to keep her job, and she became despondent. She has sought counseling at the local mental health clinic.

Select the answers that are most appropriate for this situation.

1. Karen says to the psychiatric nurse, "I am a complete failure. I'm so dumb, I can't do anything right." What is the most appropriate nursing diagnosis for Karen?

   a. Chronic low self-esteem
   b. Situational low self-esteem
   c. Defensive coping
   d. Risk for situational low self-esteem

2. Which of the following outcome criteria would be most appropriate for Karen?

   a. Karen is able to express positive aspects about herself and her life situation.
   b. Karen is able to accept constructive criticism without becoming defensive.
   c. Karen is able to develop positive interpersonal relationships.
   d. Karen is able to accept positive feedback from others.

3. Which of the following nursing interventions is best for Karen's specific problem?

   a. Encourage Karen to talk about her feeling of shame over the failure.
   b. Assist Karen to problem solve her reasons for failing the exam.
   c. Help Karen understand the importance of good self-care and personal hygiene in the maintenance of self-esteem.
   d. Explore with Karen her past successes and accomplishments.

4. The psychiatric nurse encourages Karen to express her anger. Why is this an appropriate nursing intervention?

   a. Anger is the basis for self-esteem problems.
   b. The nurse suspects that Karen was abused as a child.
   c. The nurse is attempting to guide Karen through the grief process.
   d. The nurse recognizes that Karen has long-standing repressed anger.

5. Karen is demonstrating a number of behaviors attributed to low self-esteem that were triggered by her failure of the examination. In Karen's case, failure of the exam can be considered a

   a. Focal stimulus.
   b. Contextual stimulus.
   c. Residual stimulus.
   d. Spatial stimulus.

Match the statements on the left with the descriptions on the right:

_____6. "What do you want to do tonight?" "Whatever you   a. Rigid boundary
        want to do."

_____7. Twins Jan and Jean still dress alike   b. Too flexible boundary.
        even though they are grown and married.

TABLE 18–2	Assessing the Degree of Suicidal Risk		

	Intensity of Risk		
Behavior	**Low**	**Moderate**	**High**
Anxiety	Mild	Moderate	High or panic
Depression	Mild	Moderate	Severe
Isolation; withdrawal	Some feelings of isolation; no withdrawal	Some feelings of helplessness, hopelessness, and withdrawal	Hopeless, helpless, withdrawn, and self-deprecating
Daily functioning	Fairly good in most activities	Moderately good in some activities	Not good in any activities
Resources	Several	Some	Few or none
Coping strategies being used	Generally constructive	Some that are constructive	Predominantly destructive
Significant others	Several who are available	Few or only one available	Only one or none available
Psychiatric help in past	None, or positive attitude toward	Yes, and moderately satisfied with results	Negative view of help received
Lifestyle	Stable	Moderately stable	Unstable
Alcohol or drug use	Infrequently to excess	Frequently to excess	Continual abuse
Previous suicide attempts	None, or of low lethality	One or more of moderate lethality	Multiple attempts of high lethality
Disorientation; disorganization	None	Some	Marked
Hostility	Little or none	Some	Marked
Suicidal plan	Vague, fleeting thoughts but no plan	Frequent thoughts, occasional ideas about a plan	Frequent or constant thought with a specific plan

SOURCE: From Hatton, Valente, & Rink (1984), with permission.

● **Martial Status.** Single, divorced, and widowed are at higher risk than married.
● **Socioeconomic Status.** Individuals in the highest and lowest socioeconomic classes are at higher risk than those in the middle classes.
● **Occupation.** Professional health care personnel and business executives are at highest risk.
● **Method.** Use of firearms presents a significantly higher risk than overdose of substances.
● **Religion.** Individuals who are not affiliated with any religious group are at higher risk than those who have this type of affiliation.
● **Family History.** Higher risk if individual has family history of suicide.

Presenting Symptoms/Medical–Psychiatric Diagnosis

Assessment data must be gathered regarding any psychiatric or physical condition for which the client is being treated. Mood disorders (major depression and bipolar disorders) are the most common disorders that precede suicide. Individuals with substance use disorders are also at high risk. Other psychiatric disorders in which suicide may be a risk include anxiety disorders, schizophrenia, and borderline and antisocial personality disorders (Jacobs et al., 2006). Other chronic and terminal physical illnesses have also precipitated suicidal acts.

Suicidal Ideas or Acts

How serious is the intent? Does the person have a plan? If so, does he or she have the means? How lethal are the means? Has the individual ever attempted suicide before? These are all questions that must be answered by the person conducting the suicidal assessment.

Individuals may leave both behavioral and verbal clues as to the intent of their act. Examples of behavioral clues include giving away prized possessions, getting financial affairs in order, writing suicide notes, or sudden lifts in mood (may indicate a decision to carry out the intent).

Verbal clues may be both direct and indirect. Examples of direct statements include "I want to die" or "I'm going to kill myself." Examples of indirect statements include "This is the last time you'll see me," "I won't be around much longer for the doctor to have to worry about," or "I don't have anything worth living for anymore."

Other assessments include determining whether the individual has a plan, and if so, whether he or she has the means to carry out that plan. If the person states the suicide will be carried out with a gun, does he or she have access to a gun? Bullets? If pills are planned, what kind of pills? Are they accessible?

Interpersonal Support System

Does the individual have support persons on whom he or she can rely during a crisis situation? Lack of a meaningful network of satisfactory relationships may implicate an individual at high risk for suicide during an emotional crisis.

Analysis of the Suicidal Crisis

● **The Precipitating Stressor:** Adverse life events in combination with other risk factors such as depression may lead to suicide. Life stresses accompanied by an increase in emotional disturbance include the loss of a loved person either by death or by divorce, problems in major relationships, changes in roles, or serious physical illness.
● **Relevant History:** Has the individual experienced numerous failures or rejections that would increase his or her vulnerability for a dysfunctional response to the current situation?
● **Life-Stage Issues:** The ability to tolerate losses and disappointments is often compromised if those losses and disappointments occur during various stages of life in which the individual struggles with developmental issues (e.g., adolescence, midlife).

Psychiatric/Medical/Family History

The individual should be assessed with regard to previous psychiatric treatment for depression, alcoholism, or for previous suicide attempts. Medical history should be obtained to determine presence of chronic, debilitating, or terminal illness. Is there a history of depressive disorder in the family, and has a close relative committed suicide in the past?

Coping Strategies

How has the individual handled previous crisis situations? How does this situation differ from previous ones?

Diagnosis/Outcome Identification

Nursing diagnoses for the suicidal client may include the following:

1. Risk for suicide related to feelings of hopelessness and desperation.
2. Hopelessness related to absence of support systems and perception of worthlessness.

Outcome Criteria

Outcome criteria include short- and long-term goals. Timelines are individually determined. The following criteria may be used for measurement of outcomes in the care of the suicidal client.

The client:

1. Has experienced no physical harm to self.
2. Sets realistic goals for self.
3. Expresses some optimism and hope for the future.

Planning/Implementation

Table 18–3 provides a plan of care for the hospitalized suicidal client. Nursing diagnoses are presented, along with outcome criteria, appropriate nursing interventions, and rationales for each.

Intervention with the Suicidal Client Following Discharge (or Outpatient Suicidal Client)

In some instances, it may be determined that suicidal intent is low and that hospitalization is not required. Instead, the client with suicidal ideation may be treated in an outpatient setting. Guidelines for treatment of the suicidal client on an outpatient basis include the following:

1. The person should not be left alone. Arrangements must be made for the client to stay with family or friends. If this is not possible, hospitalization should be reconsidered.
2. Establish a no-suicide contract with the client. Formulate a written contract that the client will not harm himself or herself in a stated period of time. For example, the client writes, "I will not harm myself in any way between now and the time of our next counseling session," or "I will call the suicide hotline (or go to the emergency room) if I start to feel like harming myself." When the time period of this short-term contract has lapsed, a new contract is negotiated.
3. Enlist the help of family or friends to ensure that the home environment is safe from dangerous items, such as firearms or stockpiled drugs. Give support persons the telephone number of counselor or emergency contact person in the event that the counselor is not available.
4. Appointments may need to be scheduled daily or every other day at first until the immediate suicidal crisis has subsided.
5. Establish rapport and promote a trusting relationship. It is important for the suicide counselor to become a key person in the client's support system at this time.
6. Accept the client's feelings in a nonjudgmental manner.

CLINICAL PEARL

Be direct. Talk openly and matter-of-factly about suicide. Listen actively and encourage expression of feelings, including anger.

TABLE 21–1   Effects of Psychotropic Medications on Neurotransmitters

Example of Medication	Action on Neurotransmitter and/or Receptor	Physiological Effects	Side Effects
SSRIs	Inhibit reuptake of serotonin (5-HT)	Reduces depression Controls anxiety Controls obsessions	Nausea, agitation, headache, sexual dysfunction
Tricyclic antidepressants	Inhibit reuptake of serotonin (5-HT) Inhibit reuptake of norepinephrine (NE) Block NE (α_1) receptor Block ACh receptor Block histamine (H_1) receptor	Reduces depression Relief of severe pain Prevent panic attacks	Sexual dysfunction (NE & 5-HT) Sedation, weight gain (H_1) Dry mouth, constipation, blurred vision, urinary retention (ACh) Postural hypotension and tachycardia (α_1)
MAO inhibitors	Increase NE and 5-HT by inhibiting the enzyme that degrades them (MAO-A)	Reduces depression Controls anxiety	Sedation, dizziness Sexual dysfunction Hypertensive crisis (interaction with tyramine)
Trazodone and Nefazodone	5-HT reuptake block 5-HT_2 receptor antagonism Adrenergic receptor blockade	Reduces depression Reduces anxiety	Nausea (5-HT) Sedation (5-HT_2) Orthostasis (α_1) Priapism (α_2)
SSNRIs: venlafaxine, desvenlafaxine, and duloxetine	Potent inhibitor of serotonin and norepinephrine reuptake Weak inhibitor of dopamine reuptake	Reduces depression Relieves pain of neuropathy (duloxetine) Relieves anxiety (venlafaxine)	Nausea (5-HT) ↑sweating (NE) Insomnia (NE) Tremors (NE) Sexual dysfunction (5-HT)
Bupropion	Inhibits reuptake of NE and dopamine (D)	Reduces depression Aid in smoking cessation ↓ symptoms of ADHD	Insomnia, dry mouth, tremor, seizures
Antipsychotics: phenothiazines and haloperidol	Strong D_2 receptor blockade Weaker blockade of ACh, H_1, α_1-adrenergic, and 5-HT_2 receptors	Relief of psychosis Relief of anxiety (Some) provide relief from nausea and vomiting and intractable hiccoughs	Blurred vision, dry mouth, decreased sweating, constipation, urinary retention, tachycardia (ACh) EPS (D_2) ↑plasma prolactin (D_2) Sedation; weight gain (H_1) Ejaculatory difficulty (5-HT_2) Postural hypotension (α; H_1)
Antipsychotics (Novel): clozapine, olanzepine, aripiprazole, quetiapine, risperidone, ziprasidone paliperidone	Receptor antagonism of 5-HT_1 and 5-HT_2 $D_1 - D_5$ (varies with drug) H_1 α_1-adrenergic muscarinic (ACh)	Relief of psychosis (with minimal or no EPS) Relief of anxiety Relief of acute mania	Potential with some of the drugs for mild EPS (D_2) Sedation, weight gain (H_1) Orthostasis and dizziness (α-adrenergic) Blurred vision, dry mouth, decreased sweating, constipation, urinary retention, tachycardia (ACh)
Antianxiety: benzodiazepines	Binds to BZ receptor sites on the $GABA_A$ receptor complex; increases receptor affinity for GABA	Relief of anxiety Sedation	Dependence (with longterm use) Confusion; memory impairment; motor incoordination
Antianxiety: Buspirone	5-HT_{1A} agonist D_2 agonist D_2 antagonist	Relief of anxiety	Nausea, headache, dizziness Restlessness

ACh, acetylcholine; BZ, benzodiazepine; EPS, extrapyramidal symptoms; GABA, gamma-aminobutyric acid; 5-HT, 5-hydroxytryptamine (serotonin); MAO, monoamine oxidase; NE, norepinephrine.

also block receptor sites that are unrelated to their mechanisms of action. These include α-adrenergic, histaminergic, and muscarinic cholinergic receptors. Blocking these receptors is also associated with the development of certain side effects.

Antipsychotic medications block dopamine receptors, and some affect muscarinic cholinergic, histaminergic, and α-adrenergic receptors. The "atypical" antipsychotics block a specific serotonin receptor. Benzodiazepines facilitate the transmission of the inhibitory neurotransmitter

[handwritten in margin: Stop @ Go to 321]

gamma-aminobutyric acid (GABA). The psychostimulants work by increasing norepinephrine, serotonin, and dopamine release.

Although each psychotropic medication affects neurotransmission, the specific drugs within each class have varying neuronal effects. Their exact mechanisms of action are unknown. Many of the neuronal effects occur acutely; however, the therapeutic effects may take weeks for some medications such as antidepressants and antipsychotics. Acute alterations in neuronal function do not fully explain how these medications work. Long-term neuropharmacologic reactions to increased norepinephrine and serotonin levels relate more to their mechanisms of action. Recent research suggests that the therapeutic effects are related to the nervous system's adaptation to increased levels of neurotransmitters. These adaptive changes result from a homeostatic mechanism, much like a thermostat, that regulates the cell and maintains equilibrium.

APPLYING THE NURSING PROCESS IN PSYCHOPHARMACOLOGICAL THERAPY

An assessment tool for obtaining a drug history is provided in Box 21–1. This tool may be adapted for use by staff nurses admitting clients to the hospital, or by nurse practitioners who may wish to use it with prescriptive privileges. It may also be used when a client's signature of informed consent is required prior to pharmacological therapy.

Antianxiety Agents

Background Assessment Data

Indications. Antianxiety drugs are also called *anxiolytics* and *minor tranquilizers*. They are used in the treatment of anxiety disorders, anxiety symptoms, acute alcohol withdrawal, skeletal muscle spasms, convulsive disorders, status epilepticus, and preoperative sedation. Their use and efficacy for periods greater than 4 months have not been evaluated.

Examples of commonly used antianxiety agents are presented in Table 21–2.

Action. Antianxiety drugs depress subcortical levels of the CNS, particularly the limbic system and reticular formation. They may potentiate the effects of the powerful inhibitory neurotransmitter GABA in the brain, thereby producing a calmative effect. All levels of CNS depression can be effected, from mild sedation to hypnosis to coma.

EXCEPTION: Buspirone (BuSpar) does not depress the CNS. Although its action is unknown, the drug is

	TABLE 21–2	**Antianxiety Agents**					
Chemical Class	**Generic (Trade) Name**	**Controlled Categories**	**Pregnancy Categories**	**Half-Life (hr)**	**Daily Adult Dosage Range (mg)**	**Available Forms**	
Antihistamines	Hydroxyzine (Atarax)		C	3	100–400	Tabs: 10, 25, 50, 100 Syrup: 10/5 mL	
	(Vistaril)		C	3	100–400	Caps: 25, 50, 100 Oral Susp: 25/5 mL Inj: 25, 50	
Benzodiazepines	Alprazolam (Xanax)	CIV	D	6–26	0.75–4	Tabs: 0.25, 0.5, 1.0, 2.0 Tabs ER: 0.5, 1, 2, 3 Oral Solu: 1/mL	
	Chlordiazepoxide (Librium)	CIV	D	5–30	15–100	Caps: 5, 10, 25 Inj: 100/amp	
	Clonazepam (Klonopin)	CIV	C	18–50	1.5–20	Tabs: 0.5, 1.0, 2.0 Tabs (orally disintegrating): 0.125, 0.25, 0.5, 1.0, 2.0	
	Clorazepate (Tranxene)	CIV	UK	40–50	15–60	Tabs & Caps: 3.75, 7.5, 15 Single Dose: 11.25, 22.5	
	Diazepam (Valium)	CIV	D	20–80	4–40	Tabs: 2, 5, 10 Oral Solu: 5/5 mL, 5/mL Inj: 5/mL	
	Lorazepam (Ativan)	CIV	D	10–20	2–6	Tabs: 0.5, 1.0, 2.0 Oral Solu: 2/mL Inj: 2/mL, 4/mL	
	Oxazepam (Serax)	CIV	D	5–20	30–120	Tabs: 15 Caps: 10, 15, 30	
Carbamate derivative	Meprobamate	CIV	D	6–17	400–2400	Tabs: 200, 400	
Azaspirodecanediones	Buspirone (BuSpar)		B	2–3	15–60	Tabs: 5, 7.5, 10, 15, 30	

[handwritten note: ✓ Delayed onset / Doesn't upset CNS]

believed to produce the desired effects through interactions with serotonin, dopamine, and other neurotransmitter receptors.

Contraindications/Precautions. Antianxiety drugs are contraindicated in individuals with known hypersensitivity to any of the drugs within the classification (e.g., benzodiazepines). They should not be taken in combination with other CNS depressants and are contraindicated in pregnancy and lactation, narrow-angle glaucoma, shock, and coma.

Caution should be taken in administering these drugs to elderly or debilitated clients and clients with hepatic or renal dysfunction. (The dosage usually has to be decreased.) Caution is also required with individuals who have a history of drug abuse or addiction and with those who are depressed or suicidal. In depressed clients, CNS depressants can exacerbate symptoms.

Interactions. Increased effects of antianxiety agents can occur when taken concomitantly with alcohol, barbiturates, narcotics, antipsychotics, antidepressants, antihistamines, neuromuscular blocking agents, cimetidine, or disulfiram. Increased effects can also occur with herbal depressants (e.g., kava; valerian). Decreased effects can occur with cigarette smoking and caffeine consumption.

Diagnosis

The following nursing diagnoses may be considered for clients receiving therapy with antianxiety agents:

1. Risk for injury related to seizures; panic anxiety; acute agitation from alcohol withdrawal (indications); abrupt withdrawal after long-term use; effects of intoxication or overdose.
2. Risk for activity intolerance related to side effects of sedation and lethargy.
3. Risk for acute confusion related to action of the medication on the CNS.

Planning/Implementation

The plan of care should include monitoring for the following side effects from antianxiety agents. Nursing implications related to each side effect are designated by an asterisk (*).

1. **Drowsiness, confusion, lethargy** (most common side effects)
   *Instruct the client not to drive or operate dangerous machinery while taking the medication.
2. **Tolerance; physical and psychological dependence** (does not apply to buspirone)
   *Instruct the client on long-term therapy not to quit taking the drug abruptly. Abrupt withdrawal can be life threatening. Symptoms include depression, insomnia, increased anxiety, abdominal and muscle

cramps, tremors, vomiting, sweating, convulsions, and delirium.
3. **Ability to potentiate the effects of other CNS depressants**
   *Instruct the client not to drink alcohol or take other medications that depress the CNS while taking this medication.
4. **Possibility of aggravating symptoms in depressed persons**
   *Assess the client's mood daily.
   *Take necessary precautions for potential suicide.
5. **Orthostatic hypotension**
   *Monitor lying and standing blood pressure and pulse at every nursing shift.
   *Instruct the client to arise slowly from a lying or sitting position.
6. **Paradoxical excitement** (client develops symptoms opposite of the medication's desired effect)
   *Withhold drug and notify the physician.
7. **Dry mouth**
   *Have the client take frequent sips of water, suck on ice chips or hard candy, or chew sugarless gum.
8. **Nausea and vomiting**
   *Have the client take the drug with food or milk.
9. **Blood dyscrasias**
   *Symptoms of sore throat, fever, malaise, easy bruising, or unusual bleeding should be reported to the physician immediately.
10. **Delayed onset** (buspirone only)
    *Ensure that the client understands there is a lag time of 10 days to 2 weeks between onset of therapy with buspirone and subsiding of anxiety symptoms. Client should continue to take the medication during this time.

NOTE: Buspirone is not recommended for p.r.n. administration because of this delayed therapeutic onset. There is no evidence that buspirone creates tolerance or physical dependence as do the CNS depressant anxiolytics.

Client/Family Education

The client should:
● Not drive or operate dangerous machinery. Drowsiness and dizziness can occur.
● Not stop taking the drug abruptly, as this can produce serious withdrawal symptoms, such as depression, insomnia, anxiety, abdominal and muscle cramps, tremors, vomiting, sweating, convulsions, delirium.
● (*With buspirone only*): Be aware of lag time between start of therapy and subsiding of symptoms. Relief is usually evident within 10 to 14 days. The client must take the medication regularly, as ordered, so that it has sufficient time to take effect.

- Not consume other CNS depressants (including alcohol).
- Not take nonprescription medication without approval from the physician.
- Rise slowly from sitting or lying position to prevent sudden drop in blood pressure.
- Immediately report symptoms of sore throat, fever, malaise, easy bruising, unusual bleeding, or motor restlessness to physician.
- Be aware of risks of taking this drug during pregnancy. (Congenital malformations have been associated with use during the first trimester.) The client should notify the physician of the desirability to discontinue the drug if pregnancy is suspected or planned. (*Exceptions:* Although risk is less with clonazepam, it cannot be ruled out. With buspirone, safety has been established only in animal studies.)
- Be aware of possible side effects. The client should refer to written materials furnished by healthcare providers regarding the correct method of self-administration.
- Carry a card or piece of paper at all times stating the names of medications being taken.

Outcome Criteria/Evaluation

The following criteria may be used for evaluating the effectiveness of therapy with antianxiety agents.

The client:

1. Demonstrates a reduction in anxiety, tension, and restless activity.
2. Experiences no seizure activity.
3. Experiences no physical injury.
4. Is able to tolerate usual activities without excessive sedation.
5. Exhibits no evidence of confusion.
6. Tolerates the medication without gastrointestinal distress.
7. Verbalizes understanding of the need for, side effects of, and regimen for self-administration.
8. Verbalizes possible consequences of abrupt withdrawal from the medication.

Antidepressants

Background Assessment Data

Indications. Antidepressant medications are used in the treatment of dysthymic disorder; major depression with melancholia or psychotic symptoms; depression associated with organic disease, alcoholism, schizophrenia, or mental retardation; depressive phase of bipolar disorder; and depression accompanied by anxiety. These drugs elevate mood and alleviate other symptoms associated with moderate-to-severe depression. Selected agents are also used to treat anxiety disorders, bulimia nervosa, and premenstrual dysphoric disorder. Examples of commonly used antidepressant medications are presented in Table 21–3.

Action. These drugs ultimately work to increase the concentration of norepinephrine, serotonin, and/or dopamine in the body. This is accomplished in the brain by blocking the reuptake of these neurotransmitters by the neurons (tricyclics, selective serotonin reuptake

TABLE 21–3	**Antidepressant Medications**				
Chemical Class	**Generic (Trade) Name**	**Pregnancy Categories/ Half-life (hr)**	**Daily Adult Dosage Range (mg)***	**Therapeutic Plasma Ranges**	**Available Forms (mg)**
Tricyclics	Amitriptyline (Elavil; Endep)	D/31–46	50–300	110–250 (including metabolite)	Tabs: 10, 25, 50, 75, 100, 150
	Amoxapine (Asendin)	C/8	50–300	200–500	Tabs: 25, 50, 100, 150
	Clomipramine (Anafranil)	C/19–37	25–250	80–100	Caps: 25, 50, 75
	Desipramine (Norpramin)	C/12–24	25–300	125–300	Tabs: 10, 25, 50, 75, 100, 150
	Doxepin (Sinequan)	C/8–24	25–300	100–200 (including metabolite)	Caps: 10, 25, 50, 75, 100, 150 Oral Conc: 10/mL
	Imipramine (Tofranil)	D/11–25	30–300	200–350 (including metabolite)	HCl Tabs: 10, 25, 50 Pamoate Caps: 75, 100, 125, 150
	Nortriptyline (Aventyl; Pamelor)	D/18–44	30–100	50–150	Caps: 10, 25, 50, 75 Oral Solu: 10/5 mL
	Protriptyline (Vivactil)	C/67–89	15–60	100–200	Tabs: 5, 10
	Trimipramine (Surmontil)	C/7–30	50–300	180 (including metabolite)	Caps: 25, 50, 100

Chemical Class	Generic (Trade) Name	Pregnancy Categories/ Half-life (hr)	Daily Adult Dosage Range (mg)*	Therapeutic Plasma Ranges	Available Forms (mg)
Selective Serotonin Reuptake Inhibitors	Citalopram (Celexa)	C/~35	20–40	Not well established	Tabs: 10, 20, 40 Oral Solu: 10/5 mL
	Escitalopram (Lexapro)	C/27–32	10–20	Not well established	Tabs: 5, 10, 20 Oral Solu: 5/5 mL
	Fluoxetine (Prozac; Serafem)	C/1–16 days (including metabolite)	20–80	Not well established	Tabs: 10, 20 Caps: 10, 20, 40 Caps (delayed release): 90 Oral Solu: 20/5 mL
	Fluvoxamine (Luvox)	C/13.6–15.6	50–300	Not well established	Tabs: 25, 50, 100
	Paroxetine (Paxil)	C/21	10–50 (CR: 12.5–75)	Not well established	Tabs: 10, 20, 30, 40 Oral Susp: 10/5 mL Tabs (CR): 12.5, 25, 37.5
	Sertraline (Zoloft)	C/26–104 (including metabolite)	25–200	Not well established	Tabs: 25, 50, 100 Oral Conc: 20/mL
Monoamine Oxidase Inhibitors	Isocarboxazid (Marplan)	C/Not established	20–60	Not well established	Tabs: 10
	Phenelzine (Nardil)	C/Not established	45–90	Not well established	Tabs: 15
	Tranylcypromine (Parnate)	C/2.4–2.8	30–60	Not well established	Tabs: 10
	Selegiline Transdermal System (Emsam)	C/18–25 (including metabolites)	6/24 hr – 12/24 hr patch	Not well established	Transdermal patches: 6/24 hr, 9/24 hr, 12/24 hr
Others	Bupropion (Zyban; (Wellbutrin)	B/8–24	200–450	Not well established	Tabs: 75, 100 Tabs (SR): 100, 150, 200 Tabs (XL): 150, 300
	Maprotiline (Ludiomil)	B/21–25	25–225	200–300 (incl. metabolite)	Tabs: 25, 50, 75
	Mirtazapine (Remeron)	C/20–40	15–45	Not well established	Tabs: 7.5, 15, 30, 45 Tabs (orally disintegrating): 15, 30, 45
	Trazodone†	C/4–9	150–600	800–1600	Tabs: 50, 100, 150, 300
	Nefazodone‡	C/2–4	200–600	Not well established	Tabs: 50, 100, 150, 200, 250
	Venlafaxine (Effexor)	C/3–7 (metabolite, 9–13)	75–375	Not well established	Tabs: 25, 37.5, 50, 75, 100 Caps (XR): 37.5, 75, 150
	Duloxetine (Cymbalta)	C/8–17	40–60	Not well established	Caps: 20, 30, 60
	Desvenlafaxine (Pristiq)	C/11	50–400	Not well established	Tabs: 50, 100
Psychotherapeutic Combinations	Olanzapine and fluoxetine (Symbyax)	C/(see individual drugs)	6/25–12/50	Not well established	Caps: 6/25, 6/50, 12/25, 12/50
	Chlordiazepoxide and fluoxetine (Limbitrol DS)	D/(see individual drugs)	20/50–40/100	Not well established	Tabs: 5/12.5; 10/25
	Perphenazine and amitriptyline (Etrafon)	C–D/(see individual drugs)	6/30–16/200	Not well established	Tabs: 2/10, 2/25, 4/10, 4/25, 4/50

* Dosage requires slow titration; onset of therapeutic response may be 1 to 4 weeks.
† Brand-name Desyrel is no longer being manufactured. Generic trazodone is still available and is made by several different manufacturers.
‡ Bristol Myers Squibb voluntarily removed their brand of nefazodone (Serzone) from the market in 2004. The generic equivalent is currently available through various other manufacturers.

inhibitors, and others). It also occurs when an enzyme, monoamine oxidase (MAO), that is known to inactivate norepinephrine, serotonin, and dopamine, is inhibited at various sites in the nervous system (MAO inhibitors [MAOIs]).

Contraindications/Precautions. Antidepressant drugs are contraindicated in individuals with hypersensitivity. Tricyclics are contraindicated in the acute recovery phase following myocardial infarction and in individuals with angle-closure glaucoma.

Caution should be used in administering these drugs to elderly or debilitated clients and those with hepatic, renal, or cardiac insufficiency. (The dosage usually must be decreased.) Caution is also required with psychotic clients, with clients who have benign prostatic hypertrophy, and with individuals who have a history of seizures (may decrease seizure threshold).

NOTE: As these drugs take effect, and mood begins to lift, the individual may have increased energy with which to implement a suicide plan. Suicide potential often increases as level of depression decreases. The nurse should be particularly alert to sudden lifts in mood.

Interactions

Tricyclic Antidepressants

- Increased effects of tricyclic antidepressants with **bupropion, cimetidine, haloperidol, SSRIs, and valproic acid.**
- Decreased effects of tricyclic antidepressants with **carbamazepine, barbiturates, and rifamycins.**
- Hyperpyretic crisis, convulsions, and death can occur with **MAO inhibitors.**
- Co-administration with **clonidine** may produce hypertensive crisis.
- Decreased effects of **levodopa** and **guanethidine** with tricyclic antidepressants.
- Potentiation of pressor response with direct-acting **sympathomimetics.**
- Increased anticoagulation effects with **dicumarol.**
- Increased serum levels of carbamazepines occur with concomitant use of tricyclics.
- Increased risk of seizures with concomitant use of maprotiline and **phenothiazines.**

MAO Inhibitors

- Serious, potentially fatal adverse reactions may occur with concurrent use of other **antidepressants, carbamazepine, cyclobenzaprine, bupropion, SSRIs, SARIs, buspirone, sympathomimetics, tryptophan, dextromethorphan, anesthetic agents, CNS depressants,** and **amphetamines.** Avoid using within 2 weeks of each other (5 weeks after therapy with **fluoxetine**).

- Hypertensive crisis may occur with **amphetamines, methyldopa, levodopa, dopamine, epinephrine, norepinephrine, guanethidine, guanadrel, reserpine, vasoconstrictors,** or ingestion of tyramine-containing foods (Box 21–2)
- Hypertension or hypotension, coma, convulsions, and death may occur with **opioids** (avoid use of **meperidine** within 14 to 21 days of MAO inhibitor therapy).
- Excess CNS stimulation and hypertension may occur with **methylphenidate.**
- Additive hypotension may occur with **antihypertensives, thiazide diuretics,** or **spinal anesthesia.**
- Additive hypoglycemia may occur with **insulins** or **oral hypoglycemic agents.**
- **Doxapram** may increase pressor response.
- Serotonin syndrome may occur with concomitant use of **St. John's wort.**
- Consumption of foods or beverages with high **caffeine** content increases the risk of hypertension and arrhythmias.
- Bradycardia may occur with concurrent use of MAOIs and **beta blockers.**

Selective Serotonin Reuptake Inhibitors (SSRIs)

- Toxic, sometimes fatal, reactions have occurred with concomitant use of **MAOIs.**
- Increased effects of SSRIs with **cimetidine, L-tryptophan, lithium, linezolid,** and **St. John's wort.**
- Serotonin syndrome may occur with concomitant use of SSRIs and **metoclopramide, sibutramine, tramadol,** or **5-HT-receptor agonists (triptans).**
- Concomitant use of SSRIs may increase effects of **hydantoins, tricyclic antidepressants, cyclosporine, benzodiazepines, beta blockers, methadone, carbamazepine, clozapine, olanzapine, pimozide, haloperidol, phenothiazines, St. John's wort, sumatriptan, sympathomimetics, tacrine, theophylline,** and **warfarin.**
- Concomitant use of SSRIs may decrease effects of **buspirone** and **digoxin.**
- **Lithium** levels may be increased or decreased by concomitant use of SSRIs.
- Decreased effects of SSRIs with concomitant use of **carbamazepine** and **cyproheptadine.**

Others

- Concomitant use with **MAOIs** results in serious, sometimes fatal, effects resembling neuroleptic malignant syndrome. Coadministration is contraindicated.
- Serotonin syndrome may occur when any of the following are used together: **St. John's wort, sumatriptan, sibutramine, trazodone, nefazodone, venlafaxine, duloxetine.**

BOX 21–2 Diet and Drug Restrictions for Clients on MAOI Therapy

Foods Containing Tyramine

High Tyramine Content (Avoid while on MAOI therapy)	Moderate Tyramine Content (May eat occasionally while on MAOI therapy)	Low Tyramine Content (Limited quantities permissible while on MAOI therapy)
Aged cheeses (cheddar, Swiss, Camembert, blue cheese, Parmesan, provolone, Romano, brie)	Gouda cheese, processed American cheese, mozzarella	Pasteurized cheeses (cream cheese, cottage cheese, ricotta)
Raisins, fava beans, flat Italian beans, Chinese pea pods	Yogurt, sour cream	Figs
Red wines (Chianti, burgundy, cabernet sauvignon)	Avocados, bananas	Distilled spirits (in moderation)
Smoked and processed meats (salami, bologna, pepperoni, summer sausage)	Beer, white wine, coffee, colas, tea, hot chocolate	
Caviar, pickled herring, corned beef, chicken or beef liver	Meat extracts, such as bouillon	
Soy sauce, brewer's yeast, meat tenderizer (MSG)	Chocolate	

Drugs Restrictions

Ingestion of the following substances while on MAOI Therapy could result in life-threatening hypertensive crisis. A 14-day interval is recommended between use of these drugs and an MAOI.

Other antidepressants (tricyclic, SSRIs, bupropion, mirtazapine, nefazodone, trazodone, venlafaxine)

Sympathomimetics: (epinephrine, dopamine, norepinephrine, ephedrine, pseudoephedrine, phenylephrine, phenyl-propanolamine, over-the-counter cough and cold preparations)

Stimulants (amphetamines, cocaine, diet drugs)

Antihypertensives (methyldopa, guanethidine, reserpine)

Meperidine and (possibly) other opioid narcotics (morphine, codeine)

Antiparkinsonian agents (levodopa)

SOURCES: Andreasen & Black (2006); Sadock & Sadock (2007); and Martinez, Marangell, & Martinez (2008).

- Increased effects of **haloperidol, clozapine,** and **desipramine** when used concomitantly with venlafaxine.
- Increased effects of venlafaxine with **cimetidine.**
- Increased effects of **warfarin** with venlafaxine and duloxetine.
- Increased effects of duloxetine with CYP1A2 inhibitors (e.g., fluvoxamine, quinolone antibiotics) and CYP2D6 inhibitors (e.g., fluoxetine, quinidine, paroxetine).
- Increased risk of liver injury with concomitant use of **alcohol** and duloxetine.
- Increased risk of toxicity or adverse effects from drugs extensively metabolized by CYP2D6 (e.g., **flecainide, phenothiazines, propafenone, tricyclic antidepressants, thioridazine**) when used concomitantly with duloxetine or bupropion.
- Decreased effects of bupropion and trazodone with **carbamazepine.**
- Altered anticoagulant effect of **warfarin** with bupropion, venlafaxine, duloxetine, or trazodone.

Diagnosis

The following nursing diagnoses may be considered for clients receiving therapy with antidepressant medications:

1. Risk for suicide related to depressed mood.
2. Risk for injury related to side effects of sedation, lowered seizure threshold, orthostatic hypotension, **priapism,** photosensitivity, arrhythmias, hypertensive crisis, or serotonin syndrome.
3. Social isolation related to depressed mood.
4. Risk for constipation related to side effects of the medication.

Planning/Implementation

The plan of care should include monitoring for the following side effects from antidepressant medications. Nursing implications are designated by an asterisk (*). A general profile of the side effects of antidepressant medications is presented in Table 21–4.

| TABLE 21–4 | Side Effect Profiles of Antidepressant Medications | | | | | | |

	CNS Side Effects		Cardiovascular Side Effects		Other Side Effects		
	Sedation	Insomnia/ Agitation	Orthostatic Hypotension	Cardiac Arrhythmia	Gastrointestinal Distress	Weight Gain (>6 kg)	Anticholinergic*
Amitriptyline	4+	0	4+	3+	0	4+	4+
Clomipramine	3+	0	2+	3+	2+	1+	3+
Desipramine	1+	1+	2+	2+	0	1+	1+
Doxepin	4+	0	2+	2+	0	3+	3+
Imipramine	3+	1+	4+	3+	1+	3+	3+
Nortriptyline	1+	0	2+	2+	0	1+	1+
Protriptyline	1+	1+	2+	2+	0	0	2+
Trimipramine	4+	0	2+	2+	0	3+	1+
Amoxapine	2+	2+	2+	3+	0	1+	2+
Maprotiline	4+	0	0	1+	0	2+	2+
Mirtazapine	4+	0	0	1+	0	2+	2+
Trazodone	4+	0	1+	0	1+	0	0
Nefazodone	3+	0	1+	0	1+	0	0
Bupropion	0	2+	0	1+	1+	0	0
Fluoxetine	0	2+	0	0	3+	0	0
Fluvoxamine	0	2+	0	0	3+	0	0
Paroxetine	0	2+	0	0	3+	0	0
Sertraline	0	2+	0	0	3+	0	0
Citalopram	1+	2+	0	0	3+	0	0
Escitalopram	0	2+	0	0	3+	0	0
Venlafaxine	0	2+	0	0	3+	0	0
Duloxetine	0	1+	0	0	3+	0	0
Monoamine Oxidase Inhibitors (MAOIs)	1+	2+	2+	0	1+	2+	1+

KEY:
0 = Absent or rare.
1+ = Infrequent
2+, 3+ = Relatively common.
4+ = Frequent
*Dry mouth, blurred vision, urinary hesitancy, constipation.
SOURCES: Drug Facts & Comparisons (2007); Karasu, Gelenberg, Merriam, & Wang (2006); and Schatzberg, Cole, & DeBattista (2007).

1. **May occur with all chemical classes:**
   a. Dry mouth
      *Offer the client sugarless candy, ice, frequent sips of water.
      *Strict oral hygiene is very important.
   b. Sedation
      *Request an order from the physician for the drug to be given at bedtime.
      *Request that the physician decrease the dosage or perhaps order a less sedating drug.
      *Instruct the client not to drive or use dangerous equipment while experiencing sedation.
   c. Nausea
      *Medication may be taken with food to minimize GI distress.
   d. Discontinuation syndrome
      *All classes of antidepressants have varying potentials to cause discontinuation syndromes. Abrupt withdrawal following long-term therapy with SSRIs, venlafaxine, desvenlafaxine, and duloxetine may result in dizziness, lethargy, headache, and nausea. Fluoxetine is less likely to result in withdrawal symptoms because of its long half-life. Abrupt withdrawal from tricyclics may produce hypomania, akathisia, cardiac arrhythmias, gastrointestinal upset, and panic attacks. The discontinuation syndrome associated with MAOIs includes flulike symptoms, confusion, hypomania, and worsening of depressive symptoms. All antidepressant medication should be tapered gradually to prevent withdrawal symptoms (Schatzberg, Cole, & DeBattista, 2007).

2. **Most commonly occur with tricyclics and others, such as bupropion, maprotiline, mirtazapine, trazodone, and nefazodone:**
   a. Blurred vision
      *Offer reassurance that this symptom should subside after a few weeks.
      *Instruct the client not to drive until vision is clear.
      *Clear small items from routine pathway to prevent falls.
   b. Constipation
      *Order foods high in fiber; increase fluid intake if not contraindicated; and encourage the client to increase physical exercise, if possible.

c. Urinary retention
*Instruct the client to report hesitancy or inability to urinate.
*Monitor intake and output.
*Try various methods to stimulate urination, such as running water in the bathroom or pouring water over the perineal area.

d. Orthostatic hypotension
*Instruct the client to rise slowly from a lying or sitting position.
*Monitor blood pressure (lying and standing) frequently, and document and report significant changes.
*Avoid long hot showers or tub baths.

e. Reduction of seizure threshold
*Observe clients with history of seizures closely.
*Institute seizure precautions as specified in hospital procedure manual.
*Bupropion (Wellbutrin) should be administered in doses of no more than 150 mg and should be given at least 4 hours apart. Bupropion has been associated with a relatively high incidence of seizure activity in anorexic and cachectic clients.

f. Tachycardia; arrhythmias
*Carefully monitor blood pressure and pulse rate and rhythm, and report any significant change to the physician.

g. Photosensitivity
*Ensure that client wears sunblock lotion, protective clothing, and sunglasses while outdoors.

h. Weight gain
*Provide instructions for reduced-calorie diet.
*Encourage increased level of activity, if appropriate.

3. **Most commonly occur with SSRIs:**
a. Insomnia; agitation
*Administer or instruct client to take dose early in the day.
*Instruct client to avoid caffeinated food and drinks.
*Teach relaxation techniques to use before bedtime.

b. Headache
*Administer analgesics, as prescribed.
*Request that the physician order another SSRI or another class of antidepressants

c. Weight loss (may occur early in therapy)
*Ensure that client is provided with caloric intake sufficient to maintain desired weight.
*Caution should be taken in prescribing these drugs for anorectic clients.
*Weigh client daily or every other day, at the same time, and on the same scale, if possible.
*After prolonged use, some clients may gain weight on SSRIs

d. Sexual dysfunction
*Men may report abnormal ejaculation or impotence.
*Women may experience delay or loss of orgasm.

*If side effect becomes intolerable, a switch to another antidepressant may be necessary.

e. Serotonin syndrome (may occur when two drugs that potentiate serotonergic neurotransmission are used concurrently [see "Interactions"])
*Most frequent symptoms include changes in mental status, restlessness, myoclonus, hyperreflexia, tachycardia, labile blood pressure, diaphoresis, shivering, and tremors.
*Discontinue the offending agent immediately.
*The physician will prescribe medications to block serotonin receptors, relieve hyperthermia and muscle rigidity, and prevent seizures. In severe cases, artificial ventilation may be required. The histamine-1 receptor antagonist cyproheptadine is commonly used to treat the symptoms of serotonin syndrome.
*Supportive nursing measures include monitoring vital signs, providing safety measures to prevent injury when muscle rigidity and changes in mental status are present, cooling blankets and tepid baths to assist with temperature regulation, and monitoring intake and output (Prator, 2006).
*The condition will usually resolve on its own once the offending medication has been discontinued. However, if the medication is not discontinued, the condition can progress to a more serious state and become fatal (Schatzberg, Cole, & DeBattista, 2007).

4. **Most commonly occur with MAOIs:**
a. Hypertensive crisis
*Hypertensive crisis occurs if the individual consumes foods containing tyramine while receiving MAOI therapy (see Table 21–5). (**NOTE:** Hypertensive crisis has not shown to be a problem with selegiline transdermal system at the 6 mg/24 hr dosage, and dietary restrictions at this dose is not recommended. Dietary modifications are recommended, however, at the 9 mg/24 hr and 12 mg/24 hr dosages.)
*Symptoms of hypertensive crisis include severe occipital headache, palpitations, nausea/vomiting, nuchal rigidity, fever, sweating, marked increase in blood pressure, chest pain, and coma.
*Treatment of hypertensive crisis: discontinue drug immediately; monitor vital signs; administer short-acting antihypertensive medication, as ordered by physician; use external cooling measures to control hyperpyrexia.

b. Application site reactions (with selegiline transdermal system [Emsam])
*The most common reactions include rash, itching, erythema, redness, irritation, swelling, or urticarial lesions. Most reactions resolve spontaneously, requiring no treatment. However, if reaction becomes problematic, it should be reported to the physician. Topical corticosteroids have been used in treatment.

5. **Miscellaneous side effects:**
   a. Priapism (with trazodone)
      *Priapism is a rare side effect, but it has occurred in some men taking trazodone
      *If the client complains of prolonged or inappropriate penile erection, withhold medication and notify the physician immediately.
      *Priapism can become very problematic, requiring surgical intervention, and, if not treated successfully, can result in impotence.
   b. Hepatic failure (with nefazodone)
      *Cases of life-threatening hepatic failure have been reported in clients treated with nefazodone.
      *Advise clients to be alert for signs or symptoms suggestive of liver dysfunction (e.g., jaundice, anorexia, GI complaints, or malaise) and to report them to physician immediately.

Client/Family Education

The client should:

● Continue to take the medication even though the symptoms have not subsided. The therapeutic effect may not be seen for as long as 4 weeks. If after this length of time no improvement is noted, the physician may prescribe a different medication.
● Use caution when driving or operating dangerous machinery. Drowsiness and dizziness can occur. If these side effects become persistent or interfere with activities of daily living, the client should report them to the physician. Dosage adjustment may be necessary.
● Not stop taking the drug abruptly. To do so might produce withdrawal symptoms, such as nausea, vertigo, insomnia, headache, malaise, and nightmares.
● Use sunblock lotion and wear protective clothing when spending time outdoors. The skin may be sensitive to sunburn.
● Report occurrence of any of the following symptoms to the physician immediately: sore throat, fever, malaise, yellowish skin, unusual bleeding, easy bruising, persistent nausea/vomiting, severe headache, rapid heart rate, difficulty urinating, anorexia/weight loss, seizure activity, stiff or sore neck, and chest pain.
● Rise slowly from a sitting or lying position to prevent a sudden drop in blood pressure.
● Take frequent sips of water, chew sugarless gum, or suck on hard candy if dry mouth is a problem. Good oral care (frequent brushing, flossing) is very important.
● Not consume the following foods or medications while taking MAOIs: aged cheese, wine (especially Chianti), beer, chocolate, colas, coffee, tea, sour cream, smoked and processed meats, beef or chicken liver, canned figs, soy sauce, overripe and fermented foods, pickled herring, raisins, caviar, yogurt, yeast products, broad beans, cold remedies, diet pills. To do so could cause a life-threatening hypertensive crisis.
● Avoid smoking while receiving tricyclic therapy. Smoking increases the metabolism of tricyclics, requiring an adjustment in dosage to achieve the therapeutic effect.
● Not drink alcohol while taking antidepressant therapy. These drugs potentiate the effects of each other.
● Not consume other medications (including over-the-counter medications) without the physician's approval while receiving antidepressant therapy. Many medications contain substances that, in combination with antidepressant medication, could precipitate a life-threatening hypertensive crisis.
● Notify physician immediately if inappropriate or prolonged penile erections occur while taking trazodone. If the erection persists longer than 1 hour, seek emergency room treatment. This condition is rare, but has occurred in some men who have taken trazodone. If measures are not instituted immediately, impotence can result.
● Not "double up" on medication if a dose of bupropion (Wellbutrin) is missed, unless advised to do so by the physician. Taking bupropion in divided doses will decrease the risk of seizures and other adverse effects.
● Follow the correct procedure for applying the selegiline transdermal patch:
  • Apply to dry, intact skin on upper torso, upper thigh, or outer surface of upper arm.
  • Apply approximately same time each day to new spot on skin, after removing and discarding old patch.
  • Wash hands thoroughly after applying the patch.
  • Avoid exposing application site to direct heat (e.g., heating pads, electric blankets, heat lamps, hot tub, or prolonged direct sunlight).
  • If patch falls off, apply new patch to a new site and resume previous schedule.
● Be aware of possible risks of taking antidepressants during pregnancy. Safe use during pregnancy and lactation has not been fully established. These drugs are believed to readily cross the placental barrier; if so, the fetus could experience adverse effects of the drug. Inform the physician immediately if pregnancy occurs, is suspected, or is planned.
● Be aware of the side effects of antidepressants. Refer to written materials furnished by healthcare providers for safe self-administration.
● Carry a card or other identification at all times describing the medications being taken.

Outcome Criteria/Evaluation

The following criteria may be used for evaluating the effectiveness of therapy with antidepressant medications:

The client:

1. Has not harmed self.
2. Has not experienced injury caused by side effects such as priapism, hypertensive crisis, or photosensitivity.
3. Exhibits vital signs within normal limits.
4. Manifests symptoms of improvement in mood (brighter affect, interaction with others, improvement in hygiene, clear thought and communication patterns).
5. Willingly participates in activities and interacts appropriately with others.

Mood-Stabilizing Agents

Background Assessment Data

For many years, the drug of choice for treatment and management of bipolar mania was lithium carbonate. However, in recent years, a number of investigators and clinicians in practice have achieved satisfactory results with several other medications, either alone or in combination with lithium. Table 21–5 provides information about the indication, action, and contraindications and precautions of various medications being used as mood stabilizers.

Interactions

Lithium Carbonate. Increased renal excretion of lithium may occur with acetazolamide, osmotic diuretics, and theophylline. Decreased renal excretion of lithium may occur with nonsteroidal anti-inflammatory drugs and thiazide diuretics. There is an increased risk of neurotoxicity with concurrent use of lithium and carbamazepine, haloperidol, or methyldopa. Concurrent use with fluoxetine or loop diuretics may result in increased serum lithium levels. Increased effects of neuromuscular blocking agents or tricyclic antidepressants and decreased pressor sensitivity of sympathomimetics can occur with concomitant use of lithium. Use of lithium with phenothiazines may result in neurotoxicity, decreased phenothiazine concentrations, or increased lithium concentration. Concurrent use with verapamil may result in decreased lithium levels or lithium toxicity.

Clonazepam. The effects of clonazepam may be increased with concomitant use of CNS depressants, cimetidine, hormonal contraceptives, disulfiram, fluoxetine, isoniazid, ketoconazole, metoprolol, propoxyphene, propranolol, or valproic acid. The effects of clonazepam are decreased by rifampin, barbiturates, theophylline, or phenytoin. Concomitant use may result in increased phenytoin levels and decreased efficacy of levodopa.

Carbamazepine. The effects of carbamazepine may be increased by verapamil, diltiazem, propoxyphene, erythromycin, clarithromycin, SSRIs, antidepressants, cimetidine, isonizaid, danazol, or lamotrigine. The effects of carbamazepine may be decreased by cisplatin, doxorubicin, felbamate, rifampin, barbiturates, hydantoins,

primidone, or theophylline. Concurrent use with carbamazepine may decrease levels of corticosteroids, doxycycline, felbamate, quinidine, warfarin, estrogen-containing contraceptives, cyclosporine, benzodiazepines, theophylline, lamotrigine, valproic acid, bupropion, haloperidol, olanzapine, tiagabine, topiramate, voriconazole, ziprasidone, or felbamate. Concurrent use with carbamazepine may result in increased levels of lithium and life-threatening hypertensive reaction with MAOIs.

Valproic Acid. The effects of valproic acid may be increased by chlorpromazine, cimetidine, erythromycin, felbamate, or salicylates. The effects of valproic acid may be decreased by rifampin, carbamazepine, cholestyramine, lamotrigine, phenobarbital, hydantoins, or ethosuximide. Concomitant use with valproic acid may increase the effects of tricyclic antidepressants, carbamazepine, CNS depressants, ethosuximide, lamotrigine, phenobarbital, warfarin and other antiplatelet agents, zidovudine, or hydantoins.

Lamotrigine. The effects of lamotrigine are increased by valproic acid. The effects of lamotrigine are decreased by primidone, phenobarbital, phenytoin, rifamycin, succinimides, oral contraceptives, oxcarbazepine, acetaminophen, or carbamazepine. Concomitant use with lamotrigine may result in decreased levels of valproic acid or increased levels of carbamazepine.

Gabapentin. The effects of gabapentin are increased by cimetidine, hydrocodone, or morphine. Antacids reduce the bioavailability of gabapentin. Concomitant use with gabapentin may result in decreased effects of hydrocodone.

Topiramate. The effects of topiramate may be increased with metformin. The effects of topiramate may be decreased with phenytoin, carbamazepine, or valproic acid. Concomitant use of topiramate with alcohol or other CNS depressants can potentiate CNS depression or other cognitive or neuropsychiaric adverse events. A risk of renal stone formation exists with co-administration of topiramate and carbonic anhydrase inhibitors (e.g., acetazolamide or dichlorphenamide). Concomitant use with topiramate may result in increased effects of phenytoin, metformin, or amitriptyline and decreased effects of oral contraceptives, digoxin, lithium, risperidone, and valproic acid.

Verapamil. The effects of verapamil are increased by cimetidine, ranitidine, beta blockers, or grapefruit juice. The effects of verapamil are decreased by hydantoins, rifampin, or antineoplastics. There is a risk of cardiotoxicity and decreased cardiac output with concomitant use of amiodarone. Concomitant use with verapamil may result in increased effects of beta blockers, 3-hydroxy-3-methylglutaryl coenzyme A (HMG-CoA) reductase inhibitors, imipramine, nondepolarizing muscle relaxants, prazosin, quinidine, sirolimus, tacrolimus, and theophyllines. Coadministration with verapamil may cause a reduction in lithium levels.

TABLE 21-5	Mood-Stabilizing Agents				
Classification: Generic (Trade)	**Pregnancy Category/ Half-life/ Indications**	**Mechanism of Action**	**Contraindications/ Precautions**	**Daily Adult Dosage Range/ Therapeutic Plasma Range**	**Available Forms (mg)**
Antimanic Lithium carbonate (Eskalith, Lithane; Lithobid)	D/10–50 hr/ • Prevention and treatment of manic episodes of bipolar disorder. *Unlabeled uses:* • Neutropenia • Cluster headaches (prophylaxis) • Alcohol dependence • Bulimia • Postpartum affective psychosis • Corticosteroid- induced psychosis	Not fully understood, but may enhance reuptake of norepinephrine and serotonin, decreasing the levels in the body, resulting in decreased hyper- activity (may take 1–3 weeks for symptoms to subside).	Hypersensitivity. Cardiac or renal disease, dehydra- tion; sodium depletion; brain damage; pregnancy and lactation. Caution with thyroid disorders, diabetes, urinary retention, history of seizures, and with the elderly.	Acute mania: 1800–2400 mg Maintenance: 900–1200 mg/ Acute mania: 1.0–1.5 mEq/L Maintenance: 0.6–1.2 mEq/L	Caps: 150, 300, 600 Tabs: 300 Tabs (ER): 300, 450 Tabs (CR): 450 Syrup: 8 mEq (as citrate equivalent to 300 mg lithium carbonate)/5 mL
Anticonvulsants Carbamazepine (Tegretol)	D/25–65 hr (initial); 12–17 hr (repeated doses)/ • Epilepsy • Trigeminal neuralgia *Unlabeled uses:* • Bipolar disorder • Resistant schizophrenia • Management of alcohol withdrawal • Restless legs syndrome • Postherpetic neuralgia	Action in the treatment of bipolar disorder is unclear.	Hypersensitivity. With MAOIs, lactation. Caution with elderly, liver/renal/cardiac disease, pregnancy.	200–1200 mg/ 4–12 µg/mL	Tabs: 100, 200 Tabs XR: 100, 200, 400 Caps XR: 100, 200, 300 Oral suspension: 100/5 mL 200/5 mL
Clonazepam (Klonopin)	C/18–60 hr/ • Petit mal, akinetic, and myoclonic seizures • Panic disorder *Unlabeled uses:* • Acute manic episodes • Uncontrolled leg movements during sleep • Neuralgias	Action in the treatment of bipolar disorder is unclear.	Hypersensitivity, glaucoma, liver disease, lactation. Caution in elderly, liver/renal disease, pregnancy.	0.5–20 mg/ 20–80 ng/mL	Tabs: 0.5, 1, 2
Valproic acid (Depakene; Depakote)	D/5–20 hr/ • Epilepsy • Manic episodes • Migraine prophylaxis • Adjunct therapy in schizophrenia	Action in the treatment of bipolar disorder is unclear.	Hypersensitivity; liver disease. Caution in elderly, renal/cardiac diseases, pregnancy and lactation.	5 mg per kg to 60 mg per kg/ 50–150 µg/mL	Caps: 250 Syrup: 250/5 mL Tabs (DR): 125, 250, 500 Tabs (ER): 250, 500 Caps (sprinkle): 125 Injection: 100/mL in 5 mL vial
Lamotrigine (Lamictal)	C/~33 hr/ • Epilepsy *Unlabeled use:* • Bipolar disorder	Action in the treatment of bipolar disorder is unclear.	Hypersensitivity. Caution in renal and hepatic insufficiency, pregnancy, lactation, and children < 16 years old.	100–400 mg/ No value established	Tabs: 25, 100, 150, 200 Tabs (chewable): 2, 5, 25

Classification: Generic (Trade)	Pregnancy Category/ Half-life/ Indications	Mechanism of Action	Contraindications/ Precautions	Daily Adult Dosage Range/ Therapeutic Plasma Range	Available Forms (mg)
Gabapentin (Neurontin; Gabarone)	C/5–7 hr/ • Epilepsy • Postherpetic neuralgia *Unlabeled uses:* • Bipolar disorder • Migraine prophylaxis • Neuropathic pain • Tremors associated with multiple sclerosis	Action in the treatment of bipolar disorder is unclear.	Hypersensitivity and children < 3 years. Caution in renal insufficiency, pregnancy, lactation, children, and the elderly.	900–1800 mg/ No value established	Caps: 100, 300, 400 Tabs: 100, 300, 400, 600, 800 Oral Solu: 250/5 mL
Topiramate (Topamax)	C/21 hr/ • Epilepsy • Migraine prophylaxis *Unlabeled uses:* • Bipolar disorder • Cluster headaches • Bulimia • Binge eating disorder • Weight loss in obesity	Action in the treatment of bipolar disorder is unclear.	Hypersensitivity. Caution in renal and hepatic impairment, pregnancy, lactation, children, and the elderly.	50–400 mg/ No value established	Tabs: 25, 50, 100, 200 Caps (sprinkle): 15, 25
Calcium Channel Blocker Verapamil (Calan; Isoptin)	C/3–7 hr (initially); 4.5–12 hr (repeated dosing); ~12 hr (SR); 2–5 hr (IV)/ • Angina • Arrhythmias • Hypertension *Unlabeled uses:* • Bipolar mania • Migraine headache prophylaxis	Action in the treatment of bipolar disorder is unclear.	Hypersensitivity; severe left ventricular dysfunction, heart block, hypotension, cardiogenic shock, congestive heart failure. Caution in liver or renal disease, cardiomyopathy, intracranial pressure, elderly patients, pregnancy and lactation.	80–320 mg/ 80–300 ng/ml	Tabs: 40, 80, 120 Tabs (XR; SR): 120, 180, 240 Caps SR: 120, 180, 240, 360 Caps XR: 100, 120, 180, 200, 240, 300 Injection: 2.5/mL
Antipsychotics Olanzapine (Zyprexa)	C/21–54 hr/ • Schizophrenia • Acute manic episodes • Management of bipolar disorder • Agitation associated with schizophrenia or mania *Unlabeled uses:* • Obsessive-compulsive disorder	**All antipsychotics:** Efficacy in schizophrenia is achieved through a combination of dopamine and serotonin type 2 (5-HT$_2$) antagonism. Mechanism of action in the treatment of mania is unknown.	**All antipsychotics:** Hypersensitivity, children, lactation. Caution with hepatic or cardiovascular disease, history of seizures, comatose or other CNS-depression, prostatic hypertrophy, narrow-angle glaucoma, diabetes or risk factors for diabetes, pregnancy, elderly and debilitated patients.	10–20 mg/ Not established	Tabs: 2.5, 5, 7.5, 10, 15, 20 Tabs (orally disintegrating): 5, 10, 15, 20 Powder for injection: 10 mg/vial

Continued on following page

TABLE 21–5	Mood-Stabilizing Agents *(Continued)*

Classification: Generic (Trade)	Pregnancy Category/ Half-life/ Indications	Mechanism of Action	Contraindications/ Precautions	Daily Adult Dosage Range/ Therapeutic Plasma Range	Available Forms (mg)
Olanzapine and fluoxetine (Symbyax)	C/(see individual drugs)/ • For the treatment of depressive episodes associated with bipolar disorder			6/25–12/50 mg/ Not established	Caps: 6/25, 6/50, 12/25, 12/50
Aripiprazole (Abilify)	C/ 75-94 hr (including metabolite)/ • Bipolar mania • Schizophrenia			10–30 mg/ Not established	Tabs: 5, 10, 15, 20, 30 Oral Solu: 1/mL
Chlorpromazine (Thorazine)	C/24 hr/ • Bipolar mania • Schizophrenia • Emesis/hiccoughs • Acute intermittent porphyria • Preoperative apprehension *Unlabeled uses:* • Migraine headaches			40–400 mg/ Not established	Tabs: 10, 25, 50, 100, 200 Oral concentrate: 100/mL Suppositories: 100 Injection: 25/mL
Quetiapine (Seroquel)	C/6 hr/ • Schizophrenia • Acute manic episodes			100–800 mg/ Not established	Tabs: 25, 100, 200, 300
Risperidone (Risperdal)	C/3–21 hr (including metabolite)/ • Bipolar mania • Schizophrenia *Unlabeled uses:* • Severe behavioral problems in children • Behavioral problems associated with autism • Obsessive–compulsive disorder			1–6 mg/ Not established	Tabs: 0.25, 0.5, 1, 2, 3, 4 Tabs (orally disintegrating): 0.5, 1, 2 Oral Solu: 1/mL Powder for injection: 25/vial, 37.5/vial, 50/vial
Ziprasidone (Geodon)	C/7 hr (oral); 2–4 hr (IM)/ • Bipolar mania • Schizophrenia • Acute agitation in schizophrenia			40–160 mg/ Not established	Caps: 20, 40, 60, 80 Powder for injection: 20/vial

Antipsychotics. Concomitant use of all antipsychotics with alcohol or other CNS depressants results in increased CNS depression. Coadministration with antihypertensives may result in increased hypotension. The effects of olanzapine are increased by fluvoxamine and fluoxetine and decreased by carbamazepine, omeprazole, and rifampin. The effects of aripiprazole are increased by quinidine and CYP3A4 inhibitors and decreased by carbamazepine, famotidine, and valproate. The effects of chlorpromazine are increased by beta blockers and paroxetine and decreased by centrally acting anticholinergics.

Coadministration with chlorpromazine results in increased or decreased phenytoin levels; increased effects of beta blockers, meperidine, and anticholinergic agents; and decreased effects of guanethidine and oral anticoagulants. The effects of quetiapine are increased by cimetidine or CYP3A4 inhibitors and decreased by phenytoin or thioridazine. Coadministration with quetiapine, olanzapine, ziprasidone, or risperidone results in decreased effects of levodopa and dopamine agonists. The effects of risperidone are increased by clozapine, fluoxetine, paroxetine, or ritonavir and decreased by carbamazepine. Coadministration with risperidone results in increased effects of clozapine and valproate. The effects of ziprasidone are increased by CYP3A4 inhibitors and decreased by carbamazepine. Life-threatening prolongation of QT interval can occur with coadministration of ziprasidone and quinidine, dofetilide, other class Ia and III antiarrhythmics, pimozide, sotalol, thioridazine, chlorpromazine, floquine, pentamadine, arsenic trioxide, mefloquine, dolasetron, tacrolimus, droperidol, gatifloxacin, or moxifloxacin.

Diagnosis

The following nursing diagnoses may be considered for clients receiving therapy with mood stabilizing agents:

1. Risk for injury related to manic hyperactivity.
2. Risk for self-directed or other-directed violence related to unresolved anger turned inward on the self or outward on the environment.
3. Risk for injury related to lithium toxicity.
4. Risk for activity intolerance related to side effects of drowsiness and dizziness.

Planning/Implementation

The plan of care should include monitoring for side effects of therapy with mood-stabilizing agents and intervening when required to prevent the occurrence of adverse events related to medication administration. Side effects and nursing implications for mood stabilizing agents are presented in Table 21–6.

Lithium Toxicity. The margin between the therapeutic and toxic levels of lithium carbonate is very narrow. The usual ranges of therapeutic serum concentrations are:

- For acute mania: 1.0 to 1.5 mEq/L
- For maintenance: 0.6 to 1.2 mEq/L

Serum lithium levels should be monitored once or twice a week after initial treatment until dosage and serum levels are stable, then monthly during maintenance therapy. Blood samples should be drawn 12 hours after the last dose.

Symptoms of lithium toxicity begin to appear at blood levels greater than 1.5 mEq/L and are dosage determinate. Symptoms include:

- **At serum levels of 1.5 to 2.0 mEq/L:** blurred vision, ataxia, tinnitus, persistent nausea and vomiting, severe diarrhea.
- **At serum levels of 2.0 to 3.5 mEq/L:** excessive output of dilute urine, increasing tremors, muscular irritability, psychomotor retardation, mental confusion, giddiness.
- **At serum levels above 3.5 mEq/L:** impaired consciousness, nystagmus, seizures, coma, oliguria/anuria, arrhythmias, myocardial infarction, cardiovascular collapse.

Lithium levels should be monitored prior to medication administration. The dosage should be withheld and the physician notified if the level reaches 1.5 mEq/L or at the earliest observation or report by the client of even the mildest symptom. If left untreated, lithium toxicity can be life threatening.

Lithium is similar in chemical structure to sodium, behaving in the body in much the same manner and competing at various sites in the body with sodium. If sodium intake is reduced or the body is depleted of its normal sodium (e.g., due to excessive sweating, fever, or diuresis), lithium is reabsorbed by the kidneys, increasing the possibility of toxicity. Therefore, the client must consume a diet adequate in sodium as well as 2500 to 3000 mL of fluid per day. Accurate records of intake, output, and client's weight should be kept on a daily basis.

Client/Family Education (for Lithium)

The client should:

- Take medication on a regular basis, even when feeling well. Discontinuation can result in return of symptoms.
- Not drive or operate dangerous machinery until lithium levels are stabilized. Drowsiness and dizziness can occur.
- Not skimp on dietary sodium intake. He or she should choose foods from the food pyramid and avoid "junk" foods. The client should drink 6 to 8 large glasses of water each day and avoid excessive use of beverages containing caffeine (coffee, tea, colas), which promote increased urinary output.
- Notify the physician if vomiting or diarrhea occurs. These symptoms can result in sodium loss and an increased risk of toxicity.
- Carry card or other identification noting that he or she is taking lithium.
- Be aware of appropriate diet should weight gain become a problem. Include adequate sodium and other nutrients while decreasing number of calories.
- Be aware of risks of becoming pregnant while receiving lithium therapy. Use information furnished by healthcare providers regarding methods of contraception. Notify the physician as soon as possible if pregnancy is suspected or planned.
- Be aware of side effects and symptoms associated with toxicity. Notify the physician if any of the following symptoms occur: Persistent nausea and vomiting, severe diarrhea, ataxia, blurred vision, tinnitus, excessive output of urine, increasing tremors, or mental confusion.
- Refer to written materials furnished by healthcare providers while receiving self-administered maintenance therapy. Keep appointments for outpatient follow-up; have serum lithium level checked every 1 to 2 months, or as advised by physician.

TABLE 21–6   **Side Effects and Nursing Implications of Mood-Stabilizing Agents**

Medication	Side Effects	Nursing Implications
Antimanic Lithium carbonate (Eskalith, Lithane, Lithobid)	1. Drowsiness, dizziness, headache 2. Dry mouth; thirst 3. GI upset; nausea/vomiting 4. Fine hand tremors 5. Hypotension; arrhythmias; pulse irregularities 6. Polyuria; dehydration 7. Weight gain	1. Ensure that client does not participate in activities that require alertness, or operate dangerous machinery. 2. Provide sugarless candy, ice, frequent sips of water. Ensure that strict oral hygiene is maintained. 3. Administer medications with meals to minimize GI upset. 4. Report to physician, who may decrease dosage. Some physicians prescribe a small dose of beta blocker propranolol to counteract this effect. 5. Monitor vital signs two or three times a day. Physician may decrease dose of medication. 6. May subside after initial week or two. Monitor daily intake and output and weight. Monitor skin turgor daily. 7. Provide instructions for reduced calorie diet. Emphasize importance of maintaining adequate intake of sodium.
Anticonvulsants Clonazepam (Klonopin) Carbamazepine (Tegretol) Valproic acid (Depakene; Depakote) Gabapentin (Neurontin) Lamotrigine (Lamictal) Topiramate (Topamax)	1. Nausea/vomiting 2. Drowsiness; dizziness 3. Blood dyscrasias 4. Prolonged bleeding time (with valproic acid) 5. Risk of severe rash (with lamotrigine) 6. Decreased efficacy with oral contraceptives (with topiramate)	1. May give with food or milk to minimize GI upset. 2. Ensure that client does not operate dangerous machinery or participate in activities that require alertness. 3. Ensure that client understands the importance of regular blood tests while receiving anticonvulsant therapy. 4. Ensure that platelet counts and bleeding time are determined before initiation of therapy with valproic acid. Monitor for spontaneous bleeding or bruising. 5. Ensure that client is informed that he or she must report evidence of skin rash to physician immediately. 6. Ensure that client is aware of decreased efficacy of oral contraceptives with concomitant use.
Calcium Channel Blocker Verapamil (Calan; Isoptin)	1. Drowsiness; dizziness 2. Hypotension; bradycardia 3. Nausea 4. Constipation	1. Ensure that client does not operate dangerous machinery or participate in activities that require alertness. 2. Take vital signs just before initiation of therapy and before daily administration of the medication. Physician will provide acceptable parameters for administration. Report marked changes immediately. 3. May give with food to minimize GI upset. 4. Encourage increased fluid (if not contraindicated) and fiber in the diet.
Antipsychotics Olanzapine (Zyprexa) Aripiprazole (Abilify) Chlorpromazine (Thorazine) Quetiapine (Seroquel) Risperidone (Risperdal) Ziprasidone (Geodon)	1. Drowsiness; dizziness 2. Dry mouth; constipation 3. Increased appetite; weight gain 4. ECG Changes 5. Extrapyramidal Symptoms 6. Hyperglycemia and diabetes.	1. Ensure that client does not operate dangerous machinery or participate in activities that require alertness. 2. Provide sugarless candy or gum, ice, and frequent sips of water. Provide foods high in fiber; encourage physical activity and fluid if not contraindicated. 3. Provide calorie-controlled diet; provide opportunity for physical exercise; provide diet and exercise instruction. 4. Monitor vital signs. Observe for symptoms of dizziness, palpitations, syncope, or weakness. 5. Monitor for symptoms. Administer prn medication at first sign. 6. Monitor blood glucose regularly. Observe for the appearance of symptoms of polydipsia, polyuria, polyphagia, and weakness at any time during therapy.

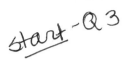
Start-Q3

Client/Family Education (for Anticonvulsants)

The client should:

- Not stop taking drug abruptly. Physician will administer orders for tapering the drug when therapy is to be discontinued.
- Report the following symptoms to the physician immediately: skin rash, unusual bleeding, spontaneous bruising, sore throat, fever, malaise, dark urine, and yellow skin or eyes.
- Not drive or operate dangerous machinery until reaction to the medication has been established.
- Avoid consuming alcoholic beverages and nonprescription medications without approval from physician.
- Carry card at all times identifying the name of medications being taken.

Client/Family Education (for Calcium Channel Blocker)

The client should:

- Take medication with meals if gastrointestinal (GI) upset occurs.
- Use caution when driving or when operating dangerous machinery. Dizziness, drowsiness, and blurred vision can occur.
- Not abruptly discontinue taking drug. To do so may precipitate cardiovascular problems.
- Report occurrence of any of the following symptoms to physician immediately: irregular heart beat, shortness of breath, swelling of the hands and feet, pronounced dizziness, chest pain, profound mood swings, severe and persistent headache.
- Rise slowly from a sitting or lying position to prevent a sudden drop in blood pressure.
- Not consume other medications (including over-the-counter medications) without physician's approval.
- Carry card at all times describing medications being taken.

Client/Family Education for Antipsychotics

This information is included in the next section on "Antipsychotic Agents."

Outcome Criteria/Evaluation

The following criteria may be used for evaluating the effectiveness of therapy with mood stabilizing agents:

The client:

1. Is maintaining stability of mood.
2. Has not harmed self or others.
3. Has experienced no injury from hyperactivity.
4. Is able to participate in activities without excessive sedation or dizziness.
5. Is maintaining appropriate weight.
6. Exhibits no signs of lithium toxicity.
7. Verbalizes importance of taking medication regularly and reporting for regular laboratory blood tests.

Antipsychotic Agents

Background Assessment Data

Antipsychotic drugs are also called *major tranquilizers* and *neuroleptics*. They were introduced into the United States in the 1950s with the phenothiazines. Other drugs in this classification soon followed. Since that time a second generation of medications has been developed. The first-generation antipsychotics are called "typical" and include the phenothiazines, haloperidol, loxapine, molindone, pimozide, and thiothixene. The second-generation antipsychotics are called "atypical" or "novel" antipsychotics and include aripiprazole, clozapine, olanzapine, quetiapine, risperidone, paliperidone, and ziprasidone.

Indications. Antipsychotics are used in the treatment of schizophrenia and other psychotic disorders. Selected agents are used in the treatment of bipolar mania (see previous section on "mood-stabilizing agents"). Others are used as antiemetics (chlorpromazine, perphenazine, prochlorperazine), in the treatment of intractable hiccoughs (chlorpromazine), and for the control of tics and vocal utterances in Tourette's disorder (haloperidol, pimozide). Examples of commonly used antipsychotic agents are presented in Table 21–7.

Action. The exact mechanism of action is not known. These drugs are thought to work by blocking postsynaptic dopamine receptors in the basal ganglia, hypothalamus, limbic system, brainstem, and medulla. Affinity also exists for cholinergic, adrenergic, and histaminic receptors. Newer medications may exert antipsychotic properties by blocking action on receptors specific to dopamine, serotonin, and other neurotransmitters, including cholinergic, adrenergic, and histaminic. Antipsychotic effects may also be related to inhibition of dopamine-mediated transmission of neural impulses at the synapses (see Chapter 4).

Contraindications/Precautions

Typical Antipsychotics. Typical antipsychotics are contraindicated in clients with known hypersensitivity (cross-sensitivity may exist among phenothiazines). They should not be used in comatose states or when CNS depression is evident; when blood dyscrasias exist; in clients with Parkinson's disease or narrow-angle glaucoma; those with liver, renal, or cardiac insufficiency; or with poorly controlled seizure disorders. Thioridazine,

TABLE 21-7 **Antipsychotic Agents**

Chemical Class	Generic (Trade Name)	Pregnancy Categories/ Half-life (hr)	Daily Dosage Range (mg)	Available Forms (mg)
Phenothiazines	Chlorpromazine (Thorazine)	C/24	40–400	Tabs: 10, 25, 50, 100, 200 Oral conc: 100/mL Supp: 100 Inj: 25/mL
	Fluphenazine (Prolixin)	C/ HCl: 18 hr Decanoate: 6.8–9.6 days	2.5–10	Tabs: 1, 2.5, 5, 10 Elixir: 2.5/5mL Conc: 5/mL Inj: 2.5/mL Inj (Decanoate): 25/mL
	Perphenazine (Trilafon)	C/ 9–12	12–64	Tabs: 2, 4, 8, 16 Oral conc: 16/5 mL
	Prochlorperazine (Compazine)	C/ 3–5 (oral) 6.9 (IV)	15–150	Tabs: 5, 10 Caps (SR): 10, 15 Supp: 2.5, 5, 25 Syrup: 5/5mL Inj: 5/mL
	Thioridazine	C/ 24	150–800	Tabs: 10, 15, 25, 50, 100, 150, 200 Conc: 30/mL, 100/mL
	Trifluoperazine (Stelazine)	C/ 18	4–40	Tabs: 1, 2, 5, 10
Phenylbutylpiperadines	Haloperidol (Haldol)	C/ ~18 (oral); ~3 wk (IM decanoate)	1–100	Tabs: 0.5, 1, 2, 5, 10, 20 Conc: 2/mL Inj: 5/mL Inj (decanoate): 50/mL, 100/mL
	Pimozide (Orap)	C/~55	1–10	Tabs: 1, 2
Thioxanthene	Thiothixene (Navane)	C/34	6–30	Caps: 1, 2, 5, 10, 20 Conc: 5/mL Inj: 10/vial
Benzisoxazoles	Risperidone (Risperdal)	C/ ~3–20	1–6	Tabs: 0.25, 0.5, 1, 2, 3, 4 Tabs (orally disintegrating): 0.5, 1, 2, 3, 4 Oral Solu: 1/mL Powder for inj: 25, 37.5, 50
	Paliperidone (Invega)	C/ 23	6–12	Tabs (ER): 3, 6, 9, 12
Dibenzepines	Loxapine (Loxitane)	C/8	20–250	Caps: 5, 10, 25, 50
	Clozapine (Clozaril)	B/8 (single dose); 12 (at steady state)	300–900	Tabs: 12.5, 25, 50, 100 Tabs (orally disintegrating): 12.5, 25, 50, 100
	Olanzapine (Zyprexa)	C/21–54	5–20	Tabs: 2.5, 5, 7.5, 10, 15, 20 Tabs (orally disintegrating:): 5, 10, 15, 20 Powder for inj: 10/vial
	Quetiapine (Seroquel)	C/~6	150–750	Tabs: 25, 50, 100, 200, 300
Dihydroindolones	Molindone (Moban)	C/12	15–225	Tabs: 5, 10, 25, 50
	Ziprasidone (Geodon)	C/~7 (oral), 2–5 (IM)	40–160	Caps: 20, 40, 60, 80 Powder for inj: 20/vial
Quinolinone	Aripiprazole (Abilify)	C/75, metabolite 94	10–30	Tabs: 5, 10, 15, 20, 30 Oral Solu: 1/mL

pimozide, haloperidol, and molindone have been shown to prolong the QT interval and are contraindicated with drugs that prolong the QT interval.

Caution should be taken in administering these drugs to clients who are elderly, severely ill, or debilitated, and to diabetic clients or clients with respiratory insufficiency, prostatic hypertrophy, or intestinal obstruction. Antipsychotics may lower seizure threshold. Individuals should avoid exposure to extremes in temperature while taking antipsychotic medication. Safety in pregnancy and lactation has not been established.

Atypical Antipsychotics. These drugs are contraindicated in hypersensitivity, comatose or severely depressed patients, patients with dementia-related psychosis, and lactation. Ziprasidone, risperidone, and paliperidone are contraindicated in patients with a history of QT prolongation or cardiac arrhythmias, recent MI, uncompensated heart failure, and concurrent use with other drugs that prolong the QT interval. Clozapine is contraindicated in patients with myeloproliferative disorders, with a history of clozapine-induced agranulocytosis or severe granulocytopenia, and in uncontrolled epilepsy.

Caution should be taken in administering these drugs to elderly or debilitated patients; patients with cardiac, hepatic, or renal insufficiency; patients with a history of seizures; patients with diabetes or risk factors for diabetes; clients exposed to temperature extremes; conditions that cause hypotension (dehydration, hypovolemia, treatment with antihypertensive medication); and in pregnancy and children (safety not established).

Interactions

Typical Antipsychotics. Additive hypotension with antihypertensive agents; additive CNS effects with CNS depressants; and additive anticholinergic effects with drugs that have anticholinergic properties. Phenothiazines may reduce effectiveness of oral anticoagulants. Concurrent use of phenothiazines or haloperidol with epinephrine or dopamine may result in severe hypotension. Additive effects of QT prolongation with haloperidol, thioridazine, pimozide, or molindone with other drugs that prolong QT interval. Pimozide is contraindicated with CYP3A inhibitors. Thioridazine is contraindicated with CYP2D6 inhibitors. Decreased therapeutic effects of haloperidol with carbamazepine; increased effects of carbamazepine.

Atypical Antipsychotics. Additive hypotension with antihypertensive agents; additive CNS effects with CNS depressants. Additive anticholinergic effects with risperidone or paliperidone and drugs that have anticholinergic properties. Additive effects of QT prolongation with ziprasidone and other drugs that prolong QT interval. Decreased effects of levodopa and dopamine agonists with ziprasidone, olanzapine, quetiapine, risperidone, or paliperidone. Increased effects of ziprasidone, clozapine, quetiapine, and aripiprazole with CYP3A4 inhibitors.

Decreased effects of ziprasidone, clozapine, olanzapine, risperidone, paliperidone, and aripiprazole with CYP1A2 inducers and increased effects with CYP1A2 inhibitors. Additive orthostatic hypotension with risperidone or paliperidone and other drugs that cause this adverse reaction.

Diagnosis

The following nursing diagnoses may be considered for clients receiving antipsychotic therapy:

1. Risk for other-directed violence related to panic anxiety and mistrust of others.
2. Risk for injury related to medication side effects of sedation, photosensitivity, reduction of seizure threshold, **agranulocytosis, extrapyramidal symptoms, tardive dyskinesia, neuroleptic malignant syndrome,** or QT prolongation.
3. Risk for activity intolerance related to medication side effects of sedation, blurred vision, and weakness.
4. Noncompliance with medication regimen related to suspiciousness and mistrust of others.

Planning/Implementation

The plan of care should include monitoring for the following side effects from antipsychotic medications. Nursing implications related to each side effect are designated by an asterisk (*). A profile of side effects comparing various antipsychotic medications is presented in Table 21–8.

1. Anticholinergic effects (see Table 21–8 for differences between typicals and atypicals)
   a. Dry mouth
      *Provide the client with sugarless candy or gum, ice, and frequent sips of water.
      *Ensure that client practices strict oral hygiene.
   b. Blurred vision
      *Explain that this symptom will most likely subside after a few weeks.
      *Advise client not to drive a car until vision clears.
      *Clear small items from pathway to prevent falls.
   c. Constipation
      *Order foods high in fiber; encourage increase in physical activity and fluid intake if not contraindicated.
   d. Urinary retention
      *Instruct client to report any difficulty urinating; monitor intake and output.
2. Nausea; GI upset (may occur with all classifications)
      *Tablets or capsules may be administered with food to minimize GI upset.
      *Concentrates may be diluted and administered with fruit juice or other liquid; they should be mixed immediately before administration.

TABLE 21–8 | **Comparison of Side Effects Among Antipsychotic Agents**

Chemical Class	Generic (Trade) Name	Extrapyramidal Symptoms	Sedation	Anticholinergic	Orthostatic Hypotension	Seizures
Phenothiazines	Chlorpromazine (Thorazine)	3	4	3	4	4
	Fluphenazine (Prolixin)	5	2	2	2	2
	Perphenazine (Trilafon)	4	2	2	2	3
	Prochlorperazine (Compazine)	4	3	2	2	4
	Thioridazine	2	4	4	4	1
	Trifluoperazine (Stelazine)	4	2	2	2	2
Thioxanthene	Thiothixene (Navane)	4	2	2	2	2
Benzisoxazoles	Risperidone (Risperdal)	1	1	1	3	1
	Paliperidone (Invega)	1	1	1	3	1
Phenylbutyl-piperadines	Haloperidol (Haldol)	5	1	1	1	1
	Pimozide (Orap)	4	3	2	2	2
Dibenzepines	Loxapine (Loxitane)	4	3	2	3	4
	Clozapine (Clozaril)	1	5	5	4	4
	Olanzapine (Zyprexa)	1	3	2	1	1
	Quetiapine (Seroquel)	1	3	2	1	1
Dihydroindolones	Molindone (Moban)	4	1	2	2	2
	Ziprasidone (Geodon)	1	2	1	1	1
Quinolinone	Aripiprazole (Abilify)	2	2	1	3	2

KEY:
1 = Very low
2 = Low
3 = Moderate
4 = High
5 = Very high

SOURCE: Adapted from Schatzberg, Cole, & DeBattista (2007); *Drug Facts and Comparisons* (2007); and Tandon & Jibson (2003).

3. Skin rash (may occur with all classifications)
 *Report appearance of any rash on skin to the physician.
 *Avoid spilling any of the liquid concentrate on skin; contact dermatitis can occur with some medications.
4. Sedation (see Table 21–8 for differences between typicals and atypicals)
 *Discuss with the physician the possibility of administering the drug at bedtime.
 *Discuss with physician a possible decrease in dosage or an order for a less sedating drug.
 *Instruct client not to drive or operate dangerous equipment while experiencing sedation.
5. Orthostatic hypotension (see Table 21–8 for differences between typicals and atypicals)

 *Instruct client to rise slowly from a lying or sitting position
 *Monitor blood pressure (lying and standing) each shift; document and report significant changes.
6. Photosensitivity (may occur with all classifications)
 *Ensure that the client wears a sunblock lotion, protective clothing, and sunglasses while spending time outdoors.
7. Hormonal effects (may occur with all classifications, but more common with typicals)
 a. Decreased libido, **retrograde ejaculation**, **gynecomastia** (men)
 *Provide explanation of the effects and reassurance of reversibility. If necessary, discuss with physician possibility of ordering alternate medication.

CORE CONCEPT

Electroconvulsive Therapy
The induction of a grand mal (generalized) seizure through the application of electrical current to the brain.

ELECTROCONVULSIVE THERAPY, DEFINED

The stimulus is applied through electrodes that are placed either bilaterally in the frontotemporal region or unilaterally on the same side as the dominant hand (Marangell, Silver, Goff, & Yudofsky, 2003). Controversy exists over optimal placement of the electrodes in terms of possible greater efficacy with bilateral placement versus the potential in some clients for less confusion and acute amnesia with unilateral placement.

The amount of electrical stimulus applied is another point of controversy among clinicians. Dose of stimulation is based on the client's seizure threshold, which is highly variable among individuals. The duration of the seizure should be at least 15 to 25 seconds (Karasu, Gelenberg, Merriam, & Wang, 2006). Movements are very minimal because of the administration of a muscle relaxant before the treatment. The tonic phase of the seizure usually lasts 10 to 15 seconds and may be identified by a rigid plantar extension of the feet. The clonic phase follows and is usually characterized by rhythmic movements of the muscles that decrease in frequency and finally disappear. Because of the muscle relaxant, movements may be observed merely as a rhythmic twitching of the toes.

Most clients require an average of 6 to 12 treatments, but some may require up to 20 treatments (Sadock & Sadock, 2007). Treatments are usually administered every other day, three times per week. Treatments are performed on an inpatient basis for those who require close observation and care (e.g., clients who are suicidal, agitated, delusional, catatonic, or acutely manic). Those at less risk may have the option of receiving therapy at an outpatient treatment facility.

HISTORICAL PERSPECTIVES

The first electroconvulsive therapy treatment was performed in April 1938 by Italian psychiatrists Ugo Cerletti and Lucio Bini in Rome. Other somatic therapies had been tried before that time, in particular **insulin coma therapy** and **pharmacoconvulsive therapy**.

Insulin coma therapy was introduced by the German psychiatrist Manfred Sakel in 1933. His therapy was used for clients with schizophrenia. The insulin injection treatments would induce a hypoglycemic coma, which Sakel claimed was effective in alleviating schizophrenic symptoms. This therapy required vigorous medical and nursing intervention through the stages of induced coma. Some fatalities occurred when clients failed to respond to efforts directed at termination of the coma. The efficacy of insulin coma therapy has been questioned, and its use has been discontinued in the treatment of mental illness.

Pharmacoconvulsive therapy was introduced in Budapest in 1934 by Ladislas Meduna (Fink, 1999). He induced convulsions with intramuscular injections of camphor in oil in clients with schizophrenia. He based his treatment on clinical observation and on his theory that there was a biological antagonism between schizophrenia and epilepsy. Thus, by inducing seizures he hoped to reduce schizophrenic symptoms. Because he discovered that camphor was unreliable for inducing seizures, he began using pentylenetetrazol (Metrazol). Some successes were reported in terms of reduction of psychotic symptoms, and, until the advent of ECT in 1938, pentylenetetrazol was the most frequently used procedure for producing seizures in psychotic clients. There was a brief resurgence of pharmacoconvulsive therapy in the late 1950s, when flurothyl (Indoklon), a potent inhalant convulsant, was introduced as an alternative for individuals who were unwilling to consent to ECT for the treatment of depression and schizophrenia. Pharmacoconvulsive therapy is no longer used in psychiatry.

Periodic recognition of the important contribution of ECT in the treatment of mental illness has been evident in the United States. An initial acceptance was observed from 1940 to 1960, followed by a 20-year period during which ECT was considered objectionable by both the psychiatric profession and the lay public. A second wave of acceptance began around 1980 and has been increasing to the present. The period of nonacceptability coincided with the introduction of tricyclic and monoamine oxidase inhibitor antidepressant drugs and ended with the realization among many psychiatrists that the widely heralded replacement of ECT with these chemical agents had failed to materialize (Abrams, 2002). Some individuals showed improvement with ECT after failing to respond to other forms of therapy.

Currently, an estimated 100,000 people in the United States and about 2 million people worldwide receive ECT treatments each year (Dukakis & Tye, 2006). The typical client is white, female, middle-aged, and from a middle- to upper-income background, receiving treatment in a private or university hospital for major depression, usually after drug therapy has proved ineffective. Largely because of the expense involved, as well as the need for a team of highly skilled medical specialists, many public hospitals are not able to offer this service to their clients.

INDICATIONS

Major Depression

ECT has been shown to be effective in the treatment of severe depression. It appears to be particularly effective in depressed clients who are also experiencing psychotic symptoms and those with psychomotor retardation and neurovegetative changes, such as disturbances in sleep, appetite, and energy. These symptoms are associated with the diagnoses of major depressive disorder, major depressive disorder with psychotic or melancholic symptoms, and bipolar disorder depression (Sadock & Sadock, 2007). ECT is not often used as the treatment of choice for depressive disorders but is considered only after a trial of therapy with antidepressant medication has proved ineffective.

Mania

ECT is also indicated in the treatment of acute manic episodes of bipolar affective disorder (Andreasen & Black, 2006). At present, it is rarely used for this purpose, having been superceded by the widespread use of antipsychotic drugs and/or lithium. However, it has been shown to be effective in the treatment of manic clients who do not tolerate or fail to respond to lithium or other drug treatment, or when life is threatened by dangerous behavior or exhaustion.

Schizophrenia

ECT can induce a remission in some clients who present with acute schizophrenia, particularly if it is accompanied by catatonic or affective (depression or mania) symptomatology (Andreasen & Black, 2006). It does not appear to be of value to individuals with chronic schizophrenic illness.

Other Conditions

ECT has also been tried with clients experiencing a variety of neuroses, obsessive–compulsive disorders, and personality disorders. Little evidence exists to support the efficacy of ECT in the treatment of these conditions.

CONTRAINDICATIONS

The only absolute contraindication for ECT is increased intracranial pressure (from brain tumor, recent cardiovascular accident, or other cerebrovascular lesion). ECT is associated with a physiological rise in cerebrospinal fluid pressure during the treatment, resulting in increased intracranial pressure that could lead to brain stem herniation (Marangell et al., 2003).

Various other conditions, not considered absolute contraindications but rendering clients at high risk for the treatment, have been identified (Andreasen & Black, 2006; Eisendrath & Lichtmacher, 2005; Marangell et al., 2003). These conditions are largely cardiovascular in nature and include myocardial infarction or cerebrovascular accident within the preceding 3 to 6 months, aortic or cerebral aneurysm, severe underlying hypertension, and congestive heart failure. Clients with cardiovascular problems are placed at risk because of the response of the body to the seizure itself. The initial vagal response results in a sinus bradycardia and drop in blood pressure. This is followed immediately by tachycardia and a hypertensive response. These changes can be life threatening to an individual with an already compromised cardiovascular system. Other factors that place clients at risk for ECT include severe osteoporosis, acute and chronic pulmonary disorders, and high-risk or complicated pregnancy.

MECHANISM OF ACTION

The exact mechanism by which ECT effects a therapeutic response is unknown. Several theories exist, but the one to which the most credibility has been given is the biochemical theory. A number of researchers have demonstrated that electric stimulation results in significant increases in the circulating levels of several neurotransmitters (Wahlund & von Rosen, 2003). These neurotransmitters include serotonin, norepinephrine, and dopamine, the same biogenic amines that are affected by antidepressant drugs. Additional evidence suggests that ECT may also result in increases in glutamate and gamma-aminobutyric acid (Grover, Mattoo, & Gupta, 2005). The results of studies relating to the mechanism underlying the effectiveness of ECT are still ongoing and continue to be controversial.

SIDE EFFECTS

The most common side effects of ECT are temporary memory loss and confusion. Critics of the therapy argue that these changes represent irreversible brain damage. Proponents insist they are temporary and reversible. Marangell and associates (2003) state, "To date, no reliable data have shown permanent memory loss caused by modern ECT." Other researchers have suggested that varying degrees of memory loss may be evident in some clients up to 6 to 7 months following ECT (Hall & Bensing, 2007; Popolos, 2007).

The controversy continues regarding the choice of unilateral versus bilateral ECT. Studies have shown that unilateral placement of the electrodes decreases the amount of memory disturbance. However, unilateral ECT often requires a higher stimulus dose or a greater number of treatments to match the efficacy of bilateral ECT in the relief of depression (Geddes, 2003).

RISKS ASSOCIATED WITH ELECTROCONVULSIVE THERAPY

Mortality

Studies indicate that the mortality rate from ECT is about 2 per 100,000 treatments (Marangell et al., 2003; Sadock & Sadock, 2007). Although the occurrence is rare, the major cause of death with ECT is from cardiovascular complications (e.g., acute myocardial infarction or cerebrovascular accident), usually in individuals with previously compromised cardiac status. Assessment and management of cardiovascular disease *prior to* treatment is vital in the reduction of morbidity and mortality rates associated with ECT.

Permanent Memory Loss

Marangell and associates (2003) state:

> The initial confusion and cognitive deficits associated with ECT treatment are usually temporary, lasting approximately 30 minutes. Whereas many patients report no problems with their memory, aside form the time immediately surrounding the ECT treatments, others report that their memory is not as good as it was before receiving ECT. To date, no reliable data have shown permanent memory loss caused by modern ECT. Prospective computed tomography and magnetic resonance imaging studies of the brain show no evidence of ECT-induced structural changes. (p. 1126)

Sackeim and associates (2007) recently reported on the results of a longitudinal study of clinical and cognitive outcomes in patients with major depression treated with ECT at seven facilities in the New York City metropolitan area. Subjects were evaluated shortly following the ECT course and 6 months later. Data revealed that cognitive deficits at the 6-month interval were directly related to type of electrode placement and electrical waveform used. Bilateral electrode placement resulted in more severe and persisting (as evaluated at the 6-month follow-up) retrograde amnesia than unilateral placement. The extent of the amnesia was directly related to the number of ECT treatments received. The researchers also found that stimulation produced by sine wave (continuous) current resulted in greater short- and long-term deficits than that produced by short-pulse wave (intermittent) current.

Brain Damage

Brain damage from ECT remains a concern for those who continue to believe in its usefulness and efficacy as a treatment for depression. Critics of the procedure remain adamant in their belief that ECT always results in some degree of immediate brain damage (Frank, 2002). However, evidence is based largely on animal studies in which the subjects received excessive electrical dosages, and the seizures were unmodified by muscle paralysis and oxygenation (Abrams, 2002). Although this is an area for continuing study, there is no evidence to substantiate that ECT produces any permanent changes in brain structure or functioning (Sadock & Sadock, 2007).

THE ROLE OF THE NURSE IN ELECTROCONVULSIVE THERAPY

Nurses play an integral role in the teaching and preparation for and administration of ECT. They provide support before, during, and after the treatment to the client and family, and assist the medical professionals who are conducting the therapy. The nursing process provides a systematic approach to the provision of care for the client receiving ECT.

Assessment

A complete physical examination must be completed by the appropriate medical professional prior to the initiation of ECT. This evaluation should include a thorough assessment of cardiovascular and pulmonary status as well as laboratory blood and urine studies. A skeletal history and radiographic assessment should also be considered.

The nurse may be responsible for ensuring that informed consent has been obtained from the client. If the depression is severe and the client is clearly unable to consent to the procedure, permission may be obtained from family or other legally responsible individual. Consent is secured only after the client or responsible individual acknowledges understanding of the procedure, including possible side effects and potential risks involved. Client and family must also understand that ECT is voluntary, and that consent may be withdrawn at any time (American Psychiatric Association, 2001; Hall & Bensing, 2007).

Nurses may also be required to assess:

- The client's mood and level of interaction with others
- Evidence of suicidal ideation, plan, and means
- Level of anxiety and fears associated with receiving ECT
- Thought and communication patterns
- Baseline memory for short- and long-term events
- Client and family knowledge of indications for, side effects of, and potential risks associated with ECT
- Current and past use of medications
- Baseline vital signs and history of allergies
- The client's ability to carry out activities of daily living

Diagnosis/Outcome Identification

Selection of appropriate nursing diagnoses for the client undergoing ECT is based on continual assessment before, during, and after treatment. Selected potential nursing diagnoses with outcome criteria for evaluation are presented in Table 22–1.

Planning/Implementation

ECT treatments are usually performed in the morning. The client is given nothing by mouth (NPO) for 6 to 8 hours before the treatment. Some institutional policies require that the client be placed on NPO status at midnight prior to the treatment day. The treatment team routinely consists of the psychiatrist, anesthesiologist, and two or more nurses.

Nursing interventions before the treatment include:

● Ensure that the physician has obtained informed consent and that a signed permission form is on the chart.
● Ensure that the most recent laboratory reports (complete blood count, urinalysis) and results of electrocardiogram (ECG) and x-ray examination are available.
● Approximately 1 hour before treatment is scheduled, take vital signs and record them. Have the client void and remove dentures, eyeglasses or contact lenses, jewelry, and hairpins. Following institutional requirements, the client should change into hospital gown or, if permitted, into own loose clothing or pajamas. Client should remain in bed with side rails up.
● Approximately 30 minutes before treatment, administer the pretreatment medication as prescribed by the physician. The usual order is for atropine sulfate or glycopyrrolate (Robinul) given intramuscularly. Either of these medications may be ordered to decrease secretions (to prevent aspiration) and counteract the effects of vagal stimulation (bradycardia) induced by the ECT.

● Stay with the client to help allay fears and anxiety. Maintain a positive attitude about the procedure, and encourage the client to verbalize feelings.

In the treatment room, the client is placed on the treatment table in a supine position. The anesthesiologist administers intravenously a short-acting anesthetic, such as thiopental sodium (Pentothal) or methohexital sodium (Brevital). A muscle relaxant, usually succinylcholine chloride (Anectine), is given intravenously to prevent severe muscle contractions during the seizure, thereby reducing the possibility of fractured or dislocated bones. Because succinylcholine paralyzes respiratory muscles as well, the client is oxygenated with pure oxygen during and after the treatment, except for the brief interval of electrical stimulation, until spontaneous respirations return (Sadock & Sadock, 2007). A blood pressure cuff may be placed on the lower leg and inflated above systolic pressure before injection of the succinylcholine. This is to ensure that the seizure activity can be observed in this one limb that is unaffected by the muscle relaxant.

An airway/bite block is placed in the client's mouth and he or she is positioned to facilitate airway patency. Electrodes are placed (either bilaterally or unilaterally) on the temples to deliver the electrical stimulation.

Nursing interventions during the treatment include:

● Ensure patency of airway. Provide suctioning if needed.
● Assist anesthesiologist with oxygenation as required.
● Observe readouts on machines monitoring vital signs and cardiac functioning.
● Provide support to the client's arms and legs during the seizure.
● Observe and record the type and amount of movement induced by the seizure.

After the treatment, the anesthesiologist continues to oxygenate the client with pure oxygen until spontaneous respirations return. Most clients awaken within 10 or 15 minutes of the treatment and are confused and

TABLE 22–1	Potential Nursing Diagnoses and Outcome Criteria for Client Receiving ECT
Nursing Diagnoses	**Outcome Criteria**
Anxiety (moderate to severe) related to impending therapy	Client verbalizes a decrease in anxiety following explanation of procedure and expression of fears.
Deficient knowledge related to necessity for and side effects or risks of ECT	Client verbalizes understanding of need for and side effects/risks of ECT following explanation.
Risk for injury related to risks associated with ECT	Client undergoes treatment without sustaining injury
Risk for aspiration related to altered level of consciousness immediately following treatment	Client experiences no aspiration during ECT
Decreased cardiac output related to vagal stimulation occurring during the ECT	Client demonstrates adequate tissue perfusion during and after treatment (absence of cyanosis or severe change in mental status).
Disturbed thought processes related to side effects of temporary memory loss and confusion	Client maintains reality orientation following ECT treatment.
Self-care deficit related to incapacitation during postictal stage	Client's self-care needs are fulfilled at all times.
Risk for activity intolerance related to post-ECT confusion and memory loss	Client gradually increases participation in therapeutic activities to the highest level of personal capability.

disoriented; however, some clients will sleep for 1 to 2 hours following the treatment. All clients require close observation in this immediate post-treatment period.

Nursing interventions in the post-treatment period include:

- Monitor pulse, respirations, and blood pressure every 15 minutes for the first hour, during which time the client should remain in bed.
- Position the client on side to prevent aspiration.
- Orient the client to time and place.
- Describe what has occurred.
- Provide reassurance that any memory loss the client may be experiencing is only temporary.
- Allow the client to verbalize fears and anxieties related to receiving ECT.
- Stay with the client until he or she is fully awake, oriented, and able to perform self-care activities without assistance.
- Provide the client with a highly structured schedule of routine activities in order to minimize confusion.

Evaluation

Evaluation of the effectiveness of nursing interventions is based on the achievement of the projected outcomes. Reassessment may be based on answers to the following questions:

- Was the client's anxiety maintained at a manageable level?
- Was the client/family teaching completed satisfactorily?
- Did the client/family verbalize understanding of the procedure, its side effects, and risks involved?
- Did the client undergo treatment without experiencing injury or aspiration?
- Has the client maintained adequate tissue perfusion during and following treatment? Have vital signs remained stable?
- With consideration to the individual client's condition and response to treatment, is the client reoriented to time, place, and situation?
- Have all of the client's self-care needs been fulfilled?
- Is the client participating in therapeutic activities to his or her maximum potential?
- What is the client's level of social interaction?

Careful documentation is an important part of the evaluation process. Some routine observations may be evaluated on flow sheets specifically identified for ECT. However, progress notes with detailed descriptions of client behavioral changes are essential to evaluate improvement and help determine the number of treatments that will be administered. Continual reassessment, planning, and evaluation will ensure that the client receives adequate and appropriate nursing care throughout the course of therapy.

SUMMARY AND KEY POINTS

- Electroconvulsive therapy (ECT) is the induction of a grand mal seizure through the application of electrical current to the brain.
- It is a safe and effective treatment alternative for individuals with depression, mania, or schizoaffective disorder who do not respond to other forms of therapy.
- ECT is contraindicated for individuals with increased intracranial pressure.
- Individuals with cardiovascular problems are at high risk for complications from ECT.
- Other factors that place clients at risk include severe osteoporosis, acute and chronic pulmonary disorders, and high-risk or complicated pregnancy.
- The exact mechanism of action of ECT is unknown, but it is thought that the electrical stimulation results in significant increases in the circulating levels of the neurotransmitters serotonin, norepinephrine, and dopamine.
- The most common side effects with ECT are temporary memory loss and confusion.
- Although it is rare, death must be considered a risk associated with ECT. When it does occur, the most common cause is cardiovascular complications.
- Other possible risks include permanent memory loss and brain damage, for which there is little or no substantiating evidence.
- The nurse assists with ECT using the steps of the nursing process before, during, and after treatment.
- Important nursing interventions include ensuring client safety, managing client anxiety, and providing adequate client education.
- Nursing input into the ongoing evaluation of client behavior is an important factor in determining the therapeutic effectiveness of ECT.

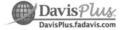

REVIEW QUESTIONS

Self-Examination/Learning Exercise

Select the answer that is most appropriate for each of the following questions

1. Electroconvulsive therapy is most commonly prescribed for:
    a. Bipolar disorder, manic.
    b. Paranoid schizophrenia.
    c. Major depression.
    d. Obsessive–compulsive disorder.

2. Which of the following best describes the average number of ECT treatments given and the timing of administration?
    a. One treatment per month for 6 months
    b. One treatment every other day for a total of 6 to 12
    c. One treatment three times per week for a total of 20 to 30
    d. One treatment every day for a total of 10 to 15

3. Which of the following conditions is considered to be the only absolute contraindication for ECT?
    a. Increased intracranial pressure
    b. Recent myocardial infarction
    c. Severe underlying hypertension
    d. Congestive heart failure

4. Electroconvulsive therapy is thought to effect a therapeutic response by
    a. Stimulation of the CNS.
    b. Decreasing the levels of acetylcholine and monoamine oxidase.
    c. Increasing the levels of serotonin, norepinephrine, and dopamine.
    d. Altering sodium metabolism within nerve and muscle cells.

5. The most common side effects of ECT are:
    a. Permanent memory loss and brain damage.
    b. Fractured and dislocated bones.
    c. Myocardial infarction and cardiac arrest.
    d. Temporary memory loss and confusion.

Situation: Sam has just been admitted to the inpatient psychiatric unit with a diagnosis of major depression. Sam has been treated with antidepressant medication for 6 months without improvement. His psychiatrist has suggested a series of ECT treatments. Sam says to the nurse on admission, "I don't want to end up like McMurphy on *One Flew Over the Cuckoo's Nest*! I'm scared!" The following questions pertain to Sam.

6. Sam's priority nursing diagnosis at this time would be:
    a. Anxiety related to deficient knowledge about ECT.
    b. Risk for injury related to risks associated with ECT.
    c. Deficient knowledge related to negative media presentation of ECT.
    d. Disturbed thought processes related to side effects of ECT.

7. Which of the following statements would be most appropriate by the nurse in response to Sam's expression of concern?
    a. "I guarantee you won't end up like McMurphy, Sam."
    b. "The doctor knows what he is doing. There's nothing to worry about."

REVIEW QUESTIONS

Self-Examination/Learning Exercise

Match the following herbs with the uses for which they have been associated

_c_ 1. Chamomile   a. For mild to moderate depression

_e_ 2. Echinacea   b. To improve memory

_f_ 3. Feverfew   c. To relieve upset stomach

_b_ 4. Ginkgo   d. For insomnia

_g_ 5. Psyllium   e. To stimulate the immune system

_a_ 6. St. John's wort   f. For migraine headache

_d_ 7. Valerian   g. For constipation

8. Which of the following applies to vitamin C?

     a. Coenzyme in protein metabolism; found in meat and dairy products
     b. Necessary in formation of DNA; found in beans and other legumes
     c. A powerful antioxidant; found in tomatoes and strawberries
     d. Necessary for blood clotting; found in whole grains and bananas

9. Which of the following applies to calcium?

     a. Coenzyme in carbohydrate metabolism; found in whole grains and citrus fruits
     b. Facilitates iron absorption; found in vegetable oils and liver
     c. Prevents night blindness; found in egg yolk and cantaloupe
     d. Important for nerve and muscle functioning; found in dairy products and oysters

10. Subluxation is a term used by chiropractic medicine to describe

     a. Displacement of vertebrae in the spine.
     b. Adjustment of displaced vertebrae in the spine.
     c. Interference with the flow of energy from the brain.
     d. Pathways along which energy flows throughout the body.

11. Nancy has been diagnosed with Dysthymic Disorder. The physician has just prescribed fluoxetine 20 mg/day. Nancy tells the nurse that she has been taking St. John's wort, but still feels depressed. Which of the following is the appropriate response by the nurse?

     a. "St. John's wort is not effective for depression."
     b. "Do not take fluoxetine and St. John's wort together."
     c. "You probably just need to increase your dose of St. John's wort."
     d. "Go ahead and take the St. John's wort with the fluoxetine. Maybe both of them together will be more helpful."

REFERENCES

Ashar, B.H., & Dobs, A.S. (2006). Complementary and alternative medicine. In *The American College of Physicians ACP Medicine*. New York: WebMD Publishing.

Avants, S.K., Margolin, A., Holford, T.R., & Kosten, T.R. (2000). A randomized controlled trial of auricular acupuncture for cocaine dependence. *Archives of Internal Medicine, 160*(15), 2305–2312.

Banks, M.R., & Banks, W.A. (2002). The effects of animal-assisted therapy on loneliness in an elderly population in long-term care facilities. *The Journals of Gerontology Series A: Biological Sciences and Medical Sciences, 57*(7), M428–M432.

Blumenthal, M. (Ed.). (1998). *The complete German Commission E monographs: Therapeutic guide to herbal medicines*. Austin, TX: American Botanical Council.

Coeytaux, R.R., Kaufman, J.S., Kaptchuk, T.J., Chen, W., Miller, W.M., Callahan, L.F., & Mann, D. (2005). A randomized, controlled trial of acupuncture for chronic daily headache. *Headache, 45*(9), 1113–1123.

Coniglione, T. (1998, June). Our doctors must begin looking at the total person. *In Balance*. Oklahoma City, OK: The Balanced Healing Medical Center.

Council for Responsible Nutrition. (2007). Historical comparison of RDIs, RDAs, and DRIs, 1968 to present. Retrieved January 30, 2007 from http://www.crnusa.org/

Council of Acupuncture and Oriental Medicine Associations (CAOMA). (2007). *Standards for acupuncture and oriental medicine.* Retrieved January 30, 2007 from http://www.acucouncil.org

DeSantis, L. (2006). Alternative and complementary healing practices. In J.T. Catalano (Ed.), *Nursing Now! Today's issues, tomorrow's trends* (4th ed.). Philadelphia: F.A. Davis.

Godenne, G. (2001). The role of pets in nursing homes . . . and psychotherapy. *The Maryland Psychiatrist, 27*(3), 5–6.

HealthGoods. (2007). *Alternative systems of medical practice: Classification of alternative medicine practices.* Retrieved January 27, 2007 from http://www.healthgoods.com/education/health_information/Alternative_Therapies/classification_alternative_medical.htm

Holt, G.A., & Kouzi, S. (2002). Herbs through the ages. In M.A. Bright (Ed.), *Holistic health and healing.* Philadelphia: F.A. Davis.

Institute of Medicine (IOM). (2005). *Complementary and alternative medicine in the United States.* Washington, DC: The National Academies Press.

Lutz, C.A., & Przytulski, K.R. (2006). *Nutrition and diet therapy: Evidence-based applications* (4th ed.). Philadelphia: F.A. Davis.

National Academy of Sciences. (2004). *Dietary Reference Intakes (DRIs) Tables.* Food and Nutrition Board, Institute of Medicine. Retrieved January 30, 2007 from http://www.iom.edu/file.asp?id=21372

National Center for Complementary and Alternative Medicine (NCCAM). (2006, December). *Get the facts: Acupuncture.* NCCAM Publication No. D003. Bethesda, MD: National Institutes of Health.

National Center for Complementary and Alternative Medicine (NCCAM). (2007, January 16). *NCCAM facts-at-a-glance and mission.* Bethesda, MD: National Institutes of Health.

PDR for Herbal Medicines (3rd ed.). (2004). Montvale, NJ: Thomson PDR.

Pranthikanti, S. (2007). Ayurvedic treatments. In J.H. Lake and D. Spiegel (Eds.), *Complementary and alternative treatments in mental health care.* Washington, DC: American Psychiatric Publishing.

Sadock, B.J., & Sadock, V.A. (2007). *Synopsis of psychiatry: Behavioral sciences/clinical psychiatry* (10th ed.). Philadelphia: Lippincott Williams & Wilkins.

Schoenen, J., Jacquy, J., & Lenaerts, M. (1998, February). Effectiveness of high-dose riboflavin in migraine prophylaxis: A randomized controlled trial. *Neurology 50,* 466–469.

Siegel, J.M., Angulo, F.J., Detels, R., Wesch, J., & Mullen, A. (1999). AIDS diagnosis and depression in the Multicenter AIDS Cohort Study: The ameliorating impact of pet ownership. *AIDS Care, 11*(2), 157–170.

Steinberg, L. (2002). Yoga. In M.A. Bright (Ed.), *Holistic health and healing.* Philadelphia: F.A. Davis.

Trivieri, L., & Anderson, J.W. (2002). *Alternative medicine: The definitive guide.* Berkeley, CA: Celestial Arts.

U.S. Department of Agriculture & U.S. Department of Health and Human Services (2005). *Dietary guidelines for Americans 2005* (6th ed.). Washington, DC: USDA & USDHHS.

Whitaker, J. (2000). Pet owners are a healthy breed. *Health & Healing 10*(10), 1–8.

Table 25–2 Care Plan for the Child with Mental Retardation

NURSING DIAGNOSIS: RISK FOR INJURY

RELATED TO: Altered physical mobility or aggressive behavior

Outcome Criteria	Nursing Interventions	Rationale
Short-/Long-Term Goal: ● Client will not experience injury.	1. Create a safe environment for the client. 2. Ensure that small items are removed from area where client will be ambulating and that sharp items are out of reach. 3. Store items that client uses frequently within easy reach. 4. Pad siderails and headboard of client with history of seizures. 5. Prevent physical aggression and acting-out behaviors by learning to recognize signs that client is becoming agitated.	1–5. Client safety is a nursing priority.

NURSING DIAGNOSIS: SELF-CARE DEFICIT

RELATED TO: Altered physical mobility or lack of maturity

Outcome Criteria	Nursing Interventions	Rationale
Short-Term Goal: ● Client will be able to participate in aspects of self-care. **Long-Term Goal:** ● Client will have all self-care needs met.	1. Identify aspects of self-care that may be within the client's capabilities. Work on one aspect of self-care at a time. Provide simple, concrete explanations. Offer positive feedback for efforts. 2. When one aspect of self-care has been mastered to the best of the client's ability, move on to another. Encourage independence but intervene when client is unable to perform.	1. Positive reinforcement enhances self-esteem and encourages repetition of desirable behaviors. 2. Client comfort and safety are nursing priorities.

NURSING DIAGNOSIS: IMPAIRED VERBAL COMMUNICATION

RELATED TO: Developmental alteration

Outcome Criteria	Nursing Interventions	Rationale
Short-Term Goal: ● Client will establish trust with caregiver and a means of communication of needs. **Long-Term Goals:** ● Client's needs are being met through established means of communication. ● If client cannot speak or communicate by other means, needs are met by caregiver's anticipation of client's needs.	1. Maintain consistency of staff assignment over time. 2. Anticipate and fulfill client's needs until satisfactory communication patterns are established. Learn (from family, if possible) special words client uses that are different from the norm. Identify nonverbal gestures or signals that client may use to convey needs if verbal communication is absent. Practice these communications skills repeatedly.	1. Consistency of staff assignments facilitates trust and the ability to understand client's actions and communications. 2. Some children with mental retardation, particularly at the severe level, can learn only by systematic habit training.

Continued on following page

Table 25-2 *(Continued)*

NURSING DIAGNOSIS: IMPAIRED SOCIAL INTERACTION

RELATED TO: Speech deficiencies or difficulty adhering to conventional social behavior

Outcome Criteria	Nursing Interventions	Rationale
Short-Term Goal: ● Client will attempt to interact with others in the presence of trusted caregiver. **Long-Term Goal:** ● Client will be able to interact with others using behaviors that are socially acceptable and appropriate to developmental level.	1. Remain with the client during initial interactions with others on the unit. 2. Explain to other clients the meaning behind some of the client's nonverbal gestures and signals. Use simple language to explain to the client which behaviors are acceptable and which are not. Establish a procedure for behavior modification with rewards for appropriate behaviors and aversive reinforcement for inappropriate behaviors.	1. The presence of a trusted individual provides a feeling of security. 2. Positive, negative, and aversive reinforcements can contribute to desired changes in behavior. These privileges and penalties are individually determined as staff learns the likes and dislikes of the client.

Although this plan of care is directed toward the individual client, it is essential that family members or primary caregivers participate in the ongoing care of the client with mental retardation. They need to receive information regarding the scope of the condition, realistic expectations and client potentials, methods for modifying behavior as required, and community resources from which they may seek assistance and support.

Evaluation

Evaluation of care given to the client with mental retardation should reflect positive behavioral changes. Evaluation is accomplished by determining if the goals of care have been met through implementation of the nursing actions selected. The nurse reassesses the plan and makes changes where required. Reassessment data may include information gathered by asking the following questions:

1. Have nursing actions providing for the client's safety been sufficient to prevent injury?
2. Have all of the client's self-care needs been fulfilled? Can he or she fulfill some of these needs independently?
3. Has the client been able to communicate needs and desires so that he or she can be understood?
4. Has the client learned to interact appropriately with others?
5. When regressive behaviors surface, can the client accept constructive feedback and discontinue the inappropriate behavior?
6. Has anxiety been maintained at a manageable level?
7. Has the client learned new coping skills through behavior modification? Does the client demonstrate evidence of increased self-esteem because of the accomplishment of these new skills and adaptive behaviors?

8. Have primary caregivers been taught realistic expectations of the client's behavior and methods for attempting to modify unacceptable behaviors?
9. Have primary caregivers been given information regarding various resources from which they can seek assistance and support within the community?

CORE CONCEPT

Pervasive Developmental Disorders
A group of disorders that are characterized by impairment in several areas of development, including social interaction skills and interpersonal communication. Included in this category are autistic disorder, Rett's disorder, childhood disintegrative disorder, and Asperger's disorder (APA, 2000).

AUTISTIC DISORDER

Clinical Findings

Autistic disorder is characterized by a withdrawal of the child into the self and into a fantasy world of his or her own creation. The child has markedly abnormal or impaired development in social interaction and communication and a markedly restricted repertoire of activity and interests (APA, 2000). Activities and interests are restricted and may be considered somewhat bizarre.

Epidemiology and Course

A recent study was conducted by the Autism and Developmental Disabilities Monitoring (ADDM) Network and

introduced in the mid-1970s. Studies on the effect of food and food-additive allergies remain controversial, largely because of the inconsistencies in the results. Striking improvement in behavior has been reported by some parents and teachers when hyperactive children are placed on a diet free of dyes and additives. Researchers in Great Britain recently reported on a study that revealed significant hyperactive behavior in 3-, 8-, and 9-year-old children who were given fruit drinks with food additives compared with children who received a placebo drink (McCann et al., 2007). Further study in this area is still required.

Another diet factor that has received much attention in its possible link to ADHD is sugar. A number of studies have been conducted in an effort to determine the effect of sugar on hyperactive behavior, and the results strongly suggest that sugar plays no role in hyperactivity.

Psychosocial Influences

Disorganized or chaotic environments or a disruption in family equilibrium may predispose some individuals to ADHD. A high degree of psychosocial stress, maternal mental disorder, paternal criminality, low socioeconomic status, poverty, growing up in an institution, and unstable foster care are factors that have been implicated (Dopheide, 2001; Voeller, 2004).

Application of the Nursing Process to ADHD

Background Assessment Data (Symptomatology)

A major portion of the hyperactive child's problems relate to difficulties in performing age-appropriate tasks. Hyperactive children are highly distractible and have extremely limited attention spans. They often shift from one uncompleted activity to another. Impulsivity, or deficit in inhibitory control, is also common.

Hyperactive children have difficulty forming satisfactory interpersonal relationships. They demonstrate behaviors that inhibit acceptable social interaction. They are disruptive and intrusive in group endeavors. They have difficulty complying with social norms. Some children with ADHD are very aggressive or oppositional, whereas others exhibit more regressive and immature behaviors. Low frustration tolerance and outbursts of temper are common.

Children with ADHD have boundless energy, exhibiting excessive levels of activity, restlessness, and fidgeting. They have been described as "perpetual motion machines," continuously running, jumping, wiggling, or squirming. They experience a greater than average number of accidents, from minor mishaps to more serious incidents that may lead to physical injury or the destruction of property. The *DSM-IV-TR* diagnostic criteria for ADHD are presented in Box 25–3.

Box 25 – 3 Diagnostic Criteria for Attention-Deficit/Hyperactivity Disorder

A. Either (1) or (2):

1. Six (or more) of the following symptoms of inattention have persisted for at least 6 months to a degree that is maladaptive and inconsistent with developmental level:

   Inattention
   (a) Often fails to give close attention to details or makes careless mistakes in school work, work, or other activities.
   (b) Often has difficulty sustaining attention in tasks or play activities.
   (c) Often does not seem to listen when spoken to directly.
   (d) Often does not follow through on instructions and fails to finish schoolwork, chores, or duties in the workplace (not because of oppositional behavior or failure to understand instructions).
   (e) Often has difficulty organizing tasks and activities.
   (f) Often avoids, dislikes, or is reluctant to engage in tasks that require sustained mental effort (such as schoolwork or homework).
   (g) Often loses things necessary for tasks or activities (e.g., toys, school assignments, pencils, books, or tools)
   (h) Is often easily distracted by extraneous stimuli.
   (i) Is often forgetful in daily activities.

2. Six (or more) of the following symptoms of hyperactivity-impulsivity have persisted for at least 6 months to a degree that is maladaptive and inconsistent with developmental level:

   Hyperactivity
   (a) Often fidgets with hands or feet or squirms in seat.
   (b) Often leaves seat in classroom or in other situations in which remaining seated is expected.
   (c) Often runs about or climbs excessively in situations in which it is inappropriate (in adolescents or adults, may be limited to subjective feelings of restlessness).
   (d) Often has difficulty playing or engaging in leisure activities quietly.
   (e) Is often "on the go" or often acts as if "driven by a motor."
   (f) Often talks excessively.

   Impulsivity
   (g) Often blurts out answers before questions have been completed.
   (h) Often has difficulty awaiting turn.
   (i) Often interrupts or intrudes on others (e.g., butts into conversations or games).

B. Some hyperactive–impulsive or inattentive symptoms that caused impairment were present before age 7 years.

C. Some impairment from the symptoms is present in two or more settings (e.g., at school or work and at home).

D. There is clear evidence of clinically significant impairment in social, academic, or occupational functioning.

E. The symptoms do not occur exclusively during the course of a pervasive developmental disorder, schizophrenia, or other psychotic disorder and are not better accounted for by another mental disorder (e.g., mood disorder, anxiety disorder, dissociative disorder, or a personality disorder).

Continued on following page

BOX 25 – 3 **Diagnostic Criteria for Attention-Deficit/Hyperactivity Disorder (*Continued*)**

Subtypes:

1. **Attention-Deficit/Hyperactivity Disorder, Combined Type:** If both criteria A1 and A2 are met for the past 6 months.
2. **Attention-Deficit/Hyperactivity Disorder, Predominantly Inattentive Type:** If criterion A1 is met but criterion A2 is not met for the past 6 months.
3. **Attention-Deficit/Hyperactivity Disorder, Predominantly Hyperactive-Impulsive Type:** If criterion A2 is met but criterion A1 is not met for the past 6 months.

SOURCE: From APA (2000), with permission.

Comorbidity

As many as two-thirds of children diagnosed with ADHD have at least one other diagnosable psychiatric disorder (Julien, 2005). Those commonly identified include oppositional defiant disorder, conduct disorder, anxiety, depression, and substance abuse. It is extremely important to identify and treat any comorbid psychiatric conditions in a child with ADHD. In some instances, as with anxiety and depression, the comorbid disorders may be treated concurrently with the symptoms of ADHD. Jenson (2005) suggests that comorbid depression and ADHD may respond to bupropion or atomoxetine as a single agent, and that individuals with comorbid anxiety and ADHD may benefit from treatment with atomoxetine.

Other disorders may require separate treatment. Wilens and Upadhyaya (2007) state, "In patients with coexisting substance use disorders and ADHD, the priority is to stabilize the addiction before treating the ADHD." Because stimulants can exacerbate mania, it is suggested that medication for ADHD be initiated only after bipolar symptoms have been controlled with a mood stabilizer (Kowatch et al., 2005). Types of conditions often seen with ADHD and their rate of comorbidity are presented in Table 25–4.

TABLE 25–4 **Type and Frequency of Comorbidity with Attention-Deficit/Hyperactivity Disorder**

Comorbidity	Rates (%)
Oppositional defiant disorder	Up to 50
Conduct disorder	~ 33
Learning disorders	20–30
Anxiety	~ 25
Depression	6–38
Bipolar disorder	11–20
Substance use	13–26

SOURCES: Jenson (2005) and Robb (2006).

Diagnosis/Outcome Identification

Based on the data collected during the nursing assessment, possible nursing diagnoses for the child with ADHD include:

● Risk for injury related to impulsive and accident-prone behavior and the inability to perceive self-harm.
● Impaired social interaction related to intrusive and immature behavior.
● Low self-esteem related to dysfunctional family system and negative feedback.
● Noncompliance with task expectations related to low frustration tolerance and short attention span.

Outcome Criteria

Outcome criteria include short- and long-term goals. Timelines are individually determined. The following criteria may be used for measurement of outcomes in the care of a child with ADHD.

The client:

1. Has experienced no physical harm.
2. Interacts with others appropriately.
3. Verbalizes positive aspects about self.
4. Demonstrates fewer demanding behaviors.
5. Cooperatives with staff in an effort to complete assigned tasks.

Planning/Implementation

Table 25–5 provides a plan of care for the child with ADHD using nursing diagnoses common to the disorder, outcome criteria, and appropriate nursing interventions and rationales.

The concept map care plan is an innovative approach to planning and organizing nursing care (see Chapter 9). It is a diagrammatic teaching and learning strategy that allows visualization of interrelationships between medical diagnoses, nursing diagnoses, assessment data, and treatments. An example of a concept map care plan for a client with ADHD is presented in Figure 25–2.

Evaluation

Evaluation of the care of a client with ADHD involves examining client behaviors following implementation of the nursing actions to determine if the goals of therapy have been achieved. Collecting data by using the following types of questions may provide appropriate information for evaluation.

1. Have the nursing actions directed at client safety been effective in protecting the child from injury?
2. Has the child been able to establish a trusting relationship with the primary caregiver?
3. Is the client responding to limits set on unacceptable behaviors?

Table 25–5   Care Plan for the Child with Attention-Deficit/Hyperactivity Disorder

NURSING DIAGNOSIS: RISK FOR INJURY

RELATED TO: Impulsive and accident-prone behavior and the inability to perceive self-harm

Outcome Criteria	Nursing Interventions	Rationale
Short-/Long-Term Goal: ● Client will be free of injury.	1. Ensure that client has a safe environment. Remove objects from immediate area on which client could injure self as a result of random, hyperactive movements. 2. Identify deliberate behaviors that put the child at risk for injury. Institute consequences for repetition of this behavior. 3. If there is risk of injury associated with specific therapeutic activities, provide adequate supervision and assistance, or limit client's participation if adequate supervision is not possible.	1. Objects that are appropriate to the normal living situation can be hazardous to the child whose motor activities are out of control. 2. Behavior can be modified with aversive reinforcement. 3. Client safety is a nursing priority.

NURSING DIAGNOSIS: IMPAIRED SOCIAL INTERACTION

RELATED TO: Intrusive and immature behavior

Outcome Criteria	Nursing Interventions	Rationale
Short-Term Goal: ● Client will interact in age-appropriate manner with nurse in one-to-one relationship within 1 week. **Long-Term Goal:** ● Client will observe limits set on intrusive behavior and will demonstrate ability to interact appropriately with others.	1. Develop a trusting relationship with the child. Convey acceptance of the child separate from the unacceptable behavior. 2. Discuss with client those behaviors that are and are not acceptable. Describe in a matter-of-fact manner the consequences of unacceptable behavior. Follow through. 3. Provide group situations for client.	1. Unconditional acceptance increases feelings of self-worth. 2. Aversive reinforcement can alter undesirable behaviors. 3. Appropriate social behavior is often learned from the positive and negative feedback of peers.

NURSING DIAGNOSIS: LOW SELF-ESTEEM

RELATED TO: Dysfunctional family system and negative feedback

Outcome Criteria	Nursing Interventions	Rationale
Short-Term Goal: ● Client will independently direct own care and activities of daily living within 1 week. **Long-Term Goal:** ● Client will demonstrate increased feelings of self-worth by verbalizing positive statements about self and exhibiting fewer demanding behaviors.	1. Ensure that goals are realistic. 2. Plan activities that provide opportunities for success. 3. Convey unconditional acceptance and positive regard. 4. Offer recognition of successful endeavors and positive reinforcement for attempts made. Give immediate positive feedback for acceptable behavior.	1. Unrealistic goals set client up for failure, which diminishes self-esteem. 2. Success enhances self-esteem. 3. Affirmation of client as worthwhile human being may increase self-esteem 4. Positive reinforcement enhances self-esteem and may increase the desired behaviors.

Continued on following page

Table 25–5 *(Continued)*

NURSING DIAGNOSIS: NONCOMPLIANCE (WITH TASK EXPECTATIONS)
RELATED TO: Low frustration tolerance and short attention span

Outcome Criteria	Nursing Interventions	Rationale
Short-Term Goal: ● Client will participate in and cooperate during therapeutic activities. **Long-Term Goal:** ● Client will be able to complete assigned tasks willingly and independently or with a minimum of assistance.	1. Provide an environment for task efforts that is as free of distractions as possible. 2. Provide assistance on a one-to-one basis, beginning with simple, concrete instructions 3. Ask client to repeat instructions to you. 4. Establish goals that allow client to complete a part of the task, rewarding each step-completion with a break for physical activity. 5. Gradually decrease the amount of assistance given, while assuring the client that assistance is still available if deemed necessary.	1. Client is highly distractible and is unable to perform in the presence of even minimal stimulation. 2. Client lacks the ability to assimilate information that is complicated or has abstract meaning. 3. Repetition of the instructions helps to determine client's level of comprehension. 4. Short-term goals are not so overwhelming to one with such a short attention span. The positive reinforcement (physical activity) increases self-esteem and provides incentive for client to pursue the task to completion. 5. This encourages the client to perform independently while providing a feeling of security with the presence of a trusted individual.

4. Is the client able to interact appropriately with others?
5. Is the client able to verbalize positive statements about self?
6. Is the client able to complete tasks independently or with a minimum of assistance? Can he or she follow through after listening to simple instructions?
7. Is the client able to apply self-control to decrease motor activity?

Psychopharmacological Intervention for ADHD

Central nervous system stimulants are sometimes given to children with ADHD. Those commonly used include dextroamphetamine (Dexedrine), methamphetamine (Desoxyn), a dextroamphetamine/amphetamine composite (Adderall), methylphenidate (Ritalin and others), and dexmethylphenidate (Focalin). The actual mechanism by which these medications improve behavior associated with ADHD is not known. In most individuals, they produce stimulation, excitability, and restlessness. In children with ADHD, the effects include an increased attention span, control of hyperactive behavior, and improvement in learning ability.

Side effects include insomnia, anorexia, weight loss, tachycardia, and temporary decrease in rate of growth and development. Physical tolerance can occur.

In 2002, the U.S. Food and Drug Administration approved atomoxetine (Strattera), a medication specific for treating ADHD. Atomoxetine is a selective norepinephrine reuptake inhibitor. The exact mechanism by which it produces its therapeutic effect in ADHD is unknown. Side effects include headache, nausea and vomiting, upper abdominal pain, dry mouth, decreased appetite, weight loss, constipation, insomnia, increased blood pressure and heart rate, and sexual dysfunction.

The antidepressant bupropion (Wellbutrin) has also been used with some success in the treatment of ADHD. It is distributed in a short- and long-lasting form. The side effects are similar to those of the stimulants: tachycardia, dizziness, shakiness, insomnia, nausea, anorexia, and weight loss. Individuals with a history of seizures or eating disorders should not take this medication.

Route and dosage information for agents used to treat ADHD is presented in Table 25–6.

Nursing Implications

● Assess the client's mental status for changes in mood, level of activity, degree of stimulation, and aggressiveness.
● Ensure that the client is protected from injury. Environmental stimuli should be kept low and environment as quiet as possible to discourage overstimulation.
● To reduce anorexia, the medication may be administered immediately after meals. The client should be weighed regularly (at least weekly) while on therapy with CNS stimulants because of the potential for anorexia and weight loss and the temporary interruption of growth and development.

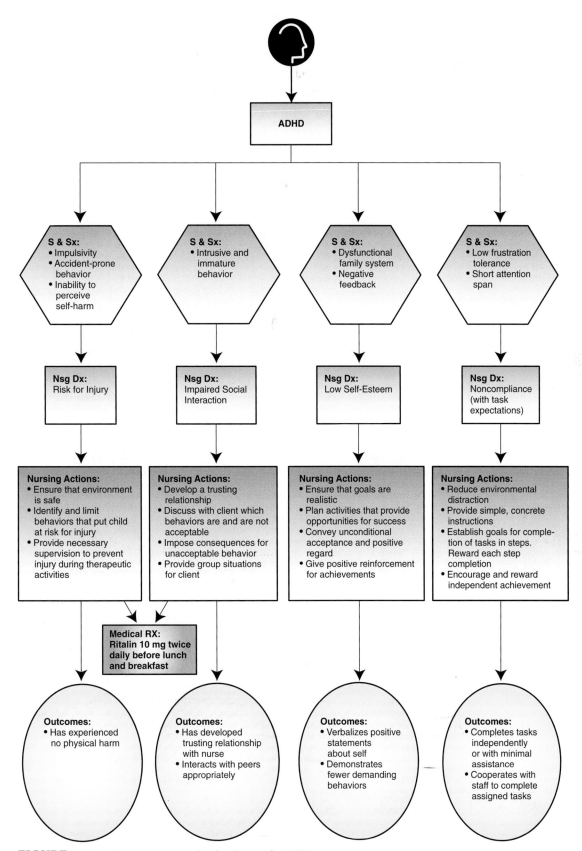

FIGURE 25–2 Concept map care plan for client with ADHD.

TABLE 25–6 Medications Used to Treat ADHD

Medication	Route and Dosage Information
Dextroamphetamine sulfate (Dexedrine; Dextrostat)	*Children 3 to 5 years:* **PO:** Initial dose: 2.5 mg/day. May increase in increments of 2.5 mg/day at weekly intervals. *Children ≥6 years:* **PO:** Initial dose: 5 mg 1 or 2 times daily. May increase in increments of 5 mg/day at weekly intervals. *Sustained-release caps* may be used for once-a-day dosage. With immediate-release tablets, give first dose on awakening and 1 or 2 additional doses at intervals of 4 to 6 hours.
Methamphetamine (Desoxyn)	5 mg once or twice daily. May increase in increments of 5 mg at weekly intervals. Usual effective dose is 20 to 25 mg/day.
Lisdexamphetamine (Vyvanse)	*Children 6 to 12 years:* **PO:** 30 mg/day given in the morning. May increase in increments of 20 mg/day at weekly intervals. Maximum recommended dosage: 70 mg.
Amphetamine/dextroamphetamine mixtures (Adderall; Adderall XR)	*Children 3 to 5 years:* **PO:** Initial dose: 2.5 mg/day. May increase in increments of 2.5 mg/day at weekly intervals. *Children ≥6 years:* Initial dose: 5 mg 1 or 2 times daily. May increase in increments of 5 mg/day at weekly intervals. *Extended-release caps: Children ≥6 years:* **PO:** Initial dose: 10 mg once daily in the morning. May increase daily dosage in increments of 10 mg at weekly intervals. Maximum dosage: 30 mg/day.
Methylphenidate (Ritalin; Ritalin-SR; Ritalin LA; Methylin; Methylin ER; Metadate ER; Metadate CD; Concerta; Daytrana)	*Immediate-release forms: Adults:* **PO:** Range 10 to 60 mg/day in divided doses 2 or 3 times/day preferably 30 to 45 min before meals. Average dose is 20 to 30 mg/day. To prevent interruption of sleep, take last dose of the day before 6 P.M. *Children ≥6 years:* **PO:** Individualize dosage. May start with low dose of 5 mg twice daily before breakfast and lunch. May increase dosage in 5- to 10-mg increments at weekly intervals. Maximum daily dosage: 60 mg. *Ritalin-SR, Methylin ER, and Metadate ER: All patients:* **PO:** May be used in place of the immediate-release tablets when the 8-hour dosage corresponds to the titrated 8-hour dosage of the immediate-release tablets. Must be swallowed whole. *Ritalin LA and Metadate CD: All patients:* **PO:** Initial dosage: 20 mg once daily in the morning. May increase dosage in 10- to 20-mg increments at weekly intervals to a maximum of 60 mg taken once daily in the morning. Capsules may be swallowed whole with liquid or opened and contents sprinkled on soft food (e.g., applesauce). Ensure that entire contents of capsule are consumed when taken in this manner. *Note:* Ritalin LA may be used in place of twice-daily regimen given once daily at same total dose, or in place of SR product at same dose. *Concerta: All patients:* **PO:** Should be taken once daily in the morning. Must be swallowed whole and not chewed, divided, or crushed. *Clients new to methylphenidate:* 18 mg once daily in the morning. May adjust dosage at weekly intervals to maximum of 54 mg/day for children 6 to 12 years, and to a maximum of 72 mg/day (not to exceed 2 mg/kg per day) for adolescents 13 to 17 years. *Clients currently using methylphenidate:* Should use following conversion table: **Previous methylphenidate dose** / **Recommended Concerta dose** 5 mg 2 or 3 times/day or 20 mg (SR) / 18 mg every morning 10 mg 2 or 3 times/day or 40 mg (SR) / 36 mg every morning 15 mg 2 or 3 times/day or 60 mg (SR) / 54 mg every morning *Daytrana: Children 6 to 12 years:* **Transdermal Patch:** Apply to hip area 2 hours before an effect is needed. Remove 9 hours after application. Dose should be individualized according to patient response and titrated according to the following schedule: Week 1 / Week 2 / Week 3 / Week 4 10 mg / 15 mg / 20 mg / 30 mg
Dexmethylphenidate (Focalin; Focalin XR)	*Adults and Children ≥6 years:* Administer doses twice daily, at least 4 hours apart. Extended release capsules are for administration once daily in the morning. *Clients new to the medication: Immediate release tabs:* Starting dose: 2.5 mg twice daily. May increase dosage in 2.5- to 5-mg increments at weekly intervals to a maximum of 20 mg/day (10 mg twice a day). *Extended-release caps:* 5 mg/day for pediatric patients and 10 mg/day for adults. May increase dosage in 5-mg increments for pediatric patients and 10-mg increments for adults at weekly intervals to a maximum of 20 mg/day. *Clients currently taking methylphenidate:* Starting dose: One-half of the dose of methylphenidate being taken. Maximum recommended dose of dexmethylphenidate: 20 mg/day (10 mg twice daily immediate-release).
Atomoxetine (Strattera)	*Adults, adolescents, and children weighing more than 70 kg (154 lb):* **PO:** Initial dose: 40 mg/day. Increase after a minimum of 3 days to a target total daily dose of 80 mg, as a single dose in the morning or 2 evenly divided doses in the morning and late afternoon or early evening. After 2 to 4 weeks, total dosage may be increased to a maximum of 100 mg, if needed. *Children weighing 70 kg (154 lb) or less:* **PO:** Initial dose: 0.5 mg/kg per day. Increase after a minimum of 3 days to a target total daily dose of about 1.2 mg/kg taken either as a single dose in the morning or two evenly divided doses in the morning and late afternoon or early evening. Maximum daily dose: 1.4 mg/kg or 100 mg daily, whichever is less.
Bupropion (Wellbutrin; Wellbutrin SR; Wellbutrin XL)	*Children: ADHD:* **PO:** 3 mg/kg per day. *Adults: Depression:* **PO:** *(immediate-release tabs):* 100 mg 2 times/day. May increase after 3 days to 100 mg given 3 times/day. For patients who do not show improvement after several weeks of dosing at 300 mg/day, an increase in dosage up to 450 mg/day may be considered. No single dose of bupropion should exceed 150 mg. To prevent the risk of seizures, administer with 4 to 6 hours between doses. *Sustained-release tabs:* Give as a single 150-mg dose in the morning. May increase to twice a day (total 300 mg), with 8 hours between doses. *Extended-release tabs:* Begin dosing at 150-mg/day, given as a single daily dose in the morning. May increase after 3 days to 300 mg/day, given as a single daily dose in the morning.

IMPLICATIONS OF RESEARCH FOR EVIDENCE-BASED PRACTICE

Frame, K., Kelly, L., & Bayley, E.: Increasing perceptions of self-worth in preadolescents diagnosed with ADHD. *Journal of Nursing Scholarship (2003), 35(3), 225–229.*

Description of the Study: The theoretical framework for this study was based on the Roy adaptation model. The sample in this study consisted of 65 preadolescents diagnosed with ADD or ADHD in an upper-middle class community in the United States. Participants were randomly assigned to either the control group or the experimental group, and all completed the Harter's Self-Perception Profile for Children instrument at the beginning of the study and 4 weeks later. This tool was designed to measure perceptions of scholastic competence, social acceptance, athletic competence, physical appearance, behavioral conduct, and global self-worth. Children in the experimental group participated in a school-nurse facilitated support group that met twice weekly for 4 weeks. In the group, the participants were assisted to learn strategies for effective interactions with their peers, teachers, and families. Interventions served to promote adaptive self-evaluations and to address the unfavorable self-perceptions of many children with ADHD.

Results of the Study: On post-testing, participants in the support group scored significantly higher than controls on each of the six subscales, with significant increases on four of the subscales, including perceived social acceptance, perceived athletic competence, perceived physical appearance, and perceived global self-worth.

Implications for Nursing Practice: This study has implications for nurses who work with children, particularly those who work with children diagnosed with ADHD. Because preadolescence is a time when children compare themselves, either positively or negatively, with their peers, group interaction is an especially significant intervention. The authors state, "The support group, with children helping children, enabled participants to engage in creative problem-solving and to develop solutions to their difficulties." This intervention was shown to promote positive perceptions and behaviors among children with ADD and ADHD. It is especially appropriate for the role of school nurse, but it is also consistent with the role of any nurse who interacts directly with children or adolescents who have similar problems.

- To prevent insomnia, the last dose should be administered at least 6 hours before bedtime. Sustained-release forms should be taken in the morning.
- In children with behavior disorders, a drug "holiday" should be attempted periodically under direction of the physician to determine effectiveness of the medication and need for continuation.
- The FDA recently issued warnings associated with CNS stimulants and atomoxetine of the risk for sudden death in patients who have cardiovascular disease. A careful personal and family history of heart disease, heart defects, or hypertension should be obtained before these medications are prescribed. Careful

monitoring of cardiovascular function during administration must be ongoing.
- Severe liver damage has been noted with atomoxetine. Any of the following side effects should be reported to the physician immediately: itching, dark urine, right upper quadrant pain, yellow skin or eyes, sore throat, fever, malaise.
- New or worsened psychiatric symptoms have been noted with CNS stimulants and atomoxetine. It is important to monitor continuously for psychotic symptoms (e.g., hearing voices, paranoid behaviors, delusions) and for manic symptoms, including aggressive and hostile behaviors.
- Over-the-counter (OTC) medications should be avoided while the child is receiving stimulant medication. Some OTC medications, particularly cold and hay fever preparations, contain sympathomimetic agents that could compound the effects of the stimulant and create a drug interaction that may be toxic to the child.
- The medication should not be withdrawn abruptly. Withdrawal should be gradual and under the direction of the physician.
- Any of the following side effects should be reported to the physician immediately: shortness of breath, chest pain, jaw/left arm pain, fainting, seizures, sudden vision changes, weakness on one side of the body, slurred speech, confusion, itching, dark urine, right upper quadrant pain, yellow skin or eyes, sore throat, fever, malaise, increased hyperactivity, believing things that are not true, or hearing voices.

 CORE CONCEPT

Disruptive Behavior Disorders
A disturbance of conduct severe enough to produce significant impairment in social, occupational, or academic functioning because of symptoms that range from oppositional defiant to moderate and severe conduct disturbances (Shahrokh & Hales, 2003).

CONDUCT DISORDER

Conduct disorder involves a repetitive and persistent pattern of behavior in which the basic rights of others or major age-appropriate societal norms or rules are violated (APA, 2000). Physical aggression is common. The *DSM-IV-TR* divides this disorder into two subtypes based on the age at onset:

1. **Childhood-Onset Type.** This subtype is defined by the onset of at least one criterion characteristic of conduct disorder before age 10. Individuals with this subtype are usually boys, frequently display physical aggression, and have disturbed peer relationships. They

may have had oppositional defiant disorder during early childhood, usually meet the full criteria for conduct disorder by puberty, and are likely to develop antisocial personality disorder in adulthood.

2. **Adolescent-Onset Type.** This subtype is defined by the absence of any criteria characteristic of conduct disorder before age 10. They are less likely to display aggressive behaviors and tend to have more normal peer relationships than those with childhood-onset type. They are also less likely to have persistent conduct disorder or develop antisocial personality disorder than those with childhood-onset type. The ratio of boys to girls is lower in adolescent-onset type than in childhood-onset type.

CORE CONCEPT

Temperament
Personality characteristics that define an individual's mood and behavioral tendencies. The sum of physical, emotional, and intellectual components that affect or determine a person's actions and reactions.

Predisposing Factors

Biological Influences

Genetics. Studies with monozygotic and dizygotic twins as well as with nontwin siblings have revealed a significantly higher number of conduct disorders among those who have family members with the disorder (APA, 2000). Although genetic factors appear to be involved in the etiology of conduct disorders, little is yet known about the actual mechanisms involved in genetic transmission. One recent study found that regions on chromosomes 19 and 2 may contain genes conferring risk to conduct disorder (Dick et al., 2004). In this study, the same region on chromosome 2 was also linked to alcohol dependence. These researchers report that childhood conduct disorder is known to be associated with the susceptibility for future alcohol problems. They have concluded that these findings suggest that some of the genes contributing to alcohol dependence in adulthood may also contribute to conduct disorder in childhood.

Temperament. The term *temperament* refers to personality traits that become evident very early in life and may be present at birth. Evidence suggests a genetic component in temperament and an association between temperament and behavioral problems later in life. Studies have shown that, without appropriate intervention, difficult temperament at age 3 has significant links to conduct disorder and movement into care or institutional life at age 17 (Bagley & Mallick, 2000).

Biochemical Factors. Researchers have investigated various chemicals as biological markers. Alterations in the neurotransmitters norepinephrine and serotonin

have been suggested by some studies (Comings et al., 2000; Searight, Rottnek, & Abby, 2001). Some investigators have examined the possibility of testosterone association with violence. One study correlates higher levels of testosterone in pubertal boys with social dominance and association with deviant peers (Rowe, Maughan, Worthman, Costello, & Angold, 2004).

Psychosocial Influences

Peer Relationships. Social groups have a significant impact on a child's development. Peers play an essential role in the socialization of interpersonal competence, and skills acquired in this manner affect the child's long-term adjustment. Studies have shown that poor peer relations during childhood were consistently implicated in the etiology of later deviance (Ladd, 1999). Aggression was found to be the principal cause of peer rejection, thus contributing to a cycle of maladaptive behavior.

Family Influences. The following factors related to family dynamics have been implicated as contributors in the predisposition to this disorder (Foley et al., 2004; Popper et al., 2003; Sadock & Sadock, 2007):

- Parental rejection
- Inconsistent management with harsh discipline
- Early institutional living
- Frequent shifting of parental figures
- Large family size
- Absent father
- Parents with antisocial personality disorder and/or alcohol dependence
- Association with a delinquent subgroup
- Marital conflict and divorce
- Inadequate communication patterns
- Parental permissiveness

Application of the Nursing Process to Conduct Disorder

Background Assessment Data (Symptomatology)

The classic characteristic of conduct disorder is the use of physical aggression in the violation of the rights of others. The behavior pattern manifests itself in virtually all areas of the child's life (home, school, with peers, and in the community). Stealing, lying, and truancy are common problems. The child lacks feelings of guilt or remorse.

The use of tobacco, liquor, or nonprescribed drugs, as well as participation in sexual activities, occurs earlier than at the expected age for the peer group. Projection is a common defense mechanism.

Low self-esteem is manifested by a "tough guy" image. Characteristics include poor frustration tolerance, irritability, and frequent temper outbursts. Symptoms of anxiety and depression are not uncommon.

Level of academic achievement may be low in relation to age and IQ.

Manifestations associated with ADHD (e.g., attention difficulties, impulsiveness, and hyperactivity) are very common in children with conduct disorder.

The *DSM-IV-TR* diagnostic criteria for conduct disorder are presented in Box 25–4.

BOX 25 – 4   Diagnostic Criteria for Conduct Disorder

A. A repetitive and persistent pattern of behavior in which the basic rights of others or major age-appropriate societal norms or rules are violated, as manifested by the presence of three (or more) of the following criteria in the past 12 months, with at least one criterion present in the past 6 months:

1. **Aggression to people and animals**
   a. Often bullies, threatens, or intimidates others.
   b. Often initiates physical fights.
   c. Has used a weapon that can cause serious physical harm to others (e.g., a bat, brick, broken bottle, knife, gun)
   d. Has been physically cruel to people.
   e. Has been physically cruel to animals.
   f. Has stolen while confronting a victim (e.g., mugging, purse snatching, extortion, armed robbery).
   g. Has forced someone into sexual activity.

2. **Destruction of property**
   a. Has deliberately engaged in fire setting with the intention of causing serious damage.
   b. Has deliberately destroyed others' property (other than by fire setting).

3. **Deceitfulness or theft**
   a. Has broken into someone else's house, building, or car.
   b. Often lies to obtain goods or favors or to avoid obligations (i.e., "cons" others)
   c. Has stolen items of nontrivial value without confronting a victim (e.g., shoplifting, but without breaking and entering; forgery).

4. **Serious violations of rules**
   a. Often stays out at night despite parental prohibitions, beginning before age 13 years.
   b. Has run away from home overnight at least twice while living in parental or parental surrogate home (or once without returning for a lengthy period).
   c. Is often truant from school, beginning before age 13 years.

B. The disturbance in behavior causes clinically significant impairment in social, academic, or occupational functioning.

C. If the individual is age 18 years or older, criteria are not met for antisocial personality disorder.

Subtypes:

1. **Childhood-Onset Type:** Onset of at least one criterion characteristic of conduct disorder before age 10 years.

2. **Adolescent-Onset Type:** Absence of any criteria characteristic of conduct disorder before age 10 years.

3. **Unspecified Onset:** Age at onset is not known.

SOURCE: From APA (2000), with permission.

Diagnosis/Outcome Identification

Based on the data collected during the nursing assessment, possible nursing diagnoses for the client with conduct disorder include:

● Risk for other-directed violence related to characteristics of temperament, peer rejection, negative parental role models, dysfunctional family dynamics.
● Impaired social interaction related to negative parental role models, impaired peer relationships leading to inappropriate social behaviors.
● Defensive coping related to low self-esteem and dysfunctional family system.
● Low self-esteem related to lack of positive feedback and unsatisfactory parent–child relationship.

Outcome Criteria

Outcome criteria include short- and long-term goals. Timelines are individually determined. The following criteria may be used for measurement of outcomes in the care of the client with conduct disorder:

The client:

1. Has not harmed self or others.
2. Interacts with others in a socially appropriate manner.
3. Accepts direction without becoming defensive.
4. Demonstrates evidence of increased self-esteem by discontinuing exploitative and demanding behaviors toward others.

Planning/Implementation

Table 25–7 provides a plan of care for the child with conduct disorder using nursing diagnoses common to the disorder, outcome criteria, and appropriate nursing interventions and rationales.

Evaluation

Following the planning and implementation of care, evaluation is made of the behavioral changes in a child with conduct disorder. This is accomplished by determining if the goals of therapy have been achieved. Reassessment, the next step in the nursing process, may be initiated by gathering information using the following questions:

1. Have the nursing actions directed toward managing the client's aggressive behavior been effective?
2. Have interventions prevented harm to others or others' property?
3. Is the client able to express anger in an appropriate manner?
4. Has the client developed more adaptive coping strategies to deal with anger and feelings of aggression?
5. Does the client demonstrate the ability to trust others? Is he or she able to interact with staff and peers in an appropriate manner?

Table 25–7	Care Plan for Child/Adolescent with Conduct Disorder

NURSING DIAGNOSIS: RISK FOR OTHER-DIRECTED VIOLENCE

RELATED TO: Characteristics of temperament, peer rejection, negative parental role models, dysfunctional family dynamics

Outcome Criteria	Nursing Interventions	Rationale
Short-Term Goal: ● Client will discuss feelings of anger with nurse or therapist. **Long-Term Goal:** ● Client will not harm others or others' property.	1. Observe client's behavior frequently through routine activities and interactions. Become aware of behaviors that indicate a rise in agitation. 2. Redirect violent behavior with physical outlets for suppressed anger and frustration. 3. Encourage client to express anger and act as a role model for appropriate expression of anger. 4. Ensure that a sufficient number of staff is available to indicate a show of strength if necessary. 5. Administer tranquilizing medication, if ordered, or use mechanical restraints or isolation room only if situation cannot be controlled with less restrictive means.	1. Recognition of behaviors that precede the onset of aggression may provide the opportunity to intervene before violence occurs. 2. Excess energy is released through physical activities inducing a feeling of relaxation. 3. Discussion of situations that create anger may lead to more effective ways of dealing with them. 4. This conveys an evidence of control over the situation and provides physical security for staff. 5. It is the client's right to expect the use of techniques that ensure safety of the client and others by the least restrictive means.

NURSING DIAGNOSIS: IMPAIRED SOCIAL INTERACTION

RELATED TO: Negative parental role models; impaired peer·relations leading to inappropriate social behavior

Outcome Criteria	Nursing Interventions	Rationale
Short-Term Goal: ● Client will interact in age-appropriate manner with nurse in one-to-one relationship within 1 week. **Long-Term Goal:** ● Client will be able to interact with staff and peers using age-appropriate, acceptable behaviors.	1. Develop a trusting relationship with the client. Convey acceptance of the person separate from the unacceptable behavior. 2. Discuss with client which behaviors are and are not acceptable. Describe in matter-of-fact manner the consequence of unacceptable behavior. Follow through. 3. Provide group situations for client.	1. Unconditional acceptance increases feeling of self-worth. 2. Aversive reinforcement can alter or extinguish undesirable behaviors. 3. Appropriate social behavior is often learned from the positive and negative feedback of peers.

NURSING DIAGNOSIS: DEFENSIVE COPING

RELATED TO: Low self-esteem and dysfunctional family system

Outcome Criteria	Nursing Interventions	Rationale
Short-Term Goal: ● Client will verbalize personal responsibility for difficulties experienced in interpersonal relationships within (time period reasonable for client).	1. Explain to client the correlation between feelings of inadequacy and the need for acceptance from others and how these feelings provoke defensive behaviors, such as blaming others for own behaviors.	1. Recognition of the problem is the first step in the change process toward resolution.

Substance-Intoxication Delirium

With this disorder, the symptoms of delirium may arise within minutes to hours after taking relatively high doses of certain drugs such as cannabis, cocaine, and hallucinogens. It may take longer periods of sustained intoxication to produce delirium symptoms with alcohol, anxiolytics, or narcotics (APA, 2000).

Substance-Withdrawal Delirium

Withdrawal delirium symptoms develop after reduction or termination of sustained, usually high-dose use of certain substances, such as alcohol, sedatives, hypnotics, or anxiolytics (APA, 2000). The duration of the delirium is directly related to the half-life of the substance involved and may last from a few hours to 2 to 4 weeks.

= antipsychotics

Delirium Due to Multiple Etiologies

This diagnosis is used when the symptoms of delirium are brought on by more than one cause. For example, the delirium may be related to more than one general medical condition or it may be a result of the combined effects of a general medical condition and substance use (APA, 2000).

CORE CONCEPT

Dementia
Dementia is defined by a loss of previous levels of cognitive, executive, and memory function in a state of full alertness (Bourgeois, Seaman, & Servis, 2008).

DEMENTIA

Clinical Findings, Epidemiology, and Course

This disorder constitutes a large and growing public health problem. Scientists estimate that 4.5 million people currently have Alzheimer's disease (AD), the most common form of dementia, and the prevalence (the number of people with the disease at any one time) doubles for every 5-year age group beyond age 65 (National Institute on Aging [NIA], 2005). The disease affects one in ten people age 65 and older, one in five ages 75 to 85, and one in two age 85 and older (Laraia, 2004). Researchers estimate that by 2050, 13.2 million Americans will have AD if current population trends continue and no preventive treatments become available

(Herbert, Scherr, Bienias, Bennett, & Evans, 2003). After heart disease and cancer, AD is the third most costly disease to society, accounting for $100 billion in yearly costs (NIA, 2005). This proliferation is not the result of an "epidemic." It has occurred because more people now survive into the high-risk period for dementia, which is middle age and beyond.

Dementia can be classified as either primary or secondary. Primary dementias are those, such as AD, in which the dementia itself is the major sign of some organic brain disease not directly related to any other organic illness. Secondary dementias are caused by or related to another disease or condition, such as human immunodeficiency virus (HIV) disease or a cerebral trauma. *stroke*

In dementia, impairment is evident in abstract thinking, judgment, and impulse control. The conventional rules of social conduct are often disregarded. Behavior may be uninhibited and inappropriate. Personal appearance and hygiene are often neglected.

Language may or may not be affected. Some individuals may have difficulty naming objects, or the language may seem vague and imprecise. In severe forms of dementia, the individual may not speak at all (**aphasia**). The client may know his or her needs but may not know how to communicate those needs to a caregiver.

Personality change is common in dementia and may be manifested by either an alteration or accentuation of premorbid characteristics. For example, an individual who was previously very socially active may become apathetic and socially isolated. A previously neat person may become markedly untidy in his or her appearance. Conversely, an individual who may have had difficulty trusting others prior to the illness may exhibit extreme fear and paranoia as manifestations of the dementia.

The reversibility of a dementia is a function of the underlying pathology and of the availability and timely application of effective treatment (APA, 2000). Truly reversible dementia occurs in only a small percentage of cases and might be more appropriately termed *temporary* dementia. Reversible dementia can occur as a result of cerebral lesions, depression, side effects of certain medications, normal pressure hydrocephalus, vitamin or nutritional deficiencies (especially B_{12} or folate), central nervous system infections, and metabolic disorders (Srikanth & Nagaraja, 2005). In most clients, dementia runs a progressive, irreversible course.

As the disease progresses, **apraxia**, which is the inability to carry out motor activities despite intact motor function, may develop. The individual may be irritable, moody, or exhibit sudden outbursts over trivial issues. The ability to work or care for personal needs independently will no longer be possible. These individuals can no longer be left alone because they do not comprehend their limitations and are therefore at serious risk for

IMPLICATIONS OF RESEARCH FOR EVIDENCE-BASED PRACTICE

Kovach, C.R., Noonan, P.E., Schlidt, A.M., & Wells, T. (2005). A model of consequences of need-driven, dementia-compromised behavior. *Journal of Nursing Scholarship*, *37*(2), 134–140.

Description of the Study: Need-driven, dementia-compromised behavior (NDB) occurs because the caregiver is unable to comprehend needs, and the person with dementia cannot make needs known. The behaviors are viewed as an attempt on the part of the person with dementia to communicate a need and as a symptom that the need is not being met. The authors extend the primary need model to encompass secondary needs when primary needs go unresolved. From an extensive literature review, the authors proposed a framework for improving understanding of the person with dementia and the consequences of behavioral symptoms and unmet needs.

Results of the Study: The experiences of people with dementia who have unmet needs is described as having "cascading effects." In people with dementia, basic needs (e.g., thirst/need for fluid) result in primary NDB (e.g., restlessness/repetitive movements), which if left unmet may result in the negative outcome of constipation and abdominal discomfort. This need for relief may lead to the secondary NDB of aggression. The authors state, "Secondary NDBs are iatrogenic outcomes of these cascading effects and the response of a vulnerable person to the recurrent and unpredictable stress of treatment targeted inappropriately or care providers who dismiss the NDB communication." Common problematic behaviors that may be associated with unmet needs include resistiveness to care, verbal complaining, restlessness, facial grimacing, aggression, crying, moaning, calling out, exiting behavior, tense body parts, and rubbing or holding a body part. Unmet needs may also influence affective status (e.g., depression or anxiety), physical status (e.g., immune suppression), and acceleration in functional status.

Implications for Nursing Practice: The authors of this study state, "The consequences of need-driven dementia-compromised behavior theory indicates that meeting needs of people with dementia will moderate the sequence of events that leads to negative outcomes." When caregivers cannot understand primary NDBs, they cannot provide anticipatory care. The anticipation and fulfillment of clients' needs is necessary to decrease the prevalence and severity of new unmet needs, thereby positively influencing comfort and quality of life for people with dementia.

accidents. Wandering away from the home or care setting often becomes a problem.

Several causes have been described for the syndrome of dementia (see section on Predisposing Factors), but AD accounts for 50 to 60 percent of all cases (Andreasen & Black, 2006). The progressive nature of symptoms associated with AD has been described according to stages (Alzheimer's Association, 2007; NIA, 2007; Stanley, Blair, & Beare, 2005):

Stage 1. No Apparent Symptoms. In the first stage of the illness, there is no apparent decline in memory.

Stage 2. Forgetfulness. The individual begins to lose things or forget names of people. Losses in short-term memory are common. The individual is aware of the intellectual decline and may feel ashamed, becoming anxious and depressed, which in turn may worsen the symptom. Maintaining organization with lists and a structured routine provide some compensation. These symptoms often are not observed by others.

Stage 3. Mild Cognitive Decline. In this stage, there is interference with work performance, which becomes noticeable to coworkers. The individual may get lost when driving his or her car. Concentration may be interrupted. There is difficulty recalling names or words, which becomes noticeable to family and close associates. A decline occurs in the ability to plan or organize.

Stage 4. Mild-to-Moderate Cognitive Decline; Confusion. At this stage, the individual may forget major events in personal history, such as his or her own child's birthday; experience declining ability to perform tasks, such as shopping and managing personal finances; or be unable to understand current news events. He or she may deny that a problem exists by covering up memory loss with **confabulation** (creating imaginary events to fill in memory gaps). Depression and social withdrawal are common.

Stage 5. Moderate Cognitive Decline; Early Dementia. In the early stages of dementia, individuals lose the ability to perform some activities of daily living (ADLs) independently, such as hygiene, dressing, and grooming, and require some assistance to manage these on an ongoing basis. They may forget addresses, phone numbers, and names of close relatives. They may become disoriented about place and time, but they maintain knowledge about themselves. Frustration, withdrawal, and self-absorption are common.

Stage 6. Moderate-to-Severe Cognitive Decline; Middle Dementia. At this stage, the individual may be unable to recall recent major life events or even the name of his or her spouse. Disorientation to surroundings is common, and the person may be unable to recall the day, season, or year. The person is unable to manage ADLs without assistance. Urinary and fecal incontinence are common. Sleeping becomes a problem. Psychomotor symptoms include wandering, obsessiveness, agitation, and aggression. Symptoms seem to worsen in the late afternoon and evening—a phenomenon termed **sundowning.** Communication becomes more difficult, with increasing loss of language skills. Institutional care is usually required at this stage.

Stage 7. Severe Cognitive Decline; Late Dementia. In the end stages of AD, the individual is unable to recognize family members. He or she most commonly is bedfast and aphasic. Problems of immobility, such as decubiti and contractures, may occur.

Stanley and associates (2005) describe the late stages of dementia in the following manner:

During late-stage dementia, the person becomes more chairbound or bedbound. Muscles are rigid, contractures may develop, and primitive reflexes may be present. The person may have very active hands and repetitive movements, grunting, or other vocalizations. There is depressed immune system function, and this impairment coupled with immobility may lead to the development of pneumonia, urinary tract infections, sepsis, and pressure ulcers. Appetite decreases and dysphagia is present; aspiration is common. Weight loss generally occurs. Speech and language are severely impaired, with greatly decreased verbal communication. The person may no longer recognize any family members. Bowel and bladder incontinence are present and caregivers need to complete most ADLs for the person. The sleep-wake cycle is greatly altered, and the person spends a lot of time dozing and appears socially withdrawn and more unaware of the environment or surroundings. Death may be caused by infection, sepsis, or aspiration, although there are not many studies examining cause of death. (p. 358)

Predisposing Factors

The disorders of dementia are differentiated by their etiology, although they share a common symptom presentation. Categories of dementia include:

1. Dementia of the Alzheimer's type
2. Vascular dementia
3. Dementia due to HIV disease
4. Dementia due to head trauma
5. Dementia due to Lewy body disease
6. Dementia due to Parkinson's disease
7. Dementia due to Huntington's disease
8. Dementia due to Pick's disease
9. Dementia due to Creutzfeldt–Jakob disease
10. Dementia due to other general medical conditions
11. Substance-induced persisting dementia
12. Dementia due to multiple etiologies

Dementia of the Alzheimer's Type

This disorder is characterized by the syndrome of symptoms identified as dementia in the *DSM-IV-TR* and in the seven stages described previously. The onset of symptoms is slow and insidious, and the course of the disorder is generally progressive and deteriorating. The *DSM-IV-TR* further categorizes this disorder as *early onset* (first symptoms occurring at age 65 or younger) or *late onset* (first symptoms occurring after age 65) and by the clinical presentation of behavioral disturbance (such as wandering or agitation) superimposed on the dementia.

Refinement of diagnostic criteria now enables clinicians to use specific clinical features to identify the disease with considerable accuracy. Examination by computerized tomography (CT) scan or magnetic resonance imaging (MRI) reveals a degenerative pathology of the brain that includes atrophy, widened cortical sulci, and

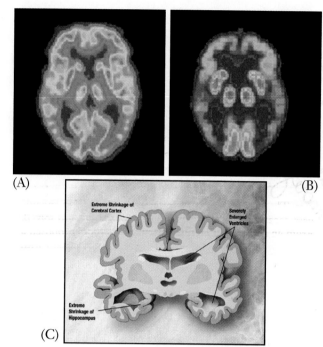

(A)   (B)

(C)

FIGURE 26–1 Changes in the Alzheimer's Brain. *A.* PET scan showing metabolic activity in a normal brain. *B.* Diminished metabolic activity in the Alzheimer's diseased brain. *C.* Late stage Alzheimer's disease with generalized atrophy and enlargement of the ventricles and sulci. (Source: Alzheimer's Disease Education & Referral Center, A Service of the National Institute on Aging. 2005. http://www.alzheimers.org/)

enlarged cerebral ventricles (Figures 26–1 and 26–2). Microscopic examinations reveal numerous neurofibrillary tangles and senile plaques in the brains of clients with AD. These changes apparently occur as a part of the normal aging process. However, in clients with AD, they are found in dramatically increased numbers and their profusion is concentrated in the hippocampus and certain parts of the cerebral cortex.

Etiology. The exact cause of AD is unknown. Several hypotheses have been supported by varying amounts and quality of data. These hypotheses include:

1. **Acetylcholine Alterations.** Research has indicated that in the brains of AD clients, the enzyme required to produce acetylcholine is dramatically reduced. The reduction seems to be greatest in the nucleus basalis of the inferior medial forebrain area (Cummings & Mega, 2003). This decrease in production of acetylcholine reduces the amount of the neurotransmitter that is released to cells in the cortex and hippocampus, resulting in a disruption of the cognitive processes. Other neurotransmitters implicated in the pathology and clinical symptoms of AD include norepinephrine, serotonin, dopamine, and the amino acid glutamate. It has been proposed that in dementia, excess glutamate leads to overstimulation of the *N*-methyl-D-aspartate (NMDA) receptors, leading to increased intracellular calcium, and subsequent neuronal degeneration and cell death.

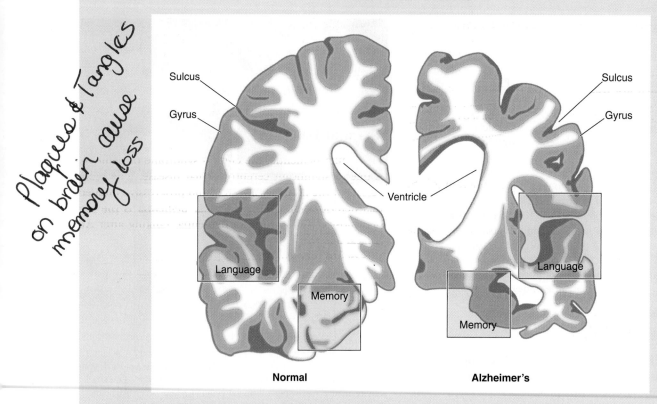

Plaques & Tangles on brain cause memory loss

FIGURE 26–2 Neurobiology of Alzheimer's Disease. (Source: American Health Assistance Foundation, [2005], with permission. http://www.ahaf.org/alzdis/about/BrainAlzheimer.htm)

Neurotransmitters

A decrease in the neurotransmitter *acetylcholine* has been implicated in the etiology of Alzheimer's disease. Cholinergic sources arise from the brain stem and the basal forebrain to supply areas of the basal ganglia, thalamus, limbic structures, hippocampus, and cerebral cortex.

Cell bodies of origin for the *serotonin* pathways lie within the raphe nuclei located in the brain stem. Those for *norepinephrine* originate in the locus ceruleus. Projections for both neurotransmitters extend throughout the forebrain, prefrontal cortex, cerebellum, and limbic system. *Dopamine* pathways arise from areas in the midbrain and project to the frontal cortex, limbic system, basal ganglia, and thalamus. Dopamine neurons in the hypothalamus innervate the posterior pituitary.

Glutamate, an excitatory neurotransmitter, has largely descending pathways with highest concentrations in the cerebral cortex. It is also found in the hippocampus, thalamus, hypothalamus, cerebellum, and spinal cord.

Areas of the Brain Affected

Areas of the brain affected by Alzheimer's disease and associated symptoms include the following:

Frontal lobe:	Impaired reasoning ability. Unable to solve problems and perform familiar tasks. Poor judgment. Inability to evaluate the appropriateness of behavior. Aggressiveness.
Parietal lobe:	Impaired orientation ability. Impaired visuospatial skills (unable to remain oriented within own environment).
Occipital lobe:	Impaired language interpretation. Unable to recognize familiar objects.
Temporal lobe:	Inability to recall words. Inability to use words correctly (language comprehension). In late stages, some clients experience delusions, and hallucinations.
Hippocampus:	Impaired memory. Short-term memory is affected initially. Later, the individual is unable to form new memories.
Amygdala:	Impaired emotions: depression, anxiety, fear, personality changes, apathy, paranoia.
Neurotransmitters:	Alterations in acetylcholine, dopamine, norepinephrine, serotonin and others may play a role in behaviors such as restlessness, sleep impairment, mood, and agitation.

Medications and Their Effects on the Brain

1. Cholinesterase inhibitors (e.g., tacrine, donepezil, rivastigmine, and galantamine) act by inhibiting acetylcholinesterase, which slows the degradation of acetylcholine, thereby increasing concentrations of the neurotransmitter in the brain. Most common side effects include dizziness, GI upset, fatigue, and headache.
2. NMDA receptor antagonists (e.g., memantine) act by blocking NMDA receptors from excessive glutamate, preventing continuous influx of calcium into the cells, and ultimately slowing down neuronal degradation. Possible side effects include dizziness, headache, and constipation.

2. **Plaques and Tangles.** As mentioned previously, an overabundance of structures called plaques and tangles appears in the brains of individuals with AD. The plaques are made of a protein called amyloid beta ($A\beta$), which are fragments of a larger protein called amyloid precursor protein (APP; Alzheimer's Disease Education & Referral Center [ADEAR], 2003). Plaques are formed when these fragments clump together and mix with molecules and other cellular matter. Tangles are formed from a special kind of cellular protein called tau protein, whose function it is to provide stability to the neuron. In AD, the tau protein is chemically altered (ADEAR, 2003). Strands of the protein become tangled together, interfering with the neuronal transport system. It is not known whether the plaques and tangles cause AD or are a consequence of the AD process. It is thought that the plaques and tangles contribute to the destruction and death of neurons, leading to memory failure, personality changes, inability to carry out ADLs, and other features of the disease (ADEAR, 2003).

3. **Head Trauma.** The etiology of AD has been associated with serious head trauma (Munoz & Feldman, 2000). Studies have shown that some individuals who had experienced head trauma had subsequently (after years) developed AD. This hypothesis is being investigated as a possible cause. Munoz and Feldman (2000) report an increased risk for AD in individuals who are both genetically predisposed and who experience traumatic head injury.

4. **Genetic Factors.** There is clearly a familial pattern with some forms of AD. Some families exhibit a pattern of inheritance that suggests possible autosomal-dominant gene transmission (Sadock & Sadock, 2007). Some studies indicate that early-onset cases are more likely to be familial than late-onset cases, and that from one third to one half of all cases may be of the genetic form. Some researchers believe that there is a link between AD and the alteration of a gene found on chromosome 21 (Munoz & Feldman, 2000; Saunders, 2001). People with Down syndrome, who carry an extra copy of chromosome 21, have been found to be unusually susceptible to AD (Lott & Head, 2005).

Some studies have linked the apolipoprotein E epsilon 4 (*ApoE ε4*) gene, found on chromosome 19, to an increased risk of late-onset AD (Poduslo & Yin, 2001). The presenilin 1 (*PS-1*) gene on chromosome 14 and the presenilin 2 (*PS-2*) gene on chromosome 1 have been associated with the onset of AD before age 65 years (Saunders, 2001).

Rogaeva and associates (2007) recently reported on the results of a study in which they describe how variants in the *SOR1* gene were found to be more common in people with late-onset AD than in healthy people the same age. These variants apparently alter the normal function of *SOR1*, reducing the amount. When *SOR1* is reduced, this paves the way for increased amounts of APP to be shunted into endosomes, where it is broken down into $A\beta$. The researchers suggest that these inherited variants of the *SOR1* gene are associated with an increased risk of AD.

Vascular Dementia

In vascular dementia, the clinical syndrome of dementia is due to significant cerebrovascular disease. The blood vessels of the brain are affected, and progressive intellectual deterioration occurs. Vascular dementia is the second most common form of dementia, ranking after AD (Black, 2005).

Vascular dementia differs from AD in that it has a more abrupt onset and runs a highly variable course. Progression of the symptoms occurs in "steps" rather than as a gradual deterioration; that is, at times the dementia seems to clear up and the individual exhibits fairly lucid thinking. Memory may seem better, and the client may become optimistic that improvement is occurring, only to experience further decline of functioning in a fluctuating pattern of progression. This irregular pattern of decline appears to be an intense source of anxiety for the client with this disorder.

In vascular dementia, clients suffer the equivalent of small strokes that destroy many areas of the brain. The pattern of deficits is variable, depending on which regions of the brain have been affected (APA, 2000). Certain focal neurological signs are commonly seen with vascular dementia, including weaknesses of the limbs, small-stepped gait, and difficulty with speech.

The disorder is more common in men than in women (APA, 2000). Arvanitakis (2000) states:

> Prognosis for patients with vascular dementia is worse than that for Alzheimer's patients. The three-year mortality rate in cases over the age of 85 years old is quoted at 67 percent as compared to 42 percent in Alzheimer's disease, and 23 percent in non-demented individuals. However, outcome is ultimately dependent on the underlying risk factors and mechanism of disease, and further studies taking these distinctions into account are warranted.

The diagnosis can be subtyped when the dementia is superimposed with symptoms of delirium, delusions, or depressed mood.

Etiology. The cause of vascular dementia is directly related to an interruption of blood flow to the brain. Symptoms result from death of nerve cells in regions nourished by diseased vessels. Various diseases and conditions that interfere with blood circulation have been implicated.

High blood pressure is thought to be one of the most significant factors in the etiology of multiple small strokes or cerebral infarcts. Hypertension leads to damage to the lining of blood vessels. This can result in rupture of the blood vessel with subsequent hemorrhage or an accumulation of fibrin in the vessel with intravascular clotting and inhibited blood flow (DeMartinis, 2005). Dementia also can result from infarcts related to occlusion of blood vessels by particulate matter that travels through the bloodstream to the brain. These emboli may be solid (e.g., clots, cellular debris, platelet aggregates), gaseous (e.g., air, nitrogen), or liquid (e.g., fat, following soft tissue trauma or fracture of long bones).

Cognitive impairment can occur with multiple small infarcts (sometimes called "silent strokes") over time or with a single cerebrovascular insult that occurs in a strategic area of the brain. An individual may have both vascular dementia and AD simultaneously. This is referred to as *mixed dementia*, the prevalence of which is likely to increase as the population ages (Langa, Foster, & Larson, 2004).

Dementia Due to Human Immunodeficiency Virus

Infection with the human immunodeficiency virus-type 1 (HIV-1) produces a dementing illness called HIV-1–associated cognitive/motor complex (also called HIV-Associated Dementia [HAD]). A less severe form, known as HIV-1–associated minor cognitive/motor disorder, also occurs. The severity of symptoms correlates with the extent of brain pathology. The immune dysfunction associated with HIV disease can lead to brain infections by other organisms, and the HIV-1 also appears to cause dementia directly. In the early stages, neuropsychiatric symptoms may be manifested by barely perceptible changes in a person's normal psychological presentation. Severe cognitive changes, particularly confusion, changes in behavior, and sometimes psychoses, are not uncommon in the later stages.

With the advent of the highly active antiretroviral therapies (HAART), incidence rates of dementia associated with HIV disease have been on the decline. However, it is possible that the prolonged life span of HIV-infected patients taking medications may actually increase the prevalence of this disorder in coming years (McArthur, 2004).

Dementia Due to Head Trauma

Serious head trauma can result in symptoms associated with the syndrome of dementia. Amnesia is the most common neurobehavioral symptom following head trauma, and a degree of permanent disturbance may persist (Bourgeois et al., 2008). Repeated head trauma, such as the type experienced by boxers, can result in *dementia pugilistica*, a syndrome characterized by emotional lability, dysarthria, ataxia, and impulsivity (Sadock & Sadock, 2007).

Dementia Due to Lewy Body Disease

[handwritten: confusion / hallucination ✕]
[handwritten: Older patient]

Clinically, Lewy body disease is fairly similar to AD; however, it tends to progress more rapidly, and there is an earlier appearance of visual hallucinations and parkinsonian features (Rabins et al., 2006). This disorder is distinctive by the presence of Lewy bodies—eosinophilic inclusion bodies—seen in the cerebral cortex and brainstem (Andreasen & Black, 2006). These patients are highly sensitive to extrapyramidal effects of antipsychotic medications. The disease is progressive and irreversible, and may account for as many as 25 percent of all dementia cases.

Dementia Due to Parkinson's Disease

Dementia is observed in as many as 60 percent of clients with Parkinson's disease (Bourgeois et al., 2008). In this disease, there is a loss of nerve cells located in the substantia nigra, and dopamine activity is diminished, resulting in involuntary muscle movements, slowness, and rigidity. Tremor in the upper extremities is characteristic. In some instances, the cerebral changes that occur in dementia of Parkinson's disease closely resemble those of AD.

Dementia Due to Huntington's Disease

Huntington's disease is transmitted as a Mendelian dominant gene. Damage is seen in the areas of the basal ganglia and the cerebral cortex. The onset of symptoms (i.e., involuntary twitching of the limbs or facial muscles; mild cognitive changes; depression and apathy) is usually between age 30 and 50 years. The client usually declines into a profound state of dementia and **ataxia**. The average duration of the disease is based on age at onset. One study concluded that juvenile-onset and late-onset clients have the shortest duration (Foroud, Gray, Ivashina, & Conneally, 1999). In this study, the median duration of the disease was 21.4 years.

Dementia Due to Pick's Disease *[handwritten: Personality may change]*

The cause of Pick's disease is unknown, but a genetic factor appears to be involved. The clinical picture is strikingly similar to that of AD. One major difference is that the initial symptom in Pick's disease is usually personality change, whereas the initial symptom in AD is memory impairment. Studies reveal that pathology of Pick's disease results from atrophy in the frontal and temporal lobes of the brain, in contrast to AD, which is more widely distributed.

[handwritten: Mad Cow Disease]

Dementia Due to Creutzfeldt–Jakob Disease

Creutzfeldt–Jakob disease is an uncommon neurodegenerative disease caused by a transmissible agent known as a "slow virus" or prion (APA, 2000). Five to 15 percent of cases have a genetic component. The clinical presentation is typical of the syndrome of dementia, along with involuntary movements, muscle rigidity, and ataxia. Symptoms may develop at any age in adults, but typically occur between ages 40 and 60 years. The clinical course is extremely rapid, with progressive deterioration and death within 1 year (Wise, Gray, & Seltzer, 1999).

Dementia Due to Other General Medical Conditions

A number of other general medical conditions can cause dementia. Some of these include endocrine conditions (e.g., hypoglycemia, hypothyroidism), pulmonary disease, hepatic or renal failure, cardiopulmonary insufficiency, fluid and electrolyte imbalances, nutritional deficiencies, frontal or temporal lobe lesions, central nervous system (CNS) or systemic infections, uncontrolled epilepsy, and other neurological conditions such as multiple sclerosis (APA, 2000).

Substance-Induced Persisting Dementia

The features associated with this type of dementia are those associated with dementias in general; however, evidence must exist from history, physical examination, or laboratory findings to show that the deficits are etiologically related to the persisting effects of substance use (APA, 2000). The term *persisting* is used to indicate that the dementia persists long after the effects of substance intoxication or substance withdrawal have subsided. The

DSM-IV-TR identifies the following types of substances with which persisting dementia is associated:

1. Alcohol
2. Inhalants
3. Sedatives, hypnotics, and anxiolytics
4. Medications
   a. Anticonvulsants
   b. Intrathecal methotrexate
5. Toxins
   a. Lead
   b. Mercury
   c. Carbon monoxide
   d. Organophosphate insecticides
   e. Industrial solvents

The diagnosis is made according to the specific etiological substance involved. For example, if the substance known to cause the dementia is alcohol, the diagnosis is Alcohol-Induced Persisting Dementia. If the exact substance presumed to be causing the dementia were unknown, the diagnosis would be Unknown Substance-Induced Persisting Dementia.

Dementia Due to Multiple Etiologies

This diagnosis is used when the symptoms of dementia are attributed to more than one cause. For example, the dementia may be related to more than one medical condition or to the combined effects of a general medical condition and the long-term use of a substance (APA, 2000).

The etiological factors associated with delirium and dementia are summarized in Box 26–1.

BOX 26–1   Etiological Factors Implicated in the Development of Delirium and/or Dementia

Biological Factors	Exogenous Factors
Hypoxia: any condition leading to a deficiency of oxygen to the brain	Birth trauma: prolonged labor, damage from use of forceps, other obstetric complications
Nutritional deficiencies: vitamins (particularly B and C); protein; fluid and electrolyte imbalances	Cranial trauma: concussion, contusions, hemorrhage, hematomas
Metabolic disturbances: porphyria; encephalopathies related to hepatic, renal, pancreatic, or pulmonary insufficiencies; hypoglycemia	Volatile inhalant compounds: gasoline, glue, paint, paint thinners, spray paints, cleaning fluids, typewriter correction fluid, varnishes, and lacquers
Endocrine dysfunction: thyroid, parathyroid, adrenal, pancreas, pituitary	Heavy metals: lead, mercury, manganese
Cardiovascular disease: stroke, cardiac insufficiency, atherosclerosis	Other metallic elements: aluminum
Primary brain disorders: epilepsy, Alzheimer's disease, Pick's disease, Huntington's disease, multiple sclerosis, Parkinson's disease	Organic phosphates: various insecticides
Infections: encephalitis, meningitis, pneumonia, septicemia, neurosyphilis (dementia paralytica), HIV disease, acute rheumatic fever, Creutzfeldt–Jakob disease	Substance abuse/dependence: alcohol, amphetamines, caffeine, cannabis, cocaine, hallucinogens, inhalants, nicotine, opioids, phencyclidine, sedatives, hypnotics, anxiolytics
Intracranial neoplasms	Other medications: anticholinergics, antihistamines, antidepressants, antipsychotics, antiparkinsonians, antihypertensives, steroids, digitalis
Congenital defects: prenatal infections, such as first-trimester maternal rubella	

CORE CONCEPT

Amnesia
The inability to retain or recall past experiences. The condition may be temporary or permanent, depending on etiology.

AMNESTIC DISORDERS

Amnestic disorders are characterized by an inability to learn new information (short-term memory deficit) despite normal attention, and an inability to recall previously learned information (long-term memory deficit). Events from the remote past often are recalled more easily than recently occurring ones. The syndrome differs from dementia in that there is no impairment in abstract thinking or judgment, no other disturbances of higher cortical function, and no personality change.

Profound amnesia may result in disorientation to place and time, but rarely to self (APA, 2000). The individual may engage in confabulation—the creation of imaginary events to fill in memory gaps.

Some individuals will continue to deny that they have a problem despite evidence to the contrary. Others may acknowledge that a problem exists, but appear unconcerned. Apathy, lack of initiative, and emotional blandness are common. The person may appear friendly and agreeable, but the emotionality is superficial.

The onset of symptoms may be acute or insidious, depending on the pathological process causing the amnestic disorder. Duration and course of the illness may be quite variable and are also correlated with extent and severity of the cause.

Predisposing Factors

Amnestic disorders share a common symptom presentation of memory impairment but are differentiated in the *DSM-IV-TR* (APA, 2000) according to etiology:

1. Amnestic disorder due to a general medical condition
2. Substance-induced persisting amnestic disorder

Amnestic Disorder Due to a General Medical Condition

In this type of amnestic disorder, evidence must exist from the history, physical examination, or laboratory findings to show that the memory impairment is the direct physiological consequence of a general medical condition (APA, 2000). The diagnosis is specified further by indicating whether the symptoms are *transient* (present for no more than 1 month) or *chronic* (present for more than 1 month).

General medical conditions that may be associated with amnestic disorder include head trauma, cerebrovascular disease, cerebral neoplastic disease, cerebral anoxia, herpes simplex encephalitis, poorly controlled insulin-dependent diabetes, and surgical intervention to the brain (Andreasen & Black, 2006; APA, 2000).

Transient amnestic syndromes can occur from cerebrovascular disease, cardiac arrhythmias, migraine, thyroid disorders, and epilepsy (Bourgeois et al., 2003).

Substance-Induced Persisting Amnestic Disorder

In this disorder, evidence must exist from the history, physical examination, or laboratory findings that the memory impairment is related to the persisting effects of substance use (e.g., a drug of abuse, a medication, or toxin exposure; APA, 2000). The term *persisting* is used to indicate that the symptoms exist long after the effects of substance intoxication or withdrawal have subsided. The *DSM-IV-TR* identifies the following substances with which amnestic disorder can be associated:

1. Alcohol
2. Sedatives, hypnotics, and anxiolytics
3. Medications
   a. Anticonvulsants
   b. Intrathecal methotrexate
4. Toxins
   a. Lead
   b. Mercury
   c. Carbon monoxide
   d. Organophosphate insecticides
   e. Industrial solvents

The diagnosis is made according to the specific etiological substance involved. For example, if the substance known to be the cause of the amnestic disorder is alcohol, the diagnosis would be Alcohol-Induced Persisting Amnestic Disorder.

APPLICATION OF THE NURSING PROCESS

Assessment

Nursing assessment of the client with delirium, dementia, or persisting amnesia is based on knowledge of the symptomatology associated with the various disorders described in the beginning of this chapter. Subjective and objective data are gathered by various members of the healthcare team. Clinicians report use of a variety of methods for obtaining assessment information.

3. Provide guidance and support for independent actions by talking her through tasks one step at a time.
4. Provide a structured schedule of activities that does not change from day to day.
5. Ensure that Carmen has snacks between meals.
6. Take Carmen to the bathroom regularly (according to her usual pattern, e.g., after meals, before bedtime, on arising)
7. To minimize nighttime wetness, offer fluids every 2 hours during the day and restrict fluids after 6:00 P.M.
8. To promote more restful nighttime sleep (and less wandering at night), reduce naps during late afternoon and encourage sitting exercises, walking, and ball toss. Carbohydrate snacks at bedtime may also be helpful.

EVALUATION

The outcome criteria identified for Carmen have been met. She has experienced no injury. She has not fallen out of bed. She continues to wander in a safe area. She can find her room by herself, but occasionally requires some assistance when she is anxious and more confused. She has some difficulty communicating her needs to the staff, but those who work with her on a consistent basis are able to anticipate her needs. All ADLs are being fulfilled, and Carmen assists with dressing and grooming, accomplishing about half on her own. Nighttime wandering has been minimized. Soft bedtime music helps to relax her.

SUMMARY AND KEY POINTS

- Cognitive disorders constitute a large and growing public health concern.
- Cognitive disorders include delirium, dementia, and amnestic disorders.
- A delirium is a disturbance of consciousness and a change in cognition that develop rapidly over a short period. Level of consciousness is often affected and psychomotor activity may fluctuate between agitated purposeless movements and a vegetative state resembling catatonic stupor.
- The symptoms of delirium usually begin quite abruptly and often are reversible and brief.
- Delirium may be caused by a general medical condition, substance intoxication or withdrawal, or ingestion of a medication or toxin.
- Dementia is a syndrome of acquired, persistent intellectual impairment with compromised function in multiple spheres of mental activity, such as memory, language, visuospatial skills, emotion or personality, and cognition.
- Symptoms of dementia are insidious and develop slowly over time. In most clients, dementia runs a progressive, irreversible course.
- Dementia may be caused by genetics, cardiovascular disease, infections, neurophysiological disorders, and other general medical conditions.
- Amnestic disorders are characterized by an inability to learn new information despite normal attention and an inability to recall previously learned information. Remote past events are often more easily recalled than recent ones.

- The onset of amnestic symptoms may be acute or insidious, depending on the pathological process causing the disorder. Duration and course of the illness may be quite variable and are also correlated with extent and severity of the cause.
- Nursing care of the client with a cognitive disorder is presented around the six steps of the nursing process.
- Objectives of care for the client experiencing an acute syndrome are aimed at eliminating the etiology, promoting client safety, and a return to the highest possible level of functioning.
- Objectives of care for the client experiencing a chronic, progressive disorder are aimed at preserving the dignity of the individual, promoting deceleration of the symptoms, and maximizing functional capabilities.
- Nursing interventions are also directed toward helping the client's family or primary caregivers learn about a chronic, progressive cognitive disorder.
- Education is provided about the disease process, expectations of client behavioral changes, methods for facilitating care, and sources of assistance and support as they struggle, both physically and emotionally, with the demands brought on by a disease process that is slowly taking their loved one away from them.

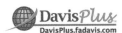 **DavisPlus**
DavisPlus.fadavis.com

For additional clinical tools and study aids, visit DavisPlus.

REVIEW QUESTIONS

Self-Examination/Learning Exercise

Mrs. G. is 67 years old. Her husband brings her to the hospital. He explains that she has become increasingly confused and forgetful. Yesterday, she started a fire in the kitchen when she put some bacon on to fry and went off and forgot it on the stove. Her husband reports that sometimes she seems okay, and sometimes she is completely disoriented. The physician has made an admitting diagnosis of dementia, etiology unknown.

Select the answer that is most appropriate for each of the following questions

1. Because the etiology of Mrs. G.'s symptoms is unknown, the physician will attempt to rule out the possibility that a reversible condition exists. An example of a treatable (reversible) form of dementia is one that is caused by:

    a. Multiple sclerosis.
    b. Multiple small brain infarcts.
    c. Electrolyte imbalances.
    d. HIV disease.

2. The physician rules out all reversible etiological factors and diagnoses Mrs. G. with Dementia of the Alzheimer's Type. The *primary* nursing intervention in working with Mrs. G. would be:

    a. Ensuring that she receives food she likes, to prevent hunger.
    b. Ensuring that the environment is safe, to prevent injury.
    c. Ensuring that she meets the other patients, to prevent social isolation.
    d. Ensuring that she takes care of her own ADLs, to prevent dependence.

3. Some medications have been indicated to decrease the agitation, violence, and bizarre thoughts associated with dementia. A drug that has been used for this is:

    a. Haloperidol (Haldol). Anti-psychotic "Atypical" brings on Extrapyramidal
    b. Tacrine (Cognex).
    c. Ergoloid (Hydergine).
    d. Diazepam (Valium). withdrawl for antidepressant

4. Even though Mrs. G. has been taking the medication identified in the previous question, her agitation increases markedly. The nurse should suspect

    a. Depression.
    b. Extrapyramidal side effects.
    c. Abdominal pain.
    d. Altered perceptions.

5. Mrs. G. has trouble sleeping and wanders around at night. Which of the following nursing actions would be *best* to promote sleep in Mrs. G.?

    a. Ask the doctor to prescribe flurazepam (Dalmane).
    b. Do not allow her to sleep at all during the day.
    c. Make Mrs. G. a cup of tea with honey before bedtime.
    d. Ensure that Mrs. G. gets regular physical exercise during the day.

6. The night nurse finds Mrs. G. wandering the hallway at 4 A.M. and trying to open the door to the side yard. Which statement by the nurse probably reflects the most accurate assessment of the situation?

    a. "That door leads out to the patio, Mrs. G. It's nighttime. You don't want to go outside now."
    b. "You look confused, Mrs. G. What is bothering you?"
    c. "This is the patio door, Mrs. G. Are you looking for the bathroom?"
    d. "Are you lonely? Perhaps you'd like to go back to your room and talk for a while."

7. In addition to disturbances in her cognition and orientation, Mrs. G. may also show changes in her

    a. Hearing, speech, and vision.
    b. Energy, creativity, and coordination.

c. Personality, speech, and mobility.
d. Appetite, affect, and attitude.

8. Mrs. G.'s daughter says to the nurse, "I read an article about Alzheimer's and it said the disease is hereditary. Does that mean I'll get it when I'm old?" The nurse bases her response on the knowledge that which of the following factors is *not* associated with increased incidence of dementia of the Alzheimer's type?
   a. Multiple small strokes *vascular*
   b. Family history of Alzheimer's disease
   c. Head trauma
   d. Advanced age

9. The physician determines that Mrs. G.'s dementia is related to cardiovascular disease and changes her diagnosis to vascular dementia. In explaining this disorder to Mrs. G.'s family, which of the following statements by the nurse is correct?
   a. "She will probably live longer than if her dementia was of the Alzheimer's type."
   b. "Vascular dementia shows stepwise progression. This is why she sometimes seems okay." *up & down*
   c. "Vascular dementia is caused by plaques and tangles that form in the brain." *Alzheim's Type*
   d. "The cause of vascular dementia is unknown."

10. Which of the following interventions is (are) most appropriate in helping Mrs. G. with her ADLs? (More than one answer may apply.)
    a. Perform ADLs for her while she is in the hospital.
    b. Provide her with a written list of activities she is expected to perform. *she has plaques & tangles*
    c. Assist her with step-by-step instructions.
    d. Tell her that if her morning care is not completed by 9:00 A.M. it will be performed for her by the nurse's aide so that Mrs. G. can attend group therapy.
    e. Encourage her and give her plenty of time to perform as many of her ADLs as possible independently.

Test Your Critical Thinking Skills

Joe, a 62-year-old accountant, began having difficulty remembering details necessary to perform his job. He was also having trouble at home, failing to keep his finances straight, and forgetting to pay bills. It became increasingly difficult for him to function properly at work, and eventually he was forced to retire. Cognitive deterioration continued, and behavioral problems soon began. He became stubborn, verbally and physically abusive, and suspicious of most everyone in his environment. His wife and son convinced him to see a physician, who recommended hospitalization for testing.

At Joe's initial evaluation, he was fully alert and cooperative but obviously anxious and fidgety. He thought he was at his accounting office and could not state what year it was. He could not say the names of his parents or siblings, nor did he know who was currently the president of the United States. He could not perform simple arithmetic calculations, write a proper sentence, or copy a drawing. He interpreted proverbs concretely and had difficulty stating similarities between related objects.

Laboratory serum studies revealed no abnormalities, but a CT scan showed marked cortical atrophy. The physician's diagnosis was Dementia of the Alzheimer's Type, Early Onset.

Answer the following questions related to Joe:

1. Identify the pertinent assessment data from which nursing care will be devised.
2. What is the primary nursing diagnosis for Joe?
3. How would outcomes be identified?

REFERENCES

Alzheimer's Association (2006). *Fact sheet: About memantine.* Retrieved February 19, 2007 from http://www.alz.org/

Alzheimer's Association. (2007). *Stages of Alzheimer's Disease.* Retrieved February 13, 2007 from http://www.alz.org/alzheimers_disease_stages_of_alzheimers.asp

Alzheimer's Disease Education & Referral Center [ADEAR]. (2003). *Alzheimer's disease: Unraveling the mystery.* NIH Publication Number: 02-3782. Washington, DC: National Institutes of Health.

American Psychiatric Association. (1994). *Diagnostic and statistical manual of mental disorders* (4th ed.). Washington, DC: American Psychiatric Publishing.

American Psychiatric Association. (2000). *Diagnostic and statistical manual of mental disorders* (4th ed.) *Text revision.* Washington, DC: American Psychiatric Publishing.

Andreasen, N.C., & Black, D.W. (2006). *Introductory textbook of psychiatry* (4th ed.). Washington, DC: American Psychiatric Publishing.

Arvanitakis, Z. (2000). *Dementia and vascular disease.* Duval County Medical Society. Retrieved February 16, 2007 from http://www.dcmsonline.org/jax-medicine/2000journals/February2000/vascdement.htm

Beers, M.H., & Jones, T.V. (Eds.). (2004). Drugs and aging. *The Merck manual of health and aging.* Whitehouse Station, NJ: Merck Research Laboratories.

Black, S.E. (2005). Vascular dementia: Stroke risk and sequelae define therapeutic approaches. *Postgraduate Medicine, 117*(1). Retrieved February 15, 2007 from http://www.postgradmed.com/issues/2005/01_05/black.htm

Bourgeois, J.A., Seaman, J.S., & Servis, M.E. (2008). Delirium, dementia, and amnestic disorders. In R.E. Hales, S.C. Yudofsky, & G.O. Gabbard (Eds.), *Textbook of psychiatry* (5th ed.). Washington, DC: American Psychiatric Publishing.

Bullock, R. (2005). Treatment of behavioural and psychiatric symptoms in dementia: Implications of recent safety warnings. *Current Medical Research and Opinion, 21*(1), 1–10.

Coelho Filho, J.M., & Birks, J. (2001). Physostigmine for dementia due to Alzheimer's disease (Cochrane Review). *The Cochrane Database of Systematic Reviews,* Issue 2. Art. No.: CD001499.

Cummings, J.L., Frank, J.C., Cherry, D., Kohatsu, N.D., Kemp, B., Hewett, L., & Mittman, B. (2002). Guidelines for managing Alzheimer's disease: Part II. Treatment. *American Family Physician, 65*(12), 2525–2534.

Cummings, J.L., & Mega, M.S. (2003). *Neuropsychiatry and behavioral neuroscience.* New York: Oxford University Press.

DeMartinis, J.E. (2005). Management of clients with hypertensive disorders. In J.M. Black & J.H. Hawks (Eds.), *Medical surgical nursing: Clinical management for positive outcomes* (7th ed.). St. Louis: Elsevier Saunders.

Eisendrath, S.J. & Lichtmacher, J.E. (2005). Psychiatric disorders. In L.M. Tierney, S.J. McPhee, & M.A. Papadakis (Eds.), *Current medical diagnosis and treatment.* New York: McGraw-Hill.

Foroud, T., Gray, J., Ivashina, J., & Conneally, P.M. (1999). Differences in duration of Huntington's disease based on age at onset. *Journal of Neurology, Neurosurgery and Psychiatry, 66,* 52–56.

Herbert, L.E., Scherr, P.A., Bienias, J.L., Bennett, D.A., & Evans, D.A. (2003). Alzheimer's disease in the U.S. population: Prevalence estimates using the 2000 census. *Archives of Neurology, 60*(8), 1119–1122.

Langa, K.M., Foster, N.L., & Larson, E.B. (2004). Mixed dementia: Emerging concepts and therapeutic implications. *Journal of the American Medical Association, 292*(23), 2901–2908.

Laraia, M.T. (2004, January/February). Memantine: First NMDA Receptor antagonist approved for the treatment of moderate to severe Alzheimer's disease. *APNA News, 16*(1), 12–13.

Lott, I.T., & Head, E. (2005). Alzheimer disease and Down syndrome: Factors in pathogenesis. *Neurobiology of Aging, 26*(3), 383–389.

Lyketsos, C.G., DelCampo, L., Steinberg, M., Miles, Q., Steele, C.D., Munro, C., Baker, A.S., Sheppard, J.E., Frangakis, C., Brandt, J., & Rabins, P.V. (2003). Treating depression in Alzheimer's disease. *Archives of General Psychiatry, 60*(7), 737–746.

McArthur, J. (2004). The Geneva Report. Update on neurology: HIV-associated dementia. Retrieved February 19, 2007 from http://www.hopkins-aids.edu/geneva/hilites_mcar_dem.html

McShane, R. (2000). Hallucinations and delusions. *The Alzheimer's Society.* Gordon House, 10 Greencoat Place, London.

Munoz, D.G., & Feldman, H. (2000). Causes of Alzheimer's disease. *Canadian Medical Association Journal, 162*(1), 65–72.

NANDA International (NANDA-I). (2007). *Nursing diagnoses: Definitions & classification 2007–2008.* Philadelphia: NANDA International.

National Institute on Aging [NIA]. (2005). *Progress Report on Alzheimer's Disease—2004–2005.* Washington, DC: National Institutes of Health, U.S. Department of Health and Human Services.

National Institute on Aging [NIA]. (2007). *Understanding stages and symptoms of Alzheimer's disease.* Retrieved February 13, 2007 from http://www.nia.nih.gov/

Poduslo, S.E., & Yin, X. (2001). A new locus on chromosome 19 linked with late-onset Alzheimer's disease. *Clinical Neuroscience and Neuropathology, 12*(17), 3759–3761.

Rabins, P., Bland, W., Bright-Long, L., Cohen, E., Katz, I., Rovner, B., Schneider, L., & Blacker, D. (2006). Practice guideline for the treatment of patients with Alzheimer's disease and other dementias of late life. *American Psychiatric Association Practice Guidelines for the Treatment of Psychiatric Disorders, Compendium 2006.* Washington, DC: American Psychiatric Association.

Reisberg, B., Doody, R., Stoffler, A., Schmitt, F., Ferris, S., & Mobius, H.J. (2003). Memantine in moderate-to-severe Alzheimer's disease. *New England Journal of Medicine, 348,* 1333–1341.

Rogaeva, E., Meng. Y., Lee, J.H., Gu, Y., Kawarai, T., Zou, F., Katayama, T., Baldwin, C.T., Cheng, R., et al. (2007). The neuronal sortilin-related receptor SOR1 is genetically associated with Alzheimer disease. *Nature Genetics, 39*(2), 168–177.

Sadock, B.J., & Sadock, V.A. (2007). *Synopsis of psychiatry: Behavioral sciences/clinical psychiatry* (10th ed.). Philadelphia: Lippincott Williams & Wilkins.

Saunders, A.M. (2001). Gene identification in Alzheimer's disease. *Pharmacogenomics, 2*(3), 239–249.

Small, G.W., Kepe, V., Ercoli, L.M., Siddarth, P., Bookheimer, S.Y., Miller, K.J., Lavretsky, H., et al. (2006). PET of brain amyloid and tau in mild cognitive impairment. *The New England Journal of Medicine, 355*(25), 2652–2663.

Srikanth, S., & Nagaraja, A.V. (2005). A prospective study of reversible dementias: Frequency, causes, clinical profile and results of treatment. *Neurology India, 53*(3), 291–294.

Stanley, M., Blair, K.A., & Beare, P.G. (2005). *Gerontological nursing: Promoting successful aging with older adults* (3rd ed.). Philadelphia: F.A. Davis.

Tariot, P.N., Farlow, M.R., Grossberg, G.T., Graham, S.M., McDonald, S., & Gergel, I. (2004). Memantine treatment in patients with moderate to severe Alzheimer disease already receiving donepezil: A randomized controlled trial. *Journal of the American Medical Association, 291,* 317–324.

Trzepacz, P., Breitbart, W., Franklin, J., Levenson, J., Martini, D.R., & Wang, P. (2006). Practice guideline for the treatment of patients with delirium. *American Psychiatric Association Practice Guidelines for the Treatment of Psychiatric Disorders, Compendium 2006.* Washington, DC: American Psychiatric Publishing.

Wise, M.G., Gray, K.F., & Seltzer, B. (1999). Delirium, dementia, and amnestic disorders. In R.E. Hales & S.C. Yudofsky (Eds.), *Essentials of clinical psychiatry.* Washington, DC: American Psychiatric Press.

@ Internet References

- Additional information about Alzheimer's disease is located at the following Web sites:
  - http://www.alz.org
  - http://www.nia.nih.gov/alzheimers
  - http://www.ninds.nih.gov/disorders/alzheimersdisease/alzheimersdisease.htm

- Information on caregiving is located at the following Web site:
  - http://www.aarp.org

- Additional information about medications to treat Alzheimer's disease is located at the following Web sites:
  - http://www.fadavis.com/townsend
  - http://www.nlm.nih.gov/medlineplus/druginformation.html
  - http://www.nimh.nih.gov/publicat/medicate.cfm

Substance-Related Disorders

CHAPTER OUTLINE

KEY WORDS

Alcoholics Anonymous
amphetamines
ascites
cannabis
codependence
detoxification
disulfiram
dual diagnosis
esophageal varices

hepatic encephalopathy
Korsakoff's psychosis
opioids
peer assistance
    programs
phencyclidine
substitution therapy
Wernicke's
    encephalopathy

CORE CONCEPTS

abuse
dependence
intoxication
withdrawal

OBJECTIVES

After reading this chapter, the student will be able to:

1. Define *abuse*, *dependence*, *intoxication*, and *withdrawal*.
2. Discuss predisposing factors implicated in the etiology of substance-related disorders.
3. Identify symptomatology and use the information in assessment of clients with various substance-use disorders and substance-induced disorders.
4. Identify nursing diagnoses common to clients with substance-use disorders and substance-induced disorders, and select appropriate nursing interventions for each.
5. Identify topics for client and family teaching relevant to substance-use

disorders and substance-induced disorders.
6. Describe relevant outcome criteria for evaluating nursing care of clients with substance-use disorders and substance-induced disorders.
7. Discuss the issue of substance-related disorders within the profession of nursing.
8. Define codependency and identify behavioral characteristics associated with the disorder.
9. Discuss treatment of codependency.
10. Describe various modalities relevant to treatment of individuals with substance-use disorders and substance-induced disorders.

Substance-related disorders are composed of two groups: the substance-use disorders (dependence and abuse) and the substance-induced disorders (intoxication, withdrawal, delirium, dementia, amnesia, psychosis, mood disorder, anxiety disorder, sexual dysfunction, and sleep disorders). This chapter discusses dependence, abuse, intoxication, and withdrawal. The remainder of the substance-induced disorders are included in the chapters with which they share symptomatology (e.g., substance-induced mood disorders are included in Chapter 29).

Drugs are a pervasive part of our society. Certain mood-altering substances are quite socially acceptable and are used moderately by many adult Americans. They include alcohol, caffeine, and nicotine. Society has even developed a relative indifference to an occasional abuse of these substances, despite documentation of their negative impact on health.

A wide variety of substances are produced for medicinal purposes. These include central nervous system (CNS) stimulants (e.g., **amphetamines**), CNS depressants (e.g., sedatives, tranquilizers), as well as numerous over-the-counter preparations designed to relieve nearly every kind of human ailment, real or imagined.

Some illegal substances have achieved a degree of social acceptance by various subcultural groups within our society. These drugs, such as marijuana and hashish, are by no means harmless, and the long-term effects are still being studied. On the other hand, the dangerous effects of other illegal substances (e.g., lysergic acid diethylamide [LSD], **phencyclidine**, cocaine, and heroin) have been well documented.

This chapter discusses the physical and behavioral manifestations and personal and social consequences related to the abuse of or dependency on alcohol, other CNS depressants, CNS stimulants, **opioids**, hallucinogens, and cannabinols. Wide cultural variations in attitudes exist regarding substance consumption and patterns of use. Substance abuse is especially prevalent among individuals between the ages of 18 and 24. Substance-related disorders are diagnosed more commonly in men than in women, but the gender ratios vary with the class of the substance (American Psychiatric Association [APA], 2000).

Codependency is described in this chapter, as are aspects of treatment for the disorder. The issue of substance impairment within the profession of nursing is also explored. Nursing care for substance abuse, dependence, intoxication, and withdrawal is presented in the context of the six steps of the nursing process. Various medical and other treatment modalities are also discussed.

SUBSTANCE-USE DISORDERS

 CORE CONCEPT

Abuse
To use wrongfully or in a harmful way. Improper treatment or conduct that may result in injury.

Substance Abuse

The *DSM-IV-TR* (APA, 2000) identifies substance abuse as a maladaptive pattern of substance use manifested by recurrent and significant adverse consequences related to repeated use of the substance. Substance abuse has also been referred to as any use of substances that poses significant hazards to health.

DSM-IV-TR Criteria for Substance Abuse

Substance abuse is described as a maladaptive pattern of substance use leading to clinically significant impairment or distress, as manifested by one (or more) of the following, occurring within a 12-month period:

1. Recurrent substance use resulting in a failure to fulfill major role obligations at work, school, or home (e.g., repeated absences or poor work performance related to substance use; substance-related absences, suspensions, or expulsions from school; neglect of children or household).
2. Recurrent substance use in situations in which it is physically hazardous (e.g., driving an automobile or operating a machine when impaired by substance use).
3. Recurrent substance-related legal problems (e.g., arrests for substance-related disorderly conduct).
4. Continued substance use despite having persistent or recurrent social or interpersonal problems caused or exacerbated by the effects of the substance (e.g., arguments with spouse about consequences of intoxication, physical fights).

 CORE CONCEPT

Dependence
A compulsive or chronic requirement. The need is so strong as to generate distress (either physical or psychological) if left unfulfilled.

Substance Dependence

Physical Dependence

Physical dependence on a substance is evidenced by a cluster of cognitive, behavioral, and physiological symptoms indicating that the individual continues use of the substance despite significant substance-related problems (APA, 2000). As the condition develops, repeated administration of the substance necessitates its continued use to prevent the unpleasant effects characteristic of the withdrawal syndrome associated with that particular drug. The development of physical dependence is promoted by the phenomenon of *tolerance*. Tolerance is defined as the need for increasingly larger or more frequent doses of a substance in order to obtain the desired effects originally produced by a lower dose.

Psychological Dependence

An individual is considered to be psychologically dependent on a substance when there is an overwhelming desire to repeat the use of a particular drug in order to produce pleasure or avoid discomfort. It can be extremely powerful, producing intense craving for a substance as well as its compulsive use.

DSM-IV-TR Criteria for Substance Dependence

At least three of the following characteristics must be present for a diagnosis of substance dependence:

1. Evidence of tolerance, as defined by either of the following:
   a. A need for markedly increased amounts of the substance to achieve intoxication or desired effects.
   b. Markedly diminished effect with continued use of the same amount of the substance.
2. Evidence of withdrawal symptoms, as manifested by either of the following:
   a. The characteristic withdrawal syndrome for the substance.
   b. The same (or a closely related) substance is taken to relieve or avoid withdrawal symptoms.
3. The substance is often taken in larger amounts or over a longer period than was intended.
4. There is a persistent desire or unsuccessful efforts to cut down or control substance use.
5. A great deal of time is spent in activities necessary to obtain the substance (e.g., visiting multiple doctors or driving long distances), use the substance (e.g., chain smoking), or recover from its effects.
6. Important social, occupational, or recreational activities are given up or reduced because of substance use.
7. The substance use is continued despite knowledge of having a persistent or recurrent physical or psychological problem that is likely to have been caused or exacerbated by the substance (e.g., current cocaine use despite recognition of cocaine-induced depression, or continued drinking despite recognition that an ulcer was made worse by alcohol consumption).

SUBSTANCE-INDUCED DISORDERS

 CORE CONCEPT

Intoxication
A physical and mental state of exhilaration and emotional frenzy or lethargy and stupor.

Substance Intoxication

Substance intoxication is defined as the development of a reversible substance-specific syndrome caused by the recent ingestion of (or exposure to) a substance (APA, 2000). The behavior changes can be attributed to the physiological effects of the substance on the CNS and develop during or shortly after use of the substance. This category does not apply to nicotine.

DSM-IV-TR Criteria for Substance Intoxication

1. The development of a reversible substance-specific syndrome caused by recent ingestion of (or exposure to) a substance.

NOTE: Different substances may produce similar or identical syndromes.

2. Clinically significant maladaptive behavior or psychological changes that are due to the effect of the substance on the CNS (e.g., belligerence, mood lability, cognitive impairment, impaired judgment, impaired social or occupational functioning) and develop during or shortly after use of the substance.
3. The symptoms are not due to a general medical condition and are not better accounted for by another mental disorder.

 CORE CONCEPT

Withdrawal
The physiological and mental readjustment that accompanies the discontinuation of an addictive substance.

Substance Withdrawal

Substance withdrawal is the development of a substance-specific maladaptive behavioral change, with physiological and cognitive concomitants, that is due to the cessation of, or reduction in, heavy and prolonged substance use (APA, 2000). Withdrawal is usually, but not always, associated with substance dependence.

DSM-IV-TR Criteria for Substance Withdrawal

1. The development of a substance-specific syndrome caused by the cessation of (or reduction in) heavy and prolonged substance use.
2. The substance-specific syndrome causes clinically significant distress or impairment in social, occupational, or other important areas of functioning.
3. The symptoms are not due to a general medical condition and are not better accounted for by another mental disorder.

CLASSES OF PSYCHOACTIVE SUBSTANCES

The following 11 classes of psychoactive substances are associated with substance-use and substance-induced disorders:

1. Alcohol
2. Amphetamines and related substances
3. Caffeine
4. **Cannabis**
5. Cocaine
6. Hallucinogens
7. Inhalants
8. Nicotine
9. Opioids
10. Phencyclidine (PCP) and related substances
11. Sedatives, hypnotics, or anxiolytics

PREDISPOSING FACTORS TO SUBSTANCE-RELATED DISORDERS

A number of factors have been implicated in the predisposition to abuse of substances. At present, there is no single theory that can adequately explain the etiology of the problem. No doubt, the interaction between various elements forms a complex collection of determinants that influence a person's susceptibility to abuse substances.

Biological Factors

Genetics

An apparent hereditary factor is involved in the development of substance-use disorders. This is especially evident with alcoholism, but less so with other substances. Children of alcoholics are three times more likely than other children to become alcoholics (Harvard Medical School, 2001). Studies with monozygotic and dizygotic twins have also supported the genetic hypothesis. Monozygotic (one egg, genetically identical) twins have a higher rate for concordance of alcoholism than dizygotic (two eggs, genetically nonidentical) twins (Andreasen & Black, 2006). Other studies have shown that biological offspring of alcoholic parents have a significantly greater incidence of alcoholism than offspring of nonalcoholic parents. This is true whether the child was reared by the biological parents or by nonalcoholic adoptive parents (Knowles, 2003).

Biochemical Aspects

A second biological hypothesis relates to the possibility that alcohol may produce morphine-like substances in the brain that are responsible for alcohol addiction. These substances are formed by the reaction of biologically active amines (e.g., dopamine, serotonin) with products of alcohol metabolism, such as acetaldehyde (Jamal et al., 2003). Examples of these morphine-like substances include tetrahydropapaveroline and salsolinol. Some tests with animals have shown that injection of small amounts of these compounds into the brain results in patterns of alcohol addiction in animals who had previously avoided even the most dilute alcohol solutions (Behavioral Neuroscience Laboratory, 2002).

Psychological Factors

Developmental Influences

The psychodynamic approach to the etiology of substance abuse focuses on a punitive superego and fixation at the oral stage of psychosexual development (Sadock & Sadock, 2007). Individuals with punitive superegos turn to alcohol to diminish unconscious anxiety and increase feelings of power and self-worth. Sadock and Sadock (2007) state, "As a form of self-medication, alcohol may be used to control panic, opioids to diminish anger, and amphetamines to alleviate depression" (p. 386).

Personality Factors

Certain personality traits have been associated with a tendency toward addictive behavior. Some clinicians believe low self-esteem, frequent depression, passivity, the inability to relax or to defer gratification, and the inability to communicate effectively are common in individuals who abuse substances. These personality characteristics cannot be called *predictive* of addictive behavior, yet for reasons not completely understood, they have been found to accompany addiction in many instances.

Substance abuse has also been associated with antisocial personality and depressive response styles. This may be explained by the inability of the individual with antisocial personality to anticipate the aversive consequences of his or her behavior. It is likely an effort on the part of the depressed person to treat the symptoms of discomfort associated with dysphoria. Achievement of relief then provides the positive reinforcement to continue abusing the substance.

Sociocultural Factors

Social Learning

The effects of modeling, imitation, and identification on behavior can be observed from early childhood onward. In relation to drug consumption, the family appears to be an important influence. Various studies have shown that children and adolescents are more likely to use substances if they have parents who provide a model for substance use. Peers often exert a great deal of influence in the life of the child or adolescent who is being encouraged to use substances for the first time. Modeling may continue to be a factor in the use of substances once the individual enters the work force, particularly in a work setting that provides plenty of leisure time with coworkers and where drinking is valued as a way to express group cohesiveness.

Conditioning

Another important learning factor is the effect of the substance itself. Many substances create a pleasurable experience that encourages the user to repeat it. Thus, it is the intrinsically reinforcing properties of addictive drugs that "condition" the individual to seek out their use again and again. The environment in which the substance is taken also contributes to the reinforcement. If the environment is pleasurable, substance use is usually increased. Aversive stimuli within an environment are thought to be associated with a decrease in substance use within that environment.

Cultural and Ethnic Influences

Factors within an individual's culture help to establish patterns of substance use by molding attitudes, influencing patterns of consumption based on cultural acceptance, and determining the availability of the substance. For centuries, the French and Italians have considered wine an essential part of the family meal, even for the children. The incidence of alcohol dependency is low, and acute intoxication from alcohol is not common. However, the possibility of chronic physiological effects associated with lifelong alcohol consumption cannot be ignored.

Historically, a high incidence of alcohol dependency has existed within the Native American culture. Death rates from alcoholism among Native Americans are more than seven times the national average (Greer, 2004). Veterans Administration records show that 45 percent of the Indian veterans were alcohol-dependent, or twice the rate for non-Indian veterans. A number of reasons have been postulated for alcohol abuse among Native Americans: a possible physical cause (difficulty metabolizing alcohol), children modeling their parents' drinking habits, unemployment and poverty, and loss of the traditional Native American religion that some believe have led to the increased use of alcohol to fill the spiritual gap (Newhouse, 1999).

The incidence of alcohol dependence is higher among northern Europeans than southern Europeans. The Finns and the Irish use excessive alcohol consumption for the release of aggression, and the English pub is known for its attraction as a social meeting place.

Incidence of alcohol dependence among Asians is relatively low. This may be a result of a possible genetic intolerance of the substance. Some Asians develop unpleasant symptoms, such as flushing, headaches, nausea, and palpitations, when they drink alcohol. Research indicates that this is because most Asians possess an isoenzyme variant that quickly converts alcohol to acetaldehyde, and lack an isoenzyme that is needed to oxidize acetaldehyde. This results in a rapid accumulation of acetaldehyde, which produces the unpleasant symptoms (Hanley, 2004).

THE DYNAMICS OF SUBSTANCE-RELATED DISORDERS

Alcohol Abuse and Dependence

A Profile of the Substance

Alcohol is a natural substance formed by the reaction of fermenting sugar with yeast spores. Although there are many alcohols, the kind in alcoholic beverages is known scientifically as ethyl alcohol and chemically as C_2H_5OH. Its abbreviation, EtOH, is sometimes seen in medical records and in various other documents and publications.

By strict definition, alcohol is classified as a food because it contains calories; however, it has no nutritional value. Different alcoholic beverages are produced by using different sources of sugar for the fermentation process. For example, beer is made from malted barley, wine from grapes or berries, whiskey from malted grains, and rum from molasses. Distilled beverages (e.g., whiskey, scotch, gin, vodka, and other "hard" liquors) derive their name from further concentration of the alcohol through a process called distillation.

The alcohol content varies by type of beverage. For example, most American beers contain 3 to 6 percent alcohol, wines average 10 to 20 percent, and distilled beverages range from 40 to 50 percent alcohol. The average-sized drink, regardless of beverage, contains a similar amount of alcohol. That is, 12 ounces of beer, 3 to 5 ounces of wine, and a cocktail with 1 ounce of whiskey all contain approximately 0.5 ounce of alcohol. If consumed at the same rate, they all would have an equal effect on the body.

Alcohol exerts a depressant effect on the CNS, resulting in behavioral and mood changes. The effects of alcohol on the CNS are proportional to the alcoholic concentration in the blood. Most states consider that an individual is legally intoxicated with a blood alcohol level of 0.08 to 0.10 percent.

The body burns alcohol at the rate of about 0.5 ounce per hour, so behavioral changes would not be expected to occur in an individual who slowly consumed only one averaged-sized drink per hour. Other factors do influence these effects, however, such as individual size and whether or not the stomach contains food at the time the alcohol is consumed. Alcohol is thought to have a more profound effect when an individual is emotionally stressed or fatigued (National Institute on Alcohol Abuse and Alcoholism [NIAAA], 2000).

Historical Aspects

The use of alcohol can be traced back to the Neolithic age. Beer and wine are known to have been used around 6400 B.C. With the introduction of distillation by the Arabs in the Middle Ages, alchemists believed that alcohol was the answer to all of their ailments. The word "whiskey," meaning "water of life," became widely known.

In America, Native Americans had been drinking beer and wine before the arrival of the first white visitors. Refinement of the distillation process made beverages with high alcohol content readily available. By the early 1800s, one renowned physician of the time, Benjamin Rush, had begun to identify the widespread excessive, chronic alcohol consumption as a disease and an addiction. The strong religious mores on which this country was founded soon led to a driving force aimed at prohibiting the sale of alcoholic beverages. By the middle of the 19th century, 13 states had passed prohibition laws. The most notable prohibition of major proportions was that in effect in the United States from 1920 to 1933. The mandatory restrictions on national social habits resulted in the creation of profitable underground markets that led to flourishing criminal enterprises. Furthermore, millions of dollars in federal, state, and local revenues from taxes and import duties on alcohol were lost. It is difficult to measure the value of this dollar loss against the human devastation and social costs that occur as a result of alcohol abuse in the United States today.

Patterns of Use/Abuse

About half of Americans 12 years of age and older report being current drinkers of alcohol (Substance Abuse and Mental Health Services Administration [SAMHSA], 2007). Of these about one fourth are binge drinkers or engage in heavy alcohol use.

Why do people drink? Drinking patterns in the United States show that people use alcoholic beverages to enhance the flavor of food with meals; at social gatherings to encourage relaxation and conviviality among the guests; and to promote a feeling of celebration at special occasions such as weddings, birthdays, and anniversaries. An alcoholic beverage (wine) is also used as part of the sacred ritual in some religious ceremonies. Therapeutically, alcohol is the major ingredient in many over-the-counter and prescription medicines that are prepared in concentrated form. Therefore, alcohol can be harmless and enjoyable—sometimes even beneficial—if

IMPLICATIONS OF RESEARCH FOR EVIDENCE BASED PRACTICE

Stevenson, J.S., & Masters, J.A. (2005). Predictors of alcohol misuse and abuse in older women. *Journal of Nursing Scholarship, 37*(4), 329–335.

Description of the Study: The purpose of this study was to determine the predictive ability of self-report questions, physical measures, and biomarkers to detect alcohol misuse and abuse among older women. Older women are not routinely screened in healthcare settings for alcohol use. Because they often have many other health concerns, healthcare providers often fail to assess these older patients for an underlying alcohol problem. The sample included 135 healthy women aged 60 and older divided into two groups: drinkers (those who consumed 12 or more standard drinks [SDs] in the past year) and nondrinkers (those who consumed no alcohol during the past year). A standard drink is identified by the National Institute on Alcohol Abuse and Alcoholism as 1.5 oz. of distilled liquor, 12 oz. of regular beer, or 5 oz. of wine. Data were gathered from an alcohol-enhanced assessment interview (the T-ACE), a physical examination, and biomarker-enhanced standard intake blood work. Biomarkers collected in this study were gamma glutamyltransferase (GGT), mean corpuscular volume (MCV), total cholesterol (TC), high-density lipoprotein (HDL), low-density lipoprotein (LDL), and the ratio of HDL to TC. Other physical data collected were systolic and diastolic blood pressures, body mass index (BMI), exercise habits, past experiences of trauma, hemoglobin (Hgb), and hematocrit (Hct).

Results of the Study: The T-ACE questionnaire discriminated strongly between the two groups. This test is similar to the CAGE questionnaire, with one exception. The question related to "guilt" is replaced with a question related to "tolerance." ("How many drinks does it take to make you feel high?"). Analyses of the biomarkers showed significant differences in MCV, HDL, Hgb, Hct, and GGT, with drinkers showing higher levels. Drinkers also were found to consume more coffee and OTC drugs, and were more likely to be (or have been) smokers and to use alcohol to fall asleep. Nutrition, trauma, and blood pressure showed no significant differences between the groups.

Implications for Nursing Practice: This study suggests a way in which to identify older women who may be at risk for problems related to alcohol abuse. Results reveal promising predictors of alcohol use and abuse that can be part of clinical data collection during intake assessments in primary care and acute care. Indications suggest that the best predictors of high-risk drinkers include the T-ACE tool (a score of 1 or higher), elevated MCV and Hgb levels, smoking or having been a smoker, drinking large amounts of coffee, using alcohol to sleep at night, and self-medicating with two or more OTC drugs on a routine basis. The authors suggest that biological markers are significant predictors because alcohol is documented to have a powerful physiological effect on women.

it is used responsibly and in moderation. Like any other mind-altering drug, however, alcohol has the potential for abuse. Indeed, it is the most widely abused drug in the United States today. The National Council on Alcoholism and Drug Dependence (2005) reports:

Alcoholism is the third leading cause of preventable death in the U.S. As the nation's number one health problem, addiction strains the health care system, the economy, harms family life and threatens public safety. One-quarter of all emergency room admissions, one-third of all suicides, and more than half of all homicides and incidents of domestic violence are alcohol-related. Heavy drinking contributes to illness in each of the top three causes of death: heart disease, cancer, and stroke. Almost half of all traffic fatalities are alcohol-related. Fetal alcohol syndrome is the leading known cause of mental retardation.

Jellinek (1952) outlined four phases through which the alcoholic's pattern of drinking progresses. Some variability among individuals is to be expected within this model of progression.

Phase I. The Prealcoholic Phase. This phase is characterized by the use of alcohol to relieve the everyday stress and tensions of life. As a child, the individual may have observed parents or other adults drinking alcohol and enjoying the effects. The child learns that use of alcohol is an acceptable method of coping with stress. Tolerance develops, and the amount required to achieve the desired effect increases steadily.

Phase II. The Early Alcoholic Phase. This phase begins with blackouts—brief periods of amnesia that occur during or immediately following a period of drinking. Now the alcohol is no longer a source of pleasure or relief for the individual but rather a drug that is *required* by the individual. Common behaviors include sneaking drinks or secret drinking, preoccupation with drinking and maintaining the supply of alcohol, rapid gulping of drinks, and further blackouts. The individual feels enormous guilt and becomes very defensive about his or her drinking. Excessive use of denial and rationalization is evident.

Phase III. The Crucial Phase. In this phase, the individual has lost control, and physiological dependence is clearly evident. This loss of control has been described as the inability to choose whether or not to drink. Binge drinking, lasting from a few hours to several weeks, is common. These episodes are characterized by sickness, loss of consciousness, squalor, and degradation. In this phase, the individual is extremely ill. Anger and aggression are common manifestations. Drinking is the total focus, and he or she is willing to risk losing everything that was once important, in an effort to maintain the addiction. By this phase of the illness, it is not uncommon for the individual to have experienced the loss of job, marriage, family, friends, and most especially, self-respect.

Phase IV. The Chronic Phase. This phase is characterized by emotional and physical disintegration. The individual is usually intoxicated more often than he or she is sober. Emotional disintegration is evidenced by profound helplessness and self-pity. Impairment in reality testing may result in psychosis. Life-threatening physical manifestations may be evident in virtually every system of the body. Abstention from alcohol results in a terrifying syndrome of symptoms that include hallucinations, tremors, convulsions, severe agitation, and panic. Depression and ideas of suicide are not uncommon.

Effects on the Body

Alcohol can induce a general, nonselective, reversible depression of the CNS. About 20 percent of a single dose of alcohol is absorbed directly and immediately into the bloodstream through the stomach wall. Unlike other "foods," it does not have to be digested. The blood carries it directly to the brain where the alcohol acts on the brain's central control areas, slowing down or depressing brain activity. The other 80 percent of the alcohol in one drink is processed only slightly slower through the upper intestinal tract and into the bloodstream. Only moments after alcohol is consumed, it can be found in all tissues, organs, and secretions of the body. Rapidity of absorption is influenced by various factors. For example, absorption is delayed when the drink is sipped, rather than gulped; when the stomach contains food, rather than being empty; and when the drink is wine or beer, rather than distilled beverages.

At low doses, alcohol produces relaxation, loss of inhibitions, lack of concentration, drowsiness, slurred speech, and sleep. Chronic abuse results in multisystem physiological impairments. These complications include (but are not limited to) those outlined in the following sections.

Peripheral Neuropathy. Peripheral neuropathy, characterized by peripheral nerve damage, results in pain, burning, tingling, or prickly sensations of the extremities. Researchers believe it is the direct result of deficiencies in the B vitamins, particularly thiamine. Nutritional deficiencies are common in chronic alcoholics because of insufficient intake of nutrients as well as the toxic effect of alcohol that results in malabsorption of nutrients. The process is reversible with abstinence from alcohol and restoration of nutritional deficiencies. Otherwise, permanent muscle wasting and paralysis can occur.

Alcoholic Myopathy. Alcoholic myopathy may occur as an acute or chronic condition. In the acute condition, the individual experiences a sudden onset of muscle pain, swelling, and weakness; a reddish tinge in the urine caused by myoglobin, a breakdown product of muscle excreted in the urine; and a rapid rise in muscle enzymes in the blood (Barclay, 2005). Muscle symptoms are usually generalized, but pain and swelling may selectively involve the calves or other muscle groups. Laboratory studies show elevations of the enzymes creatine phosphokinase (CPK), lactate dehydrogenase (LDH), aldolase, and aspartate aminotransferase (AST). The symptoms of chronic alcoholic myopathy include a gradual wasting and weakness in skeletal muscles. Neither the pain and tenderness nor the elevated muscle enzymes seen in acute myopathy are evident in the chronic condition.

Alcoholic myopathy is thought to be a result of the same B vitamin deficiency that contributes to peripheral neuropathy. Improvement is observed with abstinence from alcohol and the return to a nutritious diet with vitamin supplements.

Wernicke's Encephalopathy. Wernicke's encephalopathy represents the most serious form of thiamine deficiency in alcoholics. Symptoms include paralysis of the ocular muscles, diplopia, ataxia, somnolence, and stupor. If thiamine replacement therapy is not undertaken quickly, death will ensue.

Korsakoff's Psychosis. Korsakoff's psychosis is identified by a syndrome of confusion, loss of recent memory, and confabulation in alcoholics. It is frequently encountered in clients recovering from Wernicke's encephalopathy. In the United States, the two disorders are usually considered together and are called *Wernicke–Korsakoff syndrome*. Treatment is with parenteral or oral thiamine replacement.

Alcoholic Cardiomyopathy. The effect of alcohol on the heart is an accumulation of lipids in the myocardial cells, resulting in enlargement and a weakened condition. The clinical findings of alcoholic cardiomyopathy generally relate to congestive heart failure or arrhythmia. Symptoms include decreased exercise tolerance, tachycardia, dyspnea, edema, palpitations, and cough. Laboratory studies may show elevation of the enzymes CPK, AST, alanine aminotransferase (ALT), and LDH. Changes may be observed by electrocardiogram, and congestive heart failure may be evident on chest X-ray films (Tazbir & Keresztes, 2005).

The treatment is total permanent abstinence from alcohol. Treatment of the congestive heart failure may include rest, oxygen, digitalization, sodium restriction, and diuretics. The prognosis is encouraging if the congestive heart failure is treated in the early stages. The death rate is high among individuals with advanced symptomatology.

Esophagitis. Esophagitis—inflammation and pain in the esophagus—occurs because of the toxic effects of alcohol on the esophageal mucosal. It also occurs because of frequent vomiting associated with alcohol abuse.

Gastritis. The effects of alcohol on the stomach include inflammation of the stomach lining characterized by epigastric distress, nausea, vomiting, and distention. Alcohol breaks down the stomach's protective mucosal barrier, allowing hydrochloric acid to erode the stomach wall. Damage to blood vessels may result in hemorrhage.

Pancreatitis. Pancreatitis may be categorized as *acute* or *chronic*. Acute pancreatitis usually occurs 1 or 2 days after a binge of excessive alcohol consumption. Symptoms include constant, severe epigastric pain, nausea and vomiting, and abdominal distention. The chronic condition leads to pancreatic insufficiency resulting in steatorrhea, malnutrition, weight loss, and diabetes mellitus.

Alcoholic Hepatitis. Alcoholic hepatitis is inflammation of the liver caused by long-term heavy alcohol use. Clinical manifestations include an enlarged and tender liver, nausea and vomiting, lethargy, anorexia, elevated white blood cell count, fever, and jaundice. **Ascites** and weight loss may be evident in more severe cases. With treatment—which includes strict abstinence from alcohol, proper nutrition, and rest—the individual can experience complete recovery. Severe cases can lead to cirrhosis or **hepatic encephalopathy.**

Cirrhosis of the Liver. In the United States, alcohol abuse is the leading cause of liver cirrhosis (Mayo Foundation for Medical Education and Research, 2005). Cirrhosis is the end-stage of alcoholic liver disease and results from long-term chronic alcohol abuse. There is widespread destruction of liver cells, which are replaced by fibrous (scar) tissue. Clinical manifestations include nausea and vomiting, anorexia, weight loss, abdominal pain, jaundice, edema, anemia, and blood coagulation abnormalities. Treatment includes abstention from alcohol, correction of malnutrition, and supportive care to prevent complications of the disease. Complications of cirrhosis include:

- **Portal Hypertension.** Elevation of blood pressure through the portal circulation results from defective blood flow through the cirrhotic liver.
- **Ascites.** Ascites, a condition in which an excessive amount of serous fluid accumulates in the abdominal cavity, occurs in response to portal hypertension. The increased pressure results in the seepage of fluid from the surface of the liver into the abdominal cavity.
- **Esophageal Varices. Esophageal varices** are veins in the esophagus that become distended because of excessive pressure from defective blood flow through the cirrhotic liver. As this pressure increases, these varicosities can rupture, resulting in hemorrhage and sometimes death.
- **Hepatic Encephalopathy.** This serious complication occurs in response to the inability of the diseased liver to convert ammonia to urea for excretion. The continued rise in serum ammonia results in progressively impaired mental functioning, apathy, euphoria or depression, sleep disturbance, increasing confusion, and progression to coma and eventual death. Treatment requires complete abstention from alcohol, temporary elimination of protein from the diet, and reduction of intestinal ammonia using neomycin or lactulose (National Library of Medicine, 2007).

Leukopenia. Production, function, and movement of the white blood cells are impaired in chronic alcoholics. This condition, called leukopenia, places the individual at high risk for contracting infectious diseases as well as for complicated recovery.

Thrombocytopenia. Platelet production and survival are impaired as a result of the toxic effects of alcohol.

This places the alcoholic at risk for hemorrhage. Abstinence from alcohol rapidly reverses the deficiency.

Sexual Dysfunction. Alcohol interferes with the normal production and maintenance of female and male hormones (National Institute on Alcohol Abuse and Alcoholism [NIAAA], 2005). For women, this can mean changes in the menstrual cycles and a decreased or loss of ability to become pregnant. For men, the decreased hormone levels result in a diminished libido, decreased sexual performance, and impaired fertility (NIAAA, 2005).

Use During Pregnancy: Fetal Alcohol Syndrome

Prenatal exposure to alcohol can result in a broad range of disorders to the fetus, known as fetal alcohol spectrum disorders (FASDs), the most common of which is fetal alcohol syndrome (FAS). Fetal alcohol syndrome includes physical, mental, behavioral, and/or learning disabilities with lifelong implications. There may be problems with learning, memory, attention span, communication, vision, hearing, or a combination of these (Centers for Disease Control [CDC], 2005). Other FASDs include alcohol-related neurodevelopmental disorder (ARND) and alcohol-related birth defects (ARBD).

No amount of alcohol during pregnancy is considered safe, and alcohol can damage a fetus at any stage of pregnancy (Carmona, 2005). Therefore, drinking alcohol should be avoided by women who are pregnant or who could become pregnant. Estimates of the prevalence of FAS range from 0.2 to 1.5 per 1000 live births (CDC, 2005). The rate is five times as high among African Americans and as much as 10 to 15 times as high among Native Americans (Harvard Medical School, 2004). Maier and West (2001) state:

> The number of women who engage in heavy alcohol consumption during pregnancy surpasses the total number of children diagnosed with either FAS or ARND, meaning that not every child whose mother drank alcohol during pregnancy develops FAS or ARND. Moreover, the degree to which people with FAS or ARND are impaired differs from person to person. Several factors may contribute to this variation in the consequences of maternal drinking. These factors include, but are not limited to, the following:
>
> - Maternal drinking pattern
> - Differences in maternal metabolism
> - Differences in genetic susceptibility
> - Timing of the alcohol consumption during pregnancy
> - Variation in the vulnerability of different brain regions (p. 168)

Children with FAS may have the following characteristics or exhibit the following behaviors (CDC, 2005):

- Small size for gestational age or small stature in relation to peers

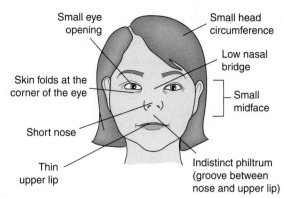

FIGURE 27–1 Facial features of FAS. (From the National Institute on Alcohol Abuse and Alcoholism of the National Institutes of Health. Washington, DC.)

- Facial abnormalities (see Figure 27–1)
- Poor coordination or delays in psychomotor development
- Hyperactive behavior
- Learning disabilities (e.g., speech and language delays)
- Mental retardation or low IQ
- Problems with daily living
- Vision or hearing problems
- Poor reasoning and judgment skills
- Sleep and sucking disturbances in infancy
- Heart and kidney defects

Neuroimaging of children with FAS shows abnormalities in the size and shape of their brains; the frontal lobes are often smaller than normal, and the corpus callosum may be damaged (Harvard Medical School, 2004). Studies show that children with FAS are often at risk for psychiatric disorders, commonly attention-deficit/hyperactivity disorder, mood disorders, anxiety disorders, eating disorders, and drug and alcohol dependence (Harvard Medical School, 2004; Wehrspann, 2006).

Children with FAS require lifelong care and treatment. There is no cure for FAS, but it can be prevented. The Surgeon General's Advisory on Alcohol Use in Pregnancy states:

> Health professionals should inquire routinely about alcohol consumption by women of childbearing age, inform them of the risks of alcohol consumption during pregnancy, and advise them not to drink alcoholic beverages during pregnancy. (Carmona, 2005, p. 1)

Alcohol Intoxication

Symptoms of alcohol intoxication include disinhibition of sexual or aggressive impulses, mood lability, impaired judgment, impaired social or occupational functioning, slurred speech, incoordination, unsteady gait, nystagmus, and flushed face. Intoxication usually occurs at blood alcohol levels between 100 and 200 mg/dL. Death has been reported at levels ranging from 400 to 700 mg/dL.

Alcohol Withdrawal

Within 4 to 12 hours of cessation of or reduction in heavy and prolonged (several days or longer) alcohol use, the following symptoms may appear: coarse tremor of hands, tongue, or eyelids; nausea or vomiting; malaise or weakness; tachycardia; sweating; elevated blood pressure; anxiety; depressed mood or irritability; transient hallucinations or illusions; headache; and insomnia. A complicated withdrawal syndrome may progress to *alcohol withdrawal delirium*. Onset of delirium is usually on the second or third day following cessation of or reduction in prolonged, heavy alcohol use. Symptoms include those described under the syndrome of delirium (Chapter 26).

Sedative, Hypnotic, or Anxiolytic Abuse and Dependence

A Profile of the Substance

The sedative-hypnotic compounds are drugs of diverse chemical structures that are all capable of inducing varying degrees of CNS depression, from tranquilizing relief of anxiety to anesthesia, coma, and even death. They are generally categorized as (1) barbiturates, (2) nonbarbiturate hypnotics, and (3) antianxiety agents. Effects produced by these substances depend on size of dose and potency of drug administered.

Table 27–1 presents a selected list of drugs included in these categories. Generic names are followed in parentheses by the trade names. Common street names for each category are also included.

Several principles have been identified that apply fairly uniformly to all CNS depressants:

1. **The effects of CNS depressants are additive with one another and with the behavioral state of the user.** For example, when these drugs are used in combination with each other or in combination with alcohol, the depressive effects are compounded. These intense depressive effects are often unpredictable and can even be fatal. Similarly, a person who is mentally depressed or physically fatigued may have an exaggerated response to a dose of the drug that would only slightly affect a person in a normal or excited state.

2. **CNS depressants are capable of producing physiological dependency.** If large doses of CNS depressants are repeatedly administered over a prolonged duration, a period of CNS hyperexcitability occurs on withdrawal of the drug. The response can be quite severe, even leading to convulsions and death.

3. **CNS depressants are capable of producing psychological dependence.** CNS depressants have the potential to generate within the individual a psychic drive for periodic or continuous administration of the drug to achieve a maximum level of functioning or feeling of well-being.

4. **Cross-tolerance and cross-dependence may exist between various CNS depressants.** Cross-tolerance is exhibited when one drug results in a lessened response to another drug. Cross-dependence is a condition in which one drug can prevent withdrawal symptoms associated with physical dependence on a different drug (Julien, 2005).

Historical Aspects

Anxiety and insomnia, two of the most common human afflictions, were treated during the 19th century with

TABLE 27–1	**Sedative, Hypnotic, and Anxiolytic Drugs**	
Categories	**Generic (Trade) Names**	**Common Street Names**
Barbiturates	Pentobarbital (Nembutal)	Yellow jackets; yellow birds
	Secobarbital (Seconal)	GBs; red birds; red devils
	Amobarbital (Amytal)	Blue birds; blue angels
	Secobarbital/amobarbital (Tuinal)	Tooies; jelly beans
	Phenobarbital	
	Butabarbital	
Nonbarbiturate Hypnotics	Chloral hydrate (Noctec)	Peter, Mickey
	Triazolam (Halcion)	Sleepers
	Flurazepam (Dalmane)	Sleepers
	Temazepam (Restoril)	Sleepers
	Quazepam (Doral)	Sleepers
Antianxiety Agents	Diazepam (Valium)	Vs (color designates strength)
	Chlordiazepoxide (Librium)	Green and whites; roaches
	Meprobamate (Miltown)	Dolls; dollies
	Oxazepam (Serax)	Candy, downers (the benzodiazepines)
	Alprazolam (Xanax)	
	Lorazepam (Ativan)	
	Clorazepate (Tranxene)	
	Flunitrazepam (Rohypnol)	Date rape drug; roofies, R-2, rope

opiates, bromide salts, chloral hydrate, paraldehyde, and alcohol (American Insomnia Association, 2005; Julien, 2005). Because the opiates were known to produce physical dependence, the bromides carried the risk of chronic bromide poisoning, and chloral hydrate and paraldehyde had an objectionable taste and smell, alcohol became the prescribed depressant drug of choice. However, some people refused to use alcohol either because they did not like the taste or for moral reasons, and others tended to take more than was prescribed. Therefore, a search for a better sedative drug continued.

Although barbituric acid was first synthesized in 1864, it was not until 1912 that phenobarbital was introduced into medicine as a sedative drug, the first of the structurally classified group of drugs called barbiturates (Julien, 2005). Since that time, more than 2500 barbiturate derivatives have been synthesized, but currently, fewer than a dozen remain in medical use. Illicit use of the drugs for recreational purposes grew throughout the 1930s and 1940s.

Efforts to create depressant medications that were not barbiturate derivatives accelerated. By the mid-1950s the market for depressants had been expanded by the appearance of the nonbarbiturates glutethimide, ethchlorvynol, methyprylon, and meprobamate. Introduction of the benzodiazepines occurred around 1960 with the marketing of chlordiazepoxide (Librium), followed shortly by its derivative diazepam (Valium). The use of these drugs, and others within their group, has grown so rapidly that they have become some of the most widely prescribed medications in clinical use today. Their margin of safety is greater than that of barbiturates and the other nonbarbiturates. Prolonged use of even moderate doses is likely to result in physical and psychological dependence, however, with a characteristic syndrome of withdrawal that can be severe.

Patterns of Use/Abuse

Sadock and Sadock (2007) report that about 15 percent of all persons in the United States have had benzodiazepines prescribed by a physician. Of all the drugs used in clinical practice, the sedative-hypnotic-antianxiety drugs are among the most widely prescribed. The *DSM-IV-TR* states:

In the United States, up to 90 percent of individuals hospitalized for medical care or surgery receive orders for sedative, hypnotic, or anxiolytic medications during their hospital stay, and more than 15 percent of American adults use these medications (usually by prescription) during any one year. (p. 291)

Two patterns of development of dependence and abuse are described. The first pattern is one of an individual whose physician originally prescribed the CNS depressant as treatment for anxiety or insomnia. Independently, the individual has increased the dosage or frequency from that which was prescribed. Use of the medication is justified on the basis of treating symptoms, but as tolerance grows, more and more of the medication is required to produce the desired effect. Substance-seeking behavior is evident as the individual seeks prescriptions from several physicians in order to maintain sufficient supplies.

The second pattern, which the *DSM-IV-TR* reports is more frequent than the first, involves young people in their teens or early 20s who, in the company of their peers, use substances that were obtained illegally. The initial objective is to achieve a feeling of euphoria. The drug is usually used intermittently during recreational gatherings. This pattern of intermittent use leads to regular use and extreme levels of tolerance. Combining use with other substances is not uncommon. Physical and psychological dependence leads to intense substance-seeking behaviors, most often through illegal channels.

Effects on the Body

The sedative-hypnotic compounds induce a general depressant effect; that is, they depress the activity of the brain, nerves, muscles, and heart tissue. They reduce the rate of metabolism in a variety of tissues throughout the body, and in general, they depress any system that uses energy (Julien, 2005). Large doses are required to produce these effects. In lower doses these drugs appear to be more selective in their depressant actions. Specifically, in lower doses these drugs appear to exert their action on the centers within the brain that are concerned with arousal (e.g., the ascending reticular activating system, in the reticular formation, and the diffuse thalamic projection system).

As stated previously, the sedative-hypnotics are capable of producing all levels of CNS depression—from mild sedation to death. The level is determined by dosage and potency of the drug used. In Figure 27–2, a continuum of the CNS depressant effects is presented to demonstrate how increasing doses of sedative-hypnotic drugs affect behavioral depression.

The primary action of sedative-hypnotics is on nervous tissue. However, large doses may have an effect on other organ systems. Following is a discussion of the physiological effects of sedative-hypnotic/anxiolytic agents.

Effects on Sleep and Dreaming. Barbiturate use decreases the amount of sleep time spent in dreaming. During drug withdrawal, dreaming becomes vivid and excessive. Rebound insomnia and increased dreaming (termed *REM rebound*) are not uncommon with abrupt withdrawal from long-term use of these drugs as sleeping aids (Julien, 2005).

Respiratory Depression. Barbiturates are capable of inhibiting the reticular activating system, resulting in respiratory depression (Sadock & Sadock, 2007). Additive

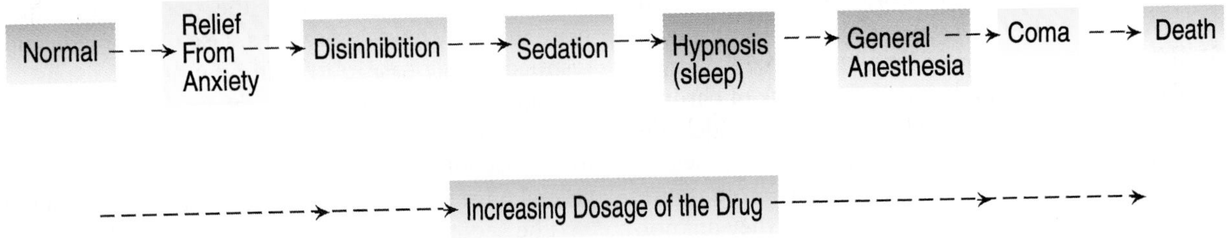

Normal - - → Relief From Anxiety - - → Disinhibition - - → Sedation - → Hypnosis (sleep) - - → General Anesthesia - - → Coma - - → Death

- - - - - - - → - - - - → Increasing Dosage of the Drug - - - - - - - → - - → →

FIGURE 27–2 Continuum of behavioral depression.

effects can occur with the concurrent use of other CNS depressants, effecting a life-threatening situation.

Cardiovascular Effects. Hypotension may be a problem with large doses. Only a slight decrease in blood pressure is noted with normal oral dosage. High dosages of barbiturates may result in decreased cardiac output, decreased cerebral blood flow, and direct impairment of myocardial contractility (Habal, 2006).

Renal Function. In doses high enough to produce anesthesia, barbiturates may suppress renal function. At the usual sedative-hypnotic dosage, however, there is no evidence that they have any direct action on the kidneys.

Hepatic Effects. The barbiturates may produce jaundice with doses large enough to produce acute intoxication. Barbiturates stimulate the production of liver enzymes, resulting in a decrease in the plasma levels of both the barbiturates and other drugs metabolized in the liver (Habal, 2006). Preexisting liver disease may predispose an individual to additional liver damage with excessive barbiturate use.

Body Temperature. High doses of barbiturates can greatly decrease body temperature. It is not significantly altered with normal dosage levels.

Sexual Functioning. CNS depressants have a tendency to produce a biphasic response. There is an initial increase in libido, presumably from the primary disinhibitory effects of the drug. This initial response is then followed by a decrease in the ability to maintain an erection.

Sedative, Hypnotic, or Anxiolytic Intoxication

The *DSM-IV-TR* (APA, 2000) describes sedative, hypnotic, or anxiolytic intoxication as the presence of clinically significant maladaptive behavioral or psychological changes that develop during, or shortly after, use of one of these substances. These maladaptive changes may include inappropriate sexual or aggressive behavior, mood lability, impaired judgment, or impaired social or occupational functioning. Other symptoms that may develop with excessive use of sedatives, hypnotics, or anxiolytics include slurred speech, incoordination, unsteady gait, nystagmus, impairment in attention or memory, and stupor or coma.

Sedative, Hypnotic, or Anxiolytic Withdrawal

Withdrawal from sedatives, hypnotics, or anxiolytics produces a characteristic syndrome of symptoms that develops after a marked decrease in or cessation of intake after several weeks or more of regular use (APA, 2000). Onset of the symptoms depends on the drug from which the individual is withdrawing. A short-acting anxiolytic (e.g., lorazepam or oxazepam) may produce symptoms within 6 to 8 hours of decreasing blood levels, whereas withdrawal symptoms from substances with longer half-lives (e.g., diazepam) may not develop for more than a week, peak in intensity during the second week, and decrease markedly during the third or fourth week (APA, 2000).

Severe withdrawal is most likely to occur when a substance has been used at high dosages for prolonged periods. However, withdrawal symptoms also have been reported with moderate dosages taken over a relatively short duration. Withdrawal symptoms associated with sedatives, hypnotics or anxiolytics include autonomic hyperactivity (e.g., sweating or pulse rate greater than 100), increased hand tremor, insomnia, nausea or vomiting, hallucinations, illusions, psychomotor agitation, anxiety, or grand mal seizures.

CNS Stimulant Abuse and Dependence

A Profile of the Substance

The CNS stimulants are identified by the behavioral stimulation and psychomotor agitation that they induce. They differ widely in their molecular structures and in their mechanisms of action. The amount of CNS stimulation caused by a certain drug depends on both the area in the brain or spinal cord that is affected by the drug and the cellular mechanism fundamental to the increased excitability.

Groups within this category are classified according to similarities in mechanism of action. The *psychomotor stimulants* induce stimulation by augmentation or potentiation of the neurotransmitters norepinephrine, epinephrine, or dopamine. The *general cellular stimulants* (caffeine and nicotine) exert their action directly on cellular activity. Caffeine inhibits the enzyme phosphodiesterase, allowing increased levels of adenosine 3', 5'-cyclic phosphate

TABLE 27–2	CNS Stimulants	
Categories	**Generic (Trade) Names**	**Common Street Names**
Amphetamines	Dextroamphetamine (Dexedrine)	Dexies, uppers, truck drivers
	Methamphetamine (Desoxyn)	Meth, speed, crystal, ice
	3,4-methylenedioxyamphetamine (MDMA)*	Adam, Ecstasy, Eve, XTC
	Amphetamine + dextroamphetamine (Adderall)	
Nonamphetamine stimulants	Phendimetrazine (Prelu-2)	Diet pills
	Benzphetamine (Didrex)	
	Diethylpropion (Tenuate)	
	Phentermine (Adipex-P; Ionamin)	
	Sibutramine (Meridia)	
	Methylphenidate (Ritalin)	Speed, uppers
	Dexmethylphenidate (Focalin)	
	Modafinil (Provigil)	
Cocaine	Cocaine hydrochloride	Coke, blow, toot, snow, lady, flake, crack
Caffeine	Coffee, tea, colas, chocolate	Java, mud, brew, cocoa
Nicotine	Cigarettes, cigars, pipe tobacco, snuff	Weeds, fags, butts, chaw, cancer sticks

*Cross-listed with the hallucinogens.

(cAMP), a chemical substance that promotes increased rates of cellular metabolism. Nicotine stimulates ganglionic synapses. This results in increased acetylcholine, which stimulates nerve impulse transmission to the entire autonomic nervous system. A selected list of drugs included in these categories is presented in Table 27–2.

The two most prevalent and widely used stimulants are caffeine and nicotine. Caffeine is readily available in every supermarket and grocery store as a common ingredient in coffee, tea, colas, and chocolate. Nicotine is the primary psychoactive substance found in tobacco products. When used in moderation, these stimulants tend to relieve fatigue and increase alertness. They are a generally accepted part of our culture; however, with increased social awareness regarding the health risks associated with nicotine, its use has become stigmatized in some circles.

The more potent stimulants, because of their potential for physiological dependency, are under regulation by the Controlled Substances Act. These controlled stimulants are available for therapeutic purposes by prescription only; however, they are also clandestinely manufactured and widely distributed on the illicit market.

Historical Aspects

Cocaine is the most potent stimulant derived from nature. It is extracted from the leaves of the coca plant, which has been cultivated in the Andean highlands of South America since prehistoric times. Natives of the region chew the leaves of the plant for refreshment and relief from fatigue.

The coca leaves must be mixed with lime to release the cocaine alkaloid. The chemical formula for the pure form of the drug was developed in 1960. Physicians began using the drug as an anesthetic in eye, nose, and throat surgeries. It has also been used therapeutically in the United States in a morphine–cocaine elixir designed to relieve the suffering associated with terminal illness. These therapeutic uses are now obsolete.

Cocaine use has achieved a degree of acceptability within some social circles. It is illicitly distributed as a white crystalline powder, often mixed with other ingredients to increase its volume and, therefore, create more profits. The drug is most commonly "snorted," and chronic users may manifest symptoms that resemble the congested nose of a common cold. The intensely pleasurable effects of the drug create the potential for extraordinary psychological dependency.

Another form of cocaine commonly used in the United States, called "crack," is a cocaine alkaloid that is extracted from its powdered hydrochloride salt by mixing it with sodium bicarbonate and allowing it to dry into small "rocks" (APA, 2000). Because this type of cocaine can be easily vaporized and inhaled, its effects have an extremely rapid onset.

Amphetamine was first prepared in 1887. Various derivatives of the drug soon followed, and clinical use of the drug began in 1927. Amphetamines were used quite extensively for medical purposes through the 1960s, but recognition of their abuse potential has sharply decreased clinical use. Today, they are prescribed only to treat narcolepsy (a rare disorder resulting in an uncontrollable desire for sleep), hyperactivity disorders in children, and in certain cases of obesity. Clandestine production of amphetamines for distribution on the illicit market has become a thriving business. In 2002, the cost to the federal government for cleaning up methamphetamine labs was over $23 million. Methamphetamine can be smoked, snorted, injected, or taken orally. The effects include an intense rush from smoking or intravenous injection to a slower onset of euphoria as a result of snorting or oral ingestion. Another form of the drug, crystal metham-phetamine, is produced by slowly recrystallizing powder methamphetamine from a solvent such as methanol, ethanol, isopropanol, or acetone (*Street Drugs*, 2005). It is a colorless, odorless, large-crystal form of *d*-metham-phetamine, and is commonly called glass or ice because of its appearance. Crystal meth is usually smoked in a glass pipe like crack cocaine.

The earliest history of caffeine is unknown and is shrouded by legend and myth. Caffeine was first discov-ered in coffee in 1820 and 7 years later in tea. Both beverages have been widely accepted and enjoyed as a "pick-me-up" by many cultures.

Tobacco was used by the aborigines from remote times. Introduced in Europe in the mid-16th century, its use grew rapidly and soon became prevalent in the Orient. Tobacco came to America with the settlement of the earliest colonies. Today, it is grown in many countries of the world, and although smoking is decreasing in most industrialized nations, it is increasing in the developing areas (APA, 2000).

Patterns of Use/Abuse

Because of their pleasurable effects, CNS stimulants have a high abuse potential. In 2006, about 2.4 million Americans were current cocaine users (SAMHSA, 2007). Use was highest among Americans ages 18 to 25.

Many individuals who abuse or are dependent on CNS stimulants began using the substance for the appetite-suppressant effect in an attempt at weight con-trol (APA, 2000). Higher and higher doses are consumed in an effort to maintain the pleasurable effects. With con-tinued use, the pleasurable effects diminish, and there is a corresponding increase in dysphoric effects. There is a persistent craving for the substance, however, even in the face of unpleasant adverse effects from the continued drug taking.

CNS stimulant abuse and dependence are usually characterized by either episodic or chronic daily, or almost daily, use. Individuals who use the substances on an episodic basis often "binge" on the drug with very high dosages followed by a day or two of recuperation. This recuperation period is characterized by extremely intense and unpleasant symptoms (called a "crash").

The daily user may take large or small doses and may use the drug several times a day or only at a specific time during the day. The amount consumed usually increases over time as tolerance occurs. Chronic users tend to rely on CNS stimulants to feel more powerful, more confi-dent, and more decisive. They often fall into a pattern of taking "uppers" in the morning and "downers," such as alcohol or sleeping pills, at night.

The average American consumes two cups of coffee (about 200 mg of caffeine) per day. Caffeine is consumed

TABLE 27–3	**Common Sources of Caffeine**
Source	**Caffeine Content (mg)**
Food and Beverages	
5–6 oz. brewed coffee	90–125
5–6 oz. instant coffee	60–90
5–6 oz. decaffeinated coffee	3
5–6 oz. brewed tea	70
5–6 oz. instant tea	45
8 oz. green tea	15–30
8–12 oz. cola drinks	60
12 oz. Red Bull energy drink	115
5–6 oz. cocoa	20
8 oz. chocolate milk	2–7
1 oz. chocolate bar	22
Prescription Medications	
APCs (aspirin, phenacetin, caffeine)	32
Cafergot	100
Darvon compound	32
Fiorinal	40
Migralam	100
Over-the-Counter Analgesics	
Anacin, Empirin, Midol, Vanquish	32
Excedrin Migraine (aspirin, acetaminophen, caffeine)	65
Over-the-Counter Stimulants	
No Doz Tablets	100
Vivarin	200
Caffedrine	250

in various amounts by 90 percent of the population. At a level of 500 to 600 mg of daily caffeine consumption, symptoms of anxiety, insomnia, and depression are not uncommon. It is also at this level that caffeine depend-ence and withdrawal can occur. Caffeine consumption is prevalent among children as well as adults. Table 27–3 lists some common sources of caffeine.

Next to caffeine, nicotine, an active ingredient in tobacco, is the most widely used psychoactive sub-stance in U.S. society. Of the U.S. population 12 years of age or older, 29.6 percent reported current use of a tobacco product in 2006 (SAMHSA, 2007). Since 1964, when the results of the first public health report on smoking were issued, the percentage of total smokers has been on the decline. However, the percentage of women and teenage smokers has declined more slowly than that of adult men. Approximately 400,000 people die annually because of tobacco use, and an estimated 60 percent of the direct healthcare costs in the United States go to treat tobacco-related illnesses (Sadock & Sadock, 2007).

Effects on the Body

The CNS stimulants are a group of pharmacological agents that are capable of exciting the entire nervous sys-tem. This is accomplished by increasing the activity or augmenting the capability of the neurotransmitter agents known to be directly involved in bodily activation and behavioral stimulation. Physiological responses vary markedly according to the potency and dosage of the drug.

Central Nervous System Effects. Stimulation of the CNS results in tremor, restlessness, anorexia, insomnia, agitation, and increased motor activity. Amphetamines, nonamphetamine stimulants, and cocaine produce increased alertness, decrease in fatigue, elation and euphoria, and subjective feelings of greater mental agility and muscular power. Chronic use of these drugs may result in compulsive behavior, paranoia, hallucinations, and aggressive behavior (*Street Drugs*, 2005).

Cardiovascular/Pulmonary Effects. Amphetamines can induce increased systolic and diastolic blood pressure, increased heart rate, and cardiac arrhythmias (*Street Drugs*, 2005). These drugs also relax bronchial smooth muscle.

Cocaine intoxication typically produces a rise in myocardial demand for oxygen and an increase in heart rate. Severe vasoconstriction may occur and can result in myocardial infarction, ventricular fibrillation, and sudden death. Inhaled cocaine can cause pulmonary hemorrhage, chronic bronchiolitis, and pneumonia. Nasal rhinitis is a result of chronic cocaine snorting.

Caffeine ingestion can result in increased heart rate, palpitations, extrasystoles, and cardiac arrhythmias. Caffeine induces dilation of pulmonary and general systemic blood vessels and constriction of cerebral blood vessels.

Nicotine stimulates the sympathetic nervous system, resulting in an increase in heart rate, blood pressure, and cardiac contractility, thereby increasing myocardial oxygen consumption and demand for blood flow (Royal College of Physicians, 2000). Contractions of gastric smooth muscle associated with hunger are inhibited, thereby producing a mild anorectic effect.

Gastrointestinal and Renal Effects. Gastrointestinal (GI) effects of amphetamines are somewhat unpredictable; however, a decrease in GI tract motility commonly results in constipation. Contraction of the bladder sphincter makes urination difficult. Caffeine exerts a diuretic effect on the kidneys. Nicotine stimulates the hypothalamus to release antidiuretic hormone, reducing the excretion of urine. Because nicotine increases the tone and activity of the bowel, it may occasionally cause diarrhea.

Most CNS stimulants induce a small rise in metabolic rate and various degrees of anorexia. Amphetamines and cocaine can cause a rise in body temperature.

Sexual Functioning. CNS stimulants apparently promote the coital urge in both men and women. Women, more than men, report that stimulants make them feel sexier and have more orgasms. In fact, some men may experience sexual dysfunction with the use of stimulants. For the majority of individuals, however, these drugs exert a powerful aphrodisiac effect.

CNS Stimulant Intoxication

CNS stimulant intoxication produces maladaptive behavioral and psychological changes that develop during, or shortly after, use of these drugs. Amphetamine and cocaine intoxication typically produces euphoria or affective blunting; changes in sociability; hypervigilance; interpersonal sensitivity; anxiety, tension, or anger; stereotyped behaviors; or impaired judgment. Physical effects include tachycardia or bradycardia, pupillary dilation, elevated or lowered blood pressure, perspiration or chills, nausea or vomiting, weight loss, psychomotor agitation or retardation, muscular weakness, respiratory depression, chest pain, cardiac arrhythmias, confusion, seizures, dyskinesias, dystonias, or coma (APA, 2000).

Intoxication from caffeine usually occurs following consumption in excess of 250 mg. Symptoms include restlessness, nervousness, excitement, insomnia, flushed face, diuresis, GI disturbance, muscle twitching, rambling flow of thought and speech, tachycardia or cardiac arrhythmia, periods of inexhaustibility, and psychomotor agitation (APA, 2000).

CNS Stimulant Withdrawal

CNS stimulant withdrawal is the presence of a characteristic withdrawal syndrome that develops within a few hours to several days after cessation of, or reduction in, heavy and prolonged use (APA, 2000). Withdrawal from amphetamines and cocaine cause dysphoria, fatigue, vivid unpleasant dreams, insomnia or hypersomnia, increased appetite, and psychomotor retardation or agitation (APA, 2000). The *DSM-IV-TR* states:

> Marked withdrawal symptoms ("crashing") often follow an episode of intense, high-dose use (a "speed run"). This "crash" is characterized by intense and unpleasant feelings of lassitude and depression, generally requiring several days of rest and recuperation. Weight loss commonly occurs during heavy stimulant use, whereas a marked increase in appetite with rapid weight gain is often observed during withdrawal. Depressive symptoms may last several days to weeks and may be accompanied by suicidal ideation. (p. 227)

The *DSM-IV-TR* does not include a diagnosis of caffeine withdrawal. However, Sadock and Sadock (2007) state that a number of well-controlled research studies indicate that caffeine withdrawal exists. They cite the following symptoms as typical: headache, fatigue, anxiety, irritability, depression, impaired psychomotor performance, nausea, vomiting, craving for caffeine, and muscle pain and stiffness.

Withdrawal from nicotine results in dysphoric or depressed mood; insomnia; irritability, frustration, or anger; anxiety; difficulty concentrating; restlessness; decreased heart rate; and increased appetite or weight gain (APA, 2000). A mild syndrome of nicotine withdrawal can appear when a smoker switches from regular cigarettes to low-nicotine cigarettes (Sadock & Sadock, 2007).

Inhalant Abuse and Dependence

A Profile of the Substance

Inhalant disorders are induced by inhaling the aliphatic and aromatic hydrocarbons found in substances such as fuels, solvents, adhesives, aerosol propellants, and paint thinners. Specific examples of these substances include gasoline, lighter fluid, glue, cleaning fluids, spray paint, and typewriter correction fluid.

Patterns of Use/Abuse

Inhalant substances are readily available, legal, and inexpensive. These three factors make inhalants the drug of choice among poor people and among children and young adults. Use may begin by ages 9 to 12 and peak in the adolescent years; it is less common after age 35 (APA, 2000). A national government survey of drug use indicated that 9.3 percent of people in the United States aged 12 years or older acknowledged ever having used inhalants (SAMHSA, 2007). The highest use was seen in the 12- to 17-year-old age group.

Methods of use include "huffing"—a procedure in which a rag soaked with the substance is applied to the mouth and nose and the vapors breathed in. Another common method is called "bagging," in which the substance is placed in a paper or plastic bag and inhaled from the bag by the user. It may also be inhaled directly from the container or sprayed in the mouth or nose.

Sadock and Sadock (2007) report that:

> Inhalant use among adolescents may be most common in those whose parents or older siblings use illegal substances. Inhalant use among adolescents is also associated with an increased likelihood of conduct disorder or antisocial personality disorder. (p. 435)

Tolerance to inhalants has been reported with heavy use. A mild withdrawal syndrome has been documented but does not appear to be clinically significant (APA, 2000).

Children with inhalant disorder may use inhalants several times a week, often on weekends and after school (APA, 2000). Adults with inhalant dependence may use the substance at varying times during each day, or they may binge on the substance during a period of several days.

Effects on the Body

Inhalants are absorbed through the lungs and reach the CNS very rapidly. Inhalants generally act as a CNS depressant (Sadock & Sadock, 2007). The effects are relatively brief, lasting from several minutes to a few hours, depending on the specific substance and amount consumed.

Central Nervous System. Inhalants can cause both central and peripheral nervous system damage, which may be permanent (APA, 2000). Neurological deficits, such as generalized weakness and peripheral neuropathies, may be evident. Other CNS effects that have been reported with heavy inhalant use include cerebral atrophy, cerebellar degeneration, and white matter lesions resulting in cranial nerve or pyramidal tract signs.

Respiratory Effects. The *DSM-IV-TR* reports the following respiratory effects with inhalant use: upper- or lower-airway irritation, including increased airway resistance; pulmonary hypertension; acute respiratory distress; coughing; sinus discharge; dyspnea; rales; or rhonchi. Rarely, cyanosis may result from pneumonitis or asphyxia. Death may occur from respiratory or cardiovascular depression.

Gastrointestinal Effects. Abdominal pain, nausea, and vomiting may occur. A rash may be present around the individual's nose and mouth. Unusual breath odors are common.

Renal System Effects. Chronic renal failure, hepatorenal syndrome, and proximal renal tubular acidosis have been reported (APA, 2000).

Inhalant Intoxication

The *DSM-IV-TR* defines inhalant intoxication as "clinically significant maladaptive behavioral or psychological changes (e.g., belligerence, assaultiveness, apathy, impaired judgment, impaired social or occupational functioning) that developed during or shortly after, use of or exposure to volatile inhalants." Two or more of the following signs are present:

1. Dizziness
2. Nystagmus
3. Incoordination
4. Slurred speech
5. Unsteady gait
6. Lethargy
7. Depressed reflexes
8. Psychomotor retardation
9. Tremor
10. Generalized muscle weakness
11. Blurred vision or diplopia
12. Stupor or coma
13. Euphoria

The symptoms are not due to a general medical condition and are not better accounted for by another mental disorder.

Opioid Abuse and Dependence

A Profile of the Substance

The term *opioid* refers to a group of compounds that includes opium, opium derivatives, and synthetic substitutes. Opioids exert both a sedative and an analgesic effect, and their major medical uses are for the relief of pain, the treatment of diarrhea, and the relief of coughing. These drugs have addictive qualities; that is, they are capable of inducing tolerance and physiological and psychological dependence.

Opioids are popular drugs of abuse in that they desensitize an individual to both psychological and physiological pain and induce a sense of euphoria. Lethargy and indifference to the environment are common manifestations.

Opioid abusers usually spend much of their time nourishing their habit. Individuals who are opioid dependent are seldom able to hold a steady job that will support their need. They must therefore secure funds from friends, relatives, or whomever they have not yet alienated with their dependency-related behavior. It is not uncommon for individuals who are opioid-dependent to resort to illegal means of obtaining funds, such as burglary, robbery, prostitution, or selling drugs.

Methods of administration of opioid drugs include oral, snorting, or smoking, and by subcutaneous, intramuscular, and intravenous injection. A selected list of opioid substances is presented in Table 27–4.

Under close supervision, opioids are indispensable in the practice of medicine. They are the most effective agents known for the relief of intense pain. They also induce a pleasurable effect on the CNS, however, which promotes their abuse. The physiological and psychological dependence that occurs with opioids, as well as the development of profound tolerance, contribute to the addict's ongoing quest for more of the substance, regardless of the means.

Historical Aspects

Opium is the Greek word for "juice." In its crude form, opium is a brownish black, gummy substance obtained from the ripened pods of the opium poppy. References to the use of opiates have been found in the Egyptian, Greek, and Arabian cultures as early as 3000 B.C. The drug became widely used both medicinally and recreationally throughout Europe during the 16th and 17th centuries. Most of the opium supply came from China, where the drug was introduced by Arabic traders in the late 17th century. Morphine, the primary active ingredient of opium, was isolated in 1803 by the European chemist Frederick Serturner. Since that time, morphine, rather than crude opium, has been used throughout the world for the medical treatment of pain and diarrhea (Julien, 2005). This process was facilitated in 1853 by the development of the hypodermic syringe, which made it possible to deliver the undiluted morphine quickly into the body for rapid relief from pain.

This development also created a new variety of opiate user in the United States: one who was able to self-administer the drug by injection. During this time, there was also a large influx of Chinese immigrants into the United States, who introduced opium smoking to this country. By the early part of the 20th century, opium addiction was widespread.

In response to the concerns over widespread addiction, in 1914 the U.S. government passed the Harrison Narcotic Act, which created strict controls on the accessibility of opiates. Until that time, these substances had been freely available to the public without a prescription. The Harrison Act banned the use of opiates for other than medicinal purposes and drove the use of heroin underground. To this day, the beneficial uses of these substances are widely acclaimed within the medical profession, but the illicit trafficking of the drugs for recreational purposes continues to resist most efforts aimed at control.

TABLE 27–4	Opioids and Related Substances	
Categories	**Generic (Trade) Names**	**Common Street Names**
Opioids of Natural Origin	Opium (ingredient in various antidiarrheal agents)	Black stuff, poppy, tar, big O
	Morphine (Astramorph)	M, white stuff, Miss Emma
	Codeine (ingredient in various analgesics and cough suppressants)	Terp, schoolboy, syrup, cody
Opioid Derivatives	Heroin	H, horse, junk, brown sugar, smack, skag, TNT, Harry
	Hydromorphone (Dilaudid)	DLs, 4s, lords, little D
	Oxycodone (Percodan; OxyContin)	Perks, perkies, Oxy, O.C.
	Hydrocodone (Vicodin)	Vike
Synthetic Opiate-like Drugs	Meperidine (Demerol)	Doctors
	Methadone (Dolophine)	Dollies, done
	Propoxyphene (Darvon)	Pinks and grays
	Pentazocine (Talwin)	Ts
	Fentanyl (Actiq; Duragesic)	Apache, China girl, China town, dance fever, goodfella, jackpot

Patterns of Use/Abuse

The development of opioid abuse and dependence may follow one of two typical behavior patterns. The first occurs in the individual who has obtained the drug by prescription from a physician for the relief of a medical problem. Abuse and dependency occur when the individual increases the amount and frequency of use, justifying the behavior as symptom treatment. He or she becomes obsessed with obtaining increasing amounts of the substance, seeking out several physicians in order to replenish and maintain supplies.

The second pattern of behavior associated with abuse and dependency of opioids occurs among individuals who use the drugs for recreational purposes and obtain them from illegal sources. Opioids may be used alone to induce the euphoric effects or in combination with stimulants or other drugs to enhance the euphoria or to counteract the depressant effects of the opioid. Tolerance develops and dependency occurs, leading the individual to procure the substance by whatever means is required to support the habit.

A recent government survey reported that there were 338,000 current heroin users aged 12 years and older in the United States in 2006 (SAMHSA, 2007). The same survey revealed an estimated 5.2 million current users of narcotic pain relievers.

Effects on the Body

Opiates are sometimes classified as *narcotic analgesics*. They exert their major effects primarily on the CNS, the eyes, and the GI tract. Chronic morphine use or acute morphine toxicity is manifested by a syndrome of sedation, chronic constipation, decreased respiratory rate, and pinpoint pupils. Intensity of symptoms is largely dose dependent. The following physiological effects are common with opioid use.

Central Nervous System. All opioids, opioid derivatives, and synthetic opioid-like drugs affect the CNS. Common manifestations include euphoria, mood changes, and mental clouding. Other common CNS effects include drowsiness and pain reduction. Pupillary constriction occurs in response to stimulation of the oculomotor nerve. CNS depression of the respiratory centers within the medulla results in respiratory depression. The antitussive response is due to suppression of the cough center within the medulla. The nausea and vomiting commonly associated with opiate ingestion is related to the stimulation of the centers within the medulla that trigger this response.

Gastrointestinal Effects. These drugs exert a profound effect on the GI tract. Both stomach and intestinal tone are increased, whereas peristaltic activity of the intestines is diminished. These effects lead to a marked decrease in the movement of food through the GI tract. This is a notable therapeutic effect in the treatment of severe diarrhea. In fact, no drugs have yet been developed that are more effective than the opioids for this purpose. However, constipation, and even fecal impaction, may be a serious problem for the chronic opioid user.

Cardiovascular Effects. In therapeutic doses, opioids have minimal effect on the action of the heart. Morphine is used extensively to relieve pulmonary edema and the pain of myocardial infarction in cardiac clients. At high doses, opioids induce hypotension, which may be caused by direct action on the heart or by opioid-induced histamine release.

Sexual Functioning. With opioids, there is decreased sexual function and diminished libido (Bruckenthal, 2001). Retarded ejaculation, impotence, and orgasm failure (in both men and women) may occur. Sexual side effects from opioids appear to be largely influenced by dosage.

Opioid Intoxication

Opioid intoxication constitutes clinically significant maladaptive behavioral or psychological changes that develop during, or shortly after, opioid use (APA, 2000). Symptoms include initial euphoria followed by apathy, dysphoria, psychomotor agitation or retardation, and impaired judgment. Physical symptoms include pupillary constriction (or dilation due to anoxia from severe overdose), drowsiness, slurred speech, and impairment in attention or memory (APA, 2000). Symptoms are consistent with the half-life of most opioid drugs, and usually last for several hours. Severe opioid intoxication can lead to respiratory depression, coma, and even death.

Opioid Withdrawal

Opioid withdrawal produces a syndrome of symptoms that develops after cessation of, or reduction in, heavy and prolonged use of an opiate or related substance. Symptoms include dysphoric mood, nausea or vomiting, muscle aches, lacrimation or rhinorrhea, pupillary dilation, piloerection, sweating, abdominal cramping, diarrhea, yawning, fever, and insomnia. With short-acting drugs such as heroin, withdrawal symptoms occur within 6 to 12 hours after the last dose, peak within 1 to 3 days, and gradually subside over a period of 5 to 7 days (APA, 2000). With longer-acting drugs such as methadone, withdrawal symptoms begin within 1 to 3 days after the last dose and are complete in 10 to 14 days (Sadock & Sadock, 2007). Withdrawal from the ultra-short-acting meperidine begins quickly, reaches a peak in 8 to 12 hours, and is complete in 4 to 5 days (Sadock & Sadock, 2007).

Hallucinogen Abuse and Dependence

A Profile of the Substance

Hallucinogenic substances are capable of distorting an individual's perception of reality. They have the ability to alter sensory perception and induce hallucinations. For this reason they have sometimes been referred to as "mind expanding." Some of the manifestations have been likened to a psychotic break. The hallucinations experienced by an individual with schizophrenia, however, are most often auditory, whereas substance-induced hallucinations are usually visual (Mack, Franklin, & Frances, 2003). Perceptual distortions have been reported by some users as spiritual, as giving a sense of depersonalization (observing oneself having the experience), or as being at peace with self and the universe. Others, who describe their experiences as "bad trips," report feelings of panic and a fear of dying or going insane. A common danger reported with hallucinogenic drugs is that of "flashbacks," or a spontaneous reoccurrence of the hallucinogenic state without ingestion of the drug. These can occur months after the drug was last taken.

Recurrent use can produce tolerance, encouraging users to resort to higher and higher dosages. No evidence of physical dependence is detectable when the drug is withdrawn; however, recurrent use appears to induce a psychological dependence to the insight-inducing experiences that a user may associate with episodes of hallucinogen use (Sadock & Sadock, 2007). This psychological dependence varies according to the drug, the dose, and the individual user. Hallucinogens are highly unpredictable in the effects they may induce each time they are used.

Many of the hallucinogenic substances have structural similarities. Some are produced synthetically; others are natural products of plants and fungi. A selected list of hallucinogens is presented in Table 27–5.

Historical Aspects

Archeological data obtained with carbon-14 dating suggest that hallucinogens have been used as part of religious ceremonies and at social gatherings by Native Americans for as long as 7000 years (Goldstein, 2002). Use of the peyote cactus as part of religious ceremonies in the southwestern part of the United States still occurs today, although this ritual use has greatly diminished.

LSD was first synthesized in 1943 by Dr. Albert Hoffman (Goldstein, 2002). It was used as a clinical research tool to investigate the biochemical etiology of schizophrenia. It soon reached the illicit market, however, and its abuse began to overshadow the research effort.

The abuse of hallucinogens reached a peak in the late 1960s, waned during the 1970s, and returned to favor in the 1980s with the so-called designer drugs (e.g., 3,4-methylene-dioxyamphetamine [MDMA] and methoxy-amphetamine [MDA]). One of the most commonly abused hallucinogens today is PCP, even though many of its effects are perceived as undesirable. A number of deaths have been directly attributed to the use of PCP, and numerous accidental deaths have occurred as a result of overdose and of the behavioral changes the drug precipitates.

Several therapeutic uses of LSD have been proposed, including the treatment of chronic alcoholism and the reduction of intractable pain such as occurs in malignant disease. A great deal more research is required regarding the therapeutic uses of LSD. At this time, there is no real evidence of the safety and efficacy of the drug in humans.

Patterns of Use/Abuse

Use of hallucinogens is usually episodic. Because cognitive and perceptual abilities are so markedly affected by

TABLE 27–5	**Hallucinogens**	
Categories	**Generic (Trade) Names**	**Common Street Names**
Naturally Occurring Hallucinogens	Mescaline (the primary active ingredient of the peyote cactus)	Cactus, mesc, mescal, half moon, big chief, bad seed, peyote
	Psilocybin and psilocin (active ingredients of *Psilocybe* mushrooms)	Magic mushroom, God's flesh, shrooms
	Ololiuqui (morning glory seeds)	Heavenly blue, pearly gates, flying saucers
Synthetic Compounds	Lysergic acid diethylamide [LSD] (synthetically produced from a fungal substance found on rye or a chemical substance found in morning glory seeds)	Acid, cube, big D, California sunshine, microdots, blue dots, sugar, orange wedges, peace tablets, purple haze, cupcakes
	Dimethyltryptamine [DMT] and diethyltryptamine [DET] (chemical analogues of tryptamine)	Businessman's trip
	2,5-Dimethoxy-4-methylamphetamine [STP, DOM]	STP (serenity, tranquility, peace)
	Phencyclidine [PCP]	Angel dust, hog, peace pill, rocket fuel
	3,4-Methylene-dioxyamphetamine [MDMA]*	XTC, Ecstasy, Adam, Eve
	Methoxy-amphetamine [MDA]	Love drug

*Cross-listed with the CNS stimulants.

these substances, the user must set aside time from normal daily activities for indulging in the consequences. According to the SAMHSA (2007) report, hallucinogens were used in the previous 30-day period before the survey in 2006 by 1.0 million persons (0.4 percent) 12 years of age or older. This number included 528,000 (0.2 percent) who had used Ecstasy.

The use of LSD does not lead to the development of physical dependence or withdrawal symptoms (Sadock & Sadock, 2007). However, tolerance does develop quickly and to a high degree. In fact, an individual who uses LSD repeatedly for a period of 3 to 4 days may develop complete tolerance to the drug. Recovery from the tolerance also occurs very rapidly (in 4 to 7 days), so that the individual is able to achieve the desired effect from the drug repeatedly and often.

PCP is usually taken episodically, in binges that can last for several days. However, some chronic users take the substance daily. Physical dependence does not occur with PCP; however, psychological dependence characterized by craving for the drug has been reported in chronic users, as has the development of tolerance. Tolerance apparently develops quickly with frequent use.

Psilocybin is an ingredient of the *Psilocybe* mushroom indigenous to the United States and Mexico. Ingestion of these mushrooms produces an effect similar to that of LSD but of a shorter duration. This hallucinogenic chemical can now be produced synthetically.

Mescaline is the only hallucinogenic compound used legally for religious purposes today by members of the Native American Church of the United States. It is the primary active ingredient of the peyote cactus. Neither physical nor psychological dependence occurs with the use of mescaline, although, as with other hallucinogens, tolerance can develop quickly with frequent use.

Among the very potent hallucinogens of the current drug culture are those that are categorized as derivatives of amphetamines. These include 2,5-dimethoxy-4-methylamphetamine (DOM, STP), MDMA (Ecstasy), and MDA. At lower doses, these drugs produce the "high" associated with CNS stimulants. At higher doses, hallucinogenic effects occur. These drugs have existed for many years but were only *rediscovered* in the mid-1980s. Because of the rapid increase in recreational use, the Drug Enforcement Agency imposed an emergency classification of MDMA as a schedule I drug in 1985. MDMA, or Ecstasy, is a synthetic drug with both stimulant and hallucinogenic qualities. It has a chemical structure similar to that of methamphetamine and mescaline, and it has become widely available throughout the world. Because of its growing popularity, the demand for this drug has led to tablets and capsules being sold as "Ecstasy," but which are not pure MDMA. Many contain drugs such as methamphetamine, PCP, amphetamine, ketamine, and *p*-methoxyamphetamine (PMA, a

stimulant with hallucinogenic properties; more toxic than MDMA). This practice has increased the dangers associated with MDMA use (*Street Drugs*, 2005).

Effects on the Body

The effects produced by the various hallucinogenics are highly unpredictable. The variety of effects may be related to dosage, the mental state of the individual, and the environment in which the substance is used. Some common effects have been reported (APA, 2000; Julien, 2005; Sadock & Sadock, 2007):

Physiological Effects

● Nausea and vomiting
● Chills
● Pupil dilation
● Increased pulse, blood pressure, and temperature
● Mild dizziness
● Trembling
● Loss of appetite
● Insomnia
● Sweating
● A slowing of respirations
● Elevation in blood sugar

Psychological Effects

● Heightened response to color, texture, and sounds
● Heightened body awareness
● Distortion of vision
● Sense of slowing of time
● All feelings magnified: love, lust, hate, joy, anger, pain, terror, despair
● Fear of losing control
● Paranoia, panic
● Euphoria, bliss
● Projection of self into dreamlike images
● Serenity, peace
● Depersonalization
● Derealization
● Increased libido

The effects of hallucinogens are not always pleasurable for the user. Two types of toxic reactions are known to occur. The first is the *panic reaction*, or "bad trip." Symptoms include an intense level of anxiety, fear, and stimulation. The individual hallucinates and fears going insane. Paranoia and acute psychosis may be evident.

The second type of toxic reaction to hallucinogens is the *flashback*. This phenomenon refers to the transient, spontaneous repetition of a previous LSD-induced experience that occurs in the absence of the substance. Various studies have reported that 15 to 80 percent of hallucinogen users report having experienced flashbacks (Sadock & Sadock, 2007).

Hallucinogen Intoxication

Symptoms of hallucinogen intoxication develop during, or shortly after (within minutes to a few hours) hallucinogen use (APA, 2000). Maladaptive behavioral or psychological changes include marked anxiety or depression, ideas of reference (a type of delusional thinking that all activity within one's environment is "referred to" [about] one's self), fear of losing one's mind, paranoid ideation, and impaired judgment. Perceptual changes occur in a state of full wakefulness and alertness and include intensification of perceptions, depersonalization, derealization, illusions, hallucinations, and synesthesias (APA, 2000). Physical symptoms include pupillary dilation, tachycardia, sweating, palpitations, blurring of vision, tremors, and incoordination (APA, 2000).

Symptoms of PCP intoxication develop within an hour of use (or less when it is smoked, snorted, or taken intravenously) (APA, 2000). Specific symptoms are dose related and include belligerence, assaultiveness, impulsiveness, unpredictability, psychomotor agitation, and impaired judgment. Physical symptoms include vertical or horizontal nystagmus, hypertension or tachycardia, numbness or diminished responsiveness to pain, ataxia, dysarthria, muscle rigidity, seizures or coma, and hyperacusis.

Cannabis Abuse and Dependence

A Profile of the Substance

Cannabis is second only to alcohol as the most widely abused drug in the United States. The major psychoactive ingredient of this class of substances is delta-9-tetrahydrocannabinol (THC). It occurs naturally in the plant *Cannabis sativa*, which grows readily in warm climates. Marijuana, the most prevalent type of cannabis preparation, is composed of the dried leaves, stems, and flowers of the plant. Hashish is a more potent concentrate of the resin derived from the flowering tops of the plant. Hash oil is a very concentrated form of THC made by boiling hashish in a solvent and filtering out the solid matter (*Street Drugs*, 2005). Cannabis products are usually smoked in the form of loosely rolled cigarettes. Cannabis can also be taken orally when it is prepared in food, but about two to three times the amount of cannabis must be ingested orally to equal the potency of that obtained by the inhalation of its smoke (Sadock & Sadock, 2007).

At moderate dosages, cannabis drugs produce effects resembling those of alcohol and other CNS depressants. By depressing higher brain centers, they release lower

centers from inhibitory influences. There has been some controversy in the past over the classification of these substances. They are not narcotics, although they are legally classified as controlled substances. They are not hallucinogens, although in very high dosages they can induce hallucinations. They are not sedative-hypnotics, although they most closely resemble these substances. Like sedative-hypnotics, their action occurs in the ascending reticular activating system.

Psychological dependence has been shown to occur with cannabis and tolerance can occur. Controversy exists about whether physiological dependence occurs with cannabis. Sadock and Sadock (2007) state:

> Withdrawal symptoms in humans are limited to modest increases in irritability, restlessness, insomnia, and anorexia and mild nausea; all these symptoms appear only when a person abruptly stops taking high doses of cannabis. (p. 418)

Common cannabis preparations are presented in Table 27–6.

Historical Aspects

Products of *Cannabis sativa* have been used therapeutically for nearly 5000 years (Julien, 2005). Cannabis was first employed in China and India as an antiseptic and an analgesic. Its use later spread to the Middle East, Africa, and Eastern Europe.

In the United States, medical interest in the use of cannabis arose during the early part of the 19th century. Many articles were published espousing its use for many and varied reasons. The drug was almost as commonly used for medicinal purposes as aspirin is today and could be purchased without a prescription in any drug store. It was purported to have antibacterial and anticonvulsant capabilities, decrease intraocular pressure, decrease pain, help in the treatment of asthma, increase appetite, and generally raise one's morale.

The drug went out of favor primarily because of the huge variation in potency within batches of medication caused by the variations in the THC content of different plants. Other medications were favored for their greater degree of solubility and faster onset of action than cannabis products. A federal law put an end to its legal use in 1937, after an association between marijuana and

TABLE 27–6	Cannabinoids	
Category	Common Preparations	Street Names
Cannabis	Marijuana	Joint, weed, pot, grass, Mary Jane, Texas tea, locoweed, MJ, hay, stick
	Hashis	Hash, bhang, ganja, charas

criminal activity became evident. In the 1960s, marijuana became the symbol of the "antiestablishment" generation, at which time it reached its peak as a drug of abuse.

Research continues in regard to the possible therapeutic uses of cannabis. It has been shown to be an effective agent for relieving the nausea and vomiting associated with cancer chemotherapy, when other antinausea medications fail. It has also been used in the treatment of chronic pain, glaucoma, multiple sclerosis, and acquired immune deficiency syndrome (Sadock & Sadock, 2007).

Advocates who praise the therapeutic usefulness and support the legalization of the cannabinoids persist within the United States today. Such groups as the Alliance for Cannabis Therapeutics (ACT) and the National Organization for the Reform of Marijuana Laws (NORML) have lobbied extensively to allow disease sufferers easier access to the drug. The medical use of marijuana has been legalized by a number of states. The U.S. Drug Enforcement Agency (USDEA; 2003) states:

Legalizing marijuana through the political process bypasses the safeguards established by the Food and Drug Administration to protect the public from dangerous or ineffective drugs. Every other prescribed drug must be tested according to scientifically rigorous protocols to ensure that it is safe and effective before it can be sold. The medical marijuana movement and its million-dollar media campaign have helped contribute to the changing attitude among our youth that marijuana use is harmless. Among marijuana's most harmful consequences is its role in leading to the use of other illegal drugs like heroin and cocaine. Long-term studies of students who use drugs show that very few young people use other illegal drugs without first trying marijuana. While not all people who use marijuana go on to use other drugs, using marijuana sometimes lowers inhibitions about drug use and exposes users to a culture that encourages use of other drugs.

A great deal more research is required to determine the long-term effects of the drug. Until results indicate otherwise, it is safe to assume that the harmful effects of the drug outweigh the benefits.

Patterns of Use/Abuse

In its 2006 National Survey on Drug Use and Health, SAMHSA (2007) reported that an estimated 20.3 million Americans 12 years of age or older were current illicit drug users, meaning they had used an illicit drug during the month before the survey interview. This estimate represents 8.3 percent of the population 12 years of age or older. Marijuana is the most commonly used illicit drug. In 2006, it was used by 73 percent of current illicit drug users. This constitutes about 14.8 million users of marijuana in the United States in the year 2006.

Many people incorrectly regard cannabis as a substance of low abuse potential. This lack of knowledge has promoted use of the substance by some individuals who believe it is harmless. Tolerance, although it tends to decline rapidly, does occur with chronic use. As tolerance develops, physical dependence also occurs, resulting in a mild withdrawal syndrome (as previously described) on cessation of drug use.

One controversy that exists regarding marijuana is whether its use leads to the use of other illicit drugs. Sadock and Sadock (2007) state:

Marijuana is the most widely used illicit drug among high school students. It has been termed a "gateway drug," because the strongest predictor of future cocaine use is frequent marijuana use during adolescence. (p. 1294)

Effects on the Body

Following is a summary of some of the effects that have been attributed to marijuana in recent years. Undoubtedly, as research continues, evidence of additional physiological and psychological effects will be made available.

Cardiovascular Effects. Cannabis ingestion induces tachycardia and orthostatic hypotension (National Institutes of Health [NIH], 2003). With the decrease in blood pressure, myocardial oxygen supply is decreased. Tachycardia in turn increases oxygen demand.

Respiratory Effects. Marijuana produces a greater amount of "tar" than its equivalent weight in tobacco. Because of the method by which marijuana is smoked—that is, the smoke is held in the lungs for as long as possible to achieve the desired effect—larger amounts of tar are deposited in the lungs, promoting deleterious effects to the lungs.

Although the initial reaction to the marijuana is bronchodilatation, thereby facilitating respiratory function, chronic use results in obstructive airway disorders (NIH, 2003). Frequent marijuana users often have laryngitis, bronchitis, cough, and hoarseness. Cannabis smoke contains more carcinogens than tobacco smoke, so lung damage and cancer are real risks for heavy users (Goldstein, 2002).

Reproductive Effects. Some studies have shown a decrease in levels of serum testosterone and abnormalities in sperm count, motility, and structure correlated with heavy marijuana use (NIH, 2003). In women, heavy marijuana use has been correlated with failure to ovulate, difficulty with lactation, and an increased risk of spontaneous abortion.

Central Nervous System Effects. Acute CNS effects of marijuana are dose related. Many people report a feeling of being "high"—the equivalent of being "drunk" on alcohol. Symptoms include feelings of euphoria, relaxed inhibitions, disorientation, depersonalization, and relaxation. At higher doses, sensory alterations may occur, including impairment in judgment of time and distance, recent memory, and learning ability. Physiological symptoms may include tremors, muscle rigidity, and conjunctival redness. Toxic effects are generally characterized by panic reactions. Very heavy usage has been shown to precipitate an acute psychosis that is self-limited and short-lived once the drug is removed from the body (Julien, 2005).

Heavy long-term cannabis use is also associated with a syndrome called *amotivational syndrome*. When this syndrome occurs, the individual is preoccupied with using the substance. Symptoms include lethargy, apathy, social and personal deterioration, and lack of motivation. This syndrome appears to be more common in countries in which the most potent preparations are used and where the substance is more freely available than it is in the United States.

Sexual Functioning. Marijuana is reported to enhance the sexual experience in both men and women. The intensified sensory awareness and the subjective slowness of time perception are thought to increase sexual satisfaction. Marijuana also enhances sexual functioning by releasing inhibitions for certain activities that would normally be restrained.

Cannabis Intoxication

Cannabis intoxication is evidenced by the presence of clinically significant maladaptive behavioral or psychological changes that develop during, or shortly after, cannabis use (APA, 2000). Symptoms include impaired motor coordination, euphoria, anxiety, a sensation of slowed time, and impaired judgment. Physical symptoms include conjunctival injection, increased appetite, dry mouth, and tachycardia. The impairment of motor skills lasts for 8 to 12 hours and interferes with the operation of motor vehicles. These effects are additive to those of alcohol, which is commonly used in combination with cannabis (Sadock & Sadock, 2007).

Tables 27–7 and 27–8 include summaries of the psychoactive substances, including symptoms of intoxication, withdrawal, use, overdose, possible therapeutic uses, and trade and common names by which they may be referred. The dynamics of substance use disorders using the Transactional Model of Stress/Adaptation are presented in Figure 27–3.

APPLICATION OF THE NURSING PROCESS

Assessment

In the preintroductory phase of relationship development, the nurse must examine his or her feelings about working with a client who abuses substances. If these behaviors are viewed as morally wrong and the nurse has internalized these attitudes from very early in life, it may be very difficult to suppress judgmental feelings. The role that alcohol or other substances has played (or plays) in the life of the nurse will most certainly affect the way in which he or she approaches interaction with the substance-abusing client.

How are attitudes examined? Some individuals may have sufficient ability for introspection to be able to recognize on their own whether they have unresolved issues related to substance abuse. For others, it may be more helpful to discuss these issues in a group situation, where insight may be gained from feedback regarding the perceptions of others.

Whether alone or in a group, the nurse may gain a greater understanding about attitudes and feelings related to substance abuse by responding to the following types of questions. As shown here, the questions are specific to alcohol, but they could be adapted for any substance.

● What are my drinking patterns?
● If I drink, why do I drink? When, where, and how much?
● If I don't drink, why do I abstain?
● Am I comfortable with my drinking patterns?
● If I decided not to drink any more, would that be a problem for me?
● What did I learn from my parents about drinking?
● Have my attitudes changed as an adult?
● What are my feelings about people who become intoxicated?
● Does it seem more acceptable for some individuals than for others?
● Do I ever use terms like "sot," "drunk," or "boozer," to describe some individuals who overindulge, yet overlook it in others?
● Do I ever overindulge myself?
● Has the use of alcohol (by myself or others) affected my life in any way?
● Do I see alcohol/drug abuse as a sign of weakness? A moral problem? An illness?

Unless nurses fully understand and accept their own attitudes and feelings, they cannot be empathetic toward clients' problems. Clients in recovery need to know they are accepted for themselves, regardless of past behaviors. Nurses must be able to separate the client from the behavior and to accept that individual with unconditional positive regard.

Assessment Tools

Nurses are often the individuals who perform the admission interview. A variety of assessment tools are appropriate for use in chemical dependency units. A nursing history and assessment tool was presented in Chapter 9 of this text. With some adaptation, it is an appropriate instrument for creating a database on clients who abuse

TABLE 27–7   Psychoactive Substances: A Profile Summary

Class of Drugs	Symptoms of Use	Therapeutic Uses	Symptoms of Overdose	Trade Names	Common Names
CNS Depressants Alcohol	Relaxation, loss of inhibitions, lack of concentration, drowsiness, slurred speech, sleep	Antidote for methanol consumption; ingredient in many pharmacological concentrates	Nausea, vomiting; shallow respirations; cold, clammy skin; weak, rapid pulse; coma; possible death	Ethyl alcohol, beer, gin, rum, vodka, bourbon, whiskey, liqueurs, wine, brandy, sherry, champagne	Booze, alcohol, liquor, drinks, cocktails, highballs, nightcaps, moonshine, white lightening, firewater
Other (barbiturates and nonbarbiturates)	Same as alcohol	Relief from anxiety and insomnia; as anticonvulsants and anesthetics	Anxiety, fever, agitation, hallucinations, disorientation, tremors, delirium, convulsions, possible death	Seconal, Nembutal, Amytal Valium Librium Noctec Miltown	Red birds, yellow birds, blue birds Blues/yellows Green & whites Mickies Downers
CNS Stimulants Amphetamines and related drugs	Hyperactivity, agitation, euphoria, insomnia, loss of appetite	Management of narcolepsy, hyperkinesia, and weight control	Cardiac arrhythmias, headache, convulsions, hypertension, rapid heart rate, coma, possible death	Dexedrine, Didrex, Tenuate, Prelu-2, Ritalin, Focalin, Meridia, Provigil	Uppers, pep pills, wakeups, bennies, eye-openers, speed, black beauties, sweet As
Cocaine	Euphoria, hyperactivity, restlessness, talkativeness, increased pulse, dilated pupils, rhinitis		Hallucinations, convulsions, pulmonary edema, respiratory failure, coma, cardiac arrest, possible death	Cocaine hydrochloride	Coke, flake, snow, dust, happy dust, gold dust, girl, cecil, C, toot, blow, crack
Opioids	Euphoria, lethargy, drowsiness, lack of motivation, constricted pupils	As analgesics; methadone in substitution therapy; heroin has no therapeutic use	Shallow breathing, slowed pulse, clammy skin, pulmonary edema, respiratory arrest, convulsions, coma, possible death	Heroin Morphine Codeine Dilaudid Demerol Dolophine Percodan Talwin Opium	Snow, stuff, H, harry, horse M, morph, Miss Emma Schoolboy Lords Doctors Dollies Perkies Ts Big O, black stuff
Hallucinogens	Visual hallucinations, disorientation, confusion, paranoid delusions, euphoria, anxiety, panic, increased pulse	LSD has been proposed in the treatment of chronic alcoholism, and in the reduction of intractable pain	Agitation, extreme hyperactivity, violence, hallucinations, psychosis, convulsions, possible death	LSD PCP Mescaline DMT STP	Acid, cube, big D Angel dust, hog, peace pill Mesc Businessman's trip Serenity and peace
Cannabinols	Relaxation, talkativeness, lowered inhibitions, euphoria, mood swings	Marijuana has been used for relief of nausea and vomiting associated with antineoplastic chemotherapy and to reduce eye pressure in glaucoma	Fatigue, paranoia, delusions, hallucinations, possible psychosis	Cannabis Hashish	Marijuana, pot, grass, joint, Mary Jane, MJ Hash, rope, Sweet Lucy

TABLE 27–8 **Summary of Symptoms Associated With the Syndromes of Intoxication and Withdrawal**

Class of Drugs	Intoxication	Withdrawal	Comments
Alcohol	Aggressiveness, impaired judgment, impaired attention, irritability, euphoria, depression, emotional lability, slurred speech, incoordination, unsteady gait, nystagmus, flushed face	Tremors, nausea/vomiting, malaise, weakness, tachycardia, sweating, elevated blood pressure, anxiety, depressed mood, irritability, hallucinations, headache, insomnia, seizures	Alcohol withdrawal begins within 4–6 hours after last drink. May progress to delirium tremens on 2nd or 3rd day. Use of Librium or Serax is common for substitution therapy.
Amphetamines and Related Substances	Fighting, grandiosity, hypervigilance, psychomotor agitation, impaired judgment, tachycardia, pupillary dilation, elevated blood pressure, perspiration or chills, nausea and vomiting.	Anxiety, depressed mood, irritability, craving for the substance, fatigue, insomnia or hypersomnia, psychomotor agitation, paranoid and suicidal ideation.	Withdrawal symptoms usually peak within 2–4 days, although depression and irritability may persist for months. Antidepressants may be used.
Caffeine	Restlessness, nervousness, excitement, insomnia, flushed face, diuresis, gastrointestinal complaints, muscle twitching, rambling flow of thought and speech, cardiac arrhythmia, periods of inexhaustibility, psychomotor agitation	Headache	Caffeine is contained in coffee, tea, colas, cocoa, chocolate, some over-the-counter analgesics, "cold" preparations, and stimulants.
Cannabis	Euphoria, anxiety, suspiciousness, sensation of slowed time, impaired judgment, social withdrawal, tachycardia, conjunctival redness, increased appetite, hallucinations	Restlessness, irritability, insomnia, loss of appetite	Intoxication occurs immediately and lasts about 3 hours. Oral ingestion is more slowly absorbed and has longer-lasting effects.
Cocaine	Euphoria, fighting, grandiosity, hypervigilance, psychomotor agitation, impaired judgment, tachycardia, elevated blood pressure, pupillary dilation, perspiration or chills, nausea/vomiting, hallucinations, delirium	Depression, anxiety, irritability, fatigue, insomnia or hypersomnia, psychomotor agitation, paranoid or suicidal ideation, apathy, social withdrawal	Large doses of the drug can result in convulsions or death from cardiac arrhythmias or respiratory paralysis.
Inhalants	Belligerence, assaultiveness, apathy, impaired judgment, dizziness, nystagmus, slurred speech, unsteady gait, lethargy, depressed reflexes, tremor, blurred vision, stupor or coma, euphoria, irritation around eyes, throat, and nose		Intoxication occurs within 5 minutes of inhalation. Symptoms last 60–90 minutes. Large doses can result in death from CNS depression or cardiac arrhythmia.
Nicotine		Craving for the drug, irritability, anger, frustration, anxiety, difficulty concentrating, restlessness, decreased heart rate, increased appetite, weight gain, tremor, headaches, insomnia	Symptoms of withdrawal begin within 24 hours of last drug use and decrease in intensity over days, weeks, or sometimes longer.
Opioids	Euphoria, lethargy, somnolence, apathy, dysphoria, impaired judgment, pupillary constriction, drowsiness, slurred speech, constipation, nausea, decreased respiratory rate and blood pressure	Craving for the drug, nausea/vomiting, muscle aches, lacrimation or rhinorrhea, pupillary dilation, piloerection or sweating, diarrhea, yawning, fever, insomnia	Withdrawal symptoms appear within 6–8 hours after last dose, reach a peak in the 2nd or 3rd day, and disappear in 7–10 days. Times are shorter with meperidine and longer with methadone.
Phencyclidine and Related Substances	Belligerence, assaultiveness, impulsiveness, psychomotor agitation, impaired judgment, nystagmus, increased heart rate and blood pressure, diminished pain response, ataxia, dysarthria, muscle rigidity, seizures, hyperacusis, delirium		Delirium can occur within 24 hours after use of phencyclidine, or may occur up to a week following recovery from an overdose of the drug.
Sedatives, Hypnotics, and Anxiolytics	Disinhibition of sexual or aggressive impulses, mood lability, impaired judgment, slurred speech, incoordination, unsteady gait, impairment in attention or memory disorientation, confusion	Nausea/vomiting, malaise, weakness, tachycardia, sweating, anxiety, irritability, orthostatic hypotension, tremor, insomnia, seizures	Withdrawal may progress to delirium, usually within 1 week of last use. Long-acting barbiturates or benzodiazepines may be used in withdrawal substitution therapy.

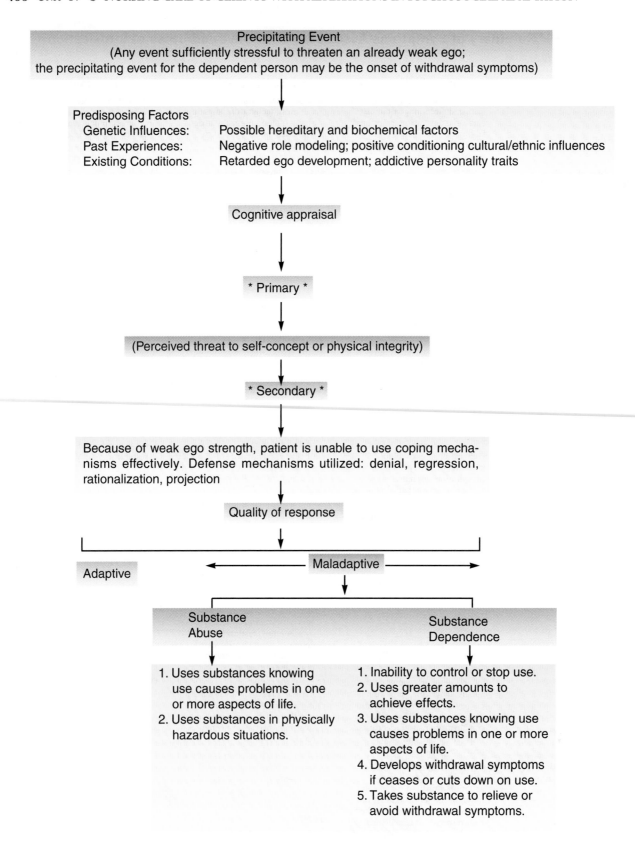

FIGURE 27–3 The dynamics of substance use disorders using the transactional model of stress/adaptation.

substances. Box 27–1 presents a drug history and assessment that could be used in conjunction with the general biopsychosocial assessment.

Box 27 – 1 Drug History and Assessment*

1. When you were growing up, did anyone in your family drink alcohol or take other kinds of drugs?
2. If so, how did the substance use affect the family situation?
3. When did you have your first drink/drugs?
4. How long have you been drinking/taking drugs on a regular basis?
5. What is your pattern of substance use?
   a. When do you use substances?
   b. What do you use?
   c. How much do you use?
   d. Where are you and with whom when you use substances?
6. When did you have your last drink/drug? What was it and how much did you consume?
7. Does using the substance(s) cause problems for you? Describe. Include family, friends, job, school, other.
8. Have you ever experienced injury as a result of substance use?
9. Have you ever been arrested or incarcerated for drinking/using drugs?
10. Have you ever tried to stop drinking/using drugs? If so, what was the result? Did you experience any physical symptoms, such as tremors, headache, insomnia, sweating, or seizures?
11. Have you ever experienced loss of memory for times when you have been drinking/using drugs?
12. Describe a typical day in your life.
13. Are there any changes you would like to make in your life? If so, what?
14. What plans or ideas do you have for seeing that these changes occur?

*To be used in conjunction with general biopsychosocial nursing history and assessment tool (Chapter 9).

The Clinical Institute Withdrawal Assessment of Alcohol Scale, Revised (CIWA-Ar) is an excellent tool that is used by many hospitals to assess risk and severity of withdrawal from alcohol. It may be used for initial assessment as well as ongoing monitoring of alcohol withdrawal symptoms. A copy of the CIWA-Ar is presented in Box 27–2

Other screening tools exist for determining whether an individual has a problem with substances. Two such tools developed by the American Psychiatric Association for the diagnosis of alcoholism include the Michigan Alcoholism Screening Test and the CAGE Questionnaire (Boxes 27–3 and 27–4). Some psychiatric units administer these surveys to all clients who are admitted to help determine if there is a secondary alcoholism problem in addition to the psychiatric problem for which the client is being admitted (sometimes called **dual diagnosis**). It would be possible to adapt these tools to use in diagnosing problems with other drugs as well.

Dual Diagnosis

If it is determined that the client has a coexisting substance disorder and mental illness, he or she may be assigned to a special program that targets both problems. Counseling for the mentally ill person who abuses substances takes a different approach than that which is directed at individuals who abuse substances but are not mentally ill. In the latter, many counselors use direct confrontation of the substance use behaviors. This approach is thought to be detrimental to the treatment of a chronically mentally ill person (Mack et al., 2003). Most dual diagnosis programs take a more supportive and less confrontational approach.

Box 27 – 2 Clinical Institute Withdrawal Assessment of Alcohol Scale, Revised (CIWA-Ar)

Date: _____   Time: _____

Patient:
Pulse or heart rate, taken for one minute: **Blood pressure:**

NAUSEA AND VOMITING — Ask "Do you feel sick to your stomach? Have you vomited?" Observation.

0 no nausea and no vomiting
1 mild nausea with no vomiting
2
3
4 intermittent nausea with dry heaves
5
6
7 constant nausea, frequent dry heaves and vomiting

TACTILE DISTURBANCES — Ask "Have you any itching, pins and needles sensations, any burning, any numbness, or do you feel bugs crawling on or under your skin?" Observation.

0 none
1 very mild itching, pins and needles, burning or numbness
2 mild itching, pins and needles, burning or numbness
3 moderate itching, pins and needles, burning or numbness
4 moderately severe hallucinations
5 severe hallucinations
6 extremely severe hallucinations
7 continuous hallucinations

Continued on following page

BOX 27 – 2 *(Continued)*

TREMOR—Arms extended and fingers spread apart. Observation.

0 no tremor
1 not visible, but can be felt fingertip to fingertip
2
3
4 moderate, with patient's arms extended
5
6
7 severe, even with arms not extended

PAROXYSMAL SWEATS — Observation.

0 no sweat visible
1 barely perceptible sweating, palms moist
2
3
4 beads of sweat obvious on forehead
5
6
7 drenching sweats

ANXIETY – Ask "Do you feel nervous?" Observation.

0 no anxiety, at ease
1 mild anxious
2
3
4 moderately anxious, or guarded, so anxiety is inferred
5
6
7 equivalent to acute panic states as seen in severe delirium or acute schizophrenic reactions

AGITATION — Observation.

0 normal activity
1 somewhat more than normal activity
2
3
4 moderately fidgety and restless
5
6
7 paces back and forth during most of the interview, or constantly thrashes about

The CIWA-Ar is not copyrighted and may be reproduced freely. This assessment for monitoring withdrawal symptoms requires approximately 5 minutes to administer. The maximum score is 67 (see instrument). Patients scoring less than 10 do not usually need additional medication for withdrawal.

AUDITORY DISTURBANCES — Ask "Are you more aware of sounds around you? Are they harsh? Do they frighten you? Are you hearing anything that is disturbing to you? Are you hearing things you know are not there?" Observation.

0 not present
1 very mild harshness or ability to frighten
2 mild harshness or ability to frighten
3 moderate harshness or ability to frighten
4 moderately severe hallucinations
5 severe hallucinations
6 extremely severe hallucinations
7 continuous hallucinations

VISUAL DISTURBANCES — Ask "Does the light appear to be too bright? Is its color different? Does it hurt your eyes? Are you seeing anything that is disturbing to you? Are you seeing things you know are not there?" Observation.

0 not present
1 very mild sensitivity
2 mild sensitivity
3 moderate sensitivity
4 moderately severe hallucinations
5 severe hallucinations
6 extremely severe hallucinations
7 continuous hallucinations

HEADACHE, FULLNESS IN HEAD — Ask "Does your head feel different? Does it feel like there is a band around your head?" Do not rate for dizziness or lightheadedness. Otherwise, rate severity.

0 not present
1 very mild
2 mild
3 moderate
4 moderately severe
5 severe
6 very severe
7 extremely severe

ORIENTATION AND CLOUDING OF SENSORIUM — Ask "What day is this? Where are you? Who am I?"

0 oriented and can do serial additions
1 cannot do serial additions or is uncertain about date
2 disoriented for date by no more than 2 calendar days
3 disoriented for date by more than 2 calendar days
4 disoriented for place/or person

Total CIWA-Ar Score_____
Rater's Initials_____
Maximum Possible Score 67

10 over need add. meds

SOURCE: Sullivan, J.T.; Sykora, K.; Schneiderman, J.; Naranjo, CA.; and Sellers, E.M. Assessment of alcohol withdrawal: The revised Clinical Institute Withdrawal Assessment for Alcohol scale (CIWA-Ar). *British Journal of Addiction,* 84:1353–1357, 1989.

Box 27 – 3   Michigan Alcoholism Screening Test (MAST)

Answer the following questions by placing an X under Yes or No. *	Yes	No
1. Do you enjoy a drink now and then?	0	0
2. Do you feel you are a normal drinker? (By normal we mean you drink less than or as much as most people.)		2
3. Have you ever awakened the morning after some drinking the night before and found that you could not remember a part of the evening?	2	
4. Does your wife, husband, parent, or other near relative ever worry or complain about your drinking?	1	
5. Can you stop drinking without a struggle after one or two drinks?		2
6. Do you ever feel guilty about your drinking?	1	
7. Do friends or relatives think you are a normal drinker?		2
8. Are you able to stop drinking when you want to?		2
9. Have you ever attended a meeting of Alcoholics Anonymous (AA)?	5	
10. Have you gotten into physical fights when drinking?	1	
11. Has your drinking ever created problems between you and your wife, husband, a parent, or other relative?	2	
12. Has your wife, husband, or another family member ever gone to anyone for help about your drinking?	2	
13. Have you ever lost friends because of your drinking?	2	
14. Have you ever gotten into trouble at work or school because of drinking?	2	
15. Have you ever lost a job because of drinking?	2	
16. Have you ever neglected your obligations, your family, or your work for 2 or more days in a row because you were drinking?	2	
17. Do you drink before noon fairly often?	1	
18. Have you ever been told you have liver trouble? Cirrhosis?	2	
19. After heavy drinking have you ever had delirium tremens (DTs) or severe shaking or heard voices or seen things that really were not there?	5	
20. Have you ever gone to anyone for help about your drinking?	5	
21. Have you ever been in a hospital because of drinking?	5	
22. Have you ever been a patient in a psychiatric hospital or on a psychiatric ward of a general hospital where drinking was part of the problem that resulted in hospitalization?	2	
23. Have you ever been seen at a psychiatric or mental health clinic or gone to any doctor, social worker, or clergyman for help with any emotional problem, where drinking was part of the problem?	2	
24. Have you ever been arrested for drunk driving, driving while intoxicated, or driving under the influence of alcoholic beverages? (If yes, how many times?_____)	2 ea	
25. Have you ever been arrested, or taken into custody, even for a few hours, because of other drunk behavior? (If yes, how many times?_____)	2 ea	

* Items are scored under the response that would indicate a problem with alcohol.
Method of scoring: 0—3 points = no problem with alcohol
                    4 points = possible problem with alcohol
                    5 or more = indicates problem with alcohol

SOURCE: From Selzer, M.L.: The Michigan alcohol screening test: The quest for a new diagnostic instrument. *American Journal of Psychiatry*
(1971), 127, 1653–1658. With permission.

Peer support groups are an important part of the treatment program. Group members offer encouragement and practical advice to each other. Psychodynamic therapy can be useful for some individuals with a dual diagnosis by delving into the personal history of how psychiatric disorders and substance abuse have reinforced one another and how the cycle can be broken (Harvard Medical School, 2003). Cognitive and behavioral therapies are helpful in training clients to monitor moods and thought patterns that lead to substance abuse. With these therapies, clients also learn to avoid substance use and to cope with cravings and the temptation to relapse (Harvard Medical School, 2003).

Box 27-4   The CAGE Questionnaire

1. Have you ever felt you should *C*ut down on your drinking?
2. Have people *A*nnoyed you by criticizing your drinking?
3. Have you ever felt bad or *G*uilty about your drinking?
4. Have you ever had a drink first thing in the morning to steady your nerves or get rid of a hangover (*E*ye-opener)?

Scoring: 2 or 3 "yes" answers strongly suggest a problem with alcohol.

SOURCE: From Mayfield, D., McLeod, G., and Hall, P. (1974), with permission.

Individuals with dual diagnoses should be encouraged to attend 12-step recovery programs (e.g., Alcoholics Anonymous or Narcotics Anonymous). Dual diagnosis clients are sometimes resistant to attending 12-step programs, and they often do better in groups specifically designed for people with psychiatric disorders.

Substance abuse groups are usually integrated into regular programming for psychiatric clients with a dual diagnosis. An individual in a psychiatric facility or day treatment program will attend a substance abuse group periodically in lieu of another scheduled activity therapy. Topics are directed toward areas that are unique to clients with a mental illness, such as mixing medications with other substances, as well as topics that are common to primary substances abusers. Individuals are encouraged to discuss their personal problems.

Mack and associates (2003) state:

The dual diagnosis patient often falls through the cracks of the treatment system. Severe psychiatric disorders often preclude full treatment in substance abuse clinics or self-help groups. The addition of other Axis I, II, and III disorders to a substance use disorder greatly complicates diagnosis and makes treatment more difficult. (p. 359)

Continued attendance at 12-step group meetings is encouraged on discharge from treatment. Family involvement is enlisted, and preventive strategies are outlined. Individual case management is common and success is often promoted by this close supervision.

Diagnosis/Outcome Identification

The next step in the nursing process is to identify appropriate nursing diagnoses by analyzing the data collected during the assessment phase. The individual who abuses or is dependent on substances undoubtedly has many unmet physical and emotional needs. Table 27–9 presents a list of client behaviors and the NANDA nursing diagnoses that correspond to those behaviors, which may be used in planning care for the client with a substance use disorder.

Outcome Criteria

The following criteria may be used for measurement of outcomes in the care of the client with substance related disorders.

The client:

1. Has not experienced physical injury.
2. Has not caused harm to self or others.

TABLE 27–9   Assigning Nursing Diagnoses to Behaviors Commonly Associated with Substance-Related Disorders

Behaviors	Nursing Diagnoses
Makes statements such as, "I don't have a problem with (substance). I can quit any time I want to." Delays seeking assistance; does not perceive problems related to use of substances; minimizes use of substances; unable to admit impact of disease on life pattern	Ineffective Denial
Abuse of chemical agents; destructive behavior toward others and self; inability to meet basic needs; inability to meet role expectations; risk taking	Ineffective Coping
Loss of weight, pale conjunctiva and mucous membranes, decreased skin turgor, electrolyte imbalance, anemia, drinks alcohol instead of eating	Imbalanced Nutrition: Less than Body Requirements/Deficient Fluid Volume
Risk factors: Malnutrition, altered immune condition, failing to avoid exposure to pathogens	Risk for Infection
Criticizes self and others, self-destructive behavior (abuse of substances as a coping mechanism), dysfunctional family background	Chronic Low Self-Esteem
Denies that substance is harmful; continues to use substance in light of obvious consequences	Deficient Knowledge
For the client withdrawing from CNS depressants: Risk factors: CNS agitation (tremors, elevated blood pressure, nausea and vomiting, hallucinations, illusions, tachycardia, anxiety, seizures)	Risk for Injury
For the client withdrawing from CNS stimulants: Risk factors: Intense feelings of lassitude and depression; "crashing," suicidal ideation	Risk for Suicide

3. Accepts responsibility for own behavior.
4. Acknowledges association between personal problems and use of substance(s).
5. Demonstrates more adaptive coping mechanisms that can be used in stressful situations (instead of taking substances).
6. Shows no signs or symptoms of infection or malnutrition.
7. Exhibits evidence of increased self-worth by attempting new projects without fear of failure and by demonstrating less defensive behavior toward others.
8. Verbalizes importance of abstaining from use of substances in order to maintain optimal wellness.

Planning/Implementation

Implementation with clients who abuse substances is a long-term process, often beginning with **detoxification** and progressing to total abstinence. The following section presents a group of selected nursing diagnoses, with short- and long-term goals and nursing interventions for each.

Some institutions are using a case management model to coordinate care (see Chapter 9 for a more detailed explanation). In case management models, the plan of care may take the form of a critical pathway.

Risk for Injury

Risk for injury is defined as "at risk for injury as a result of [internal or external] environmental conditions interacting with the individual's adaptive and defensive resources" (NANDA International [NANDA-I], 2007, p. 125).

Client Goals

Outcome criteria include short- and long-term goals. Timelines are individually determined.

Short-Term Goal
● Client's condition will stabilize within 72 hours.

Long-Term Goal
● Client will not experience physical injury.

Interventions

For the Client in Substance Withdrawal

● Assess the client's level of disorientation to determine specific requirements for safety.
● Obtain a drug history, if possible. It is important to determine the type of substance(s) used, the time and amount of last use, the length and frequency of use, and the amount used on a daily basis.
● Because subjective history is often not accurate, obtain a urine sample for laboratory analysis of substance content.

● It is important to keep the client in as quiet an environment as possible. Excessive stimuli may increase client agitation. A private room is ideal.
● Observe client behaviors frequently. If seriousness of the condition warrants, it may be necessary to assign a staff person on a one-to-one basis.
● Accompany and assist client when ambulating, and use a wheelchair for transporting the client long distances.
● Pat the headboard and side rails of the bed with thick towels to protect the client in case of a seizure.
● Suicide precautions may need to be instituted for the client withdrawing from CNS stimulants.
● Ensure that smoking materials and other potentially harmful objects are stored away from client's access.
● Frequently orient the client to reality and the surroundings.
● Monitor the client's vital signs every 15 minutes initially and less frequently as acute symptoms subside.
● Follow the medication regimen, as ordered by the physician. Common psychopharmacological intervention for substance intoxication and withdrawal is presented later in this chapter under the section entitled, "Treatment Modalities for Substance-Related Disorder."

Ineffective Denial

Ineffective denial is defined as "conscious or unconscious attempt to disavow the knowledge or meaning of an event to reduce anxiety/fear, but leading to the detriment of health" (NANDA-I, 2007, p. 67). Table 27–10 presents this nursing diagnosis in care plan format.

Client Goals

Outcome criteria include short- and long-term goals. Timelines are individually determined.

Short-Term Goal
● Client will divert attention away from external issues and focus on behavioral outcomes associated with substance use.

Long-Term Goal
● Client will verbalize acceptance of responsibility for own behavior and acknowledge association between substance use and personal problems.

Interventions

● Begin by working to develop a trusting nurse–client relationship. Be honest and keep all promises.
● Convey an attitude of acceptance to the client. Ensure that he or she understands "It is not *you* but your *behavior* that is unacceptable." An attitude of acceptance helps to promote the client's feelings of dignity and self-worth.

Table 27–10 Care Plan for the Client with a Substance-Related Disorder

NURSING DIAGNOSIS: INEFFECTIVE DENIAL
RELATED TO: Weak, underdeveloped ego
EVIDENCED BY: Statements indicating no problem with substance use

Outcome Criteria	Nursing Interventions	Rationale
Short-Term Goal ● Client will divert attention away from external issues and focus on behavioral outcomes associated with substance use. **Long-Term Goal** ● Client will verbalize acceptance of responsibility for own behavior and acknowledge association between substance use and personal problems.	1. Begin by working to develop a trusting nurse-client relationship. Be honest. Keep all promises. 2. Convey an attitude of acceptance to the client. Ensure that he or she understands "It is not you but your *behavior* that is unacceptable." 3. Provide information to correct misconceptions about substance abuse. Client may rationalize his or her behavior with statements such as, "I'm not an alcoholic. I can stop drinking any time I want. Besides, I only drink beer." Or "I only smoke pot to relax before class. So what? I know lots of people who do. Besides, you can't get hooked on pot." 4. Identify recent maladaptive behaviors or situations that have occurred in the client's life, and discuss how use of substances may have been a contributing factor. 5. Use confrontation with caring. Do not allow client to fantasize about his or her lifestyle (for example: "It is my understanding that the last time you drank alcohol, you . . ." or "The lab report shows that you were under the influence of alcohol when you had the accident that injured three people"). 6. Do not accept rationalization or projection as client attempts to make excuses for or blame his or her behavior on other people or situations. 7. Encourage participation in group activities. 8. Offer immediate positive recognition of client's expressions of insight gained regarding illness and acceptance of responsibility for own behavior.	1. Trust is the basis of a therapeutic relationship. 2. An attitude of acceptance promotes feelings of dignity and self-worth. 3. Many myths abound regarding use of specific substances. Factual information presented in a matter-of-fact, nonjudgmental way explaining what behaviors constitute substance-related disorders may help the client focus on his or her own behaviors as an illness that requires help. 4. The first step in decreasing use of denial is for client to see the relationship between substance use and personal problems. 5. Confrontation interferes with client's ability to use denial; a caring attitude preserves self-esteem and avoids putting the client on the defensive. 6. Rationalization and projection prolong denial that problems exist in the client's life because of substance use. 7. Peer feedback is often more accepted than feedback from authority figures. Peer pressure can be a strong factor as well as association with individuals who are experiencing or who have experienced similar problems. 8. Positive reinforcement enhances self-esteem and encourages repetition of desirable behaviors.

● Provide information to correct misconceptions about substance abuse. The client may rationalize his or her behavior with statements such as, "I'm not an alcoholic. I can stop drinking any time I want. Besides, I only drink beer." or "I only smoke pot to relax before class. So what? I know lots of people who do. Besides, you can't get hooked on pot." Many myths abound regarding use of specific substances. Factual information presented in a matter-of-fact, nonjudgmental way explaining what behaviors constitute substance-related disorders may help the client focus on his or her own behaviors as an illness that requires help.

- Identify recent maladaptive behaviors or situations that have occurred in the client's life, and discuss how use of substances may have been a contributing factor. The first step in decreasing use of denial is for client to see the relationship between substance use and personal problems.
- Use confrontation with caring. Do not allow client to fantasize about his or her lifestyle. (Examples: "It is my understanding that the last time you drank alcohol, you . . ." or "The lab report shows that your blood alcohol level was 250 when you were involved in that automobile accident.") Confrontation interferes with client's ability to use denial; a caring attitude preserves self-esteem and avoids putting the client on the defensive.
- Do not accept the use of rationalization or projection as client attempts to make excuses for or blame his or her behavior on other people or situations. Rationalization and projection prolong the stage of denial that problems exist in the client's life because of substance use.
- Encourage participation in group activities. Peer feedback is often more accepted than feedback from authority figures. Peer pressure can be a strong factor as well as the association with individuals who are experiencing or who have experienced similar problems.
- Offer immediate positive recognition of client's expressions of insight gained regarding illness and acceptance of responsibility for own behavior. Positive reinforcement enhances self-esteem and encourages repetition of desirable behaviors.

Ineffective Coping

Ineffective coping is defined as the "inability to form a valid appraisal of the stressors, inadequate choices of practiced responses, and/or inability to use available resources" (NANDA-I, 2007, p. 59).

Client Goals

Outcome criteria include short- and long-term goals. Timelines are individually determined.

Short-Term Goal
- Client will express true feelings about using substances as a method of coping with stress.

Long-Term Goal
- Client will be able to verbalize use of adaptive coping mechanisms, instead of substance abuse, in response to stress.

Interventions

- Spend time with the client and establish a trusting relationship.
- Set limits on manipulative behavior. Be sure that the client knows what is acceptable, what is not, and the consequences for violating the limits set. Ensure that all staff maintain consistency with this intervention. The client is unable to establish his or her own limits, so limits must be set for him or her. Unless administration of consequences for violation of limits is consistent, manipulative behavior will not be eliminated.
- Encourage the client to verbalize feelings, fears, and anxieties. Answer any questions he or she may have regarding the disorder. Verbalization of feelings in a nonthreatening environment may help the client come to terms with long-unresolved issues.
- Explain the effects of substance abuse on the body. Emphasize that the prognosis is closely related to abstinence. Many clients lack knowledge regarding the deleterious effects of substance abuse on the body.
- Explore with the client the options available to assist with stressful situations rather than resorting to substance abuse (e.g., contacting various members of Alcoholics Anonymous or Narcotics Anonymous; physical exercise; relaxation techniques; meditation). The client may have persistently resorted to chemical abuse and thus may possess little or no knowledge of adaptive responses to stress.
- Provide positive reinforcement for evidence of gratification delayed appropriately. Encourage the client to be as independent as possible in performing his or her self-care. Provide positive feedback for independent decision-making and effective use of problem-solving skills.

Dysfunctional Family Processes: Alcoholism

Dysfunctional family processes: alcoholism is defined as "psychosocial, spiritual, and physiological functions of the family unit [that] are chronically disorganized, which leads to conflict, denial of problems, resistance to change, ineffective problem solving, and a series of self-perpetuating crises" (NANDA-I, 2007, p. 81).

Client Goals

Outcome criteria include short- and long-term goals. Timelines are individually determined.

Short-Term Goals
- Family members will participate in individual family programs and support groups.
- Family members will identify ineffective coping behaviors and consequences.
- Family will initiate and plan for necessary lifestyle changes.

Long-Term Goal
- Family members will take action to change self-destructive behaviors and alter behaviors that contribute to the client's addiction.

Interventions

- Review family history; explore roles of family members, circumstances involving alcohol use, strengths, and areas of growth. Explore how family members have coped with the client's addiction (e.g., denial, repression, rationalization, hurt, loneliness, projection). Persons who enable also suffer from the same feelings as the client and use ineffective methods for dealing with the situation, necessitating help in learning new and effective coping skills.
- Determine the family's understanding of the current situation and previous methods of coping with life's problems. Assess family members' current level of functioning.
- Determine the extent of enabling behaviors being evidenced by family members; explore with each individual and client. Enabling is doing for the client what he or she needs to do for self (rescuing). People want to be helpful and do not want to feel powerless to help their loved one to stop substance use and change the behavior that is so destructive. However, the substance abuser often relies on others to cover up for his or her inability to cope with daily responsibilities.
- Provide information about enabling behavior and addictive disease characteristics for both the user and nonuser. Achieving awareness and knowledge of behaviors (e.g., avoiding and shielding, taking over responsibilities, rationalizing, and subserving) provides an opportunity for individuals to begin the process of change.
- Identify and discuss the possibility of sabotage behaviors by family members. Even though family member(s) may verbalize a desire for the individual to become substance-free, the reality of interactive dynamics is that they may unconsciously not want the individual to recover, as this would affect the family members' own role in the relationship. In addition, they may receive sympathy or attention from others (secondary gain).
- Assist the client's partner to understand that the client's abstinence and drug use are not the partner's responsibility, and that the client's use of substances may or may not change despite involvement in treatment. Partners must come to realize and accept that the only behavior they can control is their own.
- Involve the family in plans for discharge from treatment. Alcohol abuse is a family illness. Because the family has been so involved in dealing with the substance abuse behavior, family members need help adjusting to the new behavior of sobriety/abstinence. Encourage involvement with self-help associations, such as Alcoholics Anonymous, Al-Anon, Alateen, and professional family therapy. This puts client and family in direct contact with support systems necessary for continued sobriety and assists with problem resolution.

Concept Care Mapping

The concept map care plan is an innovative approach to planning and organizing nursing care (see Chapter 9). It is a diagrammatic teaching and learning strategy that allows visualization of interrelationships between medical diagnoses, nursing diagnoses, assessment data, and treatments. An example of a concept map care plan for a client with a substance-related disorder is presented in Figure 27–4.

Client/Family Education

The role of client teacher is important in the psychiatric area, as it is in all areas of nursing. A list of topics for client/family education relevant to substance-related disorders is presented in Box 27–5.

Evaluation

The final step of the nursing process involves reassessment to determine if the nursing interventions have been effective in achieving the intended goals of care. Evaluation of the client with a substance-related disorder may be accomplished by using information gathered from the following reassessment questions:

1. Has detoxification occurred without complications?
2. Is the client still in denial?
3. Does the client accept responsibility for his or her own behavior? Has he or she acknowledged a personal problem with substances?
4. Has a correlation been made between personal problems and the use of substances?
5. Does the client still make excuses or blame others for use of substances?
6. Has the client remained substance-free during hospitalization?
7. Does the client cooperate with treatment?
8. Does the client refrain from manipulative behavior and violation of limits?
9. Is the client able to verbalize alternative adaptive coping strategies to substitute for substance use? Has the use of these strategies been demonstrated? Does positive reinforcement encourage repetition of these adaptive behaviors?
10. Has nutritional status been restored? Does the client consume diet adequate for his or her size and level of activity? Is the client able to discuss the importance of adequate nutrition?
11. Has the client remained free of infection during hospitalization?
12. Is the client able to verbalize the effects of substance abuse on the body?
13. Does the client verbalize that he or she wants to recover and lead a life free of substances?

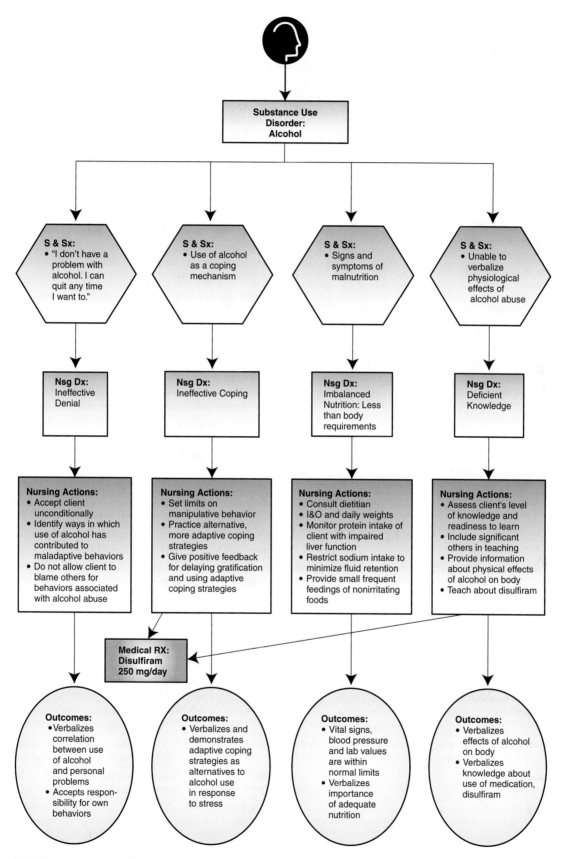

FIGURE 27–4 Concept map care plan for client with substance use disorder: alcohol.

Box 27–5 Topics for Client/Family Education Related to Substance Use Disorders

Nature of the Illness

1. Effects of (substance) on the body
   a. Alcohol
   b. Other CNS depressants
   c. CNS stimulants
   d. Hallucinogens
   e. Inhalants
   f. Opioids
   g. Cannabinols

2. Ways in which use of (substance) affects life.

Management of the Illness

1. Activities to substitute for (substance) in times of stress
2. Relaxation techniques
   a. Progressive relaxation
   b. Tense and relax
   c. Deep breathing
   d. Autogenics

3. Problem-solving skills
4. The essentials of good nutrition

Support Services

1. Financial assistance
2. Legal assistance
3. Alcoholics Anonymous (or other support group specific to another substance)
4. One-to-one support person

THE CHEMICALLY IMPAIRED NURSE

Substance abuse and dependency is a problem that has the potential for impairment in an individual's social, occupational, psychological, and physical functioning. This becomes an especially serious problem when the impaired person is responsible for the lives of others on a daily basis. Approximately 10 percent of the general population suffers from the disease of chemical dependency. It is estimated that 10 to 15 percent of nurses suffer from this disease (Raia, 2004a). Alcohol is the most widely abused drug, followed closely by narcotics.

For years, the impaired nurse was protected, promoted, transferred, ignored, or fired. These types of responses promoted the growth of the problem. Programs are needed that involve early reporting and treatment of chemical dependency as a disease, with a focus on public safety and rehabilitation of the nurse.

How does one identify the impaired nurse? It is still easiest to overlook what *might* be a problem. Denial, on the part of the impaired nurse as well as nurse colleagues, is still the strongest defense for dealing with substance-abuse problems. Some states have mandatory reporting laws that require observers to report substance-abusing

nurses to the state board of nursing. They are difficult laws to enforce, and hospitals are not always compliant with mandatory reporting. Some hospitals may choose not to report to the state board of nursing if the impaired nurse is actively seeking treatment and is not placing clients in danger.

A number of clues for recognizing substance impairment in nurses have been identified (Oklahoma Nurse Assistance Program, 2004; Raia, 2004b). They are not easy to detect and will vary according to the substance being used. There may be high absenteeism if the person's source is outside the work area, or the individual may rarely miss work if the substance source is at work. There may be an increase in "wasting" of drugs, higher incidences of incorrect narcotic counts, and a higher record of signing out drugs than for other nurses.

Poor concentration, difficulty meeting deadlines, inappropriate responses, and poor memory or recall are usually late in the disease process. The person may also have problems with relationships. Some other possible signs are irritability, tendency to isolate, elaborate excuses for behavior, unkempt appearance, impaired motor coordination, slurred speech, flushed face, lowered job performance, and frequent use of the restroom. He or she may frequently medicate other nurses' patients, and there may be patient complaints of inadequate pain control. Discrepancies in documentation may occur.

If suspicious behavior occurs, it is important to keep careful, objective records. Confrontation with the impaired nurse will undoubtedly result in hostility and denial. Confrontation should occur in the presence of a supervisor or other nurse and should include the offer of assistance in seeking treatment. If a report is made to the state board of nursing, it should be a factual documentation of specific events and actions, not a diagnostic statement of impairment.

What will the state board do? Each case is generally decided on an individual basis. A state board may deny, suspend, or revoke a license based on a report of chemical abuse by a nurse. Several state boards of nursing have passed diversionary laws that allow impaired nurses to avoid disciplinary action by agreeing to seek treatment. Some of these state boards administer the treatment programs themselves, and others refer the nurse to community resources or state nurses' association assistance programs. This may require successful completion of inpatient, outpatient, group, or individual counseling treatment program(s); evidence of regular attendance at nurse support groups or 12-step program; random negative drug screens; and employment or volunteer activities during the suspension period. When a nurse is deemed safe to return to practice, he or she may be closely monitored for several years and required to undergo random drug screenings. The nurse also may be required to practice under specifically circumscribed conditions for a designated period of time.

In 1982, the ANA House of Delegates adopted a national resolution to provide assistance to impaired nurses. Since that time, the majority of state nurses' associations have developed (or are developing) programs for nurses who are impaired by substances or psychiatric illness. The individuals who administer these efforts are nurse members of the state associations, as well as nurses who are in recovery themselves. For this reason, they are called **peer assistance programs**.

The peer assistance programs strive to intervene early, to reduce hazards to clients, and increase prospects for the nurse's recovery. Most states provide either a hot-line number that the impaired nurse or intervening colleague may call or phone numbers of peer assistance committee members, which are made available for the same purpose. Typically, a contract is drawn up detailing the method of treatment, which may be obtained from various sources, such as employee assistance programs, Alcoholics Anonymous, Narcotics Anonymous, private counseling, or outpatient clinics. Guidelines for monitoring the course of treatment are established. Peer support is provided through regular contact with the impaired nurse, usually for a period of 2 years. Peer assistance programs serve to assist impaired nurses to recognize their impairment, to obtain necessary treatment, and to regain accountability within their profession.

CODEPENDENCY

The concept of codependency arose out of a need to define the dysfunctional behaviors that are evident among members of the family of a chemically dependent person. The term has been expanded to include all individuals from families that harbor secrets of physical or emotional abuse, other cruelties, or pathological conditions. Living under these conditions results in unmet needs for autonomy and self-esteem and a profound sense of powerlessness. The codependent person is able to achieve a sense of control only through fulfilling the needs of others. Personal identity is relinquished and boundaries with the other person become blurred. The codependent person disowns his or her own needs and wants in order to respond to external demands and the demands of others. Burney (1996) refers to codependence as a dysfunctional relationship with oneself.

The traits associated with a codependent personality are varied. The *DSM-IV-TR* (APA, 2000) states that personality traits only become disorders when they are "inflexible and maladaptive and cause significant functional impairment or subjective distress." To date, no diagnostic criteria exist for the diagnosis of codependent personality disorder.

A codependent individual is confused about his or her own identity. In a relationship, the codependent person derives self-worth from that of the partner, whose feelings and behaviors determine how the codependent should feel and behave. In order for the codependent to feel good, his or her partner must be happy and behave in appropriate ways. If the partner is not happy, the codependent feels responsible for *making* him or her happy. The codependent's home life is fraught with stress. Ego boundaries are weak and behaviors are often enmeshed with those of the pathological partner. Denial that problems exist is common. Feelings are kept in control, and anxiety may be released in the form of stress-related illnesses or compulsive behaviors such as eating, spending, working, or use of substances.

Wesson (2007) describes the following behaviors characteristic of codependency. She stated that codependents:

1. Have a long history of focusing thoughts and behavior on other people.
2. Are "people pleasers" and will do almost anything to get the approval of others.
3. Seem very competent on the outside but actually feel quite needy, helpless, or perhaps nothing at all.
4. Have experienced abuse or emotional neglect as a child.
5. Are outwardly focused toward others, and know very little about how to direct their own lives from their own sense of self.

The Codependent Nurse

Certain characteristics of codependence have been associated with the profession of nursing. A shortage of nurses combined with the increasing ranks of seriously ill clients may result in nurses providing care and fulfilling everyone's needs but their own. Many healthcare workers who have been reared in homes with a chemically dependent person or otherwise dysfunctional family are at risk for having any unresolved codependent tendencies activated. Nurses who as children assumed the "fixer" role in their dysfunctional families of origin may attempt to resume that role in their caregiving professions. They are attracted to a profession in which they are needed, but they nurture feelings of resentment for receiving so little in return. Their emotional needs go unmet; however, they continue to deny that these needs exist. Instead, these unmet emotional needs may be manifested through use of compulsive behaviors, such as work or spending excessively, or addictions, such as to food or substances.

Codependent nurses have a need to be in control. They often strive for an unrealistic level of achievement. Their self-worth comes from the feeling of being needed by others and of maintaining control over their environment. They nurture the dependence of others and accept the responsibility for the happiness and contentment of others. They rarely express their true feelings, and do what is necessary to preserve harmony and maintain control. They are at high risk for physical and emotional burn out.

Treating Codependence

Cermak (1986) identified four stages in the recovery process for individuals with codependent personality.

Stage I: The Survival Stage. In this first stage, codependent persons must begin to let go of the denial that problems exist or that their personal capabilities are unlimited. This initiation of abstinence from blanket denial may be a very emotional and painful period.

Stage II: The Reidentification Stage. Reidentification occurs when the individuals are able to glimpse their true selves through a break in the denial system. They accept the label of codependent and take responsibility for their own dysfunctional behavior. Codependents tend to enter reidentification only after being convinced that it is more painful not to. They accept their limitations and are ready to face the issues of codependence.

Stage III: The Core Issues Stage. In this stage, the recovering codependent must face the fact that relationships cannot be managed by force of will. Each partner must be independent and autonomous. The goal of this stage is to detach from the struggles of life that exist because of prideful and willful efforts to control those things that are beyond the individual's power to control.

Stage IV: The Reintegration Stage. This is a stage of self-acceptance and willingness to change when codependents relinquish the power *over others* that was not rightfully theirs but reclaim the *personal* power that they do possess. Integrity is achieved out of awareness, honesty, and being in touch with one's spiritual consciousness. Control is achieved through self-discipline and self-confidence.

Self-help groups have been found to be helpful in the treatment of codependency. Groups developed for families of chemically dependent people, such as Al-Anon, may be of assistance. Groups specific to the problem of codependency also exist. Two of these groups include:

Co-Dependents Anonymous (CoDA)
P.O. Box 33577
Phoenix, AZ 85067-3577
602-277-7991

Co-Dependents Anonymous for Helping Professionals
  (CODAHP)
P.O. Box 42253
Mesa, AZ 85274-2253
602-644-8605

Both of these groups apply the Twelve Steps and Twelve Traditions developed by Alcoholics Anonymous to codependency (Box 27–6).

TREATMENT MODALITIES FOR SUBSTANCE-RELATED DISORDERS

Alcoholics Anonymous

Alcoholics Anonymous (AA) is a major self-help organization for the treatment of alcoholism. It was founded in 1935 by two alcoholics—a stockbroker, Bill Wilson, and a physician, Dr. Bob Smith—who discovered that they could remain sober through mutual support. This they accomplished not as professionals, but as peers who were able to share their common experiences. Soon they were working with other alcoholics, who in turn worked with others. The movement grew, and remarkably, individuals who had been treated unsuccessfully by professionals were able to maintain sobriety through helping one another.

Today AA chapters exist in virtually every community in the United States. The self-help groups are based on the concept of peer support—acceptance and understanding from others who have experienced the same problems in their lives. The only requirement for membership is a desire on the part of the alcoholic person to stop drinking. Each new member is assigned a support person from whom he or she may seek assistance when the temptation to drink occurs.

A survey by the General Service Office of Alcoholics Anonymous in 2004 (Alcoholics Anonymous [AA], 2005) revealed the following statistics: members ages 30 and younger comprise 10 percent of the membership and the average age of an AA members is 48; women comprise 35 percent; 89.1 percent are white, 3.2 percent are African American, 4.4 percent are Hispanic, 1.8 percent are Native American, and 1.5 percent were Asian American and other minorities. By occupation, the highest percentages included the following: 14 percent were retired; 11 percent were self-employed; 10 percent were managers or administrators; and 10 percent were in professional or technical fields.

The sole purpose of AA is to help members stay sober. When sobriety has been achieved, they in turn are expected to help other alcoholic persons. The Twelve Steps that embody the philosophy of AA provide specific guidelines on how to attain and maintain sobriety (Box 27–6).

AA accepts alcoholism as an illness and promotes total abstinence as the only cure, emphasizing that the alcoholic person can never safely return to social drinking. They encourage the members to seek sobriety, taking one day at a time. The Twelve Traditions are the statements of principles that govern the organization (Box 27–6).

AA has been the model for various other self-help groups associated with abuse or dependency problems. Some of these groups and the memberships for which they are organized are listed in Table 27–11. Nurses need to be fully and accurately informed about available self-help groups and their importance as a treatment resource on the health care continuum so that they can use them as a referral source for clients with substance-related disorders.

Pharmacotherapy

Disulfiram (Antabuse)

Disulfiram (Antabuse) is a drug that can be administered to individuals who abuse alcohol as a deterrent to

BOX 27–6 Alcoholics Anonymous

The Twelve Steps	The Twelve Traditions
1. We admitted we were powerless over alcohol—that our lives have become unmanageable. 2. Came to believe that a Power greater than ourselves could restore us to sanity. 3. Made a decision to turn our will and our lives over to the care of God as we understood Him. 4. Made a searching and fearless moral inventory of ourselves. 5. Admitted to God, to ourselves, and to another human being the exact nature of our wrongs. 6. Were entirely ready to have God remove all these defects of character. 7. Humbly asked Him to remove our shortcomings. 8. Made a list of all persons we had harmed and became willing to make amends to them all. 9. Made direct amends to such people wherever possible except when to do so would injure them or others. 10. Continued to take personal inventory and when we were wrong promptly admitted it. 11. Sought through prayer and meditation to improve our conscious contact with God as we understood Him, praying only for knowledge of His will for us and the power to carry that out. 12. Having had a spiritual awakening as the result of these steps, we tried to carry this message to alcoholics and to practice these principles in all our affairs.	1. Our common welfare should come first; personal recovery depends upon AA unity. 2. For our group purpose there is but one ultimate authority—a loving God as He may express Himself in our group conscience. Our leaders are but trusted servants; they do not govern. 3. The one requirement for AA membership is a desire to stop drinking. 4. Each group should be autonomous except in matters affecting other groups or AA as a whole. 5. Each group has but one primary purpose—to carry its message to the alcoholic who still suffers. 6. An AA group ought never endorse, finance, or lend the AA name to any related facility or outside enterprise, lest problems of money, property, and prestige divert us from our primary purpose. 7. Every AA group ought to be fully self-supporting, declining outside contributions. 8. Alcoholics Anonymous should remain forever nonprofessional, but our service centers may employ special workers. 9. Alcoholics Anonymous, as such, ought never be organized; but we may create service boards of committees directly responsible to those they serve. 10. Alcoholics Anonymous has no opinion on outside issues; hence, the Alcoholics Anonymous name ought never be drawn into public controversy. 11. Our public relations policy is based on attraction rather than promotion; we need always maintain personal anonymity at the level of press, radio, and films. 12. Anonymity is the spiritual foundation of all our traditions, ever reminding us to place principles before personalities.

The Twelve Steps and Twelve Traditions are reprinted with permission of Alcoholics Anonymous World Services, Inc. (AAWS). Permission to reprint the Twelve Steps and Twelve Traditions does not mean that AAWS has reviewed or approved the contents of this publication, or that AA necessarily agrees with the views expressed herein. AA is a program of recovery from alcoholism *only*. Use of the Twelve Steps and Twelve Traditions in connection with programs and activities which are patterned after AA, but which address other problems, or in any other non-AA context, does not imply otherwise.

TABLE 27–11 Addiction Self-Help Groups

Group	Membership
Adult Children of Alcoholics (ACOA)	Adults who grew up with an alcoholic in the home
Al-Anon	Families of alcoholics
Alateen	Adolescent children of alcoholics
Children Are People	School-age children with an alcoholic family member
Cocaine Anonymous	Cocaine addicts
Families Anonymous	Parents of children who abuse substances
Fresh Start	Nicotine addicts
Narcotics Anonymous	Narcotics addicts
Nar-Anon	Families of narcotics addicts
Overeaters Anonymous	Food addicts
Pills Anonymous	Polysubstance addicts
Potsmokers Anonymous	Marijuana smokers
Smokers Anonymous	Nicotine addicts
Women for Sobriety	Female alcoholics

drinking. Ingestion of alcohol while disulfiram is in the body results in a syndrome of symptoms that can produce a good deal of discomfort for the individual. It can even result in death if the blood alcohol level is high. The reaction varies according to the sensitivity of the individual and how much alcohol was ingested.

Disulfiram works by inhibiting the enzyme aldehyde dehydrogenase, thereby blocking the oxidation of alcohol at the stage when acetaldehyde is converted to acetate. This results in an accumulation of acetaldehyde in the blood, which is thought to produce the symptoms associated with the disulfiram–alcohol reaction. These symptoms persist as long as alcohol is being metabolized. The rate of alcohol elimination does not appear to be affected.

Symptoms of disulfiram–alcohol reaction can occur within 5 to 10 minutes of ingestion of alcohol. Mild reactions can occur at blood alcohol levels as low as 5 to 10 mg/dL. Symptoms are fully developed at approximately 50 mg/dL, and may include flushed skin, throbbing in the head and neck, respiratory difficulty, dizziness, nausea and vomiting, sweating, hyperventilation, tachycardia, hypotension, weakness, blurred vision, and confusion. With a blood alcohol level of approximately 125 to 150 mg/dL, severe reactions can occur, including respiratory depression, cardiovascular collapse, arrhythmias, myocardial infarction, acute congestive heart failure, unconsciousness, convulsions, and death.

Disulfiram should not be administered until it has been ascertained that the client has abstained from alcohol for at least 12 hours. If disulfiram is discontinued, it is important for the client to understand that the sensitivity to alcohol may last for as long as 2 weeks. Consuming alcohol or alcohol-containing substances during this 2-week period could result in the disulfiram–alcohol reaction.

The client receiving disulfiram therapy should be aware of the large number of alcohol-containing substances. These products, such as liquid cough and cold preparations, vanilla extract, after-shave lotions, colognes, mouthwash, nail polish removers, and isopropyl alcohol, if ingested or even rubbed on the skin, are capable of producing the symptoms described. The individual must read labels carefully and must inform any doctor, dentist, or other healthcare professional from whom assistance is sought that he or she is taking disulfiram. In addition, it is important that the client carry a card explaining participation in disulfiram therapy, possible consequences of the therapy, and symptoms that may indicate an emergency situation.

Obviously, the client must be assessed carefully before beginning disulfiram therapy. A thorough medical screening is performed before starting therapy, and written informed consent is usually required. The drug is contraindicated for clients who are at high risk for alcohol ingestion. It is also contraindicated for psychotic clients and clients with severe cardiac, renal, or hepatic disease.

Disulfiram therapy is not a cure for alcoholism. It provides a measure of control for the individual who desires to avoid impulse drinking. Clients receiving disulfiram therapy are encouraged to seek other assistance with their problem, such as AA or other support group, to aid in the recovery process.

Other Medications for Treatment of Alcoholism

The narcotic antagonist naltrexone (ReVia) was approved by the Food and Drug Administration (FDA) in 1994 for the treatment of alcohol dependence. Naltrexone, which was approved in 1984 for the treatment of heroin abuse, works on the same receptors in the brain that produce the feelings of pleasure when heroin or other opiates bind to them, but it does not produce the "narcotic high" and is not habit forming. Although alcohol does not bind to these same brain receptors, studies have shown that naltrexone works equally well against it (O'Malley et al., 1992; Volpicelli, Alterman, Hayashida, & O'Brien, 1992). In comparison to placebo-treated clients, subjects on naltrexone therapy showed significantly lower overall relapse rates and fewer drinks per drinking day among those clients who did resume drinking. A study with an oral form of nalmefene (Revex) produced similar results (Mason et al., 1994).

The efficacy of selective serotonin reuptake inhibitors (SSRIs) in the decrease of alcohol craving among alcohol-dependent individuals has yielded mixed results (NIAAA, 2000). A greater degree of success was observed with moderate drinkers than with heavy drinkers.

In August, 2004, the FDA approved acamprosate (Campral), which is indicated for the maintenance of abstinence from alcohol in patients with alcohol dependence who are abstinent at treatment initiation. The mechanism of action of acamprosate in maintenance of alcohol abstinence is not completely understood. It is hypothesized to restore the normal balance between neuronal excitation and inhibition by interacting with glutamate and gamma-aminobutyric acid (GABA) neurotransmitter systems. Acamprosate is ineffective in clients who have not undergone detoxification and not achieved alcohol abstinence before beginning treatment. It is recommended for concomitant use with psychosocial therapy.

Counseling

Counseling on a one-to-one basis is often used to help the client who abuses substances. The relationship is goal-directed, and the length of the counseling may vary from weeks to years. The focus is on current reality, development of a working treatment relationship, and strengthening ego assets. The counselor must be warm, kind, and nonjudgmental, yet able to set limits firmly.

REVIEW QUESTIONS

Self-Examination/Learning Exercise

Select the answer that is most appropriate for each of the following questions:

Situation: Mr. White is admitted to the hospital after an extended period of binge alcohol drinking. His wife reports that he has been a heavy drinker for a number of years. Lab reports reveal he has a blood alcohol level of 250 mg/dL. He is placed on the chemical dependency unit for detoxification.

1. When would the *first signs* of alcohol withdrawal symptoms be expected to occur?
   a. Within 12 hours after the last drink
   b. Forty-eight to 72 hours after the last drink
   c. Four to 5 days after the last drink
   d. Six to 7 days after the last drink

2. Symptoms of alcohol withdrawal include:
   a. Euphoria, hyperactivity, and insomnia
   b. Depression, suicidal ideation, and hypersomnia
   c. Diaphoresis, nausea and vomiting, and tremors
   d. Unsteady gait, nystagmus, and profound disorientation

3. Which of the following medications is the physician most likely to order for Mr. White during his withdrawal syndrome?
   a. Haloperidol (Haldol)
   b. Chlordiazepoxide (Librium)
   c. Propoxyphene (Darvon)
   d. Phenytoin (Dilantin)

Situation: Dan, age 32, has been admitted for inpatient treatment of his alcoholism. He began drinking when he was 15 years old. Through the years, the amount of alcohol he consumes has increased. He and his wife report that for the last 5 years he has consumed at least a pint of bourbon a day. He also drinks beer and wine. He has been sneaking drinks at work, and his effectiveness has started to decline. His boss has told him he must seek treatment or he will be fired. This is his second week in treatment. The first week he experienced an uncomplicated detoxification.

4. Dan states, "I don't have a problem with alcohol. I can handle my booze better than anyone I know. My boss is a jerk! I haven't missed any more days than my coworkers." The nurse's best response is:
   a. "Maybe your boss is mistaken, Dan."
   b. "You are here because your drinking was interfering with your work, Dan."
   c. "Get real, Dan! You're a boozer and you know it!"
   d. "Why do you think your boss sent you here, Dan?"

5. The defense mechanism that Dan is using is:
   a. Denial.
   b. Projection.
   c. Displacement.
   d. Rationalization.

6. Dan's drinking buddies come for a visit, and when they leave, the nurse smells alcohol on Dan's breath. Which of the following would be the best intervention with Dan at this time?
   a. Search his room for evidence.
   b. Ask, "Have you been drinking alcohol, Dan?"
   c. Send a urine specimen from Dan to the lab for drug screening.
   d. Tell Dan, "These guys cannot come to the unit to visit you again."

7. Dan begins attendance at AA meetings. Which of the statements by Dan reflects the purpose of this organization?
   a. "They claim they will help me stay sober."
   b. "I'll dry out in AA, then I can have a social drink now and then."
   c. "AA is only for people who have reached the bottom."
   d. "If I lose my job, AA will help me find another."

The following general questions relate to substance abuse.

8. From which of the following symptoms might the nurse identify a chronic cocaine user?
   a. Clear, constricted pupils
   b. Red, irritated nostrils
   c. Muscle aches
   d. Conjunctival redness

9. An individual who is addicted to heroin is likely to experience which of the following symptoms of withdrawal?
   a. Increased heart rate and blood pressure
   b. Tremors, insomnia, and seizures
   c. Incoordination and unsteady gait
   d. Nausea and vomiting, diarrhea, and diaphoresis

10. A polysubstance abuser makes the statement, "The green and whites do me good after speed." How might the nurse interpret the statement?
    a. The client abuses amphetamines and anxiolytics.
    b. The client abuses alcohol and cocaine.
    c. The client is psychotic.
    d. The client abuses narcotics and marijuana.

Test Your Critical Thinking Skills

Kelly, age 23, is a first-year law student. She is engaged to a surgical resident at the local university hospital. She has been struggling to do well in law school because she wants to make her parents, two prominent local attorneys, proud of her. She had never aspired to do anything but go into law, and that is also what her parents expected her to do.

Kelly's mid-term grades were not as high as she had hoped, so she increased the number of hours of study time, staying awake all night several nights a week to study. She started drinking large amounts of coffee to stay awake, but still found herself falling asleep as she tried to study at the library and in her apartment. As final exams approached, she began to panic that she would not be able to continue the pace of studying she felt she needed in order to make the grades she hoped for.

One of Kelly's classmates told her that she needed some "speed" to give her that extra energy to study. Her classmate said, "All the kids do it. Hardly anyone I know gets through law school without it." She gave Kelly the name of a source.

Kelly contacted the source, who supplied her with enough amphetamines to see her through final exams. Kelly was excited, because she had so much energy, did not require sleep, and was able to study the additional hours she thought she needed for the exams. However, when the results were posted, Kelly had failed two courses and would have to repeat them in summer school if she was to continue with her class in the fall. She continued to replenish her supply of amphetamines from her "contact" until he told her he could not get her anymore. She became frantic and stole a prescription blank from her fiancé and forged his name for more pills.

She started taking more and more of the medication in order to achieve the "high" she wanted to feel. Her behavior became erratic. Yesterday, her fiancé received a call from a pharmacy to clarify an order for amphetamines that Kelly had written. He insisted that she admit herself to the chemical dependency unit for detoxification.

On the unit, she appears tired, depressed, moves very slowly, and wants to sleep all the time. She keeps saying to the nurse, "I'm a real failure. I'll never be an attorney like my parents. I'm too dumb. I just wish I could die."

Answer the following questions related to Kelly:

1. What is the primary nursing diagnosis for Kelly?
2. Describe important nursing interventions to be implemented with Kelly.
3. In addition to physical safety, what would be the primary short-term goal the nurses would strive to achieve with Kelly?

REFERENCES

Alcoholics Anonymous (AA). (2005). *Alcoholics Anonymous 2004 membership survey.* Retrieved March 10, 2007 from http://www.aa.org/

American Insomnia Association. (2005). Medications: History. Retrieved March 11, 2007 from http://www.americaninsomniaassociation.org/medications.htm

Andreasen, N.C., & Black, D.W. (2006). *Introductory textbook of psychiatry* (4th ed.). Washington, DC: American Psychiatric Publishing.

Ashton, C.H. (2002). *Benzodiazepines: How they work and how to withdraw.* Newcastle upon Tyne, UK: University of Newcastle.

American Psychiatric Association. (2000). *Diagnostic and statistical manual of mental disorders* (4th ed.) *Text revision.* Washington, DC.: American Psychiatric Publishing.

Barclay, L.L. (2005). *Alcohol-related neurologic disease.* Retrieved March 11, 2007 from http://www2.vhihealthe.com/article/gale/100085011

Behavioral Neuroscience Laboratory. (2002). *Tetrahydroisoquinolines and alcohol preference in rats.* Retrieved February 14, 2002 from http://www-org.usm.edu/~neurolab/research.htm

Bruckenthal, P. (2001). *Managing nonmalignant pain: Challenges for clinicians.* Paper presented April 19–22, 2001, at the 20th Annual Meeting of the American Pain Society.

Burney, R. (1996). *Codependence—the dance of wounded souls.* Cambria, CA: Joy to You & Me Enterprises.

Carmona, R.H. (2005). *Surgeon General's Advisory on Alcohol Use in Pregnancy.* Washington, DC: U.S. Department of Health and Human Services.

Centers for Disease Control (CDC). (2005). Guidelines for identifying and referring persons with fetal alcohol syndrome. *MMWR, 54*(RR-11). Atlanta: U.S. Department of Health and Human Services.

Daly, R. (2007). Congress lets MDs treat more buprenorphine patients. *Psychiatric News, 42*(1), 4.

Goldstein, A. (2002). *Addiction: From biology to drug policy* (2nd ed.). New York: Oxford University Press.

Greer, M. (2004, October). Statistics show mental health services still needed for native populations. *APA Online, 35*(9). Retrieved March 11, 2007 from http://www.apa.org/monitor/oct04/services.html

Habal, R. (2006). Toxicity, barbiturate. Retrieved March 8, 2007 from http://www.emedicine.com/med/topic207.htm

Hanley, C.E. (2004). Navajos. In J.N. Giger & R.E. Davidhizar (Eds.), *Transcultural nursing* (4th ed.). St. Louis: C.V. Mosby.

Harvard Medical School. (2001). *Alcohol use and abuse.* Boston: Harvard Health Publications.

Harvard Medical School. (2003, September). Dual diagnosis: Part II. *Harvard Mental Health Letter, 20*(3), 1–5.

Harvard Medical School. (2004, September). Alcohol before birth. *Harvard Mental Health Letter, 21*(3), 1–8.

Jamal, M., Ameno, K., Kubota, A., Ameno, S., Zhang, X., Kumihashi, M., & Ijiri, I. (2003). In vivo formation of salsolinol induced by high acetaldehyde concentration in rat striatum employing microdialysis. *Alcohol and Alcoholism, 38*(3), 197–201.

Julien, R.M. (2005). *A primer of drug action: A comprehensive guide to actions, uses and side effects of psychoactive drugs* (10th ed.). New York: Worth.

Knowles, J.A. (2003). Genetics. In R.E. Hales & S.C. Yudofsky, (Eds.), *Textbook of clinical psychiatry* (4th ed.). Washington, DC: American Psychiatric Publishing.

Mack, A.H., Franklin, J.E., & Frances, R.J. (2003). Substance Use Disorders. In R.E. Hales & S.C. Yudofsky (Eds.), *Textbook of clinical psychiatry* (4th ed.). Washington, DC: American Psychiatric Publishing.

Maier, S.E., & West, J.R. (2001). Drinking patterns and alcohol-related birth defects. *Alcohol Research & Health, 25*(3), 168–174.

Mason, G.J., Ritvo, E.C., Morgan, R.O., Salvanto, F.R., Goldberg, G., Welch, B., & Mantero-Atienza, E. (1994). Double-blind, placebo-controlled pilot study to evaluate the efficacy and safety of oral nalmefene HCl for alcohol dependence. *Alcoholism, Clinical and Experimental Research, 18*(5), 1162–1167.

Mayo Foundation for Medical Education and Research. (2005). Cirrhosis. Retrieved March 8, 2007 from http://www.ohiohealth.com/healthreference

Najavits, L.M., & Weiss, R.D. (1994). Variations in therapist effectiveness in the treatment of patients with substance use disorders: An empirical review. *Addiction 89*(6), 679–688.

NANDA International (NANDA-I). (2007). *Nursing diagnoses: Definitions & classification 2007–2008.* Philadelphia: NANDA International.

National Council on Alcoholism and Drug Dependence. (2005). *Alcohol and drug dependence are America's number one health problem.* Retrieved March 8, 2007 from http://www.ncadd.org/facts/numberoneprob.html

National Institute on Alcohol Abuse and Alcoholism (NIAAA). (2000). *Tenth Special Report to the U.S. Congress on Alcohol and Health.* Bethesda, MD: The Institute.

National Institute on Alcohol Abuse and Alcoholism (NIAAA). (2005). Alcohol and hormones. Retrieved March 8, 2007 from http://www.niaaa.nih.gov/

National Institutes of Health (NIH) (2003). Workshop on the medical utility of marijuana. Retrieved March 8, 2007 from http://www.nih.gov/news/medmarijuana/MedicalMarijuana.htm#CLINICAL

National Library of Medicine. (2007). *Hepatic encephalopathy.* Retrieved March 6, 2007 from http://www.nlm.nih.gov/medlineplus/ency/article/000302.htm

Newhouse, E. (1999, August 22). Bane of the Blackfeet. *Great Falls Tribune.* Retrieved March 6, 2007 from http://www.gannett.com/go/difference/greatfalls/pages/part8/blackfeet.html

Oklahoma Nurse Assistance Program (ONAP). (2004). *Substance abuse employment behaviors.* Oklahoma City, OK: Oklahoma Nurses Association.

O'Malley, S.S., Jaffe, A.J., Chang, G., Schottenfeld, R.S., Meyer, R.E., & Rounsaville, B. (1992). Naltrexone and coping skills therapy for alcohol dependence: A controlled study. *Archives of General Psychiatry, 49*(11), 881–887.

Raia, S. (2004a). The problem of impaired practice. *New Jersey Nurse, 34*(6), 8.

Raia, S. (2004b). Understanding chemical dependency. *New Jersey Nurse, 34*(7), 8.

Royal College of Physicians. (2000). *Nicotine addition in Britain.* London: Royal College of Physicians.

Sadock, B.J., & Sadock, V.A. (2007). *Synopsis of psychiatry: Behavioral sciences/clinical psychiatry* (10th ed.). Philadelphia: Lippincott Williams & Wilkins.

Street Drugs. (2005). Plymouth, MN: The Publishers Group.

Substance Abuse and Mental Health Services Administration (SAMHSA). (2007). *2006 National Survey on Drug Use & Health.* Retrieved February 2, 2008 from http://www.oas.samhsa.gov/

Tazbir, J., & Keresztes, P.A. (2005). Management of clients with functional cardiac disorders. In J.M. Black & J.H. Hawks (Eds.), *Medical-surgical nursing: Clinical management for positive outcomes* (7th ed.). St. Louis: Elsevier Saunders.

U.S. Drug Enforcement Administration (USDEA). (2003). *Drug information:Cannabis.* Retrieved October 9, 2003 from http://www.dea.gov

Volpicelli, J.R., Alterman, A.I., Hayashida, M., & O'Brien, C.P. (1992). Naltrexone in the treatment of alcohol dependence. *Archives of General Psychiatry, 49*(11), 876–880.

Wehrspann, B. (2006). ADHD related to fetal alcohol syndrome. *Medscape Psychiatry & Mental Health.* Retrieved March 7, 2007 from http://www.medscape.com/viewarticle/546475

Wesson, N. (2007). *Codependence: What is it? How do I know if I am codependent?* Retrieved March 10, 2007 from http://www.wespsych.com/codepend.html

CLASSICAL REFERENCES

Cermak, T.L. (1986). Diagnosing *and treating co-dependence*. Center City, MN: Hazelton Publishing.

Jellinek, E.M. (1952). Phases of alcohol addiction. *Quarterly Journal of Studies on Alcohol, 13*, 673–684.

Mayfield, D., McLeod, G., & Hall, P. (1974). The CAGE questionnaire: Validation of a new alcoholism screening instrument. *American Journal of Psychiatry, 131*, 1121–1123.

Seltzer, M.L. (1971). The Michigan Alcoholism Screening Test: The quest for a new diagnostic instrument. *American Journal of Psychiatry, 127*, 1653–1658.

@ Internet References

- Additional information on addictions is located at the following Web sites:
  - http://www.samhsa.gov/index.aspx
  - http://www.ccsa.ca/CCSA/EN/Topics
  - http://www.well.com/user/woa/
  - http://www.apa.org/about/division/div50.html

- Additional information on self-help organizations is located at the following Web sites:
  - http://www.ca.org (Cocaine Anonymous)
  - http://www.aa.org (Alcoholics Anonymous)
  - http://www.na.org (Narcotics Anonymous)
  - http://www.al-anon.org

- Additional information about medications for treatment of alcohol and drug dependence is located at the following Web sites:
  - http://www.fadavis.com/Townsend
  - http://www.nlm.nih.gov/medlineplus/
  - http://www.nimh.nih.gov/publicat/medicate.cfm

Schizophrenia and Other Psychotic Disorders

CHAPTER OUTLINE

KEY TERMS

anhedonia
associative looseness
autism
catatonic
circumstantiality
clang association
delusions
echolalia
echopraxia
hallucinations
illusion

magical thinking
neologism
neuroleptics
paranoia
perseveration
religiosity
social skills training
tangentiality
waxy flexibility
word salad

CORE CONCEPT

psychosis

OBJECTIVES

After reading this chapter, the student will be able to:

1. Discuss the concepts of schizophrenia and related psychotic disorders.
2. Identify predisposing factors in the development of these disorders.
3. Describe various types of schizophrenia and related psychotic disorders.
4. Identify symptomatology associated with these disorders and use this information in client assessment.
5. Formulate nursing diagnoses and outcomes of care for clients with schizophrenia and other psychotic disorders.

6. Identify topics for client and family teaching relevant to schizophrenia and other psychotic disorders.
7. Describe appropriate nursing interventions for behaviors associated with these disorders.
8. Describe relevant criteria for evaluating nursing care of clients with schizophrenia and related psychotic disorders.
9. Discuss various modalities relevant to treatment of schizophrenia and related psychotic disorders.

The term *schizophrenia* was coined in 1908 by the Swiss psychiatrist Eugen Bleuler. The word was derived from the Greek "skhizo" (split) and "phren" (mind).

Over the years, much debate has surrounded the concept of schizophrenia. Various definitions of the disorder have evolved, and numerous treatment strategies have been proposed, but none have proven to be uniformly effective or sufficient.

Although the controversy lingers, two general factors appear to be gaining acceptance among clinicians. The first is that schizophrenia is probably not a homogeneous disease entity with a single cause but results from a variable combination of genetic predisposition, biochemical dysfunction, physiological factors, and psychosocial stress. The second factor is that there is not now and probably never will be a single treatment that cures the disorder. Instead, effective treatment requires a comprehensive, multidisciplinary effort, including pharmacotherapy and various forms of psychosocial care, such as living skills and **social skills training**, rehabilitation, and family therapy.

Of all the mental illnesses that cause suffering in society, schizophrenia probably is responsible for lengthier hospitalizations, greater chaos in family life, more exorbitant costs to individuals and governments, and more fears than any other. Because it is such an enormous threat to life and happiness and because its causes are an unsolved puzzle, it has probably been studied more than any other mental disorder.

Potential for suicide is a major concern among patients with schizophrenia. Radomsky, Haas, Mann, and Sweeney (1999) report that suicide is the primary cause of premature death among individuals with the disorder. They estimate that approximately 10 percent of patients with schizophrenia die by suicide. Other studies estimate evidence of suicidal ideation in individuals with schizophrenia to be in the range of 40 to 55 percent and attempted suicide to be in the range of 20 to 50 percent (Addington, 2006).

Ho, Black, and Andreasen (2003) have stated:

Schizophrenia is perhaps the most enigmatic and tragic disease that psychiatrists treat, and perhaps also the most devastating. It is one of the leading causes of disability among young adults. Schizophrenia strikes at a young age so that, unlike patients with cancer or heart disease, patients with schizophrenia usually live many years after onset of the disease and continue to suffer its effects, which prevent them from leading fully normal lives—attending school, working, having a close network of friends, marrying, or having children. Apart from its effect on individuals and families, schizophrenia creates a huge economic burden for society. A study at the National Institute of Mental Health calculated the total cost of schizophrenia in 1991 at $65 billion. Despite its emotional and economic costs, schizophrenia has yet to receive sufficient recognition as a major health concern or the necessary research support to investigate its causes, treatments, and prevention. (p. 379)

This chapter explores various theories of predisposing factors that have been implicated in the development of

schizophrenia. Symptomatology associated with different diagnostic categories of the disorder is discussed. Nursing care is presented in the context of the six steps of the nursing process. Various dimensions of medical treatment are explored.

NATURE OF THE DISORDER

 CORE CONCEPT

Psychosis

A severe mental condition in which there is disorganization of the personality, deterioration in social functioning, and loss of contact with, or distortion of, reality. There may be evidence of hallucinations and delusional thinking. Psychosis can occur with or without the presence of organic impairment.

Perhaps no psychological disorder is more crippling than schizophrenia. Characteristically, disturbances in thought processes, perception, and affect invariably result in a severe deterioration of social and occupational functioning.

In the United States, the lifetime prevalence of schizophrenia is about 1 percent (Sadock & Sadock, 2007). Symptoms generally appear in late adolescence or early adulthood, although they may occur in middle or late adult life (American Psychiatric Association [APA], 2000). Some studies have indicated that symptoms occur earlier in men than in women. The premorbid personality often indicates social maladjustment or schizoid or other personality disturbances (Ho, Black, & Andreasen, 2003). This premorbid behavior is often a predictor in the pattern of development of schizophrenia, which can be viewed in four phases.

Phase I: The Premorbid Phase

The premorbid phase is marked by a period of normal functioning, although events can occur that contribute to the development of the subsequent illness (Lehman et al., 2006). A number of factors have been identified as premorbid indicators of psychosis, which may be divided into two categories: (1) early precursors of etiological interest and (2) personality and behavioral measurements signaling latent mental illness (Olin & Mednick, 1996). Early precursors of etiological interest include family psychiatric history, perinatal and obstetric complications, and neurobehavioral deficits (e.g., poor motor coordination). Premorbid personality and behavioral measurements that have been noted include being very shy and withdrawn, having poor peer relationships, doing poorly in school, and demonstrating antisocial behavior. Olin and Mednick (1996) state:

Most schizophrenia patients are not distinguishable from their peers in childhood. Deviant behaviors tend to become more prominent in adolescence, a time of life that may present more socially challenging situations. Sex differences in social adjustment have also been noted, with males showing more antisocial behaviors and females showing more passivity and withdrawal. (p. 228)

Phase II: The Prodromal Phase

The prodrome of an illness refers to certain signs and symptoms that precede the characteristic manifestations of the acute, fully developed illness. The prodromal phase of schizophrenia begins with a change from premorbid functioning and extends until the onset of frank psychotic symptoms. This phase can be as brief as a few weeks or months, but most studies indicate that the average length of the prodromal phase is between 2 and 5 years. Lehman and associates (2006) state:

> During the prodromal phase the person experiences substantial functional impairment and nonspecific symptoms such as a sleep disturbance, anxiety, irritability, depressed mood, poor concentration, fatigue, and behavioral deficits such as deterioration in role functioning and social withdrawal. Positive symptoms such as perceptual abnormalities, ideas of reference, and suspiciousness develop late in the prodromal phase and herald the imminent onset of psychosis. (pp. 625–626)

Recognition of the behaviors associated with the prodromal phase provides an opportunity for early intervention with a possibility for improvement in long-term outcomes. Current treatment guidelines suggest therapeutic interventions that offer support with identified problems, cognitive therapies to minimize functional impairment, family interventions to improve coping, and involvement with schools to reduce the possibility of failure. Perkins (2004) states, "Pharmacologic intervention targeting the prodromal symptoms is not recommended, given the uncertain risk-benefit ratio" (p. 289).

Phase III: Schizophrenia

In the active phase of the disorder, psychotic symptoms are prominent. Following are criteria from the *DSM-IV-TR* (APA, 2000) that are used to confirm a diagnosis of schizophrenia:

1. **Characteristic Symptoms:** Two (or more) of the following, each present for a significant portion of time during a 1-month period (or less if successfully treated):
   a. **Delusions**
   b. **Hallucinations**
   c. Disorganized speech (e.g., frequent derailment or incoherence)
   d. Grossly disorganized or **catatonic behavior**
   e. Negative symptoms (i.e., affective flattening, alogia, or avolition)
2. **Social/Occupational Dysfunction:** For a significant portion of the time since the onset of the disturbance, one or more major areas of functioning such as work, interpersonal relationships, or self-care are markedly below the level achieved before the onset (or when the onset is in childhood or adolescence, failure to achieve expected level of interpersonal, academic, or occupational achievement).
3. **Duration:** Continuous signs of the disturbance persist for at least 6 months. This 6-month period must include at least 1 month of symptoms (or less if successfully treated) that meet criterion 1 (i.e., active-phase symptoms) and may include periods of prodromal or residual symptoms. During these prodromal or residual periods, the signs of the disturbance may be manifested by only negative symptoms or two or more symptoms listed in criterion 1 present in an attenuated form (e.g., odd beliefs, unusual perceptual experiences).
4. **Schizoaffective and Mood Disorder Exclusion:** Schizoaffective disorder and mood disorder with psychotic features have been ruled out because (1) no major depressive, manic, or mixed episodes have occurred concurrently with the active-phase symptoms; or (2) if mood episodes have occurred during active-phase symptoms, their total duration has been brief relative to the duration of the active and residual periods.
5. **Substance/General Medical Condition Exclusion:** The disturbance is not due to the direct physiological effects of a substance (e.g., a drug of abuse, a medication) or a general medical condition.
6. **Relationship to a Pervasive Developmental Disorder:** If there is a history of autistic disorder or another pervasive developmental disorder, the additional diagnosis of schizophrenia is made only if prominent delusions or hallucinations are also present for at least 1 month (or less if successfully treated).

Phase IV: Residual Phase

Schizophrenia is characterized by periods of remission and exacerbation. A residual phase usually follows an active phase of the illness. During the residual phase, symptoms of the acute stage are either absent or no longer prominent. Negative symptoms may remain, and flat affect and impairment in role functioning are common. Residual impairment often increases between episodes of active psychosis.

Prognosis

A return to full premorbid functioning is not common (APA, 2000). However, several factors have been associated with a more positive prognosis, including good premorbid adjustment, later age at onset, female gender, abrupt onset of symptoms precipitated by a stressful event (as opposed to gradual insidious onset of symptoms), associated mood disturbance, brief duration of active-phase symptoms, good interepisode functioning, minimal residual symptoms, absence of structural brain abnormalities, normal neurological functioning, a family history of mood disorder, and no family history of schizophrenia (Andreasen & Black, 2006; APA, 2000).

PREDISPOSING FACTORS

The cause of schizophrenia is still uncertain. Most likely, no single factor can be implicated in the etiology; rather, the disease probably results from a combination of influences that include biological, psychological, and environmental factors.

Biological Influences

Refer to Chapter 4 for a more thorough review of the biological implications of psychiatric illness.

Genetics

The body of evidence for genetic vulnerability to schizophrenia is growing. Studies show that relatives of individuals with schizophrenia have a much higher probability of developing the disease than does the general population. Whereas the lifetime risk for developing schizophrenia is about 1 percent in most population studies, the siblings or offspring of an identified client have a 5 to 10 percent risk of developing schizophrenia (Andreasen & Black, 2006).

How schizophrenia is inherited is uncertain. No definitive biological marker has as yet been found. Studies are ongoing to determine which genes are important in vulnerability to schizophrenia, and whether one or many genes are implicated. Some individuals have a strong genetic link to the illness, whereas in others the illness may have only a weak genetic basis. This theory gives further credence to the notion of multiple causations.

Twin Studies. The rate of schizophrenia among monozygotic (identical) twins is four to five times that of dizygotic (fraternal) twins and approximately 50 times that of the general population (Sadock & Sadock, 2007). Identical twins reared apart have the same rate of development of the illness as do those reared together. Because in about half of the cases only one of a pair of monozygotic twins develops schizophrenia, some investigators believe environmental factors interact with genetic ones.

Adoption Studies. In studies conducted by both American and Danish investigators, adopted children born to mothers with schizophrenia were compared with adopted children whose mothers had no psychiatric disorder. Children who were born to mothers with schizophrenia were more likely to develop the illness than the comparison control groups (Ho, Black & Andreasen, 2003). Studies also indicate that children born to nonschizophrenic parents, but reared by parents afflicted with the illness, do not seem to suffer more often from schizophrenia than general controls. These findings provide additional evidence for the genetic basis of schizophrenia.

Biochemical Influences

The oldest and most thoroughly explored biological theory in the explanation of schizophrenia attributes a pathogenic role to abnormal brain biochemistry. Notions of a "chemical disturbance" as an explanation for insanity were suggested by some theorists as early as the mid-19th century.

The Dopamine Hypothesis. This theory suggests that schizophrenia (or schizophrenia-like symptoms) may be caused by an excess of dopamine-dependent neuronal activity in the brain (see Figure 28–1). This excess activity may be related to increased production or release of the substance at nerve terminals, increased receptor sensitivity, too many dopamine receptors, or a combination of these mechanisms (Sadock & Sadock, 2007).

Pharmacological support for this hypothesis exists. Amphetamines, which increase levels of dopamine, induce psychotomimetic symptoms. The **neuroleptics** (e.g., chlorpromazine or haloperidol) lower brain levels of dopamine by blocking dopamine receptors, thus reducing the schizophrenic symptoms, including those induced by amphetamines.

Postmortem studies of brains of schizophrenic individuals have reported a significant increase in the average number of dopamine receptors in approximately two thirds of the brains studied. This suggests that an increased dopamine response may not be important in *all* schizophrenic clients. Clients with acute manifestations (e.g., delusions and hallucinations) respond with greater efficacy to neuroleptic drugs than do clients with chronic manifestations (e.g., apathy, poverty of ideas, and loss of drive). The current position, in terms of the dopamine hypothesis, is that manifestations of acute schizophrenia may be related to increased numbers of dopamine receptors in the brain and respond to neuroleptic drugs that block these receptors. Manifestations of chronic schizophrenia are probably unrelated to numbers of dopamine receptors, and neuroleptic drugs are unlikely to be as effective in treating these chronic symptoms.

Other Biochemical Hypotheses. Various other biochemicals have been implicated in the predisposition to schizophrenia. Abnormalities in the neuronal activity of the neurotransmitters norepinephrine, serotonin, acetylcholine, and gamma-aminobutyric acid and in the neuroregulators, such as prostaglandins and endorphins, have been suggested.

Physiological Influences

A number of physical factors of possible etiological significance have been identified in the medical literature. However, their specific mechanisms in the implication of schizophrenia are unclear.

Viral Infection. Sadock and Sadock (2007) report that epidemiological data indicate a high incidence of schizophrenia after prenatal exposure to influenza. They state:

Other data supporting a viral hypothesis are an increased number of physical anomalies at birth, an increased rate of pregnancy and birth complications, seasonality of birth consistent with viral infection, geographical clusters of adult cases, and seasonality of hospitalizations. (p. 469)

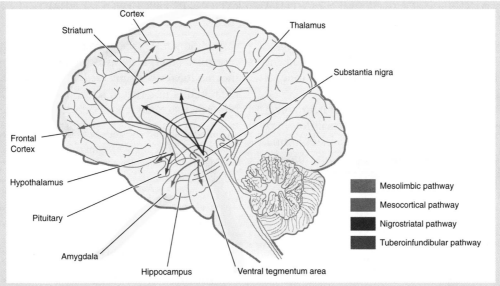

FIGURE 28–1 Neurobiology of schizophrenia.

Neurotransmitters

A number of neurotransmitters have been implicated in the etiology of schizophrenia. These include dopamine, norepinephrine, serotonin, glutamate, and GABA. The dopaminergic system has been most widely studied and closely linked to the symptoms associated with the disease.

Areas of the Brain Affected

● Four major dopaminergic pathways have been identified:
  • *Mesolimbic pathway*: Originates in the ventral tegmentum area and projects to areas of the limbic system, including the nucleus accumbens, amygdala, and hippocampus. The mesolimbic pathway is associated with functions of memory, emotion, arousal, and pleasure. Excess activity in the mesolimbic tract has been implicated in the positive symptoms of schizophrenia (e.g., hallucinations, delusions).
  • *Mesocortical pathway:* Originates in the ventral tegmentum area and has projections into the cortex. The mesocortical pathway is concerned with cognition, social behavior, planning, problem solving, motivation, and reinforcement in learning. Negative symptoms of schizophrenia (e.g., flat affect, apathy, lack of motivation, and anhedonia) have been associated with diminished activity in the mesocortical tract.
  • *Nigrostriatal pathway:* Originates in the substantia nigra and terminates in the striatum of the basal ganglia. This pathway is associated with the function of motor control. Degeneration in this pathway is associated with Parkinson's disease and involuntary psychomotor symptoms of schizophrenia.
  • *Tuberoinfundibular pathway:* Originates in the hypothalamus and projects to the pituitary gland. It is associated with endocrine function, digestion, metabolism, hunger, thirst, temperature control, and sexual arousal. Implicated in certain endocrine abnormalities associated with schizophrenia.
● Two major groups of dopamine receptors and their highest tissue locations include:
  • The D_1 family:
     D_1 receptors: basal ganglia, nucleus accumbens, and cerebral cortex
     D_5 receptors: hippocampus and hypothalamus, with lower concentrations in the cerebral cortex and basal ganglia
  • The D_2 family:
     D_2 receptors: basal ganglia, anterior pituitary, cerebral cortex, limbic structures
     D_3 receptors: limbic regions, with lower concentrations in basal ganglia
     D_4 receptors: frontal cortex, hippocampus, amygdala

Antipsychotic Medications

Type	Receptor Affinity	Associated Side Effects

Conventional (typical) antipsychotics:
  Phenothiazines
  Haloperidol
	Strong D_2 (dopamine)
	Varying degrees of affinity for:
	  (cholinergic) ACh
		EPS, hyperprolactinemia, Neuroleptic Malignant Syndrome
		
		Anticholinergic effects

Provide relief of psychosis,
  improvement in positive symptoms,
  worsening of negative symptoms.
	α_1 (norepinephrine)
	H_1 (histamine)
	Weak 5-HT (serotonin)
		Tachycardia, tremors, insomnia, postural hypotension
		Weight gain, sedation
		Low potential for ejaculatory difficulty

Novel (atypical) antipsychotics:
  Clozapine, Olanzapine, Quetiapine,
  Aripiprazole, Risperidone,
  Ziprasidone, Paliperidone
	Strong 5-HT
	Low to Moderate D_2
	Varying degrees of affinity for:
	  Ach
		Sexual dysfunction, GI disturbance, headache
		Low potential for EPS
		
		Anticholinergic effects

Provide relief of psychosis,
  improvement in positive symptoms,
  improvement in negative symptoms.
	α adrenergic
	H_1
		Tachycardia, tremors, insomnia, postural hypotension
		Weight gain, sedation

Another study found an association between viral infections of the central nervous system during childhood and adult onset schizophrenia (Rantakallio, Jones, Moring, & Von Wendt, 1997).

Anatomical Abnormalities. With the use of neuroimaging technologies, structural brain abnormalities have been observed in individuals with schizophrenia. Ventricular enlargement is the most consistent finding; however, sulci enlargement and cerebellar atrophy are also reported. Ho, Black, and Andreasen (2003) state:

> There is substantial evidence to suggest that ventricular enlargement is associated with poor premorbid functioning, negative symptoms, poor response to treatment, and cognitive impairment. CT scan abnormalities may have some clinical significance, but they are not diagnostically specific; similar abnormalities are seen in other disorders such as Alzheimer's disease or alcoholism. (p. 405)

Magnetic resonance imaging (MRI) provides a greater ability to image in multiple planes. Studies with MRI have revealed a possible decrease in cerebral and intracranial size in clients with schizophrenia. Studies have also revealed a decrease in frontal lobe size, but this has been less consistently replicated. MRI has been used to explore possible abnormalities in specific subregions such as the amygdala, hippocampus, temporal lobes, and basal ganglia in the brains of people with schizophrenia.

Histological Changes. Cerebral changes in schizophrenia have also been studied at the microscopic level. A "disordering" or disarray of the pyramidal cells in the area of the hippocampus has been suggested (Jonsson, Luts, Guldberg-Kjaer, & Brun, 1997). This disarray of cells has been compared to the normal alignment of the cells in the brains of clients without the disorder. Some researchers have hypothesized that this alteration in hippocampal cells occurs during the second trimester of pregnancy and may be related to an influenza virus infection acquired by the mother during this period. Further research is required to determine the possible link between this birth defect and the development of schizophrenia.

Physical Conditions. Some studies have reported a link between schizophrenia and epilepsy (particularly temporal lobe), Huntington's disease, birth trauma, head injury in adulthood, alcohol abuse, cerebral tumor (particularly in the limbic system), cerebrovascular accidents, systemic lupus erythematosus, myxedema, parkinsonism, and Wilson's disease.

Psychological Influences

Early conceptualizations of schizophrenia focused on family relationship factors as major influences in the development of the illness, probably in light of the conspicuous absence of information related to a biological connection. These early theories implicated poor parent–child relationships and dysfunctional family systems as the cause of schizophrenia, but they no longer hold any credibility. Researchers now focus their studies in terms of schizophrenia as a brain disorder. Nevertheless, Sadock and Sadock (2007) state:

> Clinicians should consider both the psychosocial and biological factors affecting schizophrenia. The disorder affects individual patients, each of whom has a unique psychological makeup. Although many psychodynamic theories about the pathogenesis of schizophrenia seem outdated, perceptive clinical observations can help contemporary clinicians understand how the disease may affect a patient's psyche. (p. 474)

Environmental Influences

Sociocultural Factors

Many studies have been conducted that have attempted to link schizophrenia to social class. Indeed epidemiological statistics have shown that greater numbers of individuals from the lower socioeconomic classes experience symptoms associated with schizophrenia than do those from the higher socioeconomic groups (Ho, Black, & Andreasen, 2003). Explanations for this occurrence include the conditions associated with living in poverty, such as congested housing accommodations, inadequate nutrition, absence of prenatal care, few resources for dealing with stressful situations, and feeling hopeless to change one's lifestyle of poverty.

An alternative view is that of the *downward drift hypothesis*, which suggests that, because of the characteristic symptoms of the disorder, individuals with schizophrenia have difficulty maintaining gainful employment and "drift down" to a lower socioeconomic level (or fail to rise out of a lower socioeconomic group). Proponents of this view consider poor social conditions as a consequence rather than a cause of schizophrenia.

Stressful Life Events

Studies have been conducted in an effort to determine whether psychotic episodes may be precipitated by stressful life events. There is no scientific evidence to indicate that stress causes schizophrenia. It is very probable, however, that stress may contribute to the severity and course of the illness. It is known that extreme stress can precipitate psychotic episodes. Stress may indeed precipitate symptoms in an individual who possesses a genetic vulnerability to schizophrenia.

Stressful life events may be associated with exacerbation of schizophrenic symptoms and increased rates of relapse.

The Transactional Model

The etiology of schizophrenia remains unclear. No single theory or hypothesis has been postulated that substantiates a clear-cut explanation for the disease. Indeed, it seems the more research that is conducted, the more evidence is compiled to support the concept of multiple causation in the development of schizophrenia. The most current theory seems to be that schizophrenia is a biologically based disease, the onset of which is influenced by factors within the environment (either internal or external). The dynamics of schizophrenia using the Transactional Model of Stress/Adaptation are presented in Figure 28–2.

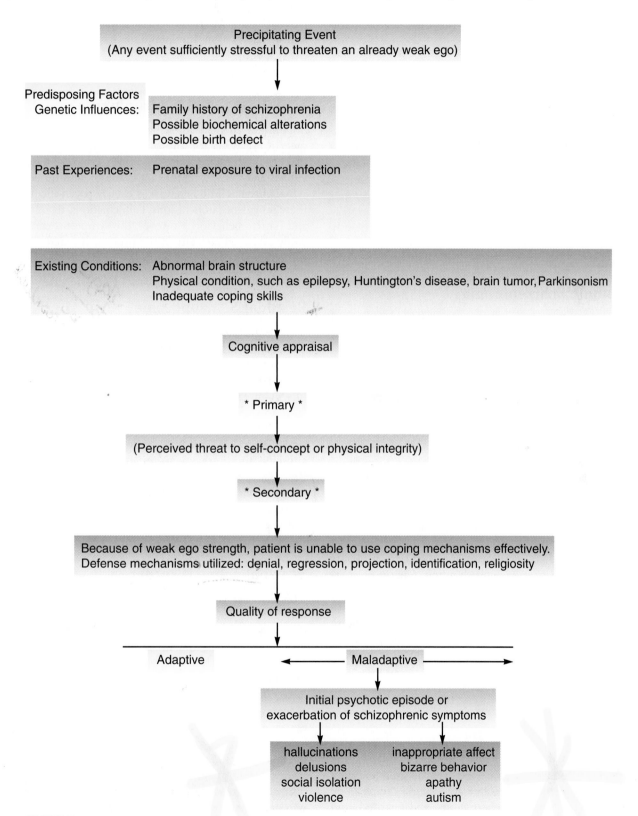

FIGURE 28–2 The dynamics of schizophrenia using the Transactional Model of Stress/Adaptation.

TYPES OF SCHIZOPHRENIA AND OTHER PSYCHOTIC DISORDERS

The *DSM-IV*-TR (APA, 2000) identifies various types of schizophrenia and other psychotic disorders. Differential diagnosis is made according to the total symptomatic clinical picture presented.

Disorganized Schizophrenia

This type previously was called *hebephrenic schizophrenia.* Onset of symptoms is usually before age 25, and the course is commonly chronic. Behavior is markedly regressive and primitive. Contact with reality is extremely poor. Affect is flat or grossly inappropriate, often with periods of silliness and incongruous giggling. Facial grimaces and bizarre mannerisms are common, and communication is consistently incoherent. Personal appearance is generally neglected, and social impairment is extreme.

Catatonic Schizophrenia

Catatonic schizophrenia is characterized by marked abnormalities in motor behavior and may be manifested in the form of *stupor* or *excitement.*

Catatonic stupor is characterized by extreme psychomotor retardation. The individual exhibits a pronounced decrease in spontaneous movements and activity. Mutism (i.e., absence of speech) is common, and negativism (i.e., an apparently motiveless resistance to all instructions or attempts to be moved) may be evident. **Waxy flexibility** may be exhibited. This term describes a type of "posturing," or voluntary assumption of bizarre positions, in which the individual may remain for long periods. Efforts to move the individual may be met with rigid bodily resistance.

Catatonic excitement is manifested by a state of extreme psychomotor agitation. The movements are frenzied and purposeless, and are usually accompanied by continuous incoherent verbalizations and shouting. Clients in catatonic excitement urgently require physical and medical control because they are often destructive and violent to others, and their excitement may cause them to injure themselves or to collapse from complete exhaustion.

The illness, which was relatively common in the past, has become quite rare since the advent of antipsychotic medications for use in psychiatry.

Paranoid Schizophrenia

Paranoid schizophrenia is characterized mainly by the presence of delusions of persecution or grandeur and auditory hallucinations related to a single theme. The individual is often tense, suspicious, and guarded, and may be argumentative, hostile, and aggressive. Onset of symptoms is usually later (perhaps in the late 20s or 30s), and less regression of mental faculties, emotional response, and behavior is seen than in the other subtypes of schizophrenia. Social impairment may be minimal, and there is some evidence that prognosis, particularly with regard to occupational functioning and capacity for independent living, is promising (APA, 2000).

Undifferentiated Schizophrenia

Sometimes clients with schizophrenic symptoms do not meet the criteria for any of the subtypes, or they may meet the criteria for more than one subtype. These individuals may be given the diagnosis of undifferentiated schizophrenia. The behavior is clearly psychotic; that is, there is evidence of delusions, hallucinations, incoherence, and bizarre behavior. However, the symptoms cannot be easily classified into any of the previously listed diagnostic categories.

Residual Schizophrenia

This diagnostic category is used when the individual has a history of at least one previous episode of schizophrenia with prominent psychotic symptoms. Residual schizophrenia occurs in an individual who has a chronic form of the disease and is the stage that follows an acute episode (prominent delusions, hallucinations, incoherence, bizarre behavior, and violence). In the residual stage, there is continuing evidence of the illness, although there are no prominent psychotic symptoms. Residual symptoms may include social isolation, eccentric behavior, impairment in personal hygiene and grooming, blunted or inappropriate affect, poverty of or overly elaborate speech, illogical thinking, or apathy.

Schizoaffective Disorder

This disorder is manifested by schizophrenic behaviors, with a strong element of symptomatology associated with the mood disorders (depression or mania). The client may appear depressed, with psychomotor retardation and suicidal ideation, or symptoms may include euphoria, grandiosity, and hyperactivity. However, the decisive factor in the diagnosis of schizoaffective disorder is the presence of characteristic schizophrenic symptoms. For example, in addition to the dysfunctional mood, the individual exhibits bizarre delusions, prominent hallucinations, incoherent speech, catatonic behavior, or blunted or inappropriate affect. The prognosis for schizoaffective disorder is generally better than that for other schizophrenic disorders but worse than that for mood disorders alone (Andreasen & Black, 2006).

"Brief Psychotic Disorder"

The essential feature of this disorder is the sudden onset of psychotic symptoms that may or may not be preceded by a severe psychosocial stressor. These symptoms last at least 1 day but less than 1 month, and there is an eventual full return to the premorbid level of functioning (APA, 2000). The individual experiences emotional turmoil or overwhelming perplexity or confusion. Evidence of impaired reality testing may include incoherent speech, delusions, hallucinations, bizarre behavior, and disorientation. Individuals with preexisting personality disorders (most commonly, histrionic, narcissistic, paranoid, schizotypal, and borderline personality disorders) appear to be susceptible to this disorder (Sadock & Sadock, 2007).

Schizophreniform Disorder

The essential features of this disorder are identical to those of schizophrenia, with the exception that the duration, including prodromal, active, and residual phases, is at least 1 month but less than 6 months (APA, 2000). If the diagnosis is made while the individual is still symptomatic but has been so for less than 6 months, it is qualified as "provisional." The diagnosis is changed to schizophrenia if the clinical picture persists beyond 6 months.

Schizophreniform disorder is thought to have a good prognosis if at least two of the following features are present:

1. Onset of prominent psychotic symptoms within 4 weeks of first noticeable change in usual behavior or functioning
2. Confusion or perplexity at the height of the psychotic episode
3. Good premorbid social and occupational functioning
4. Absence of blunted or flat affect (APA, 2000)

Delusional Disorder

The essential feature of this disorder is the presence of one or more nonbizarre delusions that persist for at least 1 month (APA, 2000). If present at all, hallucinations are not prominent, and apart from the delusions, behavior is not bizarre. The subtype of delusional disorder is based on the predominant delusional theme.

Erotomanic Type — "Brad Pitt Loves Me"

With this type of delusion, the individual believes that someone, usually of a higher status, is in love with him or her. Famous persons are often the subjects of erotomanic delusions. Sometimes the delusion is kept secret, but some individuals may follow, contact, or otherwise try to pursue the object of their delusion.

Grandiose Type — Thinks — I Am God

Individuals with grandiose delusions have irrational ideas regarding their own worth, talent, knowledge, or power. They may believe that they have a special relationship with a famous person, or even assume the identity of a famous person (believing that the actual person is an imposter). Grandiose delusions of a religious nature may lead to assumption of the identity of a deity or religious leader.

Jealous Type

The content of jealous delusions centers on the idea that the person's sexual partner is unfaithful. The idea is irrational and without cause, but the individual with the delusion searches for evidence to justify the belief. The sexual partner is confronted (and sometimes physically attacked) regarding the imagined infidelity. The imagined "lover" of the sexual partner may also be the object of the attack. Attempts to restrict the autonomy of the sexual partner in an effort to stop the imagined infidelity are common.

Persecutory Type

In persecutory delusions, which are the most common type, individuals believe they are being malevolently treated in some way. Frequent themes include being conspired against, cheated, spied on, followed, poisoned or drugged, maliciously maligned, harassed, or obstructed in the pursuit of long-term goals (APA, 2000). The individual may obsess about and exaggerate a slight rebuff (either real or imagined) until it becomes the focus of a delusional system. Repeated complaints may be directed at legal authorities, lack of satisfaction from which may result in violence toward the object of the delusion.

Somatic Type

Individuals with somatic delusions believe they have some physical defect, disorder, or disease. The *DSM-IV-TR* (APA, 2000) identifies the most common types of somatic delusions as those in which the individual believes that he or she:

1. Emits a foul odor from the skin, mouth, rectum, or vagina.
2. Has an infestation of insects in or on the skin.
3. Has an internal parasite.
4. Has misshapen and ugly body parts.
5. Has dysfunctional body parts.

Shared Psychotic Disorder "Nell — w/ Jody Foster"

The essential feature of this disorder, also called *folie à deux*, is a delusional system that develops in a second person as a result of a close relationship with another person who already has a psychotic disorder with prominent delusions (APA, 2000). The person with the primary delusional disorder is usually the dominant person in the relationship, and the delusional thinking is gradually imposed on the more passive partner. This occurs within the context of a long-term close relationship, particularly when the couple has been socially isolated from other people. The course is usually chronic, and is more common in women than in men.

Psychotic Disorder Due to a General Medical Condition

The essential features of this disorder are prominent hallucinations and delusions that can be directly attributed to a general medical condition (APA, 2000). The diagnosis is not made if the symptoms occur during the course of a delirium or chronic, progressing dementia. A number of medical conditions can cause psychotic symptoms. Common ones identified by the *DSM-IV-TR* (APA, 2000) are presented in Table 28–1.

Substance-Induced Psychotic Disorder

The essential features of this disorder are the presence of prominent hallucinations and delusions that are judged to be directly attributable to the physiological effects of a substance (i.e., a drug of abuse, a medication, or toxin exposure; APA, 2000). The diagnosis is made in the absence of reality testing and when history, physical examination, or laboratory findings indicate use of substances. When reality testing has been retained in the

TABLE 28–2	Substances that May Cause Psychotic Disorders
Drugs of Abuse	Alcohol
	Amphetamines and related substances
	Cannabis
	Cocaine
	Hallucinogens
	Inhalants
	Opioids
	Phencyclidine and related substances
	Sedatives, hypnotics, and anxiolytics
Medications	Anesthetics and analgesics
	Anticholinergic agents
	Anticonvulsants
	Antidepressant medication
	Antihistamines
	Antihypertensive agents
	Cardiovascular medications
	Antimicrobial medications
	Antiparkinsonian agents
	Chemotherapeutic agents
	Corticosteroids
	Disulfiram
	Gastrointestinal medications
	Muscle relaxants
	Nonsteroidal anti-inflammatory agents
Toxins	Anticholinesterase
	Organophosphate insecticides
	Nerve gases
	Carbon monoxide
	Carbon dioxide
	Volatile substances (e.g., fuel or paint)

presence of substance-induced psychotic symptoms, the diagnosis would be substance-related disorder (Sadock & Sadock, 2007). Substances identified by the *DSM-IV-TR* (APA, 2000) that are believed to induce psychotic disorders are presented in Table 28–2.

APPLICATION OF THE NURSING PROCESS

Background Assessment Data

In the first step of the nursing process, the nurse gathers a database from which nursing diagnoses are derived and a plan of care is formulated. This first step of the nursing process is extremely important because without an accurate assessment, problem identification, objectives of care, and outcome criteria cannot be accurately determined.

Assessment of the client with schizophrenia may be a complex process, based on information gathered from a number of sources. Clients in an acute episode of their illness are seldom able to make a significant contribution to their history. Data may be obtained from family members, if possible; from old records, if available; or from other individuals who have been in a position to report on the progression of the client's behavior.

TABLE 28–1	General Medical Conditions that May Cause Psychotic Symptoms
Neurological Conditions	Neoplasms
	Cerebrovascular disease
	Huntington's disease
	Epilepsy
	Auditory nerve injury
	Deafness
	Migraine headache
	CNS infections
Endocrine Conditions	Hyperthyroidism
	Hypothyroidism
	Hyperparathyroidism
	Hypoparathyroidism
	Hypoadrenocorticism
Metabolic Conditions	Hypoxia
	Hypercarbia
	Hypoglycemia
Autoimmune Disorders	Systemic lupus erythematosus
Others	Fluid or electrolyte imbalances
	Hepatic or renal diseases

- Antipsychotic medications remain the mainstay of treatment for psychotic disorders. Atypical antipsychotics have become the first-line of therapy, and treat both positive and negative symptoms of schizophrenia. They have a more favorable side-effect profile than the conventional (typical) antipsychotics.
- Individuals with schizophrenia require long-term integrated treatment with pharmacological and other interventions. Some of these include individual psychotherapy, group therapy, behavior therapy, social skills training, milieu therapy, family therapy, and assertive community treatment. For the majority of clients, the most effective treatment appears to be a combination of psychotropic medication and psychosocial therapy.
- Families generally require support and education about psychotic illnesses. The focus is on coping with the diagnosis, understanding the illness and its course, teaching about medication, and learning ways to manage symptoms.

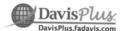

DavisPlus.fadavis.com **For additional clinical tools and study aids, visit DavisPlus.**

REVIEW QUESTIONS

Self-Examination/Learning Exercise

Situation: Tony, age 20 years, quit college 2 months ago and returned to live at his parents' home. He has become increasingly withdrawn, suspicious, and isolated since his return, and his parents have taken him to the emergency department. His parents report that he has been looking at them strangely as if he did not know them, refusing to talk to anyone, spending a lot of time in his room alone, refusing all help. The father brought the client to the hospital against his will following a verbal argument during the course of which the client attempted to stab the father with a kitchen knife. The father had successfully subdued him and removed the weapon. On arrival at the emergency department, the client was agitated and exhibiting acutely psychotic symptoms. He reports that "they" told him to kill his father before his father kills him. Verbalizations are often incoherent. Affect is flat, and he continuously scans the environment. He is admitted to the psychiatric unit with a diagnosis of schizophreniform disorder, provisional.

Based on the above situation, select the answer that is most appropriate for each of the following questions:

1. The *initial* nursing intervention for Tony is to:
   a. Give him an injection of Thorazine.
   b. Ensure a safe environment for him and others.
   c. Place him in restraints.
   d. Order a nutritious diet for him.

2. The primary goal in working with Tony would be to:
   a. Promote interaction with others.
   b. Decrease his anxiety and increase trust.
   c. Improve his relationship with his parents.
   d. Encourage participation in therapy activities.

3. Orders from the physician include 100 mg of chlorpromazine (Thorazine) STAT and then 50 mg bid; 2 mg benztropine (Cogentin) bid p.r.n. Why is chlorpromazine ordered?
   a. To reduce extrapyramidal symptoms
   b. To prevent neuroleptic malignant syndrome
   c. To decrease psychotic symptoms
   d. To induce sleep

4. Benztropine was ordered on a p.r.n. basis. Which of the following assessments by the nurse would convey a need for this medication?
   a. The client's level of agitation increases.
   b. The client complains of a sore throat.
   c. The client's skin has a yellowish cast.
   d. The client develops tremors and a shuffling gait.

5. Tony begins to tell the nurse about how the CIA is looking for him and will kill him if they find him. The most appropriate response by the nurse is:
   a. "That's ridiculous, Tony. No one is going to hurt you."
   b. "The CIA isn't interested in people like you, Tony."
   c. "Why do you think the CIA wants to kill you?"
   d. "I know you believe that, Tony, but it is hard for me to believe."

6. Tony's belief about the CIA is an example of a:
   a. Delusion of persecution.
   b. Delusion of reference.
   c. Delusion of control or influence.
   d. Delusion of grandeur.

7. Tony tilts his head to the side, stops talking in midsentence, and listens intently. The nurse recognizes from these signs that Tony is likely experiencing:
   a. Somatic delusions.
   b. Catatonic stupor.

    c. Auditory hallucinations.

    d. Pseudoparkinsonism.

8. The most appropriate nursing intervention for the symptom just described is to:

    a. Ask the client to describe his physical symptoms.

    b. Ask the client to describe what he is hearing.

    c. Administer a dose of benztropine.

    d. Call the physician for additional orders.

9. Should Tony suddenly become aggressive and violent on the unit, which of the following approaches would be best for the nurse to use *first*?

    a. Provide large motor activities to relieve Tony's pent-up tension.

    b. Administer a dose of p.r.n. Thorazine to keep Tony calm.

    c. Call for sufficient help to control the situation safely.

    d. Convey to Tony that his behavior is unacceptable and will not be permitted.

10. Tony and his parents attend a weekly family therapy group. The primary focus of this type of group is:

    a. To discuss concrete problem solving and adaptive behaviors for coping with stress.

    b. To introduce the family to others with the same problem.

    c. To keep the client and family in touch with the healthcare system.

    d. To promote family interaction and increase understanding of the illness.

Test Your Critical Thinking Skills

Sara, a 23-year-old single woman, has just been admitted to the psychiatric unit by her parents. They explain that over the past few months she has become more and more withdrawn. She stays in her room alone, but lately has been heard talking and laughing to herself.

Sara left home for the first time at age 18 to attend college. She performed well during her first semester, but when she returned after Christmas, she began to accuse her roommate of stealing her possessions. She started writing to her parents that her roommate wanted to kill her and that her roommate was turning everyone against her. She said she feared for her life. She started missing classes and stayed in her bed most of the time. Sometimes she locked herself in her closet. Her parents took her home, and she was hospitalized and diagnosed with paranoid schizophrenia. She has since been maintained on antipsychotic medication while taking a few classes at the local community college.

Sara tells the admitting nurse that she quit taking her medication 4 weeks ago because the pharmacist who fills the prescriptions is plotting to have her killed. She believes he is trying to poison her. She says she got this information from a television message. As Sara speaks, the nurse notices that she sometimes stops in midsentence and listens; sometimes she cocks her head to the side and moves her lips as though she is talking.

Answer the following questions related to Sara:

1. From the assessment data, what would be the most immediate nursing concern in working with Sara?
2. What is the nursing diagnosis related to this concern?
3. What interventions must be accomplished before the nurse can be successful in working with Sara?

REFERENCES

Addington, D.E. (2006). Reducing suicide risk in patients with schizophrenia. *Medscape Psychiatry & Mental Health.* Retrieved March 18, 2007 from http://www.medscape.com/viewprogram/5616

American Psychiatric Association. (2000). *Diagnostic and statistical manual of mental disorders* (4th ed.) *Text revision.* Washington, DC: American Psychiatric Publishing.

Andreasen, N.C., & Black, D.W. (2006). *Introductory textbook of psychiatry* (4th ed.). Washington, DC: American Psychiatric Publishing.

Asen, E. (2002). Outcome research in family therapy: Family intervention for psychosis. *Advances in Psychiatric Treatment, 8,* 230–238.

Assertive Community Treatment Association (ACTA). (2007). *ACT Model.* Retrieved March 18, 2007 from http://www.actassociation.org/actModel

Dixon, L.B., & Lehman, A.F. (1995). Family interventions for schizophrenia. National Institute of Mental Health. *Schizophrenia Bulletin, 21*(4), 631–643.

Ho, B.C., Black, D.W., & Andreasen, N.C. (2003). Schizophrenia and other psychotic disorders. In R.E. Hales & S.C. Yudofsky (Eds.). *Textbook of clinical psychiatry* (4th ed.). Washington, DC: American Psychiatric Publishing.

Jonsson, S.A., Luts, A., Guldberg-Kjaer, N., & Brun, A. (1997). Hippocampal pyramidal cell disarray correlates negatively to cell number: Implications for the pathogenesis of schizophrenia. *European Archives of Psychiatry and Clinical Neuroscience, 247*(3), 120–127.

Lehman, A.F., Lieberman, J.A., Dixon, L.B., McGlashan, T.H., Miller, A.L., Perkins, D.O., & Kreyenbuhl, J. (2006). Practice guideline for the treatment of patients with schizophrenia, 2nd edition. *American Psychiatric Association practice guidelines for the treatment of psychiatric disorders, Compendium 2006.* Washington, DC: American Psychiatric Publishing.

Medscape Psychiatry. (2008). *Conventional antipsychotic medications linked to increased cordiovascular death in elderly patients.* Retrieved August 29, 2008 from http://www.medscape.com/viewarticle/579799

The Merck Manual of Diagnosis and Therapy (MMDT). (2005). Schizophrenia. Retrieved March 18, 2007 from http://www.merck.com/

Mueser, K.T., Bond, G.R., & Drake, R.E. (2001). Community-based treatment of schizophrenia and other severe mental disorders: Treatment outcomes. *Medscape Psychiatry & Mental Health eJournal, 6*(1). Retrieved March 18, 2007 from http://www.medscape.com/viewarticle/430529

NANDA International (NANDA-I). (2007). *Nursing diagnoses: Definitions & classification 2007–2008.* Philadelphia: NANDA-I.

National Alliance for the Mentally Ill (NAMI). (2007). *Assertive Community Treatment (ACT).* Retrieved March 18, 2007 from http://www.nami.org/

Olin, S.S., & Mednick, S.A. (1996). Risk factors of psychosis: Identifying vulnerable populations premorbidly. *Schizophrenia Bulletin, 22*(2), 223–240.

Perkins, D.O. (2004). Evaluating and treating the prodromal stage of schizophrenia. *Current Psychiatry Reports, 6*(4), 289–295.

Radomsky, E.D., Haas, G.L., Mann, J.J., & Sweeney, J.A. (1999). Suicidal behavior in patients with schizophrenia and other psychotic disorders. *American Journal of Psychiatry, 156*(10), 1590–1595.

Rantakallio, P., Jones, P., Moring, J., & Von Wendt, L. (1997). Association between central nervous system infections during childhood and adult onset schizophrenia and other psychoses: A 28–year follow-up. *International Journal of Epidemiology, 26,* 837–843.

Sadock, B.J., & Sadock, V.A. (2007). *Synopsis of psychiatry: Behavioral sciences/clinical psychiatry* (10th ed.). Philadelphia: Lippincott Williams & Wilkins.

Safier, E. (1997). Our families, the context of our lives. *Menninger Perspective, 28*(1), 4–9.

@ Internet References

● Additional information about schizophrenia is located at the following Web sites:

- http://www.schizophrenia.com
- http://www.nimh.nih.gov
- http://schizophrenia.nami.org
- http://mentalhealth.com
- http://www.narsad.org/

● Additional information about medications to treat schizophrenia may be located at the following Web sites:

- http://www.medicinenet.com/medications/article.htm
- http://www.fadavis.com/townsend
- http://www.nlm.nih.gov/medlineplus

Mood Disorders

CHAPTER OUTLINE

KEY TERMS

bipolar disorder
cognitive therapy
cyclothymic
    disorder
delirious mania
dysthymic disorder

hypomania
melancholia
postpartum depression
premenstrual
    dysphoric disorder
tyramine

CORE CONCEPTS

depression
mania
mood

OBJECTIVES

After reading this chapter, the student will be able to:

1. Recount historical perspectives of mood disorders.
2. Discuss epidemiological statistics related to mood disorders.
3. Describe various types of mood disorders.
4. Identify predisposing factors in the development of mood disorders.
5. Discuss implications of depression related to developmental stage.
6. Identify symptomatology associated with mood disorders and use this information in client assessment.
7. Formulate nursing diagnoses and goals of care for clients with mood disorders.
8. Identify topics for client and family teaching relevant to mood disorders.
9. Describe appropriate nursing interventions for behaviors associated with mood disorders.
10. Describe relevant criteria for evaluating nursing care of clients with mood disorders.
11. Discuss various modalities relevant to treatment of mood disorders.

Depression is likely the oldest and still one of the most frequently diagnosed psychiatric illnesses. Symptoms of depression have been described almost as far back as there is evidence of written documentation.

An occasional bout with the "blues," a feeling of sadness or downheartedness, is common among healthy people and considered to be a normal response to everyday disappointments in life. These episodes are short-lived as the individual adapts to the loss, change, or failure (real or perceived) that has been experienced. Pathological depression occurs when adaptation is ineffective.

CORE CONCEPT

Mood
Also called *affect*. Mood is a pervasive and sustained emotion that may have a major influence on a person's perception of the world. Examples of mood include depression, joy, elation, anger, and anxiety. *Affect* is described as the emotional reaction associated with an experience (Taber's, 2005).

This chapter focuses on the consequences of complicated grieving as it is manifested by mood disorders, which can be classified as either depressive or bipolar. A historical perspective and epidemiological statistics related to mood disorders are presented. Predisposing factors that have been implicated in the etiology of mood disorders provide a framework for studying the dynamics of depression and **bipolar disorder**.

The implications of mood disorders relevant to individuals of various developmental stages are discussed. An explanation of the symptomatology is presented as background knowledge for assessing the client with a mood disorder. Nursing care is described in the context of the six steps of the nursing process. Various medical treatment modalities are explored.

CORE CONCEPT

Depression
An alteration in mood that is expressed by feelings of sadness, despair, and pessimism. There is a loss of interest in usual activities, and somatic symptoms may be evident. Changes in appetite and sleep patterns are common.

CORE CONCEPT

Mania
An alteration in mood that is expressed by feelings of elation, inflated self-esteem, grandiosity, hyperactivity, agitation, and accelerated thinking and speaking. Mania can occur as a biological (organic) or psychological disorder, or as a response to substance use or a general medical condition.

HISTORICAL PERSPECTIVE

Many ancient cultures (e.g., Babylonian, Egyptian, Hebrew) have believed in the supernatural or divine origin of depression and mania. The Old Testament states in the Book of Samuel that King Saul's depression was inflicted by an "evil spirit" sent from God to "torment" him.

A clearly nondivine point of view regarding depressive and manic states was held by the Greek medical community from the 5th century BC through the 3rd century AD. This represented the thinking of Hippocrates, Celsus, and Galen, among others. They strongly rejected the idea of divine origin and considered the brain as the seat of all emotional states. Hippocrates believed that melancholia was caused by an excess of black bile, a heavily toxic substance produced in the spleen or intestine, which affected the brain. Melancholia is a severe form of depressive disorder in which symptoms are exaggerated, and interest or pleasure in virtually all activities is lost.

During the Renaissance, several new theories evolved. Depression was viewed by some as being the result of obstruction of vital air circulation, excessive brooding, or helpless situations beyond the client's control. These strong emotions of depression and mania were reflected in major literary works of the time, including Shakespeare's *King Lear*, *Macbeth*, and *Hamlet*.

In the 19th century, the definition of mania was narrowed down from the concept of total madness to that of a disorder of affect and action. The old notion of melancholia was refurnished with meaning, and emphasis was placed on the primary affective nature of the disorder. Finally, an introduction was made to the possibility of an alternating pattern of affective symptomatology associated with the disorders.

Contemporary thinking has been shaped a great deal by the works of Sigmund Freud, Emil Kraepelin, and Adolf Meyer. Having evolved from these early 20th-century models, current thinking about mood disorders generally encompasses the intrapsychic, behavioral, and biological perspectives. These various perspectives support the notion of multiple causation in the development of mood disorders.

EPIDEMIOLOGY

Major depression is one of the leading causes of disability in the United States. It affects almost 10 percent of the population, or 19 million Americans, in a given year (International Society for Mental Health Online, 2004). During their lifetime, 10 to 25 percent of women and 5 to 12 percent of men will become clinically depressed. This preponderance has led to the consideration of depression by some researchers as "the common cold of psychiatric disorders" and this generation as an "age of melancholia."

Bipolar disorder affects approximately 5.7 million American adults, or about 2.6 percent of the U.S. population age 18 and older, in a given year (National Institute of Mental Health [NIMH], 2006).

Gender

Studies indicate that the incidence of depressive disorder is higher in women than it is in men by about 2 to 1. The incidence of bipolar disorder is roughly equal, with a ratio of women to men of 1.2 to 1.

IMPLICATIONS OF RESEARCH FOR EVIDENCE-BASED PRACTICE

Peden, A.R., Rayens, M.K., Hall, L.A., & Grant, E. (2004). Negative Thinking and the Mental Health of Low-Income Single Mothers. *Journal of Nursing Scholarship, (36)4, 337–344.*

Description of the Study: The aims of this study were to: (1) examine the prevalence of a high level of depressive symptoms in low-income, single mothers with children 2 to 6 years of age, (2) evaluate the relationships of personal sociodemographic characteristics with self-esteem, chronic stressors, negative thinking, and depressive symptoms, and (3) determine whether negative thinking mediates the effects of self-esteem and chronic stressors on depressive symptoms. Single mothers are a particularly high-risk group for clinical depression because of life circumstances such as poverty, low self-esteem, and few social resources. The average age of the mothers in the study was 27 years. The ethnicity of the sample was approximately half Caucasian and half African American. The majority had never been married; most were employed, but had annual incomes at or below $15,000. The Beck Depression Inventory was used to measure symptoms of depression; The Crandell Cognitions Inventory was used to measure negative thoughts; and the Rosenberg Self-Esteem Scale was used to measure self-worth and self-acceptance.

Results of the Study: More than 75 percent of the mothers scored somewhere in the mild to high range for depression. Negative thinking mediated the effect of self-esteem on depressive symptoms and partially mediated the effect of chronic stressors. Those subjects who were employed measured higher self-esteem, less negative thinking, fewer chronic stressors, and less depression. No differences in predictors of depression were found between Caucasian and African American mothers in this study.

Implications for Nursing Practice: The results of this study suggest the importance of intervening to address negative thinking among low-income single mothers to help them lessen their stress and decrease their risk of depression. The authors state, "Depression may interfere with parenting and participation in educational and employment opportunities, significantly undermining the quality of life in these families. A number of studies have indicated that mothers' depression may also negatively influence their children's behavior." Psychiatric nurses may employ cognitive-behavioral strategies to help women minimize negative thinking. Strategies such as writing affirmations and use of positive self-talk have been supported in nursing research. Targeting the symptom of negative thinking, which can be modified, may serve to break the links of chronic stressors and low self-esteem to depressive symptoms, resulting in improved mental health for the mother and the subsequent well-being of her children.

Age

Several studies have shown that the incidence of depression is higher in young women and has a tendency to decrease with age. The opposite has been found in men, with the prevalence of depressive symptoms being lower in younger men and increasing with age. This occurrence may be related to gender differences in social roles and economic and social opportunities and the shifts that occur with age. The construction of gender stereotypes, or *gender socialization*, promotes typical female characteristics, such as helplessness, passivity, and emotionality, which are associated with depression. In contrast, some studies have suggested that "masculine" characteristics are associated with higher self-esteem and less depression. Studies have also shown that widowhood has a stronger effect on depression for men than for women. Possible causes include the fact that widowhood is a more usual component of the life cycle for women (Lee, Willetts, & Seccombe, 1998). Other contributors to the stronger effect of widowhood for men included men's shorter average time since widowhood, lower frequency of church attendance, stronger dislike of domestic labor, and lessened ability to assist their children (Lee, DeMaris, Bavin, & Sullivan, 2001). The average age at onset for a first manic episode is the early twenties (NIMH, 2006).

Social Class

Results of studies have indicated an inverse relationship between social class and report of depressive symptoms. Bipolar disorder appears to occur more frequently among the higher socioeconomic classes (Sadock & Sadock, 2007).

Race and Culture

Studies have shown no consistent relationship between race and affective disorder. One problem encountered in reviewing racial comparisons has to do with the socioeconomic class of the race being investigated. Sample populations of nonwhite clients are many times predominantly from a lower socioeconomic class and are often compared with white populations from middle and upper social classes.

Other studies suggest a second problematic factor in the study of racial comparisons. Clinicians tend to underdiagnose mood disorders and to overdiagnose schizophrenia in clients who have racial or cultural backgrounds different from their own (Sadock & Sadock, 2007). This misdiagnosis may result from language barriers between clients and physicians who are unfamiliar with cultural aspects of nonwhite clients' language and behavior.

The *Merck Manual of Diagnosis and Therapy* (2005) states:

Cultural factors seem to modify the clinical manifestations of mood disorders. For example, physical complaints, worry, tension, and irritability are more common manifestations in lower socioeconomic classes; guilty ruminations and self-reproach are more characteristic of depression in Anglo-Saxon cultures; and mania tends to manifest itself more floridly in some Mediterranean and African countries and among black Americans.

Recent findings from the National Study of American Life, a survey of mental health among blacks in the United States, reveal that depression is more prevalent in whites than it is in blacks, but that depression tends to be more severe, persistent, and disabling in blacks, and they are less likely to be treated (Williams et al., 2007). Even among blacks whose symptoms were rated severe or very severe, only 48.5 percent of African Americans and 21.9 percent of Caribbean blacks received any treatment at all. The authors conclude that these findings highlight the importance of identifying high-risk subgroups in racial populations and the need for targeting cost-effective interventions to them.

Marital Status

The highest incidence of depressive symptoms has been indicated in individuals without close interpersonal relationships and in persons who are divorced or separated (Sadock & Sadock, 2007). When gender and marital status is considered together, the differences reveal lowest rates of depressive symptoms among married men, and the highest in married women and single men. Sadock and Sadock (2007) state:

> Bipolar I disorder is more common in divorced and single persons than among married persons, but this difference may reflect the early onset and the resulting marital discord that are characteristic of the disorder. (p. 529)

Seasonality

A number of studies have examined seasonal patterns associated with mood disorders. These studies have revealed two prevalent periods of seasonal involvement: one in the spring (March, April, and May) and one in the fall (September, October, and November). This pattern tends to parallel the seasonal pattern for suicide, which shows a large peak in the spring and a smaller one in October (Davidson, 2005). A number of etiologies associated with this trend have been postulated (Hakko, 2000). Some of these include the following:

● A meteorological factor, associating drastic temperature and barometric pressure changes to human mental instability
● Sociodemographic variables, such as the seasonal increase in social intercourse (e.g., increased social activity with the commencement of an academic year)
● Biochemical variables. There may be seasonal variations in various peripheral and central aspects of

serotonergic function involved in depression and suicide.

TYPES OF MOOD DISORDERS

The *DSM-IV-TR* (American Psychiatric Association [APA], 2000) describes the essential feature of these disorders as a disturbance of mood, characterized by a full or partial manic or depressive syndrome that cannot be attributed to another mental disorder. Mood disorders are classified under two major categories: depressive disorders and bipolar disorders.

Depressive Disorders

Major Depressive Disorder

This disorder is characterized by depressed mood or loss of interest or pleasure in usual activities. Evidence will show impaired social and occupational functioning that has existed for at least 2 weeks, no history of manic behavior, and symptoms that cannot be attributed to use of substances or a general medical condition.

Major depressive disorder may be further classified as follows:

1. **Single Episode or Recurrent.** A *single episode* specifier is used for an individual's first diagnosis of depression. *Recurrent* is specified when the history reveals two or more episodes of depression.
2. **Mild, Moderate, or Severe.** These categories are identified by the number and severity of symptoms.
3. **With Psychotic Features.** The impairment of reality testing is evident. The individual experiences delusions or hallucinations.
4. **With Catatonic Features.** This category identifies the presence of psychomotor disturbances, such as severe **psychomotor retardation**, with or without the presence of waxy flexibility or stupor, or excessive motor activity. The individual may also manifest symptoms of negativism, mutism, echolalia, or echopraxia.
5. **With Melancholic Features.** This is a typically severe form of major depressive episode. Symptoms are exaggerated. Even temporary reactivity to usually pleasurable stimuli is absent. History reveals a good response to antidepressant or other somatic therapy.
6. **Chronic.** This classification applies when the current episode of depressed mood has been evident continuously for at least the past 2 years.
7. **With Seasonal Pattern.** This diagnosis indicates the presence of depressive symptoms during the fall or winter months. This diagnosis is made when the number of seasonal depressive episodes is substantially higher than the number of nonseasonal episodes that have occurred over the individual's lifetime (APA, 2000). This disorder has previously been identified in the literature as seasonal affective disorder (SAD).

8. **With Postpartum Onset.** This specifier is used when symptoms of major depression occur within 4 weeks postpartum.

The *DSM-IV-TR* diagnostic criteria for major depressive disorder are presented in Box 29–1.

Box 29 – 1 Diagnostic Criteria for Major Depressive Disorder

A. Five (or more) of the following symptoms have been present during the same 2-week period and represent a change from previous functioning; at least one of the symptoms is either (1) depressed mood, or (2) loss of interest or pleasure.
  1. Depressed mood most of the day, nearly every day, as indicated by either subjective report (e.g., feels sad or empty) or observation made by others (e.g., appears tearful).
     NOTE: In children and adolescents, can be irritable mood.
  2. Markedly diminished interest or pleasure in all, or almost all, activities most of the day, nearly every day (as indicated either by subjective account or observation made by others).
  3. Significant weight loss when not dieting or weight gain (e.g., a change of more than 5% of body weight in a month), or a decrease or increase in appetite nearly every day.
     NOTE: In children, consider failure to make expected weight gains.
  4. Insomnia or hypersomnia nearly every day.
  5. Psychomotor agitation or retardation nearly every day (observable by others, not merely subjective feelings of restlessness or being slowed down).
  6. Fatigue or loss of energy nearly every day.
  7. Feelings of worthlessness or excessive or inappropriate guilt (which may be delusional) nearly every day (not merely self-reproach or guilt about being sick).
  8. Diminished ability to think or concentrate, or indecisiveness, nearly every day (either by subjective account or as observed by others).
  9. Recurrent thoughts of death (not just fear of dying), recurrent suicidal ideation without a specific plan, or a suicide attempt or a specific plan for committing suicide.
B. There has never been a manic episode, a mixed episode, or a hypomanic episode that was not substance or treatment induced or due to the direct physiological effects of a general medical condition.
C. The symptoms cause clinically significant distress or impairment in social, occupational, or other important areas of functioning.
D. The symptoms are not due to the direct physiological effects of a substance (e.g., a drug of abuse, a medication) or a general medical condition (e.g., hypothyroidism).
E. The symptoms are not better accounted for by bereavement (i.e., after the loss of a loved one), the symptoms persist for longer than 2 months or are characterized by marked functional impairment, morbid preoccupation with worthlessness, suicidal ideation, psychotic symptoms, or psychomotor retardation.

SOURCE: American Psychiatric Association (2000), with permission.

Dysthymic Disorder

Characteristics of this mood disturbance are similar to, if somewhat milder than, those ascribed to major depressive disorder. Individuals with **dysthymic disorder** describe their mood as sad or "down in the dumps" (APA, 2000). There is no evidence of psychotic symptoms. The essential feature is a chronically depressed mood (or possibly an irritable mood in children or adolescents) for most of the day, more days than not, for at least 2 years (1 year for children and adolescents).

Dysthymic disorder may be further classified as:

1. **Early Onset.** Identifies cases of dysthymic disorder when the onset occurs before age 21 years.
2. **Late Onset.** Identifies cases of dysthymic disorder when the onset occurs at age 21 years or older.

The *DSM-IV-TR* diagnostic criteria for dysthymic disorder are presented in Box 29–2.

Box 29 – 2 Diagnostic Criteria for Dysthymic Disorder

A. Depressed mood for most of the day, more days than not, as indicated either by subjective account or observation by others, for at least 2 years. NOTE: In children and adolescents, mood can be irritable and duration must be at least 1 year.
B. Presence, while depressed, of two (or more) of the following:
  1. Poor appetite or overeating
  2. Insomnia or hypersomnia
  3. Low energy or fatigue
  4. Low self-esteem
  5. Poor concentration or difficulty making decisions
  6. Feelings of hopelessness
C. During the 2-year period (1 year for children or adolescents) of the disturbance, the person has never been without the symptoms in A or B for more than 2 months at a time.
D. No major depressive disorder has been present during the first 2 years of the disturbance (1 year for children and adolescents).
E. There has never been a manic, mixed or hypomanic episode, and criteria have never been met for cyclothymic disorder.
F. The disturbance does not occur exclusively during the course of a chronic psychotic disorder, such as schizophrenia or delusional disorder.
G. The symptoms are not due to the direct physiological effects of a substance (e.g., a drug of abuse, a medication) or a general medical condition (e.g., hypothyroidism).
H. The symptoms cause clinically significant distress or impairment in social, occupational, or other important areas of functioning.

Specify if:
  Early onset: Before age 21 years.
  Late onset: Age 21 years or older.

SOURCE: American Psychiatric Association (2000), with permission.

Premenstrual Dysphoric Disorder

The *DSM-IV-TR* (APA, 2000) does not include **premenstrual dysphoric disorder** as an official diagnostic category, but provides a set of research criteria to promote further study of the disorder. The essential features include markedly depressed mood, marked anxiety, mood swings, and decreased interest in activities during the week prior to menses and subsiding shortly after the onset of menstruation (APA, 2000). The *DSM-IV-TR* research criteria for premenstrual dysphoric disorder are presented in Box 29–3.

Bipolar Disorders

A bipolar disorder is characterized by mood swings from profound depression to extreme euphoria (mania), with intervening periods of normalcy. Delusions or hallucinations may or may not be a part of the clinical picture, and onset of symptoms may reflect a seasonal pattern.

During a manic episode, the mood is elevated, expansive, or irritable. The disturbance is sufficiently severe to cause marked impairment in occupational functioning or in usual social activities or relationships with others or to require hospitalization to prevent harm to self or others. Motor activity is excessive and frenzied. Psychotic features may be present.

A somewhat milder degree of this clinical symptom picture is called **hypomania**. Hypomania is not severe enough to cause marked impairment in social or occupational functioning or to require hospitalization, and it does not include psychotic features. The *DSM-IV-TR* diagnostic criteria for mania are presented in Box 29–4.

The diagnostic picture for depression associated with bipolar disorder is identical to that described for major depressive disorder, with one addition: the client must have a history of one or more manic episodes.

When the symptom presentation includes rapidly alternating moods (sadness, irritability, euphoria) accompanied by symptoms associated with both depression and mania, the individual is given a diagnosis of *bipolar disorder*, mixed. This disturbance is severe enough to cause marked impairment in social or occupational functioning or to require hospitalization. Psychotic features may be evident.

 BOX 29–3   Research Criteria for Premenstrual Dysphoric Disorder

A. In most menstrual cycles during the past year, five (or more) of the following symptoms were present for most of the time during the last week of the luteal phase, began to remit within a few days after the onset of the follicular phase, and were absent in the week postmenses, with at least one of the symptoms being 1, 2, 3, or 4:
1. Markedly depressed mood, feelings of hopelessness, or self-deprecating thoughts
2. Marked anxiety, tension, feelings of being "keyed up," or "on edge"
3. Marked affective lability (e.g., feeling suddenly sad or tearful or increased sensitivity to rejection)
4. Persistent and marked anger or irritability or increased interpersonal conflicts
5. Decreased interest in usual activities (e.g., work, school, friends, hobbies)
6. Subjective sense of difficulty in concentrating
7. Lethargy, easy fatigability, or marked lack of energy
8. Marked change in appetite, overeating, or specific food cravings
9. Hypersomnia or insomnia
10. A subjective sense of being overwhelmed or out of control
11. Other physical symptoms, such as breast tenderness or swelling, headaches, joint or muscle pain, a sensation of "bloating," weight gain

B. The disturbance markedly interferes with work or school or with usual social activities and relationships with others (e.g., avoidance of social activities, decreased productivity and efficiency at work or school).
C. The disturbance is not merely an exacerbation of the symptoms of another disorder, such as major depressive disorder, panic disorder, dysthymic disorder, or a personality disorder (although it may be superimposed on any of these disorders).
D. Criteria A, B, and C must be confirmed by prospective daily ratings during at least two consecutive symptomatic cycles.

SOURCE: American Psychiatric Association (2000), with permission.

BOX 29–4   Diagnostic Criteria for Manic Episode

A. A distinct period of abnormally and persistently elevated, expansive, or irritable mood, lasting 1 week (or any duration if hospitalization is necessary).
B. During the period of mood disturbance, three (or more) of the following symptoms have persisted (four if the mood is only irritable) and have been present to a significant degree:
1. Inflated self-esteem or grandiosity
2. Decreased need for sleep (e.g., feels rested after only 3 hours of sleep)
3. More talkative than usual or pressure to keep talking
4. Flight of ideas or subjective experience that thoughts are racing
5. Distractibility (i.e., attention too easily drawn to unimportant or irrelevant external stimuli)
6. Increase in goal-directed activity (either socially, at work or school, or sexually) or psychomotor agitation
7. Excessive involvement in pleasurable activities that have a high potential for painful consequences (e.g., engaging in unrestrained buying sprees, sexual indiscretions, or foolish business investments)
C. The mood disturbance is sufficiently severe to cause marked impairment in occupational functioning or in usual social activities or relationships with others, or to necessitate hospitalization to prevent harm to self or others, or there are psychotic features.
D. The symptoms are not due to the direct physiological effects of a substance (e.g., a drug of abuse, a medication, or other treatment) or a general medical condition (e.g., hyperthyroidism).

SOURCE: American Psychiatric Association (2000), with permission.

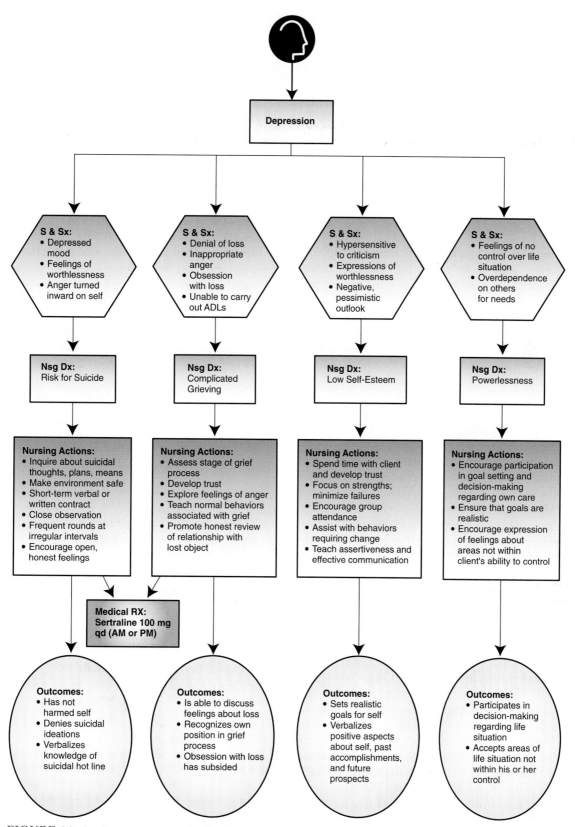

FIGURE 29–4 Concept map care plan for client with depression.

BIPOLAR DISORDER (MANIA)

The exact etiology of bipolar disorder has yet to be determined. Scientific evidence supports a chemical imbalance in the brain, although the cause of the imbalance remains unclear. Theories that consider a combination of hereditary factors and environmental triggers (stressful life events) appear to hold the most credibility.

Predisposing Factors

Biological Theories

Genetics

Research suggests that bipolar disorder strongly reflects an underlying genetic vulnerability. Evidence from family, twin, and adoption studies exists to support this observation.

Twin Studies. Twin studies have indicated a concordance rate for bipolar disorder among monozygotic twins at 60 to 80 percent compared to 10 to 20 percent in dizygotic twins. Because monozygotic twins have identical genes and dizygotic twins share only approximately half their genes, this is strong evidence that genes play a major role in the etiology.

Family Studies. Family studies have shown that if one parent has bipolar disorder, the risk that a child will have the disorder is around 28 percent (Dubovsky, Davies, & Dubovsky, 2003). If both parents have the disorder, the risk is two to three times as great. This has also been shown to be the case in studies of children born to parents with bipolar disorder who were adopted at birth and reared by adoptive parents without evidence of the disorder. These results strongly indicate that genes play a role separate from that of the environment.

Biochemical Influences

Biogenic Amines. Early studies have associated symptoms of depression with a functional deficiency of norepinephrine and dopamine and mania with a functional excess of these amines. The neurotransmitter serotonin appears to remain low in both states. One study at the University of Michigan using a presynaptic marker and positron emission tomography revealed an increased density in the amine-releasing cells in the brains of people with bipolar disorder compared to control subjects (Zubieta et al., 2000). It was hypothesized that these excess cells result in the altered brain chemistry that is associated with the symptoms of bipolar disorder. Some support of this neurotransmitter hypothesis has been demonstrated by the effects of neuroleptic drugs that influence the levels of these biogenic amines to produce the desired effect.

Electrolytes. Some studies have suggested possible alterations in normal electrolyte transfer across cell membranes in bipolar disorder resulting in elevated levels of intracellular calcium. The link between disruption of calcium regulation and symptoms of bipolar disorder may be substantiated by the effectiveness of calcium channel blockers (e.g., verapamil; amlodipine) in some cases of refractory bipolar illness (Soreff & McInnes, 2006).

Physiological Influences

Neuroanatomical Factors. Right-sided lesions in the limbic system, temporobasal areas, basal ganglia, and thalamus have been shown to induce secondary mania. Magnetic resonance imaging studies have revealed enlarged third ventricles and subcortical white matter and periventricular hyperintensities in clients with bipolar disorder (Dubovsky et al., 2003).

Medication Side Effects. Certain medications used to treat somatic illnesses have been known to trigger a manic response. The most common of these are the steroids frequently used to treat chronic illnesses such as multiple sclerosis and systemic lupus erythematosus (SLE). Some clients whose first episode of mania occurred during steroid therapy have reported spontaneous recurrence of manic symptoms years later. Amphetamines, antidepressants, and high doses of anticonvulsants and narcotics also have the potential for initiating a manic episode (Dubovsky et al., 2003).

Psychosocial Theories

The credibility of psychosocial theories has declined in recent years. Conditions such as schizophrenia and bipolar disorder are being viewed as diseases of the brain with biological etiologies. The etiology of these illnesses remains unclear, however, and it is possible that both biological and psychosocial factors (such as environmental stressors) are influential (NIMH, 2007).

The Transactional Model

Bipolar disorder most likely results from an interaction between genetic, biological, and psychosocial determinants. Kaplan and Sadock, (1998) state:

> The causative factors (of mood disorders) can be artificially divided into biological, genetic, and psychosocial, but this division is artificial because the three realms likely interact among themselves. Psychosocial and genetic factors can affect biological factors, such as concentrations of a certain neurotransmitter. Biological and psychosocial factors can also affect gene expression, and biological and genetic factors can affect a person's response to psychosocial factors. (p. 524)

The transactional model takes into consideration these various etiological influences, as well as those associated with past experiences, existing conditions, and the individual's perception of the event. Figure 29–5 depicts the dynamics

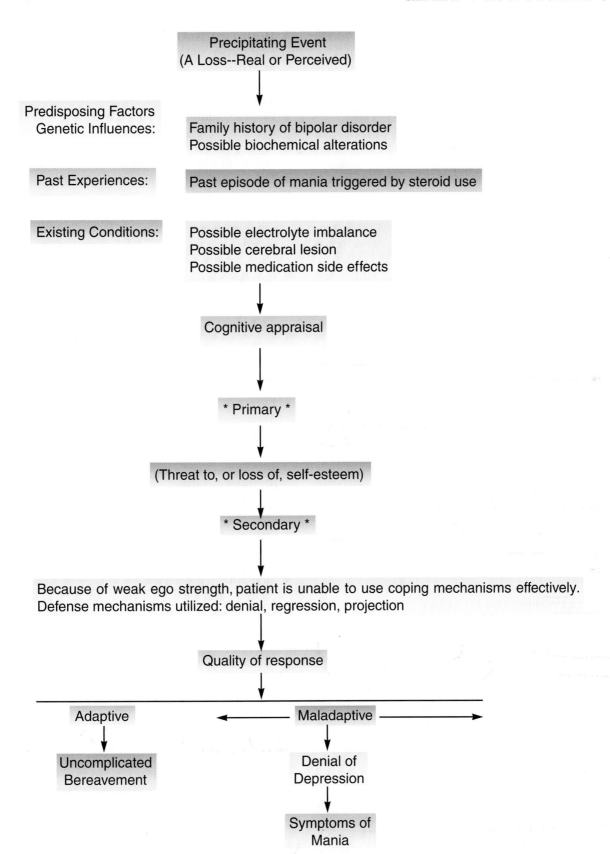

FIGURE 29–5 The dynamics of bipolar disorder, mania, using the Transactional Model of Stress/Adaptation.

of bipolar disorder, mania, using the Transactional Model of Stress/Adaptation.

Developmental Implications

Childhood and Adolescence

The lifetime prevalence of pediatric and adolescent bipolar disorders is estimated to be about 1 percent, but children and adolescents are often difficult to diagnose (Correll, 2007). The developmental courses and symptom profiles of psychiatric disorders in children are unique from those of adults; therefore, approaches to diagnosis and treatment cannot merely rely on strategies examined and implemented in a typical adult population.

A working group sponsored by the Child and Adolescent Bipolar Foundation (CABF) has developed consensus guidelines for the diagnosis and treatment of children with bipolar disorder. These guidelines were presented in the March 2005 issue of the *Journal of the American Academy of Child and Adolescent Psychiatry* and address diagnosis, comorbidity, acute treatment, and maintenance treatment (Kowatch et al., 2005).

Symptoms of bipolar disorder are often difficult to assess in children, and they may also present with comorbid conduct disorders or attention-deficit/hyperactivity disorder (ADHD). Because there is a genetic component and children of bipolar adults are at higher risk, family history may be particularly important (Allen, 2003). To differentiate between occasional spontaneous behaviors of childhood and behaviors associated with bipolar disorder, the Consensus Group recommends that clinicians use the FIND (frequency, intensity, number, and duration) strategy (Kowatch et al., 2005):

- Frequency: Symptoms occur most days in a week.
- Intensity: Symptoms are severe enough to cause extreme disturbance in one domain or moderate disturbance in two or more domains.
- Number: Symptoms occur three or four times a day.
- Duration: Symptoms occur 4 or more hours a day.

The symptoms associated with mania in children and adolescents are as follows. Regarding these symptoms, Kowatch and associates (2005) state:

> For any of these symptoms to be counted as a manic symptom, they must exceed the FIND threshold. Additionally, they must occur in concert with other manic symptoms because no one symptom is diagnostic of mania. (p. 215)

- **Euphoric/Expansive Mood.** Extremely happy, silly, or giddy.
- **Irritable Mood.** Hostility and rage, often over trivial matters. The irritability may be accompanied by aggressive and/or self-injurious behavior.
- **Grandiosity.** Believing that his or her abilities are better than everyone else's.

- **Decreased Need for Sleep.** May sleep only 4 or 5 hours per night and wake up fresh and full of energy the next day. Or he or she may get up in the middle of the night and wander around the house looking for things to do.
- **Pressured Speech.** Rapid speech that is loud, intrusive, and difficult to interrupt.
- **Racing Thoughts.** Topics of conversation change rapidly, in a manner confusing to anyone listening.
- **Distractibility.** To consider distractibility a manic symptom, it needs to reflect a change from baseline functioning, needs to occur in conjunction with a "manic" mood shift, and cannot be accounted for exclusively by another disorder, particularly ADHD (Kowatch et al., 2005). Distractibility during a manic episode may be reflected in a child who is normally a B or C student and is unable to focus on any school lessons.
- **Increase in Goal-Directed Activity/Psychomotor Agitation.** A child who is not usually highly productive, during a manic episode becomes very project oriented, increasing goal-directed activity to an obsessive level. Psychomotor agitation represents a distinct change from baseline behavior.
- **Excessive Involvement in Pleasurable or Risky Activities.** Children with bipolar disorder are often hypersexual, exhibiting behavior that has an erotic, pleasure-seeking quality about it (Kowatch et al., 2005). Adolescents may seek out sexual activity multiple times in a day.
- **Psychosis.** In addition to core symptoms of mania, psychotic symptoms, including hallucinations and delusions, are frequently present in children with bipolar disorder (Geller et al., 2002; Kafantaris, Dicker, Coletti, & Kane, 2001).
- **Suicidality.** Although not a core symptom of mania, children with bipolar disorder are at risk of suicidal ideation, intent, plans, and attempts during a depressed or mixed episode or when psychotic (Geller et al., 2002).

Treatment Strategies

Psychopharmacology

Monotherapy with the traditional mood stabilizers (e.g., lithium, divalproex, carbamazepine) or atypical antipsychotics (e.g., olanzapine, quetiapine, risperidone) was determined to be the first-line treatment (Kowatch et al., 2005). In the event of inadequate response to initial monotherapy, an alternate monotherapeutic agent is suggested. Augmentation with a second medication is indicated when monotherapy fails.

ADHD has been identified as the most common comorbid condition in children and adolescents with bipolar disorder. Because stimulants can exacerbate mania (Allen, 2003), it is suggested that medication for ADHD be initiated only after bipolar symptoms have been controlled with a mood stabilizer (Kowatch et al., 2005). Nonstimulant medications indicated for ADHD (e.g., atomoxetine, bupropion, the tricyclic antidepressants) may also induce switches to mania or hypomania.

Bipolar disorder in children and adolescents appears to be a chronic condition with a high risk of relapse (Kowatch et al., 2005). Maintenance therapy is with the same medications used to treat acute symptoms, although few research studies exist that deal with long-term maintenance of bipolar disorder in children. The Consensus Group recommends that medication tapering or discontinuation be considered after remission has been achieved for a minimum of 12 to 24 consecutive months. It was acknowledged, however, that some clients may require long-term or even lifelong pharmacotherapy (Kowatch et al., 2005).

Family Interventions

Although pharmacologic treatment is acknowledged as the primary method of stabilizing an acutely ill bipolar client, adjunctive psychotherapy has been recognized as playing an important role in preventing relapses and improving adjustment. Allen (2003) suggests that involving the family in post-episode stabilization of bipolar disorder is important and helps family members:

● Integrate their experience of the mood disorder.
● Know the symptoms of bipolar disorder and what precipitates episodes.
● Understand the client's vulnerability to future episodes.

Family support is also important in helping the client accept the necessity of ongoing medication administration. Family dynamics and attitudes can play a crucial role in the outcome of a client's recovery. Interventions with family members must include education that promotes understanding that at least part of the client's negative behaviors are attributable to an illness that must be managed, as opposed to being willful and deliberate.

Studies show that family-focused psychoeducational treatment (FFT) is an effective method of reducing relapses and increasing medication adherence in bipolar clients (Miklowitz, George, Richards, Simoneau, & Suddath, 2003). FFT includes sessions that deal with psychoeducation about bipolar disorder (i.e., symptoms, early recognition, etiology, treatment, self-management), communication training, and problem-solving skills training. Allen (2003) states:

> There are several important goals of FFT, which include: improving communication within the family, teaching the family to recognize the early warning signs of a relapse, teaching the family how to respond to these warning signs, and educating them regarding the necessary treatments. This education helps families gain some control over the conflict that occurs in the post-episode phases.

There is evidence to suggest that the addition of psychosocial therapy enhances the effectiveness of psychopharmacological therapy in the maintenance of bipolar disorder in children and adolescents.

APPLICATION OF THE NURSING PROCESS TO BIPOLAR DISORDER (MANIA)

Background Assessment Data

Symptoms of manic states can be described according to three stages: hypomania, acute mania, and **delirious mania**. Symptoms of mood, cognition and perception, and activity and behavior are presented for each stage.

Stage I: Hypomania

At this stage the disturbance is not sufficiently severe to cause marked impairment in social or occupational functioning or to require hospitalization (APA, 2000).

Mood. The mood of a hypomanic person is cheerful and expansive. There is an underlying irritability that surfaces rapidly when the person's wishes and desires go unfulfilled, however. The nature of the hypomanic person is very volatile and fluctuating.

Cognition and Perception. Perceptions of the self are exalted—ideas of great worth and ability. Thinking is flighty, with a rapid flow of ideas. Perception of the environment is heightened, but the individual is so easily distracted by irrelevant stimuli that goal-directed activities are difficult.

Activity and Behavior. Hypomanic individuals exhibit increased motor activity. They are perceived as being very extroverted and sociable, and because of this they attract numerous acquaintances. They lack the depth of personality and warmth to formulate close friendships, however. They talk and laugh a great deal, usually very loudly and often inappropriately. Increased libido is common. Some individuals experience anorexia and weight loss. The exalted self-perception leads some hypomanic individuals to engage in inappropriate behaviors, such as phoning the President of the United States, or buying huge amounts on a credit card without having the resources to pay.

Stage II: Acute Mania

Symptoms of acute mania may be a progression in intensification of those experienced in hypomania, or they may be manifested directly. Most individuals experience marked impairment in functioning and require hospitalization.

Mood. Acute mania is characterized by euphoria and elation. The person appears to be on a continuous "high." However, the mood is always subject to frequent variation, easily changing to irritability and anger or even to sadness and crying.

Cognition and Perception. Cognition and perception become fragmented and often psychotic in acute mania. Rapid thinking proceeds to racing and disjointed thinking (flight of ideas) and may be manifested by a continuous flow of accelerated, pressured speech (loquaciousness), with abrupt changes from topic to topic. When flight of ideas is severe, speech may be disorganized and incoherent. Distractibility becomes all-pervasive. Attention can be diverted by even the smallest of stimuli. Hallucinations and delusions (usually paranoid and grandiose) are common.

Activity and Behavior. Psychomotor activity is excessive. Sexual interest is increased. There is poor impulse control, and the individual who is normally discreet may become socially and sexually uninhibited. Excessive spending is common. Individuals with acute mania have the ability to manipulate others to carry out their wishes, and if things go wrong, they can skillfully project responsibility for the failure onto others. Energy seems inexhaustible, and the need for sleep is diminished. They may go for many days without sleep and still not feel tired. Hygiene and grooming may be neglected. Dress may be disorganized, flamboyant, or bizarre, and the use of excessive make-up or jewelry is common.

Stage III: Delirious Mania

Delirious mania is a grave form of the disorder characterized by severe clouding of consciousness and an intensification of the symptoms associated with acute mania. This condition has become relatively rare since the availability of antipsychotic medication.

Mood. The mood of the delirious person is very labile. He or she may exhibit feelings of despair, quickly converting to unrestrained merriment and ecstasy or becoming irritable or totally indifferent to the environment. Panic anxiety may be evident.

Cognition and Perception. Cognition and perception are characterized by a clouding of consciousness, with accompanying confusion, disorientation, and sometimes stupor. Other common manifestations include religiosity, delusions of grandeur or persecution, and auditory or visual hallucinations. The individual is extremely distractible and incoherent.

Activity and Behavior. Psychomotor activity is frenzied and characterized by agitated, purposeless movements. The safety of these individuals is at stake unless this activity is curtailed. Exhaustion, injury to self or others, and eventually death could occur without intervention.

Diagnosis/Outcome Identification

Using information collected during the assessment, the nurse completes the client database, from which the selection of appropriate nursing diagnoses is determined. Table 29–3 presents a list of client behaviors and the NANDA nursing diagnoses that correspond to those behaviors, which may be used in planning care for the client with bipolar mania.

Outcome Criteria

The following criteria may be used for measuring outcomes in the care of the manic client.

The client:

1. Exhibits no evidence of physical injury.
2. Has not harmed self or others.
3. Is no longer exhibiting signs of physical agitation.
4. Eats a well-balanced diet with snacks to prevent weight loss and maintain nutritional status.
5. Verbalizes an accurate interpretation of the environment.
6. Verbalizes that hallucinatory activity has ceased and demonstrates no outward behavior indicating hallucinations.
7. Accepts responsibility for own behaviors.
8. Does not manipulate others for gratification of own needs.
9. Interacts appropriately with others.
10. Is able to fall asleep within 30 minutes of retiring.
11. Is able to sleep 6 to 8 hours per night without medication.

TABLE 29–3 Assigning Nursing Diagnoses to Behaviors Commonly Associated with Bipolar Mania	
Behaviors	**Nursing Diagnoses**
Extreme hyperactivity; increased agitation and lack of control over purposeless and potentially injurious movements	Risk for Injury
Manic excitement, delusional thinking, hallucinations, impulsivity	Risk for Violence: Self-Directed or Other-Directed
Loss of weight, amenorrhea, refusal or inability to sit still long enough to eat	Imbalanced Nutrition: Less than Body Requirements
Delusions of grandeur and persecution; inaccurate interpretation of the environment	Disturbed Thought Processes
Auditory and visual hallucinations; disorientation	Disturbed Sensory-Perception
Inability to develop satisfying relationships, manipulation of others for own desires, use of unsuccessful social interaction behaviors	Impaired Social Interaction
Difficulty falling asleep, sleeping only short periods	Insomnia

Planning/Implementation

The following section presents a group of selected nursing diagnoses, with short- and long-term goals and nursing interventions for each.

Some institutions are using a case management model to coordinate care (see Chapter 9 for a more detailed explanation). In case management models, the plan of care may take the form of a critical pathway.

Risk for Violence: Self-Directed or Other-Directed

Risk for self- or other-directed violence is defined as "at risk for behaviors in which an individual demonstrates that he or she can be physically, emotionally, and/or sexually harmful either to self or to others" (NANDA-I, 2007, pp. 240–243). **NOTE:** Please refer to Chapter 17 for additional concepts related to anger and aggression management.

Client Goals

Outcome criteria include short- and long-term goals. Timelines are individually determined.

Short-Term Goals
- Within [a specified time], client will recognize signs of increasing anxiety and agitation and report to staff (or other care provider) for assistance with intervention.
- Client will not harm self or others.

Long-Term Goal
- Client will not harm self or others.

Interventions

- Maintain low level of stimuli in client's environment (low lighting, few people, simple decor, low noise level). Anxiety level rises in a stimulating environment. A suspicious, agitated client may perceive individuals as threatening.
- Observe the client's behavior frequently. Do this while carrying out routine activities so as to avoid creating suspiciousness in the individual. Close observation is necessary so that intervention can occur if required to ensure client (and others') safety.
- Remove all dangerous objects from the client's environment so that in his or her agitated, confused state the client may not use them to harm self or others.
- Intervene at the first sign of increased anxiety, agitation, or verbal or behavioral aggression. Offer empathetic response to the client's feelings: "You seem anxious (or frustrated, or angry) about this situation. How can I help?" Validation of the client's feelings conveys a caring attitude and offering assistance reinforces trust.
- It is important to maintain a calm attitude toward the client. As the client's anxiety increases, offer some alternatives: to participate in a physical activity (e.g., punching bag, physical exercise), talking about the situation, taking some antianxiety medication. Offering alternatives to the client gives him or her a feeling of some control over the situation.
- Have sufficient staff available to indicate a show of strength to the client if it becomes necessary. This shows the client evidence of control over the situation and provides some physical security for staff.
- If client is not calmed by "talking down" or by medication, use of mechanical restraints may be necessary. The avenue of the "least restrictive alternative" must be selected when planning interventions for a violent client. Restraints should be used only as a last resort, after all other interventions have been unsuccessful, and the client is clearly at risk of harm to self or others.
- If restraint is deemed necessary, ensure that sufficient staff is available to assist. Follow protocol established by the institution. The Joint Commission on Accreditation of Healthcare Organizations (JCAHO) requires that the physician reissue a new order for restraints every 4 hours for adults and every 1 to 2 hours for children and adolescents.
- JCAHO requires that the client in restraints be observed at least every 15 minutes to ensure that circulation to extremities is not compromised (check temperature, color, pulses); to assist the client with needs related to nutrition, hydration, and elimination; and to position the client so that comfort is facilitated and aspiration can be prevented. Some institutions may require continuous one-to-one monitoring of restrained clients, particularly those who are highly agitated, and for whom there is a high risk of self- or accidental injury.
- As agitation decreases, assess the client's readiness for restraint removal or reduction. Remove one restraint at a time while assessing the client's response. This minimizes the risk of injury to client and staff.

Impaired Social Interaction

Impaired social interaction is defined as "insufficient or excessive quantity or ineffective quality of social exchange" (NANDA-I, 2007, p. 204). Table 29–4 presents this nursing diagnosis in care plan format.

Client Goals

Outcome criteria include short- and long-term goals. Timelines are individually determined.

Short-Term Goal
- Client will verbalize which of his or her interaction behaviors are appropriate and which are inappropriate within 1 week.

Table 29–4	Care Plan for the Client Experiencing a Manic Episode	

NURSING DIAGNOSIS: IMPAIRED SOCIAL INTERACTION

RELATED TO: Delusional thought processes (grandeur and/or persecution); underdeveloped ego and low self-esteem

EVIDENCED BY: Inability to develop satisfying relationships and manipulation of others for own desires

Outcome Criteria	Nursing Interventions	Rationale
Short-Term Goal ● The client will verbalize which of his or her interaction behaviors are appropriate and which are inappropriate within 1 week. **Long-Term Goal** ● The client will demonstrate use of appropriate interaction skills as evidenced by lack of, or marked decrease in, manipulation of others to fulfill own desires.	1. Recognize the purpose manipulative behaviors serve for the client: to reduce feelings of insecurity by increasing feelings of power and control. 2. Set limits on manipulative behaviors. Explain to the client what is expected and what the consequences are if the limits are violated. Terms of the limitations must be agreed on by all staff who will be working with the client. 3. Do not argue, bargain, or try to reason with the client. Merely state the limits and expectations. Confront the client as soon as possible when interactions with others are manipulative or exploitative. Follow through with established consequences for unacceptable behavior. 4. Provide positive reinforcement for non-manipulative behaviors. Explore feelings and help the client seek more appropriate ways of dealing with them. 5. Help the client recognize that he or she must accept the consequences of own behaviors and refrain from attributing them to others. 6. Help the client identify positive aspects about self, recognize accomplishments, and feel good about them.	1. Understanding the motivation behind the manipulation may facilitate acceptance of the individual and his or her behavior. 2. The client is unable to establish own limits, so this must be done for him or her. Unless administration of consequences for violation of limits is consistent, manipulative behavior will not be eliminated. 3. Because of the strong id influence on client's behavior, he or she should receive immediate feedback when behavior is unacceptable. Consistency in enforcing the consequences is essential if positive outcomes are to be achieved. Inconsistency creates confusion and encourages testing of limits. 4. Positive reinforcement enhances self-esteem and promotes repetition of desirable behaviors. 5. The client must accept responsibility for own behaviors before adaptive change can occur. 6. As self-esteem is increased, client will feel less need to manipulate others for own gratification.

Long-Term Goal

● Client will demonstrate use of appropriate interaction skills as evidenced by lack of, or marked decrease in, manipulation of others to fulfill own desires.

Interventions

● Recognize the purpose these behaviors serve for the client: to reduce feelings of insecurity by increasing feelings of power and control. Understanding the motivation behind the manipulation may help to facilitate acceptance of the individual and his or her behavior.

● Set limits on manipulative behaviors. Explain to the client what is expected and what the consequences are if the limits are violated. Terms of the limitations must be agreed on by all staff who will be working with the client. The client is unable to establish own limits, so this must be done for him or her. Unless administration of consequences for violation of limits is consistent, manipulative behavior will not be eliminated.

● Do not argue, bargain, or try to reason with the client. Merely state the limits and expectations. Individuals with mania can be very charming in their efforts to fulfill their own desires. Confront the client as soon as possible when interactions with others are manipulative or exploitative. Follow through with established consequences for unacceptable behavior. Because of the strong id influence on client's behavior, he or she should receive immediate feedback when behavior is unacceptable. Consistency in enforcing the consequences is essential if positive outcomes are to be achieved. Inconsistency creates confusion and encourages testing of limits.

● Provide positive reinforcement for nonmanipulative behaviors. Explore feelings, and help the client seek more appropriate ways of dealing with them.

- Help the client recognize that he or she must accept the consequences of own behaviors and refrain from attributing them to others. The client must accept responsibility for own behaviors before adaptive change can occur.
- Help the client identify positive aspects about self, recognize accomplishments, and feel good about them. As self-esteem is increased, the client will feel less need to manipulate others for own gratification.

Feeding Self-Care Deficit/Insomnia

Feeding self-care deficit is defined as "impaired ability to perform or complete feeding activities (NANDA-I, 2007, p. 185). *Insomnia* is defined as "a disruption in amount and quality of sleep that impairs functioning" (NANDA-I, 2007, p. 127).

Client Goals

Outcome criteria include short- and long-term goals. Timelines are individually determined.

Short-Term Goals

- Client will consume sufficient finger foods and between-meal snacks to meet recommended daily allowances of nutrients.
- Within 3 days, with the aid of a sleeping medication, client will sleep 4 to 6 hours without awakening.

Long-Term Goals

- Client will exhibit no signs or symptoms of malnutrition.
- By time of discharge from treatment, client will be able to acquire 6 to 8 hours of uninterrupted sleep without medication.

Interventions

- In collaboration with the dietitian, determine the number of calories required to provide adequate nutrition for maintenance or realistic (according to body structure and height) weight gain. Determine client's likes and dislikes, and try to provide favorite foods, if possible. The client is more likely to eat foods that he or she particularly enjoys.
- Provide the client with high-protein, high-calorie, nutritious finger foods and drinks that can be consumed "on the run." Because of the hyperactive state, the client has difficulty sitting still long enough to eat a meal. The likelihood is greater that he or she will consume food and drinks that can be carried around and eaten with little effort. Have juice and snacks available on the unit at all times. Nutritious intake is required on a regular basis to compensate for increased caloric requirements due to the hyperactivity.
- Maintain an accurate record of intake, output, and calorie count. Weigh the client daily. Administer vitamin and mineral supplements, as ordered by the physician. Monitor laboratory values, and report significant changes to the physician. It is important to carefully monitor the data that provides an objective assessment of the client's nutritional status.
- Assess the client's activity level. He or she may ignore or be unaware of feelings of fatigue. Observe for signs such as increasing restlessness; fine tremors; slurred speech; and puffy, dark circles under eyes. The client could collapse from exhaustion if hyperactivity is uninterrupted and rest is not achieved.
- Monitor sleep patterns. Provide a structured schedule of activities that includes established times for naps or rest. Accurate baseline data are important in planning care to help the client with this problem. A structured schedule, including time for short naps, will help the hyperactive client achieve much-needed rest.
- Client should avoid intake of caffeinated drinks, such as tea, coffee, and colas. Caffeine is a CNS stimulant and may interfere with the client's achievement of rest and sleep.
- Before bedtime, provide nursing measures that promote sleep, such as back rub; warm bath; warm, nonstimulating drinks; soft music; and relaxation exercises.
- Administer sedative medications, as ordered, to assist client achieve sleep until normal sleep pattern is restored.

Concept Care Mapping

The concept map care plan is an innovative approach to planning and organizing nursing care (see Chapter 9). It is a diagrammatic teaching and learning strategy that allows visualization of interrelationships between medical diagnoses, nursing diagnoses, assessment data, and treatments. An example of a concept map care plan for a client with bipolar disorder, mania, is presented in Figure 29–6.

Client/Family Education

The role of client teacher is important in the psychiatric area, as it is in all areas of nursing. A list of topics for client/family education relevant to bipolar disorder is presented in Box 29–7.

Evaluation of Care for the Manic Client

In the final step of the nursing process, a reassessment is conducted to determine if the nursing actions have been successful in achieving the objectives of care. Evaluation of the nursing actions for the manic client may be facilitated by gathering information using the following types of questions.

1. Has the individual avoided personal injury?
2. Has violence to client or others been prevented?
3. Has agitation subsided?
4. Have nutritional status and weight been stabilized? Is the client able to select foods to maintain adequate nutrition?

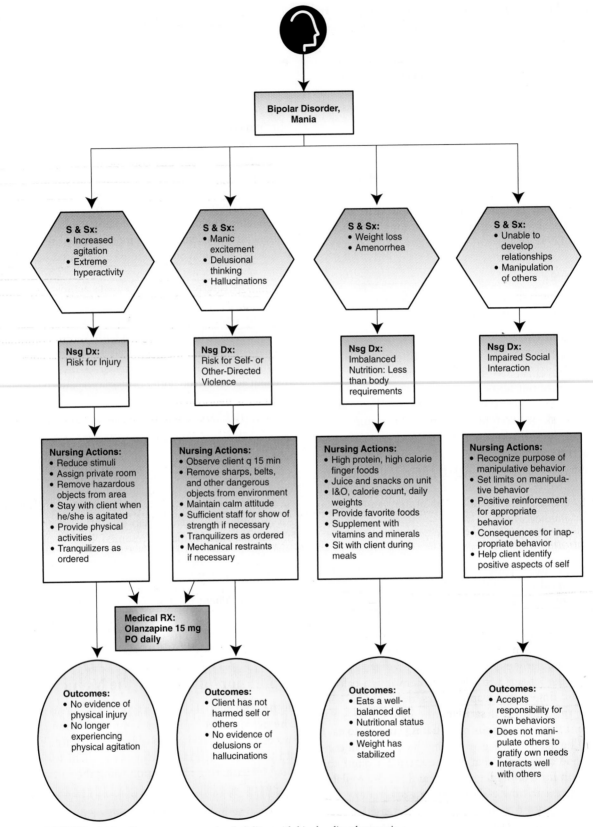

FIGURE 29–6 Concept map care plan for client with bipolar disorder, mania.

BOX 29 – 7 Topics for Client/Family Education Related to Bipolar Disorder

Nature of the Illness

1. Causes of bipolar disorder
2. Cyclic nature of the illness
3. Symptoms of depression
4. Symptoms of mania

Management of the Illness

1. Medication management
   a. Lithium
   b. Others
      1) Carbamazepine
      2) Valproic acid
      3) Clonazepam
      4) Verapamil
      5) Lamotrigine
      6) Gabapentin
      7) Topiramate
      8) Oxcarbazepine
      9) Olanzapine
      10) Risperidone
      11) Chlorpromazine
      12) Aripiprazole
      13) Quetiapine
      14) Ziprasidone
   c. Side effects
   d. Symptoms of lithium toxicity
   e. Importance of regular blood tests
   f. Adverse effects
   g. Importance of not stopping medication, even when feeling well
2. Assertive techniques
3. Anger management

Support Services

1. Crisis hotline
2. Support groups
3. Individual psychotherapy
4. Legal and/or financial assistance

5. Have delusions and hallucinations ceased? Is the client able to interpret the environment correctly?
6. Is the client able to make decisions about own self-care? Has hygiene and grooming improved?
7. Is behavior socially acceptable? Is client able to interact with others in a satisfactory manner? Has the client stopped manipulating others to fulfill own desires?
8. Is the client able to sleep 6 to 8 hours per night and awaken feeling rested?
9. Does the client understand the importance of maintenance medication therapy? Does he or she understand that symptoms may return if medication is discontinued?
10. Can the client taking lithium verbalize early signs of lithium toxicity? Does he or she understand the necessity for monthly blood level checks?

TREATMENT MODALITIES FOR MOOD DISORDERS

Individual Psychotherapy

For Depression

Research has documented both the importance of close and satisfactory attachments in the prevention of depression and the role of disrupted attachments in the development of depression. With this concept in mind, interpersonal psychotherapy focuses on the client's current interpersonal relations. Interpersonal psychotherapy with the depressed person proceeds through the following phases and interventions:

Phase I. During the first phase, the client is assessed to determine the extent of the illness. Complete information is then given to the individual regarding the nature of depression, symptom pattern, frequency, clinical course, and alternative treatments. If the level of depression is severe, interpersonal psychotherapy has been shown to be more effective if conducted in combination with antidepressant medication. The client is encouraged to continue working and participating in regular activities during therapy. A mutually agreeable therapeutic contract is negotiated.

Phase II. Treatment at this phase focuses on helping the client resolve complicated grief reactions. This may include resolving the ambivalence with a lost relationship, serving as a temporary substitute for the lost relationship, and assistance with establishing new relationships. Other areas of treatment focus may include interpersonal disputes between the client and a significant other, difficult role transitions at various developmental life cycles, and correction of interpersonal deficits that may interfere with the client's ability to initiate or sustain interpersonal relationships.

Phase III. During the final phase of interpersonal psychotherapy, the therapeutic alliance is terminated. With emphasis on reassurance, clarification of emotional states, improvement of interpersonal communication, testing of perceptions, and performance in interpersonal settings, interpersonal psychotherapy has been successful in helping depressed persons recover enhanced social functioning.

For Mania

Manic clients traditionally have been difficult candidates for psychotherapy. They form a therapeutic relationship easily because they are eager to please and grateful for the therapist's interest. However, the relationship often tends to remain shallow and rigid. Some reports have indicated that psychotherapy (in conjunction with medication maintenance treatment) and counseling may indeed be useful with these individuals. Goldberg and Hoop (2004) state:

> Interpersonal and social rhythm therapy is a form of interpersonal therapy tailored to bipolar patients. In addition to focusing on grief, role conflicts, role transitions, and interpersonal deficiencies, it includes psychoeducation about bipolar disorder and encourages treatment adherence. Studies have suggested that bipolar patients receiving the treatment were more often euthymic [stable mood] than patients receiving only clinical management.

Group Therapy for Depression and Mania

Group therapy forms an important dimension of multimodal treatment of the manic or depressed client. Once an acute phase of the illness is passed, groups can provide an atmosphere in which individuals may discuss issues in their lives that cause, maintain, or arise out of having a serious affective disorder. The element of peer support provides a feeling of security, as troublesome or embarrassing issues are discussed and resolved. Some groups have other specific purposes, such as helping to monitor medication-related issues or serving as an avenue for promoting education related to the affective disorder and its treatment.

Support groups help members gain a sense of perspective on their condition and tangibly encourage them to link up with others who have common problems. A sense of hope is conveyed when the individual is able to see that he or she is not alone or unique in experiencing affective illness.

Self-help groups offer another avenue of support for the depressed or manic client. These groups are usually peer led and are not meant to substitute for, or compete with, professional therapy. They offer supplementary support that frequently enhances compliance with the medical regimen. Examples of self-help groups are the Depression and Bipolar Support Alliance (DBSA), Depressives Anonymous, Manic and Depressive Support Group, Recovery Inc., and New Images for Widows. Although self-help groups are not psychotherapy groups, they do provide important adjunctive support experiences, which often have therapeutic benefit for participants.

Family Therapy for Depression and Mania

The ultimate objectives in working with families of clients with mood disorders are to resolve the symptoms and initiate or restore adaptive family functioning. As with group therapy, the most effective approach appears to be with a combination of psychotherapeutic and pharmacotherapeutic treatments. Some studies with bipolar disorder have shown that behavioral family treatment combined with medication substantially reduces relapse rate compared with medication therapy alone.

Sadock and Sadock (2007) state:

> Family therapy is indicated if the disorder jeopardizes the patient's marriage or family functioning or if the mood disorder is promoted or maintained by the family situation. Family therapy examines the role of the mood-disordered member in the overall psychological well-being of the whole family; it also examines the role of the entire family in the maintenance of the patient's symptoms. (p. 555).

Cognitive Therapy for Depression and Mania

In cognitive therapy, the individual is taught to control thought distortions that are considered to be a factor in the development and maintenance of mood disorders. In the cognitive model, depression is characterized by a triad of negative distortions related to expectations of the environment, self, and future. The environment and activities within it are viewed as unsatisfying, the self is unrealistically devalued, and the future is perceived as hopeless. In the same model, mania is characterized by exaggeratedly positive cognitions and perceptions. The individual perceives the self as highly valued and powerful. Life is experienced with overstated self-assurance, and the future is viewed with unrealistic optimism.

The general goals in cognitive therapy are to obtain symptom relief as quickly as possible, to assist the client in identifying dysfunctional patterns of thinking and behaving, and to guide the client to evidence and logic that effectively tests the validity of the dysfunctional thinking. Therapy focuses on changing "automatic thoughts" that occur spontaneously and contribute to the distorted affect. Examples of automatic thoughts in depression include:

1. **Personalizing**: "I'm the only one who failed."
2. **All or nothing**: "I'm a complete failure."
3. **Mind reading**: "He thinks I'm foolish."
4. **Discounting positives**: "The other questions were so easy. Any dummy could have gotten them right."

Examples of automatic thoughts in mania include:

1. **Personalizing**: "She's this happy only when she's with me." Grand.
2. **All or nothing**: "Everything I do is great."
3. **Mind reading**: "She thinks I'm wonderful."
4. **Discounting negatives**: "None of those mistakes are really important."

The client is asked to describe evidence that both supports and disputes the automatic thought. The logic underlying the inferences is then reviewed with the client. Another technique involves evaluating what would most likely happen if the client's automatic thoughts were true. Implications of the consequences are then discussed.

Clients should not become discouraged if one technique seems not to be working. No single technique works with all clients. He or she should be reassured that any of a number of techniques may be used, and both therapist and client may explore these possibilities.

Finally, the use of cognitive therapy does not preclude the value of administering medication. Particularly in the treatment of mania, cognitive therapy should be considered a secondary treatment to pharmacological treatment. Cognitive therapy alone has offered encouraging results in the treatment of depression. In fact, the results of several studies with depressed clients show that in some cases cognitive therapy may be equally or even more effective than antidepressant medication (Rupke, Blecke, & Renfrow, 2006).

Electroconvulsive Therapy for Depression and Mania

(handwritten: ~~are~~ Grand mal seizure)

Electroconvulsive therapy (ECT) is the induction of a grand mal (generalized) seizure through the application of electrical current to the brain. ECT is effective with clients who are acutely suicidal and in the treatment of severe depression, particularly in those clients who are also experiencing psychotic symptoms and those with psychomotor retardation and neurovegetative changes, such as disturbances in sleep, appetite, and energy. It is often considered for treatment only after a trial of therapy with antidepressant medication has proved ineffective.

Episodes of acute mania are occasionally treated with ECT, particularly when the client does not tolerate or fails to respond to lithium or other drug treatment, or when life is threatened by dangerous behavior or exhaustion (see Chapter 22 for a detailed discussion of ECT).

Transcranial Magnetic Stimulation

(handwritten: no Grand mal seizure)

Transcranial magnetic stimulation (TMS) is one of the newer technologies that is being used to treat depression. It is also being studied in the treatment of mania, schizophrenia, obsessive–compulsive disorder, posttraumatic stress disorder, and others, but the large majority of research has been focused on the effect of TMS on major depression (Pridmore, Khan, Reid, & George, 2001). TMS involves the use of very short pulses of magnetic energy to stimulate nerve cells in the brain, similar to the electrical activity observed with ECT. However, unlike ECT, the electrical waves generated by TMS do not result in generalized seizure activity (Rosenbaum & Judy, 2004). The waves are passed through a coil placed on the scalp to areas of the brain involved in mood regulation. Some clinicians believe that TMS holds a great deal of promise in the treatment of depression, whereas others remain skeptical. In rare instances, seizures have been triggered with the use of TMS therapy (Rosenbaum & Judy, 2004). In a recent study at King's College in London, researchers compared the efficacy of TMS with ECT in the treatment of severe depression (Eranti et al., 2007). They concluded that ECT was substantially more effective for the short-term treatment of depression, and they indicated the need for further intense clinical evaluation of TMS.

Light Therapy for Depression

Between 15 and 25 percent of people with recurrent depressive disorder exhibit a seasonal pattern whereby symptoms are exacerbated during the winter months and subside during the spring and summer (Thase, 2007). The *DSM-IV-TR* identifies this disorder as Major Depressive Disorder with Seasonal Pattern. It has commonly been known as Seasonal Affective Disorder (SAD). Bright light therapy has been suggested as a first-line treatment for winter "blues" and as an adjunct in chronic major depressive disorder or dysthymia with seasonal exacerbations (Karasu, Gelenberg, Merriam, & Wang, 2006).

SAD is thought to be related to the presence of the hormone melatonin, which is produced by the pineal gland. Melatonin plays a role in the regulation of biological rhythms for sleep and activation. It is produced during the cycle of darkness and shuts off in the light of day. During the months of longer darkness hours, there is increased production of melatonin, which seems to trigger the symptoms of SAD in susceptible people.

Light therapy, or exposure to light, has been shown to be an effective treatment for SAD. The light therapy is administered by a 10,000-lux light box, which contains white fluorescent light tubes covered with a plastic screen that blocks ultraviolet rays. The individual sits in front of the box with the eyes open (although they should not look directly into the light). Therapy usually begins with 10- to 15-minute sessions, and gradually progress to 30 to 45 minutes. Some people notice improvement rapidly, within a few days, whereas others may take several weeks to feel better. Side effects appear to be dosage related, and include headache, eyestrain, nausea, irritability, photophobia (eye sensitivity to light), insomnia (when light therapy is used late in the day), and (rarely) hypomania (Terman & Terman, 2005). Light therapy and antidepressants have shown comparable efficacy in studies of SAD treatment. One recent study compared the efficacy of light therapy for SAD to daily treatment with 20 mg of fluoxetine (Lam et al., 2006). The authors concluded that, "Light treatment showed earlier response onset and lower rate of some adverse events relative to fluoxetine, but there were no other significant differences in outcome between light therapy and antidepressant medication" (p. 805).

Psychopharmacology

For Depression

Historical Aspects

Antidepressant medication had a serendipitous beginning. In the early 1950s, patients with tuberculosis were being treated with the monoamine oxidase inhibitor (MAOI) iproniazid. Although the drug proved ineffective for tuberculosis, it was found that patients exhibited a sustained elevation of mood while taking the medication (Schatzberg, Cole, & DeBattista, 2007). Following the initial enthusiasm about MAOIs, they fell into relative disuse for nearly two decades because of a perceived poor risk-to-benefit ratio.

The tricyclic antidepressants (TCAs) had a similar introduction. In the late 1950s, imipramine was being investigated as a treatment for schizophrenia, and although it did not relieve psychotic symptoms, it appeared to elevate mood. For almost 50 years, the TCAs have been widely used to treat depression. Since the initial discovery of their antidepressant properties, they have been subjected to hundreds of controlled trials, and their efficacy in treating depressive illness is now firmly established.

The success of these first two groups of antidepressants led the pharmaceutical industry to search for compounds with similar efficacy and fewer side effects than the MAOIs and the TCAs. A detailed discussion of antidepressant medication is provided in Chapter 21; an overview is presented here. A summary of medications used in the treatment of depression is presented in Table 29–5.

CLINICAL PEARL

All antidepressants carry an FDA black box warning for increased risk of suicidality in children and adolescents.

Selective Serotonin Reuptake Inhibitors

The selective serotonin reuptake inhibitors (SSRIs) are the most widely used class of antidepressants. They act by selectively inhibiting the central nervous system (CNS) neuronal uptake of serotonin (5-HT). Examples include citalopram (Celexa), escitalopram (Lexapro), fluoxetine (Prozac; Sarafem), fluvoxamine (Luvox), paroxetine (Paxil), and sertraline (Zoloft). They have a more favorable safety and side-effect profile than the MAOIs and the TCAs, and have also proved to have a broad spectrum of activity in a variety of psychiatric disorders (Schatzberg et al., 2007).

Side Effects. SSRIs have a lower incidence of anticholinergic and cardiotoxic side effects than the TCAs. The most common side effects with SSRIs include headache, insomnia or somnolence, nausea, anorexia, diarrhea, and dry mouth. Sexual dysfunction (impotence or anorgasmia) may be the most troubling adverse effect for clients. An uncommon, but potentially life-threatening, effect of SSRIs, called serotonin syndrome, may occur if they are taken concurrently with other medications that increase levels of serotonin (e.g., MAOIs, tryptophan, amphetamines, other antidepressants, buspirone, lithium, dopamine agonists, and the 5-HT_1 receptor agonists for migraine [the "triptan" drugs]). Symptoms of serotonin syndrome include confusion, agitation, tachycardia, hypertension, nausea, abdominal pain, myoclonus, muscle rigidity, fever, sweating, and tremor. If left untreated, it can progress to rhabdomyolysis, cardiovascular collapse, coma, and death. Treatment involves discontinuation of the offending drugs, monitoring vital signs, use of cooling blankets, and supporting vital functions. Cyproheptadine and dantrolene may be prescribed.

TABLE 29–5 Medications Used in the Treatment of Depression

Chemical Class	Generic (Trade) Name	Daily Adult Dosage Range (mg)*	Side Effects
Tricyclics (TCAs)	Amitriptyline	50–300	With all TCAs:
	Clomipramine (Anafranil)	25–250	Dry mouth, drowsiness, blurred vision, urinary
	Desipramine (Norpramin)	25–300	retention, constipation, arrhythmias,
	Doxepin (Sinequan)	25–300	tachycardia, changes in AV conduction,
	Imipramine (Tofranil)	30–300	lowered seizure threshold, nausea and
	Nortriptyline (Aventyl; Pamelor)	30–100	vomiting, photosensitivity, blood dyscrasias,
	Protriptyline (Vivactil)	15–60	exacerbation of mania, orthostatic hypotension.
	Trimipramine (Surmontil)	50–300	
Selective Serotonin Reuptake Inhibitors (SSRIs)	Citalopram (Celexa)	20–60	With all SSRIs:
	Fluoxetine (Prozac; Serafem)	20–80	Headache, insomnia, nausea, diarrhea,
	Fluvoxamine (Luvox)	50–300	constipation, sexual dysfunction, somnolence,
	Escitalopram (Lexapro)	10–20	agitation, dry mouth, asthenia, serotonin
	Paroxetine (Paxil)	10–50	syndrome (if taken concurrently with other
	Sertraline (Zoloft)	50–200	medications that increase levels of serotonin)
Monoamine Oxidase Inhibitors (MAOIs)	Isocarboxazid (Marplan)	20–60	With all MAOIs:
	Phenelzine (Nardil)	45–90	Dizziness, headache, orthostatic hypotension,
	Tranylcypromine (Parnate)	30–60	constipation, nausea, dry mouth, tachycardia,
	Selegiline Transdermal System (Emsam)	6 mg/24 hr– 12 mg/24 hr	palpitations, hypomania
Heterocyclics	Bupropion (Zyban; Wellbutrin)	200–450	With heterocyclics:
	Maprotiline	50–225	Dry mouth, sedation, dizziness, tachycardia,
	Mirtazapine (Remeron)	15–45	headache, nausea/vomiting, constipation,
	Trazodone (Desyrel)	150–600	priapism (trazodone), seizures (maprotiline;
	Nefazodone	200–600	bupropion); hepatic failure (warning with
	Amoxapine	50–600	nefazodone); NMS and tardive dyskinesia (with amoxapine)
Serotonin-Norepinephrine Reuptake Inhibitors (SNRIs)	Venlafaxine (Effexor)	75–375	With SNRIs:
	Duloxetine (Cymbalta)	40–60	Nausea, dry mouth, constipation, dizziness, somnolence, insomnia, headache, sexual dysfunction

*Dosage requires slow titration; onset of therapeutic response may be 1–4 weeks.

causes priapisms

Heterocyclics

Heterocyclic antidepressants include amoxapine, maprotiline, mirtazapine (Remeron), trazodone (Desyrel), nefazodone, and bupropion (Wellbutrin). They inhibit the reuptake of norepinephrine and serotonin, and bupropion also inhibits the reuptake of dopamine. Trazodone and nefazodone inhibit neuronal reuptake of serotonin and act as antagonists at central 5-HT$_2$ receptors.

Side Effects. Common side effects include drowsiness, fatigue, dry mouth, headache, constipation, and nausea. Tachycardia can occur with bupropion, amoxapine, and maprotiline. There is a risk of seizures with bupropion and maprotiline, and trazodone has been associated with the occurrence of priapism. Amoxapine has a potential for causing neuroleptic malignant syndrome and tardive dyskinesia, and nefazodone carries a black box warning of potential for life-threatening hepatic failure.

Serotonin–Norepinephrine Reuptake Inhibitors

The serotonin–norepinephrine reuptake inhibitors (SNRIs) include venlafaxine (Effexor) and duloxetine (Cymbalta). They are potent inhibitors of neuronal serotonin and norepinephrine reuptake, and weak inhibitors of dopamine reuptake. These drugs may be more effective than the SSRIs in treating severe and melancholic depression. They have also been shown to be effective in approximately 35 percent of patients with treatment-refractory depression (Schatzberg et al, 2007).

Side Effects. Common side effects include nausea, dizziness, insomnia, hypertension, dry mouth, constipation, nervousness, and sexual dysfunction.

Tricyclic Antidepressants

The TCAs include amitriptyline, clomipramine (Anafranil), desipramine (Norpramine), doxepin (Sinequan), imipramine (Tofranil), nortriptyline (Aventyl; Pamelor), protriptyline (Vivactil), and trimipramine (Surmontil). TCAs are now considered second- or third-line agents for major depressive disorder (Schatzberg et al., 2007). They have a very narrow margin of safety, resulting in intracardiac slowing and arrhythmias with overdose.

Side Effects. Common side effects with TCAs include anticholinergic (dry mouth, blurred vision, constipation, urinary hesitancy), cardiovascular (orthostatic hypotension, palpitations, arrhythmia, conduction slowing, hypertension), CNS (tremors, headache, dizziness, drowsiness), and other effects (weight gain, photosensitivity, sexual dysfunction).

Monoamine Oxidase Inhibitors

The monoamine oxidase inhibitors (MAOIs) include isocarboxazid (Marplan), phenelzine (Nardil), tranylcypromine (Parnate), and selegiline transdermal system (Emsam). MAOIs are considered to be third-line agents for major depressive disorder. Because of their unfavorable side-effect profile, they are now prescribed only after several trials with other antidepressants have failed. However, there are those who respond better to MAOIs than to any other class of antidepressant. They are lethal in overdose, with reports of the occurrence of hypertensive crisis, stroke, and myocardial infarction (Schatzberg et al., 2007).

Side Effects. Common side effects of MAOIs include dizziness, headache, insomnia/somnolence, orthostatic hypotension, weight gain, dry mouth, blurred vision, nausea, sexual dysfunction, and disturbances in cardiac rate and rhythm. The greatest concern with using MAOIs is the potential for hypertensive crisis, which is considered a medical emergency. Hypertensive crisis occurs in clients receiving MAOI therapy who consume foods or drugs high in **tyramine** content. Typically, symptoms develop within 2 hours after ingestion of a food or drug high in tyramine, and include severe occipital and/or temporal pounding headaches with occasional photophobia. Sensations of choking, palpitations, and a feeling of "dread" are common. Marked systolic and diastolic hypertension occurs, sometimes with neck stiffness.

CLINICAL PEARL

All antidepressants have varying potentials to cause discontinuation syndromes. Symptoms such as dizziness, headache, nausea, cramping, sweating, malaise, paresthesia, and rebound depression or hypomania have occurred. All antidepressant medication should be tapered gradually to prevent withdrawal symptoms.

For Mania

Lithium Carbonate

Lithium carbonate was the first drug approved by the U.S. Food and Drug Administration (FDA) for acute manic episodes and for maintenance therapy to prevent or diminish the intensity of subsequent manic episodes. Its mode of action in the control of manic symptoms is unclear. It has also been indicated for treatment of bipolar depression (see Chapter 21 for a detailed discussion of lithium carbonate).

Side Effects. Common side effects of lithium therapy include drowsiness, dizziness, headache, dry mouth, thirst, gastrointestinal upset, fine hand tremors, pulse irregularities, polyuria, and weight gain. In initiating lithium therapy with an acutely manic individual, physicians commonly order an antipsychotic as well. Because normalization of symptoms with lithium may not be achieved for 1 to 3 weeks, the antipsychotic medication is used to calm the excessive hyperactivity of the manic client until the lithium reaches therapeutic level.

Lithium Toxicity. The therapeutic level of lithium carbonate is 1.0 to 1.5 mEq/L for acute mania and 0.6 to 1.2 mEq/L for maintenance therapy. There is a narrow margin between the therapeutic and toxic levels. Lithium levels should be drawn weekly until the therapeutic level is reached, and then monthly during maintenance therapy. Because lithium toxicity is a life-threatening condition, monitoring of lithium levels is critical. The initial signs of lithium toxicity include ataxia, blurred vision, severe diarrhea, persistent nausea and vomiting, and tinnitus. Symptoms intensify as toxicity increases and include excessive output of dilute urine, psychomotor retardation, mental confusion, tremors and muscular irritability, seizures, impaired consciousness, oliguria or anuria, arrhythmias, coma, and eventually death.

Pretreatment assessments should include adequacy of renal functioning because 95 percent of ingested lithium is eliminated via the kidneys. Use of lithium during pregnancy is not recommended. Results of studies have indicated a greater number of cardiac anomalies in babies born to mothers who consumed lithium, particularly in the first trimester.

Anticonvulsants

A number of anticonvulsant agents are being used in the treatment of bipolar disorder. Examples include carbamazepine (Tegretol), clonazepam (Klonopin), valproic acid (Depakote), lamotrigine (Lamictal), gabapentin (Neurontin), oxcarbazepine (Trileptal), and topiramate (Topamax). Their mechanism of action in the treatment of bipolar disorder is unclear.

Side Effects. Common side effects of the anticonvulsants include the following: clonazepam (drowsiness, ataxia, blood dyscrasias, dependence and tolerance

[C-IV]), carbamazepine (drowsiness, ataxia, nausea, vomiting, blood dyscrasias), valproic acid (drowsiness, dizziness, weight gain, nausea, vomiting, prolonged bleeding time), gabapentin (drowsiness, dizziness, ataxia, nystagmus, tremor), lamotrigine (ataxia, dizziness, headache, nausea, vomiting, photosensitivity, and risk of severe potentially life-threatening rash), topiramate (drowsiness, dizziness, fatigue, ataxia, impaired concentration, nervousness, vision changes, nausea, weight loss, and decreased efficacy with oral contraceptives), and oxcarbazepine (headache, dizziness, somnolence, ataxia, tremor, nausea, and vomiting).

Antipsychotics

Several antipsychotic medications have been approved by the FDA for the treatment of bipolar mania. These include chlorpromazine and the newer atypical antipsychotics olanzapine, risperidone, aripiprazole, ziprasidone, and quetiapine. Chlorpromazine is gradually becoming obsolete in the treatment of bipolar mania due to the more favorable side effect profile of the atypical antipsychotics. Depending on the severity of the symptoms, these medications may be used alone or in combination with lithium. Another atypical antipsychotic, clozapine, has also been used in the treatment of acute mania; however, its usefulness is limited by the potential for seizures and agranulocytosis (Goldberg & Hoop, 2004). Detailed information for antipsychotic agents may be found in Chapter 21.

A summary of medications used in the treatment of bipolar mania is presented in Table 29–6.

TABLE 29–6	**Medications Used in the Treatment of Bipolar Mania**	
Classification: Generic (Trade) Name	**Daily Adult Dosage Range (mg)**	**Side Effects**
Antimanic		
Lithium carbonate (Eskalith, Lithane; Lithobid)	Acute mania: 1800–2400 Maintenance: 900–1200	Drowsiness, dizziness, headache, dry mouth, thirst, GI upset, nausea and vomiting, fine hand tremors, hypotension, arrhythmias, polyuria, weight gain.
Anticonvulsants		
Clonazepam (Klonopin)	0.75–16	Nausea and vomiting, somnolence, dizziness, blood dyscrasias, diplopia, headache, prolonged bleeding time (with valproic acid), risk of severe rash (with lamotrigine), decreased efficacy with oral contraceptives (with topiramate).
Carbamazepine (Tegretol)	200–1200	
Valproic acid (Depakene; Depakote)	500–1500	
Gabapentin (Neurontin)	900–1800	
Lamotrigine (Lamictal)	100–200	
Topiramate (Topamax)	50–400	
Oxcarbazepine (Trileptal)	600–1200	
Calcium Channel Blocker		
Verapamil (Calan; Isoptin)	80–320	Drowsiness, dizziness, hypotension, bradycardia, nausea, constipation
Antipsychotics		
Chlorpromazine (Thorazine)	75–400	Drowsiness, dizziness, dry mouth, constipation, increased appetite, weight gain, ECG changes, hyperglycemia, headache (aripiprazole, risperidone, quetiapine), extrapyramidal symptoms (chlorpromazine, risperidone)
Olanzapine (Zyprexa)	5–20	
Aripiprazole (Abilify)	10–30	
Quetiapine (Seroquel)	400–800	
Risperidone (Risperdal)	1–6	
Ziprasidone (Geodon)	40–160	

CASE STUDY AND SAMPLE CARE PLAN

NURSING HISTORY AND ASSESSMENT

Sam is a 45-year-old white man admitted to the psychiatric unit of a general medical center by his family physician, Dr. Jones, who reported that Sam had become increasingly despondent over the last month. His wife reported that he had made statements such as, "Life is not worth living," and "I think I could just take all those pills Dr. Jones prescribed at one time; then it would all be over." Sam says he loves his wife and children and does not want to hurt them, but feels they no longer need him. He states, "They would probably be better off without me." His wife appears to be very concerned about his condition, though in his despondency, he seems oblivious to her feelings. His mother (a widow) lives in a neighboring state, and he sees her infrequently. His father was an alcoholic and physically abused Sam and his siblings. He admits that he is somewhat bitter toward his mother for allowing him and his siblings to "suffer from the physical and emotional brutality of their father." His siblings and their families live in distant states, and he sees them rarely, during holiday gatherings.

Sam earned a college degree while working full-time at night to pay his way. He is employed in the administration department of a large corporation. Over the last 12 years, Sam has watched as a number of his peers were promoted to management positions. Sam has been considered for several of these positions but has never been selected. Last month a management position became available for which Sam felt he was qualified. He applied for this position, believing he had a good chance of being promoted. However, when the announcement was made, the position had been given to a younger man who had been with the company only 5 years. Sam seemed to accept the decision, but over the last few weeks he has become more and more withdrawn. He speaks to very few people at the office and is falling more and more behind in his work. At home, he eats very little, talks to family members only when they ask a direct question, withdraws to his bedroom very early in the evening, and does not come out until time to leave for work the next morning. Today, he refused to get out of bed or to go to work. His wife convinced him to talk to their family doctor, who admitted him to the hospital. The referring psychiatrist diagnosed Sam with Major Depressive Disorder.

NURSING DIAGNOSES/OUTCOME IDENTIFICATION

From the assessment data, the nurse develops the following nursing diagnoses for Sam:

1. **Risk for Suicide** related to depressed mood and expressions of having nothing to live for.
   a. **Short-Term Goals:**
      - Sam will seek out staff when ideas of suicide occur.
      - Sam will maintain a short-term contract not to harm himself.
   b. **Long-Term Goal:**
      - Sam will not harm himself during his hospitalization.
2. **Complicated Grieving** related to unresolved losses (job promotion and unsatisfactory parent–child relationships) evidenced by anger turned inward on self and desire to end his life.
   a. **Short-Term Goal:**
      - Sam will verbalize anger toward boss and parents within 1 week.
   b. **Long-Term Goal:**
      - Sam will verbalize his position in the grief process and begin movement in the progression toward resolution by discharge from treatment.

PLANNING/IMPLEMENTATION

Risk for suicide

The following nursing interventions have been identified for Sam:

1. Ask Sam directly, "Have you thought about killing yourself? If so, what do you plan to do? Do you have the means to carry out this plan?"
2. Create a safe environment. Remove all potentially harmful objects from immediate access (sharp objects, straps, belts, ties, glass items).
3. Formulate a short-term verbal contract with Sam that he will not harm himself during the next 24 hours. When that contract expires, make another. Continue with this intervention until Sam is discharged.
4. Secure a promise from Sam that he will seek out a staff member if thoughts of suicide emerge.
5. Encourage verbalizations of honest feelings. Through exploration and discussion, help him to identify symbols of hope in his life (participating in activities he finds satisfying outside of his job).
6. Allow Sam to express angry feelings within appropriate limits. Encourage use of the exercise room and punching bag each day. Help him to identify the true source of his anger, and work on adaptive coping skills for use outside the hospital (e.g., jogging, exercise club available to employees of his company).
7. Identify community resources that he may use as a support system and from whom he may request help if feeling suicidal (e.g., suicidal or crisis hotline; psychiatrist or social worker at community mental health center; hospital "HELP" line).
8. Introduce the client to support and education groups for adult children of alcoholics (ACOA).
9. Spend time with Sam. This will help him to feel safe and secure while conveying the message that he is a worthwhile person.

Complicated Grieving

1. Sam is fixed in the anger stage of the grieving process. Discuss with him behaviors associated with

Continued on following page

CASE STUDY AND SAMPLE CARE PLAN *(Continued)*

this stage, so that he may come to realize why he is feeling this way.

2. Develop a trusting relationship with Sam. Show empathy and caring. Be honest and keep all promises.

3. Convey an accepting attitude—one in which he is not afraid to express feelings openly.

4. Allow him to verbalize feelings of anger. The initial expression of anger may be displaced on to the healthcare provider. Do not become defensive if this should occur. Assist him to explore these angry feelings so that they may be directed toward the intended persons (boss, parents).

5. Assist Sam to discharge pent-up anger through participation in large motor activities (brisk walks, jogging, physical exercises, volleyball, punching bag, exercise bike, or other equipment).

6. Explain normal stages of grief, and the behaviors associated with each stage. Help Sam to understand that feelings such as guilt and anger toward his boss and parents are appropriate and acceptable during this stage of the grieving process. Help him also to understand that he must work through these feelings and move past this stage in order to eventually feel better. Knowledge of acceptability of the feelings associated with normal grieving may help to relieve some of the guilt that these responses generate. Knowing why he is experiencing these feelings may also help to resolve them.

7. Encourage Sam to review the relationship with his parents. With support and sensitivity, point out the reality of the situation in areas in which misrepresentations are expressed. Explain common roles and behaviors of members in an alcoholic family. Sam must give up the desire for an idealized family and accept the reality of his childhood situation and the effect it has had on his adult life, before the grief process can be completed.

8. Assist Sam in problem solving as he attempts to determine methods for more adaptive coping. Suggest alternatives to anger turned inward on the self when negative thinking sets in (e.g., thought-stopping techniques [Chapter 15]). Provide positive feedback for strategies identified and decisions made.

9. Encourage Sam to reach out for spiritual support during this time in whatever form is desirable to him. Assess spiritual needs (see Chapter 6), and assist as necessary in the fulfillment of those needs. Sam may find comfort in religious rituals with which he is familiar.

EVALUATION

The outcome criteria identified for Sam have been met. He sought out staff when feelings of suicide surfaced. He maintained an active no-suicide contract. He has not harmed himself in any way. He verbalizes no further thought of suicide and expresses hope for the future. He is able to verbalize names of resources outside the hospital from whom he may request help if thoughts of suicide return. He is able to verbalize normal stages of the grief process and behaviors associated with each stage. He is able to identify his own position in the grief process and express honest feelings related to the loss of his job promotion and satisfactory parent–child relationships. He is no longer manifesting exaggerated emotions and behaviors related to complicated grieving and is able to carry out self-care activities independently.

SUMMARY AND KEY POINTS

- Depression is one of the oldest recognized psychiatric illnesses that is still prevalent today. It is so common, in fact, that it has been referred to as the "common cold of psychiatric disorders."

- The cause of depressive disorders is not entirely known. A number of factors, including genetics, biochemical influences, and psychosocial experiences likely enter into the development of the disorder.

- Secondary depression occurs in response to other physiological disorders.

- Symptoms of depression occur along a continuum according to the degree of severity from transient to severe.

- The disorder occurs in all developmental levels, including childhood, adolescence, senescence, and during the puerperium.

- Bipolar disorder is manifested by mood swings from profound depression to extreme elation and euphoria.

- Genetic influences have been strongly implicated in the development of bipolar disorder. Various other physiological factors, such as biochemical and electrolyte alterations, as well as cerebral structural changes, have been implicated. Side effects of certain medications may also induce symptoms of mania. No single theory can explain the etiology of bipolar disorder, and it is likely that the illness is caused by a combination of factors.

- Symptoms of mania may be observed on a continuum of three phases, each identified by the degree of severity: phase I, hypomania; phase II, acute mania; and phase III, delirious mania.

- The symptoms of bipolar disorder may occur in children and adolescents, as well as adults.

- Treatment of mood disorders includes individual therapy, group and family therapy, cognitive therapy, electroconvulsive therapy, light therapy, transcranial magnetic stimulation, and psychopharmacology.

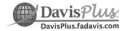

REVIEW QUESTIONS

Self-Examination/Learning Exercise

Situation: Margaret, age 68, was brought to the emergency department of a large regional medical center by her sister-in-law, who stated, "She does nothing but sit and stare into space. I can't get her to eat or anything!" On assessment, it was found that 6 months ago Margaret's husband of 45 years had died of a massive myocardial infarction. They had no children and had been inseparable. Since her husband's death, Margaret has visited the cemetery every day, changing the flowers often on his grave. She has not removed any of his clothes from the closet or chest of drawers. His shaving materials still occupy the same space in the bathroom. Over the months, Margaret has become more and more socially isolated. She refuses invitations from friends, preferring instead to make her daily trips to the cemetery. She has lost 15 pounds and her sister-in-law reports that there is very little food in the house. Today she said to her sister-in-law, "I don't really want to live anymore. My life is nothing without Frank." Her sister-in-law became frightened and, with forceful persuasion, was able to convince Margaret she needed to see a doctor. Margaret is admitted to the psychiatric unit.

Based on the above situation, select the answer that is most appropriate for each of the following questions:

1. The *priority* nursing diagnosis for Margaret would be:
   a. Imbalanced nutrition: less than body requirements.
   b. Complicated grieving.
   c. Risk for suicide.
   d. Social isolation

2. The physician orders sertraline (Zoloft) 50 mg bid for Margaret. After 3 days of taking the medication, Margaret says to the nurse, "I don't think this medicine is doing any good. I don't feel a bit better." What is the most appropriate response by the nurse?
   a. "Cheer up, Margaret. You have so much to be happy about."
   b. "Sometimes it takes a few weeks for the medicine to bring about an improvement in symptoms."
   c. "I'll report that to the physician, Margaret. Maybe he will order something different."
   d. "Try not to dwell on your symptoms, Margaret. Why don't you join the others down in the dayroom?"

After being stabilized on her medication, Margaret was released from the hospital with directions to continue taking the sertraline as ordered. A week later, her sister-in-law found Margaret in bed and was unable to awaken her. An empty prescription bottle was by her side. She was revived in the emergency department and transferred to the psychiatric unit in a state of severe depression. The physician determines that ECT may help Margaret. Consent is obtained.

3. About 30 minutes before the first treatment, the nurse administers atropine sulfate 0.4 mg IM. The rationale for this order is:
   a. To decrease secretions and increase heart rate.
   b. To relax muscles.
   c. To produce a calming effect.
   d. To induce anesthesia.

4. When Margaret is in the treatment room, the anesthesiologist administers thiopental sodium (Pentothal) followed by IV succinylcholine (Anectine). The purposes of these medications are to:
   a. Decrease secretions and increase heart rate.
   b. Prevent nausea and induce a calming effect.
   c. Minimize memory loss and stabilize mood.
   d. Induce anesthesia and relax muscles.

5. After three ECTs, Margaret's mood begins to lift and she tells the nurse, "I feel so much better, but I'm having trouble remembering some things that happened this last week." The nurse's best response would be:

   a. "Don't worry about that. Nothing important happened."
   b. "Memory loss is just something you have to put up with in order to feel better."
   c. "Memory loss is a side effect of ECT, but it is only temporary. Your memory should return within a few weeks."
   d. "Forget about last week, Margaret. You need to look forward from here."

A year later, Margaret presents in the emergency department, once again accompanied by her sister-in-law. This time Margaret is agitated, pacing, demanding, and speaking very loudly. "I didn't want to come here! My sister-in-law is just jealous, and she's trying to make it look like I'm insane!" Upon assessment, the sister-in-law reports that Margaret has become engaged to a 25-year-old construction worker to whom she has willed her sizable inheritance and her home. Margaret loudly praises her fiancé's physique and sexual abilities. She has been spending large sums of money on herself and giving her fiancé $500 a week. The sister-in-law tells the physician, "I know it is Margaret's business what she does with her life, but I'm really worried about her. She is losing weight again. She eats very little and almost never sleeps. I'm afraid she's going to just collapse!" Margaret is once again admitted to the psychiatric unit.

6. The *priority* nursing diagnosis for Margaret is:

   a. Imbalanced nutrition: less than body requirements related to not eating.
   b. Risk for injury related to hyperactivity.
   c. Disturbed sleep pattern related to agitation.
   d. Ineffective coping related to denial of depression.

7. One way to promote adequate nutritional intake for Margaret is to:

   a. Sit with her during meals to ensure that she eats everything on her tray.
   b. Have her sister-in-law bring all her food from home because she knows Margaret's likes and dislikes.
   c. Provide high-calorie, nutritious finger foods and snacks that Margaret can eat "on the run."
   d. Tell Margaret that she will be on room restriction until she starts gaining weight.

8. The physician orders lithium carbonate 600 mg tid for Margaret. There is a narrow margin between the therapeutic and toxic levels of lithium. The therapeutic range for acute mania is:

   a. 1.0 to 1.5 mEq/L.
   b. 10 to 15 mEq/L.
   c. 0.5 to 1.0 mEq/L.
   d. 5 to 10 mEq/L.

9. After an appropriate length of time, the physician determines that Margaret does not respond satisfactorily to lithium therapy. He changes her medication to another drug that has been found to be effective in the treatment of bipolar mania. This drug is:

   a. Molindone (Moban).
   b. Paroxetine (Paxil).
   c. Carbamazepine (Tegretol).
   d. Tranylcypromine (Parnate).

10. Margaret's statement, "My sister-in-law is just jealous, and she's trying to make it look like I'm insane!" is an example of:

   a. A delusion of grandeur.
   b. A delusion of persecution.
   c. A delusion of reference.
   d. A delusion of control or influence.

Test Your Critical Thinking Skills

Alice, age 29, had been working in the typing pool of a large corporation for 6 years. Her immediate supervisor recently retired and Alice was promoted to supervisor, in charge of 20 people in the department. Alice was flattered by the promotion but anxious about the additional responsibility of the position. Shortly after the promotion, she overheard two of her former coworkers saying, "Why in the world did they choose her? She's not the best one for the job. I know *I* certainly won't be able to respect her as a boss!" Hearing these comments added to Alice's anxiety and self-doubt.

Shortly after Alice began her new duties, her friends and coworkers noticed a change. She had a great deal of energy and worked long hours on her job. She began to speak very loudly and rapidly. Her roommate noticed that Alice slept very little, yet seldom appeared tired. Every night she would go out to bars and dances. Sometimes she brought men she had just met home to the apartment, something she had never done before. She bought lots of clothes and make-up and had her hair restyled in a more youthful look. She failed to pay her share of the rent and bills but came home with a brand new convertible. She lost her temper and screamed at her roommate to "Mind your own business!" when asked to pay her share.

She became irritable at work, and several of her subordinates reported her behavior to the corporate manager. When the manager confronted Alice about her behavior, she lost control, shouting, cursing, and striking out at anyone and anything that happened to be within her reach. The security officers restrained her and took her to the emergency department of the hospital, where she was admitted to the psychiatric unit. She had no previous history of psychiatric illness.

The psychiatrist assigned a diagnosis of Bipolar I disorder and wrote orders for olanzapine (Zyprexa) 15 mg PO STAT, olanzapine 15 mg PO qd, and lithium carbonate 600 mg qid.

Answer the following questions related to Alice:

1. What are the most important considerations with which the nurse who is taking care of Alice should be concerned?
2. Why was Alice given the diagnosis of Bipolar I disorder?
3. The doctor should order a lithium level drawn after 4 to 6 days. For what symptoms should the nurse be on the alert?
4. Why did the physician order olanzapine in addition to the lithium carbonate?

REFERENCES

Administration on Aging. (2007). A profile of older Americans: 2006. Washington, DC: U.S. Department of Health and Human Services.

Allen, M.H. (2003). Approaches to the treatment of mania. *Medscape Psychiatry*. Retrieved March 15, 2007 from http://www.medscape.com/viewprogram/2639_pnt

American Psychiatric Association. (2000). *Diagnostic and statistical manual of mental disorders* (4th ed.) *Text Revision*. Washington, DC: American Psychiatric Association.

Azoulary, L., Blais, L., Koren, G., LeLorier, J. & Berard, A. (2008). Isotretinoin and the risk of depression in patients with acne vulgaris: A case-crossover study. *The Journal of Clinical Psychiatry, 69*, 526–532.

Cartwright, L. (2004). Emergencies of survival: Moral spectatorship and the new vision of the child in postwar child psychoanalysis. *Journal of Visual Culture, 3*(1), 35–49.

Correll, C.U. (2007). Current understanding in the development of bipolar disorder in pediatric patients. *Medscape Psychiatry*. Retrieved February 7, 2008 from http://www.medscape.com/viewarticle/566531

Davidson, L. (2005). *Suicide and season*. New York: American Foundation for Suicide Prevention.

Dubovsky, S.L., Davies, R., & Dubovsky, A.M. (2003). Mood disorders. In R.E. Hales & S.C. Yudofsky (Eds.), *Textbook of clinical psychiatry* (4th ed.). Washington, DC: American Psychiatric Publishing.

Eranti, S., Mogg, A., Pluck, G., Landau, S., Purvis, R., Brown, R.G., Howard, R., Knapp, M., Philpot, M., Rabe-Hesketh, S., Romeo, R., Rothwell, J., Edwards, D., & McLoughlin, D.M. (2007). A randomized, controlled trial with 6-month follow-up of repetitive transcranial magnetic stimulation and electroconvulsive therapy for severe depression. *American Journal of Psychiatry, 164*(1), 73–81.

Frackiewicz, E.J., & Shiovitz, T.M. (2001). Evaluation and management of premenstrual syndrome. *Journal of the American Pharmaceutical Association, 41*(3), 437–447.

Geller, B., Zimerman, B., Williams, M., Delbello, M.P., Frazier, J., & Beringer, L. (2002). Phenomenology of prepubertal and early adolescent bipolar disorder: Examples of elated mood, grandiose behaviors, decreased need for sleep, racing thoughts, and hypersexuality. *Journal of Child and Adolescent Psychopharmacology, 12*, 3–9.

Goldberg, J.F., & Hoop, J. (2004). Bipolar depression: Long-term challenges for the clinician. *Medscape Psychiatry*. Retrieved March 15, 2007 from http://www.medscape.com/viewprogram/3350

Hakko, H. (2000). *Seasonal variation of suicides and homicides in Finland*. Oulu, Finland: University of Oulu.

Harvard Medical School. (2002, February). Depression in Children—Part I. *The Harvard Mental Health Letter*. Boston, MA: Harvard Medical School Publications Group.

International Society for Mental Health Online [ISMHO]. (2004). *All about depression*. Retrieved March 15, 2007 from http://www.allaboutdepression.com/gen_01.html#3

Kafantaris, V., Dicker, R., Coletti, D.J., & Kane, J.M. (2001). Adjunctive antipsychotic treatment is necessary for adolescents with psychotic mania. *Journal of Child and Adolescent Psychopharmacology, 11*, 409–413.

Kaplan, H.I., & Sadock, B.J. (1998). *Synopsis of psychiatry: Behavioral sciences/clinical psychiatry* (8th ed.). Baltimore: Williams & Wilkins.

Karasu, T.B., Gelenberg, A., Merriam, A., & Wang, P. (2006). Practice guideline for the treatment of patients with major depressive disorder (2nd ed.). *American Psychiatric Association Practice Guidelines for the Treatment of Psychiatric Disorders, Compendium 2006*. Washington, DC: American Psychiatric Publishing.

Kowatch, R.A., Fristad, M., Birmaher, B., Wagner, K.D., Findling, R.L., & Hellander, M. (2005). Treatment guidelines for children and adolescents with bipolar disorder. *Journal of the American Academy of Child and Adolescent Psychiatry, 44*(3), 213–235.

Lam, R.W., Levitt, A.J., Levitan, R.D., Enns, M.W., Morehouse, R., Michalak, E.E., & Tam, E.M. (2006). The Can-SAD Study: A randomized controlled trial of the effectiveness of light therapy and fluoxetine in patients with winter seasonal affective disorder. *The American Journal of Psychiatry, 163*(5), 805–812.

Lee, G.R., DeMaris, A., Bavin, S., & Sullivan, R. (2001). Gender differences in the depressive effect of widowhood in later life. *The Journals of Gerontology Series B: Psychological Sciences and Social Sciences, 56*, S56–S61.

Lee, G.R., Willetts, M.C., & Seccombe, K. (1998). Widowhood and depression: Gender differences. *Research on Aging, 20*(5), 611–630.

Mehta, A., & Sheth, S. (2006). Postpartum depression: How to recognize and treat this common condition. *Medscape Psychiatry & Mental Health, 11*(1): Online.

Merck Manual of Diagnosis and Therapy. (2005). Mood Disorders. Retrieved March 14, 2007 from http://www.merck.com/

Miklowitz, D.J., George, E.L., Richards, J.A., Simoneau, T.L., & Suddath, R.L. (2003). A randomized study of family-focused psychoeducation and pharmacotherapy in the outpatient management of bipolar disorder. *Archives of General Psychiatry, 60*(9), 904–912.

NANDA International (NANDA-I). (2007). *Nursing diagnoses: Definitions & classification 2007–2008*. Philadelphia: NANDA-I.

National Center for Health Statistics. (2007, March 15). Deaths: Leading causes for 2003. *National Vital Statistics Reports, 55*(10), 1–93.

National Institute of Mental Health (NIMH). (2006). *Mental disorders in America: The numbers count*. Bethesda, MD: National Institutes of Health.

National Institute of Mental Health (NIMH). (2007). *Different families, different characteristics—Different kinds of bipolar disorder?* Science Update. Retrieved March 15, 2007 from http://www.nimh.nih.gov/press/bp-familiality.cfm

Pridmore, S., Khan, U.A., Reid, P., & George, M.S. (2001). Transcranial magnetic stimulation in depression: An overview. *The German Journal of Psychiatry, 4*, 43–50.

Rosenbaum, J.F., & Judy, A.E. (2004). New brain stimulation therapies for depression. *Medscape Psychiatry & Mental Health*. Retrieved March 23, 2007 from http://wwwmedscape.com/viewarticle/480897

Rupke, S.J., Blecke, D., & Renfrow, M. (2006). Cognitive therapy for depression. *American Family Physician, 73*(1), 83–86.

Sadock, B.J., & Sadock, V.A. (2007). *Synopsis of psychiatry: Behavioral sciences/clinical psychiatry* (10th ed.). Philadelphia: Lippincott Williams & Wilkins

Schatzberg, A.F., Cole, J.O., & DeBattista, C. (2007). *Manual of clinical psychopharmacology* (6th ed.). Washington, DC: American Psychiatric Publishing.

Schimelpfening, N. (2002). *A vitamin a day keeps depression away*. Retrieved March 15, 2007 from http://depression.about.com/library/weekly/aa051799.htm

Slattery, D.A., Hudson, A.L., & Nutt, D.J. (2004). Invited review: The evolution of antidepressant mechanisms. *Fundamental & Clinical Pharmacology, 18*(1), 1–21.

Soreff, S., & McInnes, L.A. (2006). Bipolar affective disorder. *E-medicine: Psychiatry*. Retrieved March 15, 2007 from http://www.emedicine.com/med/topic229.htm

Taber's Cyclopedic Medical Dictionary (20th ed.). (2005). Philadelphia: FA Davis.

Tempfer, T.C. (2006). Depression in children: Developmental perspectives. Highlights of the National Association of Pediatric Nurse Practitioners 27th Annual Conference. Retrieved March 23, 2007 from http://www.medscape.com/viewprogram/5458

Terman, M., & Terman, J.S. (2005). Light therapy for seasonal and nonseasonal depression: Efficacy, protocol, safety, and side effects. *CNS Spectrums, 10*(8), 647–663.

Thase, M.E. (2007). The new "blue light" intervention for seasonal affective disorder (SAD). *Medscape Psychiatry & Mental Health*. Retrieved January 31, 2007 from http://www.medscape.com/viewarticle/550845

U.S. Department of Health and Human Services. (2007). *Health, United States, 2006*. Hyattsville, MD: National Center for Health Statistics.

Williams, D.R., Gonzalez, H.M., Neighbors, H., Nesse, R., Abelson, J.M., Sweetman, J., & Jackson, J.S. (2007). Prevalence and distribution of major depressive disorder in African Americans, Caribbean Blacks, and Non-Hispanic Whites: Results from the National Survey of American Life. *Archives of General Psychiatry, 64*(3), 305–315.

Zubieta, J.K., Huguelet, P., Koeppe, R.A., Kilbourn, M.R., Carr, J.M., Giordani, B.J., & Frey, K.A. (2000). High vesicular monoamine transporter binding in asymptomatic bipolar I disorder: Sex differences and cognitive correlates. *American Journal of Psychiatry*, 157, 1619–1628.

CLASSICAL REFERENCES

Beck, A.T., Rush, A.J., Shaw, B.F., & Emery, G. (1979). *Cognitive theory of depression*. New York: Guilford Press.

Freud, S. (1957). *Mourning and melancholia*, Vol. 14 (standard ed.). London: Hogarth Press. (Original work published 1917.)

Seligman, M.E.P. (1973). Fall into helplessness. *Psychology Today, 7*, 43–48.

@ Internet References

- Additional information about mood disorders, including psychosocial and pharmacological treatment of these disorders, is located at the following Web sites:
  - http://www.pslgroup.com/depression.htm
  - http://depression.miningco.com/
  - http://www.ndmda.org
  - http://www.fadavis.com/townsend
  - http://www.mentalhealth.com/html
  - http://www.mhsource.com/bipolar
  - http://www.mhsource.com/depression
  - http://www.mental-health-matters.com/
  - http://www.mentalhelp.net
  - http://www.nlm.nih.gov/medlineplus

of Greek or Latin can produce a phobia classification, thereby making possibilities for the list almost infinite.

The *DSM-IV-TR* identifies subtypes of the most common specific phobias. They include the following:

1. **Animal type.** This subtype would be identified as part of the diagnosis if the fear is of animals or insects.
2. **Natural environment type.** Examples of this subtype include objects or situations that occur within the natural environment, such as heights, storms, or water.
3. **Blood-injection-injury type.** This diagnosis should be specified if the fear is of seeing blood or an injury or of receiving an injection or other invasive medical or dental procedure.
4. **Situational type.** This subtype is designated if the fear is of a specific situation, such as public transportation, tunnels, bridges, elevators, flying, driving, or enclosed places.
5. **Other type.** This category covers all other excessive or irrational fears. It may include fear of contracting a serious illness, fear of situations that might lead to vomiting or choking, fear of loud noises, or fear of driving.

The *DSM-IV-TR* diagnostic criteria for specific phobia are presented in Box 30–3.

Box 3 0 – 3 Diagnostic Criteria for Specific Phobia

A. Marked and persistent fear that is excessive or unreasonable, cued by the presence or anticipation of a specific object or situation (e.g., flying, heights, animals, receiving an injection, seeing blood).
B. Exposure to the phobic stimulus almost invariably provokes an immediate anxiety response, which may take the form of a situationally bound or situationally predisposed panic attack. **NOTE:** In children, the anxiety may be expressed by crying, tantrums, freezing, or clinging.
C. The person recognizes that the fear is excessive or unreasonable. **NOTE:** In children, this feature may be absent.
D. The phobic situation(s) is avoided or else is endured with intense anxiety or distress.
E. The avoidance, anxious anticipation, or distress in the feared situation(s) interferes significantly with the person's normal routine, occupational (academic) functioning, or social activities or relationships, or there is marked distress about having the phobia.
F. In individuals under 18 years, the duration is at least 6 months.
G. The anxiety, panic attacks, or phobic avoidance associated with the specific object or situation are not better accounted for by another mental disorder.

The diagnosis may be further specified as:
   Animal type
   Natural environment type (e.g., heights, storms, water)
   Blood-injection-injury type
   Situational type (e.g., airplanes, elevators, enclosed places)
   Other type

SOURCE: American Psychiatric Association (2000), with permission.

Predisposing Factors to Phobias

The cause of phobias is unknown. However, various theories exist that may offer insight into the etiology.

Psychoanalytical Theory

Freud believed that phobias developed when a child experiences normal incestuous feelings toward the opposite-sex parent (Oedipal/Electra complex) and fears aggression from the same-sex parent (castration anxiety). To protect themselves, these children *repress* this fear of hostility from the same-sex parent, and *displace* it onto something safer and more neutral, which becomes the phobic stimulus. The phobic stimulus becomes the symbol for the parent, but the child does not realize this.

Modern-day psychoanalysts believe in the same concept of phobic development, but believe that castration anxiety is not the sole source of phobias. They believe that other unconscious fears may also be expressed in a symbolic manner as phobias. For example, a female child who was sexually abused by an adult male family friend when he was taking her for a ride in his boat grew up with an intense, irrational fear of all water vessels. Psychoanalytical theory postulates that fear of the man was repressed and displaced onto boats. Boats became an unconscious symbol for the feared person, but one that the young girl viewed as safer since her fear of boats prevented her from having to confront the real fear.

Learning Theory

Classic conditioning in the case of phobias may be explained as follows: a stressful stimulus produces an "unconditioned" response of fear. When the stressful stimulus is repeatedly paired with a harmless object, eventually the harmless object alone produces a "conditioned" response: fear. This becomes a phobia when the individual consciously avoids the harmless object to escape fear.

Some learning theorists hold that fears are conditioned responses and, thus, they are learned by imposing rewards for appropriate behaviors. In the instance of phobias, when the individual avoids the phobic object, he or she escapes fear, which is indeed a powerful reward.

Phobias also may be acquired by direct learning or imitation (modeling) (e.g., a mother who exhibits fear toward an object will provide a model for the child, who may also develop a phobia toward the same object).

Cognitive Theory

Cognitive theorists espouse that anxiety is the product of faulty cognitions or anxiety-inducing self-instructions. Two types of faulty thinking have been investigated: negative self-statements and irrational beliefs. Cognitive theorists believe that some individuals engage in negative and irrational thinking that produces anxiety reactions. The individual begins to seek out avoidance behaviors to prevent the anxiety reactions, and phobias result.

Somewhat related to the cognitive theory is the involvement of locus of control. Johnson and Sarason (1978) suggested that individuals with internal locus of control and those with external locus of control might respond differently to life change. These researchers proposed that locus of control orientation may be an important variable in the development of phobias. Individuals with an external control orientation experiencing anxiety attacks in a stressful period are likely to mislabel the anxiety and attribute it to external sources (e.g., crowded areas) or to a disease (e.g., heart attack). They may perceive the experienced anxiety as being outside of their control. Figure 30–3 depicts a graphic model of the relationship between locus of control and the development of phobias.

Biological Aspects

Temperament. Children experience fears as a part of normal development. Most infants are afraid of loud noises. Common fears of toddlers and preschoolers include strangers, animals, darkness, and fears of being separated from parents or attachment figures. During the school-age years, there is fear of death and anxiety about school achievement. Fears of social rejection and sexual anxieties are common among adolescents.

Innate fears represent a part of the overall characteristics or tendencies with which one is born that influence how he or she responds throughout life to specific situations. Innate fears usually do not reach phobic intensity but may have the capacity for such development if reinforced by events in later life. For example, a 4-year-old girl is afraid of dogs. By age 5, however, she has overcome her fear and plays with her own dog and the neighbors'

dogs without fear. Then, when she is 19, she is bitten by a stray dog and develops a dog phobia.

Life Experiences

Certain early experiences may set the stage for phobic reactions later in life. Some researchers believe that phobias, particularly specific phobias, are symbolic of original anxiety-producing objects or situations that have been repressed. Examples include:

1. A child who is punished by being locked in a closet develops a phobia for elevators or other closed places.
2. A child who falls down a flight of stairs develops a phobia for high places.
3. A young woman who, as a child, survived a plane crash in which both her parents were killed has a phobia of airplanes.

Transactional Model of Stress/Adaptation. The etiology of phobic disorders is most likely influenced by multiple factors. In Figure 30–4, a graphic depiction of this theory of multiple causation is presented in the Transactional Model of Stress-Adaptation.

 CORE CONCEPT

Obsessions
Unwanted, intrusive, persistent ideas, thoughts, impulses, or images that cause marked anxiety or distress. The most common ones include repeated thoughts about contamination, repeated doubts, a need to have things in a particular order, aggressive or horrific impulses, and sexual imagery (APA, 2000).

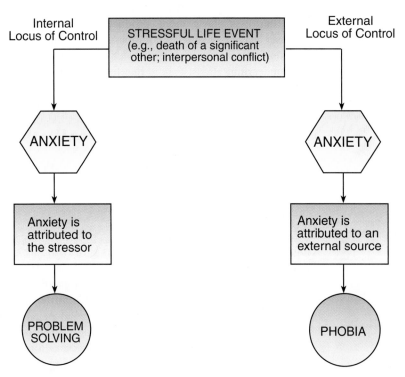

FIGURE 30–3 Locus of control as a variable in the etiology of phobias.

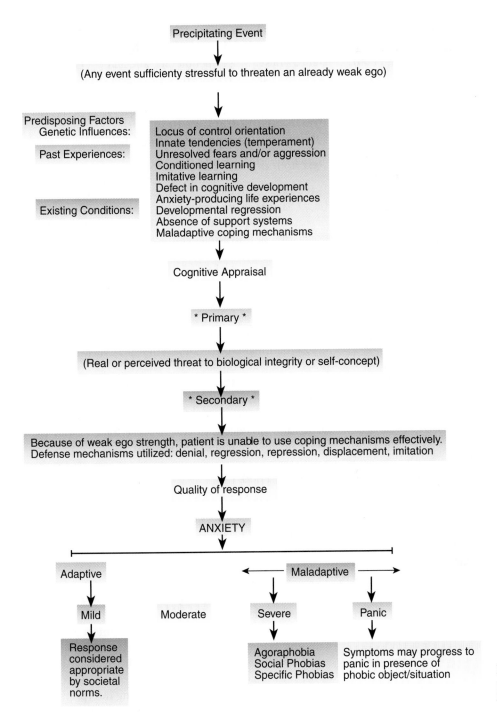

FIGURE 30–4 The dynamics of phobic disorder using the Transactional Model of Stress/Adaptation.

CORE CONCEPT

Compulsions

Unwanted repetitive behavior patterns or mental acts (e.g., praying, counting, repeating words silently) that are intended to reduce anxiety, not to provide pleasure or gratification (APA, 2000). They may be performed in response to an obsession or in a stereotyped fashion.

Obsessive–Compulsive Disorder

Background Assessment Data

The *DSM-IV-TR* describes obsessive–compulsive disorder (OCD) as recurrent obsessions or compulsions that are severe enough to be time consuming or to cause marked distress or significant impairment (APA, 2000). The individual recognizes that the behavior is excessive or unreasonable but, because of the feeling of relief from discomfort that it promotes, is compelled to continue the act.

The most common compulsions involve washing and cleaning, counting, checking, requesting or demanding assurances, repeating actions, and ordering (APA, 2000). The *DSM-IV-TR* diagnostic criteria for OCD are presented in Box 30–4.

The disorder is equally common among men and women. It may begin in childhood, but more often begins in adolescence or early adulthood. The course is usually chronic, and may be complicated by depression or substance abuse. Single people are affected by OCD more often than are married people (Sadock & Sadock, 2007).

Box 30 – 4 Diagnostic Criteria for Obsessive–Compulsive Disorder

A. Either obsessions or compulsions:
   Obsessions as defined by 1, 2, 3, and 4:
   1. Recurrent and persistent thoughts, impulses, or images that are experienced at some time during the disturbance as intrusive and inappropriate and that cause marked anxiety or distress.
   2. The thoughts, impulses, or images are not simply excessive worries about real-life problems.
   3. The person attempts to ignore or suppress such thoughts, impulses, or images, or to neutralize them with some other thought or action.
   4. The person recognizes that the obsessional thoughts, impulses, or images are a product of his or her own mind (not imposed from without as in thought insertion).

   Compulsions as defined by 1 and 2:
   1. Repetitive behaviors (e.g., hand washing, ordering, checking) or mental acts (e.g., praying, counting, repeating words silently) that the person feels driven to perform in response to an obsession, or according to rules that must be applied rigidly.
   2. The behaviors or mental acts are aimed at preventing or reducing distress or preventing some dreaded event or situation; however, these behaviors or mental acts either are not connected in a realistic way with what they are designed to neutralize or prevent or are clearly excessive.

B. At some point during the course of the disorder, the person has recognized that the obsessions or compulsions are excessive or unreasonable. **NOTE:** This does not apply to children.
C. The obsessions or compulsions cause marked distress, are time consuming (take more than 1 hr a day), or significantly interfere with the person's normal routine, occupational (or academic) functioning, or usual social activities or relationships.
D. If another axis I disorder is present, the content of the obsessions or compulsions is not restricted to it (e.g., preoccupation with food in the presence of an eating disorder; hair pulling in the presence of trichotillomania; concern with appearance in the presence of body dysmorphic disorder; preoccupation with having a serious illness in the presence of hypochondriasis; preoccupation with sexual urges or fantasies in the presence of a paraphilia; or guilty ruminations in the presence of major depressive disorder).
E. This disturbance is not due to the direct physiological effects of a substance (e.g., drug of abuse, a medication) or a general medical condition.

SOURCE: American Psychiatric Association (2000), with permission.

Predisposing Factors to Obsessive–Compulsive Disorder

Psychoanalytical Theory

Psychoanalytical theorists propose that individuals with OCD have weak, underdeveloped egos (for any of a variety of reasons: unsatisfactory parent–child relationship, conditional love, or provisional gratification). The psychoanalytical concept views clients with OCD as having regressed to earlier developmental stages of the infantile superego—the harsh, exacting, punitive characteristics which now reappear as part of the psychopathology. Regression to the preoedipal anal-sadistic phase, combined with use of specific ego defense mechanisms (isolation, undoing, displacement, reaction formation), produces the clinical symptoms of obsessions and compulsions (Sadock & Sadock, 2007). Aggressive impulses (common during the anal-sadistic developmental phase) are channeled into thoughts and behaviors that prevent the feelings of aggression from surfacing and producing intense anxiety fraught with guilt (generated by the punitive superego).

Learning Theory

Learning theorists explain obsessive–compulsive behavior as a conditioned response to a traumatic event. The traumatic event produces anxiety and discomfort, and the individual learns to prevent the anxiety and discomfort by avoiding the situation with which they are associated. This type of learning is called *passive avoidance* (staying away from the source). When passive avoidance is not possible, the individual learns to engage in behaviors that provide relief from the anxiety and discomfort associated with the traumatic situation. This type of learning is called *active avoidance* and describes the behavior pattern of the individual with OCD (Sadock & Sadock, 2007).

According to this classic conditioning interpretation, a traumatic event should mark the beginning of the obsessive–compulsive behaviors. However, in a significant number of cases, the onset of the behavior is gradual and the clients relate the onset of their problems to life stress in general rather than to one or more traumatic events.

Biological Aspects

Recent findings suggest that neurobiological disturbances may play a role in the pathogenesis and maintenance of OCD.

Neuroanatomy. Abnormalities in various regions of the brain have been implicated in the neurobiology of OCD. Functional neuroimaging techniques have shown abnormal metabolic rates in the basal ganglia and orbitofrontal cortex of individuals with the disorder (Hollander & Simeon, 2008).

Physiology. Electrophysiological, sleep electroencephalogram, and neuroendocrine studies have suggested that there are commonalities between depressive disorders and OCD (Sadock & Sadock, 2007). Neuroendocrine commonalities were suggested in studies in which about one third of OCD clients show nonsuppression on the dexamethasone-suppression test and decreased growth hormone secretion with clonidine infusions.

Biochemical Factors. A number of studies have implicated the neurotransmitter serotonin as influential in the etiology of obsessive–compulsive behaviors. Drugs that have been used successfully in alleviating the symptoms of OCD are clomipramine and the selective serotonin reuptake inhibitors (SSRIs), all of which are believed to block the neuronal reuptake of serotonin, thereby potentiating serotonergic activity in the central nervous system (see Figure 30–1).

Transactional Model of Stress/Adaptation

The etiology of obsessive–compulsive disorder is most likely influenced by multiple factors. In Figure 30–5, a graphic depiction of this theory of multiple causation is presented in the Transactional Model of Stress/Adaptation.

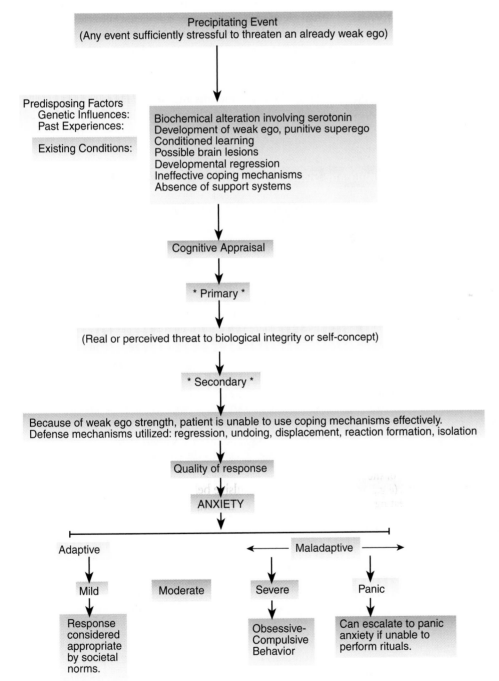

FIGURE 30–5 The dynamics of obsessive–compulsive disorder using the Transactional Model of Stress/Adaptation.

Posttraumatic Stress Disorder

Background Assessment Data

Posttraumatic stress disorder (PTSD) is described by the *DSM-IV-TR* as the development of characteristic symptoms following exposure to an extreme traumatic stressor involving a personal threat to physical integrity or to the physical integrity of others. The symptoms may occur after learning about unexpected or violent death, serious harm, or threat of death or injury of a family member or other close associate (APA, 2000). These symptoms are not related to common experiences such as uncomplicated bereavement, marital conflict, or chronic illness, but are associated with events that would be markedly distressing to almost anyone. The individual may experience the trauma alone or in the presence of others. Examples of some experiences that may produce this type of response include participation in military combat, experiencing violent personal assault, being kidnapped or taken hostage, being tortured, being incarcerated as a prisoner of war, experiencing natural or manmade disasters, surviving severe automobile accidents, or being diagnosed with a life-threatening illness (APA, 2000).

Characteristic symptoms include re-experiencing the traumatic event, a sustained high level of anxiety or arousal, or a general numbing of responsiveness. Intrusive recollections or nightmares of the event are common. Some individuals may be unable to remember certain aspects of the trauma.

Symptoms of depression are common with this disorder and may be severe enough to warrant a diagnosis of a depressive disorder. In the case of a life-threatening trauma shared with others, survivors often describe painful guilt feelings about surviving when others did not or about the things they had to do to survive (APA, 2000). Substance abuse is common.

The full symptom picture must be present for more than 1 month and cause significant interference with social, occupational, and other areas of functioning. If the symptoms have not been present for more than 1 month, the diagnosis assigned is acute stress disorder (APA, 2000).

The disorder can occur at any age. Symptoms may begin within the first 3 months after the trauma, or there may be a delay of several months or even years. The *DSM-IV-TR* diagnostic criteria for PTSD are presented in Box 30–5.

Box 3 0 – 5   Diagnostic Criteria for Posttraumatic Stress Disorder

A. The person has been exposed to a traumatic event in which both of the following were present:
   1. The person experienced, witnessed, or was confronted with an event or events that involved actual or threatened death or serious injury, or a threat to the physical integrity of self or others.
   2. The person's response involved intense fear, helplessness, or horror.

   NOTE: In children, this may be expressed instead by disorganized or agitated behavior.

B. The traumatic event is persistently re-experienced in one (or more) of the following ways:
   1. Recurrent and intrusive distressing recollections of the event, including images, thoughts, or perceptions.

   NOTE: In young children, repetitive play may occur in which themes or aspects of the trauma are expressed.

   2. Recurrent distressing dreams of the event. **NOTE**: In children, there may be frightening dreams without recognizable content.
   3. Acting or feeling as if the traumatic event were recurring (includes a sense of reliving the experience, illusions, hallucinations, and dissociative flashback episodes, including those that occur on awakening or when intoxicated).

   NOTE: In young children, trauma-specific reenactment may occur.

   4. Intense psychological distress at exposure to internal or external cues that symbolize or resemble an aspect of the traumatic event.
   5. Physiological reactivity on exposure to internal or external cues that symbolize or resemble an aspect of the traumatic event.

C. Persistent avoidance of stimuli associated with the trauma and numbing of general responsiveness (not present before the trauma), as indicated by three (or more) of the following:
   1. Efforts to avoid thoughts or feelings associated with the trauma
   2. Efforts to avoid activities, places, or people that arouse recollections of the trauma
   3. Inability to recall an important aspect of the trauma
   4. Markedly diminished interest or participation in significant activities
   5. Feeling of detachment or estrangement from others
   6. Restricted range of affect (e.g., unable to have loving feelings)
   7. Sense of a foreshortened future (e.g., does not expect to have a career, marriage, children, or a normal life span)

D. Persistent symptoms of increased arousal (not present before the trauma), as indicated by two (or more) of the following:
   1. Difficulty falling or staying asleep
   2. Irritability or outbursts of anger
   3. Difficulty concentrating
   4. Hypervigilance
   5. Exaggerated startle response

E. Duration of the disturbance more than 1 month
F. Disturbance that causes clinically significant distress or impairment in social, occupational, or other important areas of functioning
   Specify if acute (symptoms less than 3 months), chronic (symptoms 3 months or more), or delayed onset (onset of symptoms at least 6 months after the stressor).

SOURCE: American Psychiatric Association (2000), with permission.

REVIEW QUESTIONS

Self-Examination/Learning Exercise

Select the answer that is most appropriate for each of the following questions.

Situation: Ms. T. has been diagnosed with agoraphobia.

1. Which behavior would be most characteristic of this disorder?

   a. Ms. T. experiences panic anxiety when she encounters snakes.
   b. Ms. T. refuses to fly in an airplane.
   c. Ms. T. will not eat in a public place.
   d. Ms. T. stays in her home for fear of being in a place from which she cannot escape.

2. The therapist who works with Ms. T. would likely choose which of the following therapies for her?

   a. 10 mg Valium qid
   b. Group therapy with other agoraphobic individuals.
   c. Facing her fear in gradual step progression
   d. Hypnosis

3. Should the therapist choose to use implosion therapy, Ms. T. would be:

   a. Taught relaxation exercises.
   b. Subjected to graded intensities of the fear.
   c. Instructed to stop the therapeutic session as soon as anxiety is experienced.
   d. Presented with massive exposure to a variety of stimuli associated with the phobic object/situation.

Situation: Sandy is a 29-year-old woman who has been admitted to the psychiatric unit with a diagnosis of obsessive–compulsive disorder. She spends many hours during the day and night washing her hands.

4. The most likely reason Sandy washes her hands so much is that it:

   a. Relieves her anxiety.
   b. Reduces the probability of infection.
   c. Gives her a feeling of control over her life.
   d. Increases her self-concept.

5. The *initial* care plan for Sandy would include which of the following nursing interventions?

   a. Keep Sandy's bathroom locked so she cannot wash her hands all the time.
   b. Structure Sandy's schedule so that she has plenty of time for washing her hands.
   c. Put Sandy in isolation until she promises to stop washing her hands so much.
   d. Explain Sandy's behavior to her, since she is probably unaware that it is maladaptive.

6. On Sandy's fourth hospital day, she says to the nurse, "I'm feeling better now. I feel comfortable on this unit, and I'm not ill-at-ease with the staff or other patients anymore." In light of this change, which nursing intervention is most appropriate?

   a. Give attention to the ritualistic behaviors each time they occur and point out their inappropriateness.
   b. Ignore the ritualistic behaviors, and they will be eliminated for lack of reinforcement.
   c. Set limits on the amount of time Sandy may engage in the ritualistic behavior.
   d. Continue to allow Sandy all the time she wants to carry out the ritualistic behavior.

Situation: John is a 28-year-old high-school science teacher whose Army Reserve unit was called to fight in Iraq. John did not want to fight. He admits that he joined the reserves to help pay off his college loans. In Iraq, he participated in combat and witnessed the wounding of several from his unit, as well as the death of his best friend. He has been experiencing flashbacks, intrusive recollections, and nightmares. His wife reports he is afraid to go to sleep, and his work is suffering. Sometimes he just sits as though he is in a trance. John is diagnosed with PTSD.

7. John says to the nurse, "I can't figure out why God took my buddy instead of me." From this statement, the nurse assesses which of the following in John?

   a. Repressed anger.
   b. Survivor's guilt.
   c. Intrusive thoughts.
   d. Spiritual distress.

8. John experiences a nightmare during his first night in the hospital. He explains to the nurse that he was dreaming about gunfire all around and people being killed. The nurse's most appropriate *initial* intervention is:

    a. Administer alprazolam as ordered p.r.n. for anxiety.
    b. Call the physician and report the incident.
    c. Stay with John and reassure him of his safety.
    d. Have John listen to a tape of relaxation exercises.

9. Which of the following therapy regimens would most appropriately be ordered for John?

    a. Paroxetine and group therapy
    b. Diazepam and implosion therapy
    c. Alprazolam and behavior therapy
    d. Carbamazepine and cognitive therapy

10. Which of the following may be influential in the predisposition to PTSD?

    a. Unsatisfactory parent–child relationship.
    b. Excess of the neurotransmitter serotonin.
    c. Distorted, negative cognitions.
    d. Severity of the stressor and availability of support systems.

Test Your Critical Thinking Skills

Sarah, age 25, was taken to the emergency department by her friends. They were at a dinner party when Sarah suddenly clasped her chest and started having difficulty breathing. She complained of nausea and was perspiring profusely. She had calmed down some by the time they reached the hospital. She denied any pain, and electrocardiogram and laboratory results were unremarkable.

Sarah told the admitting nurse that she had a history of these "attacks." She began having them in her sophomore year of college. She knew her parents had expectations that she should follow in their footsteps and become an attorney. They also expected her to earn grades that would promote acceptance by a top Ivy League university. Sarah experienced her first attack when she made a "B" in English during her third semester of college. Since that time, she has experienced these symptoms sporadically, often in conjunction with her perception of the need to excel. She graduated with top honors from Harvard.

Last week Sarah was promoted within her law firm. She was assigned her first solo case of representing a couple whose baby had died at birth and who were suing the physician for malpractice. She has experienced these panic symptoms daily for the past week, stating, "I feel like I'm going crazy!"

Sarah is transferred to the psychiatric unit. The psychiatrist diagnoses panic disorder without agoraphobia.

Answer the following questions related to Sarah:

1. What would be the priority nursing diagnosis for Sarah?
2. What is the priority nursing intervention with Sarah?
3. What medical treatment might you expect the physician to prescribe?

REFERENCES

American Psychiatric Association (APA). (2000). *Diagnostic and statistical manual of mental disorders* (4th ed.) *Text revision.* Washington DC: American Psychiatric Association.

Daniels, C.Y., & Yerkes, S. (2006). Panic disorder. Retrieved March 25, 2007 from http://www.emedicine.com/med/topic1725.htm

Epstein, S. (1991). Beliefs and symptoms in maladaptive resolutions of the traumatic neurosis. In D. Ozer, J.M. Healy, Jr., & A.J. Stewart (Eds.), *Perspectives on personality* (Vol. 3). London: Jessica Kingsley.

Hageman, I., Anderson, H.S., & Jergensen, M.B. (2001). Post-traumatic stress disorder: A review of psychobiology and pharmacotherapy. *ACTA Psychiatrica Scandinavica, 104,* 411–422.

Harvard Medical School. (2001, March). Panic disorder. *The Harvard Mental Health Letter.* Boston, MA: Harvard Medical School Publications Group.

Hermida, T., & Malone, D. (2004). Anxiety disorders. The Cleveland Clinic, Department of Psychiatry and Psychology. Retrieved March 25, 2007 from http://www.clevelandclinicmeded.com/diseasemanagement/psychiatry/anxiety/anxiety.htm

Hollander, E. & Simeon, D. (2008). Anxiety Disorders. In R.E. Hales, S.C. Yudofsky, & G.O. Gabbard (Eds.), *Textbook of psychiatry* (5th ed.). Washington, DC:American Psychiatric Publishing.

Johnson, M. (1994, May/June). Stage fright. From *Performing Songwriter 1*(6). Retrieved March 25, 2007 from http://www.mjblue.com/pfright.html

NANDA International (NANDA-I). (2007). *Nursing diagnoses: Definitions & classification 2007–2008.* Philadelphia: NANDA-I.

National Mental Health Association (NMHA). (2005). *Children with emotional disorders in the juvenile justice system.* Alexandria, VA: NMHA.

Sadock, B.J., & Sadock, V.A. (2007). *Synopsis of psychiatry: Behavioral sciences/clinical psychiatry* (10th ed.). Philadelphia: Lippincott Williams & Wilkins.

Shahrokh, N.C., & Hales, R.E. (2003). *American psychiatric glossary.* Washington, DC: American Psychiatric Publishing.

CLASSICAL REFERENCES

Freud, S. (1959). On the grounds for detaching a particular syndrome from neurasthenia under the description 'anxiety neurosis.' In *The standard edition of the complete psychological works of Sigmund Freud* (Vol. 3). London: Hogarth Press. (Original work published 1895).

Johnson, J.H., & Sarason, I.B. (1978). Life stress, depression and anxiety: Internal-external control as moderator variable. *Journal of Psychosomatic Research, 22,* 205–208.

 Internet References

- Additional information about anxiety disorders and medications to treat these disorders is located at the following Web sites:
  - http://www.adaa.org
  - http://www.mentalhealth.com

- http://www.psychweb.com/disorders/index.htm
- http://www.nimh.nih.gov/
- http://www.anxietynetwork.com/pdhome.html
- http://www.psychiatrymatters.md/
- http://www.fadavis.com/townsend

31
CHAPTER

Somatoform and Dissociative Disorders

CHAPTER OUTLINE

KEY TERMS

anosmia
aphonia
depersonalization
derealization
fugue
hypochondriasis

integration
la belle indifference
primary gain
pseudocyesis
secondary gain
tertiary gain

CORE CONCEPTS

amnesia
dissociation
hysteria
somatization

OBJECTIVES

After reading this chapter, the student will be able to:

1. Discuss historical aspects and epidemiological statistics related to somatoform and dissociative disorders.
2. Describe various types of somatoform and dissociative disorders and identify symptomatology associated with each; use this information in client assessment.
3. Identify predisposing factors in the development of somatoform and dissociative disorders.
4. Formulate nursing diagnoses and goals of care for clients with somatoform and dissociative disorders.
5. Describe appropriate nursing interventions for behaviors associated with somatoform and dissociative disorders.
6. Evaluate the nursing care of clients with somatoform and dissociative disorders.
7. Discuss various modalities relevant to treatment of somatoform and dissociative disorders.

Somatoform disorders are characterized by physical symptoms suggesting medical disease, but without demonstrable organic pathology or known pathophysiological mechanism to account for them. They are classified as mental disorders because pathophysiological processes are not demonstrable or understandable by means of existing laboratory procedures, and there is either evidence or strong presumption that psychological factors are the major cause of the symptoms. It is now well documented that a large proportion of clients in general medical outpatient clinics and private medical offices do not have organic disease requiring medical treatment. It is likely that many of these clients have somatoform disorders, but they do not perceive themselves as having a psychiatric problem and thus do not seek treatment from psychiatrists.

Dissociative disorders are defined by a disruption in the usually integrated functions of consciousness, memory, identity, or perception (American Psychiatric Association [APA], 2000). Dissociative responses occur when anxiety becomes overwhelming and the personality becomes disorganized. Defense mechanisms that normally govern consciousness, identity, and memory break down, and behavior occurs with little or no participation on the part of the conscious personality. Four types of dissociative disorders are described by the *DSM-IV-TR*: dissociative amnesia, dissociative fugue, dissociative identity disorder, and depersonalization disorder.

This chapter focuses on disorders characterized by severe anxiety that has been repressed and is being expressed in the form of physiological symptoms and dissociative behaviors. Historical and epidemiological statistics are presented. Predisposing factors that have been implicated in the etiology of these responses provide a framework for studying the dynamics of somatoform and dissociative disorders. An explanation of the symptomatology of these disorders is presented as background knowledge for assessing the client, and nursing care is described in the context of the nursing process. Additional treatment modalities are explored.

HISTORICAL ASPECTS

CORE CONCEPT

Hysteria
A polysymptomatic disorder that usually begins in adolescence (rarely after the 20s), chiefly affects women, and is characterized by recurrent multiple somatic complaints that are unexplained by organic pathology. It is thought to be associated with repressed anxiety.

Historically, somatoform disorders have been identified as *hysterical neuroses*. The concept of hysteria is at least 4000 years old and probably originated in Egypt. The name has been in use since the time of Hippocrates.

Over the years, symptoms of hysterical neuroses have been associated with witchcraft, demonology, and sorcery; dysfunction of the nervous system; and unexpressed emotion. Somatoform disorders are thought to occur in response to repressed severe anxiety. Freud observed that, under hypnosis, clients with hysterical neurosis could recall past memories and emotional experiences that would relieve their symptoms. This led to his proposal that unexpressed emotion can be "converted" into physical symptoms.

CORE CONCEPT

Dissociation
The splitting off of clusters of mental contents from conscious awareness, a mechanism central to hysterical conversion and dissociative disorder (Shahrokh & Hales, 2003).

Freud (1962) viewed dissociation as a type of repression, an active defense mechanism used to remove threatening or unacceptable mental contents from conscious awareness. He also described the defense of splitting of the ego in the management of incompatible mental contents. Despite the fact that the study of dissociative processes dates back to the 19th century, scientists still know remarkably little about the phenomena. Questions still remain unanswered: Are dissociative disorders psychopathological processes or ego-protective devices? Are dissociative processes under voluntary control, or are they a totally unconscious effort? Maldonado and Spiegel (2008) state:

> [These disorders] have much to teach us about the way humans adapt to traumatic stress, and about information processing in the brain. (p. 665)

EPIDEMIOLOGICAL STATISTICS

The lifetime prevalence of somatization disorder in the general population is estimated to be 0.2 to 2 percent in women and 0.2 percent in men (Sadock & Sadock, 2007). Tendencies toward somatization are apparently more common in those who are poorly educated and from the lower socioeconomic classes.

Lifetime prevalence rates of conversion disorder vary widely. Statistics within the general population have ranged from 5 to 30 percent. The disorder occurs more frequently in women than in men and more frequently in adolescents and young adults than in other age groups. A higher prevalence exists in lower socioeconomic groups, rural populations, and among those with less education (Sadock & Sadock, 2007).

Hypochondriasis affects 1 to 5 percent of the general population (APA, 2000). The disorder is equally common among men and women, and the most common age at onset is in early adulthood.

Pain is likely the most frequent presenting complaint in medical practice today. Pain disorder (previously called *somatoform pain disorder*) is diagnosed more frequently in women than in men by about 2 to 1. Its onset can occur at any age, with the peak ages at onset in the 40s and 50s. It is commonly associated with other psychiatric disorders, particularly affective and anxiety disorders (Sadock & Sadock, 2007).

Body dysmorphic disorder is rare, although it may be more common than once believed. In the practices of plastic surgery and dermatology, reported rates of body dysmorphic disorder range from 6 to 15 percent (APA, 2000). Psychiatrists see only a small fraction of the cases. A profile of these clients reveals that they are usually in the late teens or 20s and unmarried. Comorbidity with another psychiatric disorder, such as major depression, anxiety disorder, or even a psychotic disorder, is not uncommon with body dysmorphic disorder (Sadock & Sadock, 2007).

Dissociative syndromes are statistically quite rare, but when they do occur they may present very dramatic clinical pictures of severe disturbances in normal personality functioning. Dissociative amnesia is relatively rare, occurring most frequently under conditions of war or during natural disasters. However, in recent years, there has been an increase in the number of reported cases, possibly attributed to increased awareness of the phenomenon, and identification of cases that were previously undiagnosed (APA, 2000). It appears to be equally common in women and men (Sadock & Sadock, 2007). Dissociative amnesia can occur at any age but is difficult to diagnose in children because it is easily confused with inattention or oppositional behavior.

Dissociative fugue is also rare and occurs most often under conditions of war, natural disasters, or intense psychosocial stress. Information regarding gender distribution and familial patterns of occurrence is not available.

Estimates of the prevalence of dissociative identity disorder (DID) vary widely. Historically, it was thought to be quite rare; however, the number of reported cases has grown rapidly in the past few decades. The disorder occurs from three to nine times more frequently in women than in men, and onset likely occurs in childhood, although manifestations of the disorder may not be recognized until much later (APA, 2000). Clinical symptoms usually are not recognized until late adolescence or early adulthood, although they have probably existed for a number of years before diagnosis. There appears to be some evidence that the disorder is more common in first-degree biological relatives of people with the disorder than in the general population.

The prevalence of severe episodes of depersonalization disorder is unknown, although single brief episodes of depersonalization may occur at some time in as many as half of all adults, particularly in the event of severe psychosocial stress (APA, 2000). Symptoms usually begin in adolescence or early adulthood. The disorder is chronic, with periods of remission and exacerbation. The incidence of depersonalization disorder is high under conditions of sustained traumatization, such as in military combat or prisoner-of-war camps. It has also been reported in many individuals who endure near-death experiences.

IMPLICATIONS OF RESEARCH FOR EVIDENCE-BASED PRACTICE

Brunner, R., Parzer, P., Schuld, V., & Resch, F. Dissociative symptomatology and traumatogenic factors in adolescent psychiatric patients. *The Journal of Nervous and Mental Disease* (2000, February); 188(2), 71–77.

Description of the Study: This study describes the relationship between different types of childhood trauma to the degree of dissociative experiences. Subjects were 198 consecutively admitted adolescent psychiatric patients, 11 to 19 years old (89 inpatients and 109 outpatients). All patients completed the Adolescent Dissociative Experiences Scale (ADES), a self-administered questionnaire with 30 items that quantifies the frequency of dissociative experiences on an 11-point scale ranging from 0 (never) to 10 (always). The instrument has been shown to discriminate patients with dissociative disorders from patients in several other diagnostic categories, as well as from adolescents in the general population. Subjects' therapists were asked to complete the Checklist of Traumatic Childhood Events, based on assessments, client self-reports, and reports by caregivers and custodial and social services. The checklist covered four main areas of traumatic experiences: sexual abuse, physical abuse, neglect, and stressful life events. Each area was further categorized by experiences considered from minor to severe. Examples of these abuse extremes included:

● Sexual: From sexualized communication to fondling to masturbation to penetration
● Physical: From being hit with a hand to punching, kicking, lacerations, burns, fractures
● Neglect: From physical and educational neglect to social/environmental neglect to emotional and psychological involvement (rejection; hostility)
● Stressful life events: From loss related to family members to physical/mental illness of family members to "others" (e.g., personal physical illness, witnessing an accident or violence, institutional placement)

Results of the Study: All mean scores by traumatized adolescents were elevated in comparison to those of the control (nontraumatized) group. Increased dissociative symptomatology was unrelated to the degree of severity of sexual abuse experiences. Interestingly, the study found an increased amount of dissociative symptomatology associated with minor forms of physical abuse, as compared to the severe forms. Only severe forms of stressful life events contributed significantly to a higher degree of dissociative experiences. The study revealed that emotional neglect appears to be the best predictor of dissociative symptoms.

Implications for Nursing Practice: The authors state: "In contrast to the current psychopathogenic model of dissociation which maintains that particularly severe traumatic events lead to dissociative symptomatology, moderate but chronic emotional stress may be equal or even more important in the development of dissociation." This is important information for the nursing database. Nurses should be aware that even less severe forms of abuse and neglect may have a significant impact on the development of dissociative psychopathology in adolescents.

APPLICATION OF THE NURSING PROCESS

Background Assessment Data: Types of Somatoform Disorders

Somatization Disorder

 CORE CONCEPT

Somatization
The process by which psychological needs are expressed in the form of physical symptoms. Somatization is thought to be associated with repressed anxiety.

Somatization disorder is a syndrome of multiple somatic symptoms that cannot be explained medically and are associated with psychosocial distress and long-term seeking of assistance from healthcare professionals. Symptoms may be vague, dramatized, or exaggerated in their presentation. The disorder is chronic, with symptoms beginning before age 30. The symptoms are identified as pain (in at least four different sites), gastrointestinal symptoms (e.g., nausea, vomiting, diarrhea), sexual symptoms (e.g., irregular menses, erectile or ejaculatory dysfunction), and symptoms suggestive of a neurological condition (e.g., paralysis, blindness, deafness) (APA, 2000). Anxiety and depression are frequently manifested, and suicidal threats and attempts are not uncommon.

The disorder usually runs a fluctuating course, with periods of remission and exacerbation. Clients often receive medical care from several physicians, sometimes concurrently, leading to the possibility of dangerous combinations of treatments (APA, 2000). They have a tendency to seek relief through overmedicating with prescribed analgesics or antianxiety agents. Drug abuse and dependence are common complications of somatization disorder. When suicide results, it is usually in association with substance abuse (Sadock & Sadock, 2007).

It has been suggested that, in somatization disorder, there may be some overlapping of personality characteristics and features associated with histrionic personality disorder. These symptoms include heightened emotionality, impressionistic thought and speech, seductiveness, strong dependency needs, and a preoccupation with symptoms and oneself.

The *DSM-IV-TR* diagnostic criteria for somatization disorder are presented in Box 31–1.

Pain Disorder

The essential feature of pain disorder is severe and prolonged pain that causes clinically significant distress or impairment in social, occupational, or other important

---

BOX 31–1 Diagnostic Criteria for Somatization Disorder

A. A history of many physical complaints beginning before age 30 years that occur over a period of several years and result in treatment being sought or significant impairment in social, occupational, or other important areas of functioning.

B. Each of the following criteria must have been met, with individual symptoms occurring at any time during the course of the disturbance:
1. *Four Pain Symptoms*: A history of pain related to at least four different sites or functions (e.g., head, abdomen, back, joints, extremities, chest, rectum, during menstruation, during sexual intercourse, or during urination).
2. *Two Gastrointestinal Symptoms*: A history of at least two gastrointestinal symptoms other than pain (e.g., nausea, bloating, vomiting other than during pregnancy, diarrhea, or intolerance of several different foods).
3. *One Sexual Symptom*: A history of at least one sexual or reproductive symptom other than pain (e.g., sexual indifference, erectile or ejaculatory dysfunction, irregular menses, excessive menstrual bleeding, vomiting throughout pregnancy).
4. *One Pseudoneurological Symptom*: A history of at least one symptom of deficit suggesting a neurological condition not limited to pain (e.g., conversion symptoms such as impaired coordination or balance, paralysis or localized weakness, difficulty swallowing or lump in throat, aphonia, urinary retention, hallucinations, loss of touch or pain sensation, double vision, blindness, deafness, seizures; dissociative symptoms such as amnesia; or loss of consciousness other than fainting).

C. Either 1 or 2:
1. After appropriate investigation, each of the symptoms in criterion B cannot be fully explained by a known general medical condition or the direct effects of a substance (e.g., a drug or abuse, a medication).
2. When there is a related general medical condition, the physical complaints or resulting social or occupational impairment are in excess of what would be expected from the history, physical examination, or laboratory findings.

D. The symptoms are not intentionally produced or feigned (as in factitious disorder or malingering).

SOURCE: American Psychiatric Association (2000), with permission.

---

areas of functioning (APA, 2000). This diagnosis is made when psychological factors have been judged to have a major role in the onset, severity, exacerbation, or maintenance of the pain, even when the physical examination reveals pathology that is associated with the pain. Psychological implications in the etiology of the pain complaint may be evidenced by the correlation of a stressful situation with the onset of the symptom. Additional psychological implications may be supported by the facts that (1) appearance of the pain enables the client to avoid some unpleasant activity [**primary gain**] and (2) the pain promotes emotional support or attention that the client might not otherwise receive [**secondary gain**].

Characteristic behaviors include frequent visits to physicians in an effort to obtain relief, excessive use of analgesics, and requests for surgery (Sadock & Sadock, 2007). Symptoms of depression are common and often severe enough to warrant a diagnosis of major depression. Dependence on addictive substances is a common complication of pain disorder. The *DSM-IV-TR* diagnostic criteria for this disorder are presented in Box 31–2.

Hypochondriasis

Hypochondriasis may be defined as an unrealistic or inaccurate interpretation of physical symptoms or sensations, leading to preoccupation and fear of having a serious disease. The fear becomes disabling and persists despite appropriate reassurance that no organic pathology can be detected. Occasionally medical disease may be present, but in the individual with hypochondriasis, the symptoms are excessive in relation to the degree of pathology.

The preoccupation may be with a specific organ or disease (e.g., cardiac disease), with bodily functions (e.g., peristalsis or heartbeat), or even with minor physical alterations (e.g., a small sore or an occasional cough) (APA, 2000). Individuals with hypochondriasis may become convinced that a rapid heart rate indicates they have heart disease or that the small sore is skin cancer. They are profoundly preoccupied with their bodies and are totally aware of even the slightest change in feeling or sensation. Their response to these small changes, however, is usually unrealistic and exaggerated.

Individuals with hypochondriasis often have a long history of "doctor shopping" and are convinced that they are not receiving the proper care. Anxiety and depression are common, and obsessive–compulsive traits frequently accompany the disorder. Social and occupational functioning may be impaired because of the disorder.

Preoccupation with the fear of serious disease may interfere with social or occupational functioning. Some individuals are able to function appropriately on the job, however, while limiting their physical complaints to non-work time.

Individuals with hypochondriasis are so totally convinced that their symptoms are related to organic pathology that they adamantly reject, and are often irritated by, any implication that stress or psychosocial factors play any role in their condition. They are so apprehensive and fearful that they become alarmed at the slightest intimation of serious illness. Even reading about a disease or hearing that someone they know has been diagnosed with an illness precipitates alarm on their part.

The *DSM-IV-TR* diagnostic criteria for hypochondriasis are presented in Box 31–3.

BOX 31–2 Diagnostic Criteria for Pain Disorder

A. Pain in one or more anatomical sites is the predominant focus of the clinical presentation and is of sufficient severity to warrant clinical attention.
B. The pain causes clinically significant distress or impairment in social, occupational, or other important areas of functioning.
C. Psychological factors are judged to have an important role in the onset, severity, exacerbation, or maintenance of the pain.
D. The symptom or deficit is not intentionally produced or feigned (as in factitious disorder or malingering).
E. The pain is not better accounted for by a mood, anxiety, or psychotic disorder and does not meet criteria for dyspareunia.

May be coded as:

Pain Disorder Associated with Psychological Factors:

Psychological factors are judged to have the major role in the onset, severity, exacerbation, or maintenance of the pain.

Acute: Duration of less than 6 months.
Chronic: Duration of 6 months or longer.

Pain Disorder Associated with Both Psychological Factors and a General Medical Condition

Both psychological factors and a general medical condition are judged to have important roles in the onset, severity, exacerbation, or maintenance of the pain.

Acute: Duration of less than 6 months.
Chronic: Duration of 6 months or longer.

Pain Disorder Associated with a General Medical Condition

A general medical condition has a major role in the onset, severity, exacerbation, or maintenance of the pain.

SOURCE: American Psychiatric Association (2000), with permission.

BOX 31–3 Diagnostic Criteria for Hypochondriasis

A. Preoccupation with fears of having, or the idea that one has, a serious disease, based on the person's misinterpretation of bodily symptoms.
B. The preoccupation persists despite appropriate medical evaluation and reassurance.
C. The belief in criterion A is not of delusional intensity (as in delusional disorder, somatic type) and is not restricted to a circumscribed concern about appearance (as in body dysmorphic disorder).
D. The preoccupation causes clinically significant distress or impairment in social, occupational, or other important areas of functioning.
E. The duration of the disturbance is at least 6 months.
F. The preoccupation is not better accounted for by generalized anxiety disorder, obsessive-compulsive disorder, panic disorder, a major depressive episode, separation anxiety, or another somatoform disorder.

SOURCE: American Psychiatric Association (2000), with permission.

Conversion Disorder

Conversion disorder is a loss of or change in body function resulting from a psychological conflict, the physical symptoms of which cannot be explained in terms of any known medical disorder or pathophysiological mechanism. Clients are unaware of the psychological basis and are therefore unable to control their symptoms.

Conversion symptoms affect voluntary motor or sensory functioning suggestive of neurological disease and are therefore sometimes called "pseudoneurological" (APA, 2000). Examples include paralysis, **aphonia**, seizures, coordination disturbance, difficulty swallowing, urinary retention, akinesia, blindness, deafness, double vision, **anosmia**, loss of pain sensation, and hallucinations. **Pseudocyesis** (false pregnancy) is a conversion symptom and may represent a strong desire to be pregnant.

Precipitation of conversion symptoms must be explained by psychological factors, and this may be evidenced by the presence of primary or secondary gain. When an individual achieves *primary gain*, the conversion symptoms enable the individual to avoid difficult situations or unpleasant activities about which he or she is anxious. Conversion symptoms promote *secondary gain* for the individual as a way to obtain attention or support that might not otherwise be forthcoming.

The symptom usually occurs after a situation that produces extreme psychological stress for the individual. The symptom appears suddenly, and often the person expresses a relative lack of concern that is out of keeping with the severity of the impairment (APA, 2000). This lack of concern is identified as **la belle indifference** and is often a clue to the physician that the problem may be psychological rather than physical. Other individuals, however, may present symptoms in a dramatic or histrionic fashion (APA, 2000).

Most symptoms of conversion disorder resolve spontaneously within a few weeks. About 20 to 25 percent of clients will experience a recurrence of symptoms within 1 year of the first episode (Sadock & Sadock, 2007). Symptoms of blindness, aphonia, and paralysis are associated with good prognosis, whereas seizures and tremor are associated with poorer prognosis (APA, 2000). The *DSM-IV-TR* diagnostic criteria for conversion disorder are presented in Box 31–4.

Body Dysmorphic Disorder

This disorder, formerly called dysmorphophobia, is characterized by the exaggerated belief that the body is deformed or defective in some specific way. The most common complaints involve imagined or slight flaws of the face or head, such as thinning hair, acne,

---

Box 31–4 Diagnostic Criteria for Conversion Disorder

A. One or more symptoms or deficits affecting voluntary motor or sensory function that suggest a neurological or other general medical condition.
B. Psychological factors are judged to be associated with the symptom or deficit because the initiation or exacerbation of the symptom or deficit is preceded by conflicts or other stressors.
C. The symptom or deficit is not intentionally produced or feigned (as in factitious disorder or malingering).
D. The symptom or deficit cannot, after appropriate investigation, be fully explained by a general medical condition, by the direct effects of a substance, or as a culturally sanctioned behavior or experience.
E. The symptom or deficit causes clinically significant distress or impairment in social, occupational, or other important areas of functioning or warrants medical evaluation.
F. The symptom or deficit is not limited to pain or sexual dysfunction, does not occur exclusively during the course of somatization disorder, and is not better accounted for by another mental disorder.
   Specify type of symptom or deficit:
      With motor symptom or deficit
      With sensory symptom or deficit
      With seizures or convulsions
      With mixed presentation

SOURCE: American Psychiatric Association (2000), with permission.

---

wrinkles, scars, vascular markings, facial swelling or asymmetry, or excessive facial hair (APA, 2000). Other complaints may have to do with some aspect of the nose, ears, eyes, mouth, lips, or teeth. Some clients may present with complaints involving other parts of the body, and in some instances a true defect is present. The significance of the defect is unrealistically exaggerated, however, and the person's concern is grossly excessive.

Symptoms of depression and characteristics associated with obsessive–compulsive personality are common in individuals with body dysmorphic disorder. Social and occupational impairment may occur because of the excessive anxiety experienced by the individual in relation to the imagined defect. The person's medical history may reflect numerous visits to plastic surgeons and dermatologists in an unrelenting drive to correct the imagined defect. He or she may undergo unnecessary surgical procedures toward this effort.

This disorder has been closely associated with delusional thinking, and the *DSM-IV-TR* suggests that if the perceived body defect is in fact of delusional intensity, the appropriate diagnosis would be delusional disorder, somatic type (APA, 2000). Traits associated with schizoid, obsessive–compulsive, and narcissistic personality disorders are not uncommon (Sadock & Sadock, 2007). The *DSM-IV-TR* diagnostic

Box 31–5 Diagnostic Criteria for Body Dysmorphic Disorder

A. Preoccupation with an imagined defect in appearance. If a slight physical anomaly is present, the person's concern is markedly excessive.
B. The preoccupation causes clinically significant distress or impairment in social, occupational, or other important areas of functioning.
C. The preoccupation is not better accounted for by another mental disorder (e.g., dissatisfaction with body shape and size in anorexia nervosa).

SOURCE: American Psychiatric Association (2000), with permission.

criteria for body dysmorphic disorder are presented in Box 31–5.

The etiology of body dysmorphic disorder is unknown. In some clients the belief is due to another more pervasive psychiatric disorder, such as schizophrenia. A high incidence of comorbidity with major mood disorder and anxiety disorder and the responsiveness of the condition to the serotonin-specific drugs may indicate some involvement of the serotonergic system.

Body dysmorphic disorder has been classified as one of several *monosymptomatic hypochondriacal syndromes*. Each of these syndromes is characterized by a single hypochondriacal belief about one's body. Body dysmorphic disorder is one of the most common such syndromes. Others include delusions of parasitosis (i.e., false belief that one is infested with some parasite or vermin) and of bromosis (i.e., false belief that one is emitting an offensive body odor).

Body dysmorphic disorder has also been defined as the fear of some physical defect thought to be noticeable to others although the client appears normal. These interpretations suggest that the disorder may be related to predisposing factors similar to those associated with hypochondriasis or phobias. The psychodynamic view suggests that unresolved emotional conflict is displaced onto a body part through symbolization and projection (Sadock & Sadock, 2007). Repression of morbid anxiety is undoubtedly an underlying factor, and it is very likely that multiple factors are involved in the predisposition to body dysmorphic disorder.

Predisposing Factors Associated with Somatoform Disorders

Genetic

Studies have shown an increased incidence of somatization disorder, conversion disorder, and hypochondriasis in first-degree relatives, implying a possible inheritable predisposition (Sadock & Sadock, 2007; Soares & Grossman, 2007; Yutzy, 2003).

Biochemical

Decreased levels of serotonin and endorphins may play a role in the etiology of pain disorder. Serotonin is probably the main neurotransmitter involved in inhibiting the firing of afferent pain fibers. The deficiency of endorphins seems to correlate with an increase of incoming sensory (pain) stimuli (Sadock & Sadock, 2007).

Psychodynamic

Some psychodynamicists view hypochondriasis as an ego defense mechanism. Physical complaints are the expression of low self-esteem and feelings of worthlessness, because it is easier to feel something is wrong with the body than to feel something is wrong with the self. Another view of hypochondriasis (as well as pain disorder) is related to a defense against guilt. The individual views the self as "bad," based on real or imagined past misconduct, and views physical suffering as the deserved punishment required for atonement.

The psychodynamic theory of conversion disorder proposes that emotions associated with a traumatic event that the individual cannot express because of moral or ethical unacceptability are "converted" into physical symptoms. The unacceptable emotions are repressed and converted to a somatic hysterical symptom that is symbolic in some way of the original emotional trauma.

Family Dynamics

Some families have difficulty expressing emotions openly and resolving conflicts verbally. When this occurs, the child may become ill, and a shift in focus is made from the open conflict to the child's illness, leaving unresolved the underlying issues that the family cannot confront openly. Thus, somatization by the child brings some stability to the family, as harmony replaces discord and the child's welfare becomes the common concern. The child in turn receives positive reinforcement for the illness.

Learning Theory

Somatic complaints are often reinforced when the sick role relieves the individual from the need to deal with a stressful situation, whether it be within society or within the family. The sick person learns that he or she may avoid stressful obligations, postpone unwelcome challenges, and is excused from troublesome duties (primary gain); becomes the prominent focus of attention because of the illness (secondary gain); or relieves conflict within the family as concern is shifted to the ill person and away from the real issue (**tertiary gain**). These types of positive reinforcements virtually guarantee repetition of the response.

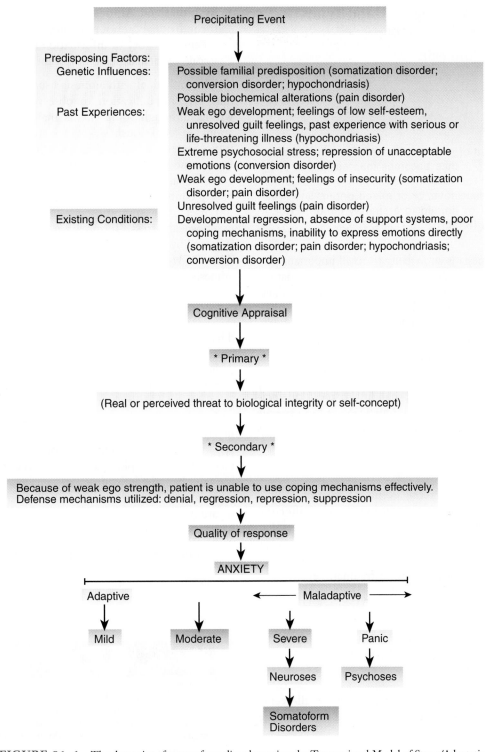

FIGURE 31–1 The dynamics of somatoform disorders using the Transactional Model of Stress/Adaptation.

Past experience with serious or life-threatening physical illness, either personal or that of close family members, can predispose an individual to hypochondriasis. Once an individual has experienced a threat to biological integrity, he or she may develop a fear of recurrence. The fear of recurring illness generates an exaggerated response to minor physical changes, leading to hypochondriacal behaviors.

Transactional Model of Stress/Adaptation

The etiology of somatoform disorders is most likely influenced by multiple factors. In Figure 31–1, a graphic depiction of this theory of multiple causation is presented in the transactional model of stress/adaptation.

Background Assessment Data: Types of Dissociative Disorders

Dissociative Amnesia

CORE CONCEPT

Amnesia
Pathologic loss of memory; a phenomenon in which an area of experience becomes inaccessible to conscious recall. The loss in memory may be organic, emotional, dissociative, or of mixed origin, and may be permanent or limited to a sharply circumscribed period of time (Shahrokh & Hales, 2003).

Dissociative amnesia is an inability to recall important personal information, usually of a traumatic or stressful nature, that is too extensive to be explained by ordinary forgetfulness and is not due to the direct effects of substance use or a neurological or other general medical condition (APA, 2000). Five types of disturbance in recall have been described. In the following examples, the individual is involved in a traumatic automobile accident in which a loved one is killed.

1. **Localized Amnesia.** The inability to recall all incidents associated with the traumatic event for a specific time period following the event (usually a few hours to a few days).

   Example:

   The individual cannot recall events of the automobile accident and events occurring during a period after the accident (a few hours to a few days).

2. **Selective Amnesia.** The inability to recall only certain incidents associated with a traumatic event for a specific period after the event.

   Example:

   The individual may not remember events leading to the impact of the accident but may remember being taken away in the ambulance.

3. **Continuous Amnesia.** The inability to recall events occurring after a specific time up to and including the present.

   Example:

   The individual cannot remember events associated with the automobile accident and anything that has occurred since. That is, the individual cannot form new memories although he or she is apparently alert and aware.

4. **Generalized Amnesia.** The rare phenomenon of not being able to recall anything that has happened during the individual's entire lifetime, including personal identity.

5. **Systematized Amnesia.** With this type of amnesia, the individual cannot remember events that relate to a specific category of information (e.g., one's family) or to one particular person or event.

The individual with amnesia usually appears alert and may give no indication to observers that anything is wrong, although some clients may present with alterations in consciousness, conversion symptoms, or in trance states (Sadock & Sadock, 2007). Clients suffering from amnesia are often brought to general hospital emergency departments by police who have found them wandering confusedly around the streets.

Onset of an amnestic episode usually follows severe psychosocial stress. Termination is typically abrupt and followed by complete recovery. Recurrences are unusual. The *DSM-IV-TR* diagnostic criteria for dissociative amnesia are presented in Box 31–6.

Dissociative Fugue

The characteristic feature of dissociative **fugue** is a sudden, unexpected travel away from home or customary place of daily activities, with inability to recall some or all of one's past (APA, 2000). An individual in a fugue state cannot recall personal identity and often assumes a new identity.

Individuals in a fugue state do not appear to be behaving in any way out of the ordinary. Contacts with other people are minimal. The assumed identity may be simple and incomplete or complex and elaborate. If a complex identity is established, the individual may engage in intricate interpersonal and occupational activities. A divergent perception regarding the assumption of a new identity in dissociative fugue is reported by Maldonado and Spiegel (2008):

> It was thought that the assumption of a new identity was typical of dissociative fugue. However, [studies have] documented that in most cases there is a loss of personal identity but no clear assumption of a new identity. (p. 678)

Box 31 – 6   Diagnostic Criteria for Dissociative Amnesia

A. The predominant disturbance is one or more episodes of inability to recall important personal information, usually of a traumatic or stressful nature, that is too extensive to be explained by ordinary forgetfulness.

B. The disturbance does not occur exclusively during the course of dissociative identity disorder, dissociative fugue, posttraumatic stress disorder, acute stress disorder, or somatization disorder and is not due to the direct physiological effect of a substance (e.g., a drug of abuse, a medication) or a neurological or other general medical condition (e.g., amnestic disorder due to head trauma).

C. The symptoms cause clinically significant distress or impairment in social, occupational, or other important areas of functioning.

SOURCE: American Psychiatric Association (2000), with permission.

Box 31–7 Diagnostic Criteria for Dissociative Fugue

A. The predominant disturbance is sudden, unexpected travel away from home or one's customary place of work, with inability to recall one's past.
B. Confusion about personal identity or assumption of a new identity (partial or complete).
C. The disturbance does not occur exclusively during the course of dissociative identity disorder and is not due to the direct physiological effects of a substance (e.g., a drug of abuse, a medication) or a general medical condition (e.g., temporal lobe epilepsy).
D. The symptoms cause clinically significant distress or impairment in social, occupational, or other important areas of functioning.

SOURCE: American Psychiatric Association (2000), with permission.

Clients with dissociative fugue often are picked up by the police when they are found wandering in a somewhat confused and frightened condition after emerging from the fugue in unfamiliar surroundings. They are usually presented to emergency departments of general hospitals. On assessment, they are able to provide details of their earlier life situation but have no recall from the beginning of the fugue state. Information from other sources usually reveals that the occurrence of severe psychological stress or excessive alcohol use precipitated the fugue behavior.

Duration is usually brief—that is, hours to days or more rarely, months—and recovery is rapid and complete. Recurrences are not common. The *DSM-IV-TR* diagnostic criteria for dissociative fugue are presented in Box 31–7.

Dissociative Identity Disorder

Dissociative identity disorder (DID) was formerly called multiple personality disorder. This disorder is characterized by the existence of two or more personalities in a single individual. Only one of the personalities is evident at any given moment, and one of them is dominant most of the time over the course of the disorder. Each personality is unique and composed of a complex set of memories, behavior patterns, and social relationships that surface during the dominant interval. The transition from one personality to another is usually sudden, often dramatic, and usually precipitated by stress. The *DSM-IV-TR* (APA, 2000) states:

The time required to switch from one identity to another is usually a matter of seconds but, less frequently, may be gradual. Behavior that may be frequently associated with identity switches include rapid blinking, facial changes, changes in voice or demeanor, or disruption in the individual's train of thought. (p. 527)

Before therapy, the original personality usually has no knowledge of the other personalities, but when there are two or more subpersonalities, they are usually aware of each other's existence. Most often, the various subpersonalities have different names, but they may be unnamed and may be of a different gender, race, and age. The various personalities are almost always quite disparate and may even appear to be the exact opposite of the original personality. For example, a normally shy, socially withdrawn, faithful husband may become a gregarious womanizer and heavy drinker with the emergence of another personality.

Generally, there is amnesia for the events that took place when another personality was in the dominant position, and clients report "gaps" in autobiographical histories. Sometimes, however, one personality does not experience such amnesia and retains complete awareness of the existence, qualities, and activities of the other personalities. Subpersonalities that are amnestic for the other subpersonalities experience the periods when others are dominant as "lost time" or blackouts. They may "wake up" in unfamiliar situations with no idea where they are, how they got there, or who the people around them are. They may frequently be accused of lying when they deny remembering or being responsible for events or actions that occurred while another personality controlled the body.

Dissociative identity disorder is not always incapacitating. Some individuals with DID maintain responsible positions, complete graduate degrees, and are successful spouses and parents before diagnosis and while in treatment. Before they are diagnosed with DID, many individuals are misdiagnosed with depression, borderline and antisocial personality disorders, schizophrenia, epilepsy, or bipolar disorder. The *DSM-IV-TR* diagnostic criteria for dissociative identity disorder are presented in Box 31–8.

Box 31–8 Diagnostic Criteria for Dissociative Identity Disorder

A. The presence of two or more distinct personality states (each with its own relatively enduring pattern of perceiving, relating to, and thinking about the environment and self).
B. At least two of these identities or personality states recurrently take control of the person's behavior.
C. Inability to recall important personal information that is too extensive to be explained by ordinary forgetfulness.
D. The disturbance is not due to the direct physiological effects of a substance (e.g., blackouts or chaotic behavior during alcohol intoxication) or a general medical condition (e.g., complex partial seizures). Note: In children, the symptoms are not attributable to imaginary playmates or other fantasy play.

SOURCE: American Psychiatric Association (2000), with permission.

Depersonalization Disorder

Depersonalization disorder is characterized by a temporary change in the quality of self-awareness, which often takes the form of feelings of unreality, changes in body image, feelings of detachment from the environment, or a sense of observing oneself from outside the body. Depersonalization (a disturbance in the perception of oneself) is differentiated from **derealization**, which describes an alteration in the perception of the external environment. Both of these phenomena also occur in a variety of psychiatric illnesses such as schizophrenia, depression, anxiety states, and organic mental disorders. As previously stated, the symptom of depersonalization is very common. It is estimated that approximately half of all adults experience transient episodes of depersonalization (APA, 2000). The diagnosis of depersonalization disorder is made only if the symptom causes significant distress or impairment in functioning.

The *DSM-IV-TR* describes this disorder as the persistence or recurrence of episodes of depersonalization characterized by a feeling of detachment or estrangement from one's self (APA, 2000). There may be a mechanical or dreamlike feeling or a belief that the body's physical characteristics have changed. If derealization is present, objects in the environment are perceived as altered in size or shape. Other people in the environment may seem automated or mechanical.

These altered perceptions are experienced as disturbing, and are often accompanied by anxiety, depression, fear of going insane, obsessive thoughts, somatic complaints, and a disturbance in the subjective sense of time (APA, 2000). The disorder occurs more often in women than it does in men, and is a disorder of younger people, rarely occurring in individuals older than 40 years of age (Andreasen & Black, 2006). The *DSM-IV-TR* diagnostic criteria for depersonalization disorder are presented in Box 31–9.

Box 3 1 – 9 Diagnostic Criteria for Depersonalization Disorder

A. Persistent or recurrent experiences of feeling detached from, and as if one is an outside observer of, one's mental processes or body (e.g., feeling like one is in a dream).
B. During the depersonalization experience, reality testing remains intact.
C. The depersonalization causes clinically significant distress or impairment in social, occupational, or other important areas of functioning.
D. The depersonalization experience does not occur exclusively during the course of another mental disorder, such as schizophrenia, panic disorder, acute stress disorder, or another dissociative disorder, and is not due to the direct physiological effects of a substance (e.g., a drug of abuse, a medication) or a general medical condition (e.g., temporal lobe epilepsy).

SOURCE: American Psychiatric Association (2000), with permission.

Predisposing Factors Associated with Dissociative Disorders

Genetics

The *DSM-IV-TR* suggests that DID is more common in first-degree relatives of people with the disorder than in the general population. The disorder is often seen in more than one generation of a family.

Neurobiological

Some clinicians have suggested a possible correlation between neurological alterations and dissociative disorders. Although available information is inadequate, it is possible that dissociative amnesia and dissociative fugue may be related to neurophysiological dysfunction. Areas of the brain that have been associated with memory include the hippocampus, amygdala, fornix, mammillary bodies, thalamus, and frontal cortex. Brunet, Holowka, and Laurence (2003) state:

> Given the intimate relationship between dissociation, memory, and trauma, researchers have begun to investigate the brain structures and neurochemical systems that mediate functions. Several substances such as sodium-lactate, yohimbine, and metachlorophenylpiperazine have been shown to elicit dissociative symptoms in patients with PTSD or panic disorder, but not in normal controls. Such findings suggest a role for the locus coeruleus/noradrenergic system, which is implicated in fear and arousal regulation and influence a number of cortical structures such as the prefrontal, sensory and parietal cortex, the hippocampus, the hypothalamus, the amygdala, and the spinal cord. Still the relationship between trauma exposure, cortisol, hippocampus damage, memory, and dissociation is tentative at best, and remains to be thoroughly investigated. (p. 26)

Some studies have suggested a possible link between DID and certain neurological conditions, such as temporal lobe epilepsy and severe migraine headaches. Electroencephalographic abnormalities have been observed in some clients with DID.

Psychodynamic Theory

Freud (1962) believed that dissociative behaviors occurred when individuals repressed distressing mental contents from conscious awareness. He believed that the unconscious was a dynamic entity in which repressed mental contents were stored and unavailable to conscious recall. Current psychodynamic explanations of dissociation are based on Freud's concepts. The repression of mental contents is perceived as a coping mechanism for protecting the client from emotional pain that has arisen from either disturbing external circumstances or anxiety-provoking internal urges and feelings (Maldonado & Spiegel, 2008). In the case of depersonalization, the pain and anxiety are expressed as feelings of unreality or detachment from the environment of the painful situation.

Psychological Trauma

A growing body of evidence points to the etiology of DID as a set of traumatic experiences that overwhelms the individual's capacity to cope by any means other than dissociation. These experiences usually take the form of severe physical, sexual, or psychological abuse by a parent or significant other in the child's life. The most widely accepted explanation for DID is that it begins as a survival strategy that serves to help children cope with the horrifying sexual, physical, or psychological abuse. In this traumatic environment, the child uses dissociation to become a passive victim of the cruel and unwanted experience. He or she creates a new being who is able to endure the overwhelming pain of the cruel reality, while the primary self can then escape awareness of the pain. Each new personality has as its nucleus a means of responding without anxiety and distress to various painful or dangerous stimuli.

Transactional Model of Stress/Adaptation

The etiology of dissociative disorders is most likely influenced by multiple factors. In Figure 31–2, a graphic

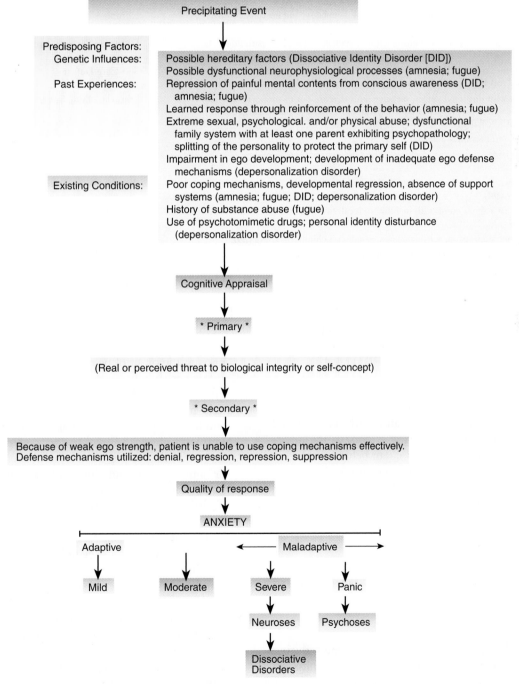

FIGURE 31–2 The dynamics of dissociative disorders using the Transactional Model of Stress/Adaptation.

TABLE 31–1 Assigning Nursing Diagnoses to Behaviors Commonly Associated with Somatoform and Dissociative Disorders	
Behaviors	**Nursing Diagnoses**
Verbalization of numerous physical complaints in the absence of any pathophysiological evidence; focus on the self and physical symptoms (*Somatization disorder*)	Ineffective Coping
History of "doctor shopping" for evidence of organic pathology to substantiate physical symptoms; statements such as, "I don't know why the doctor put me on the psychiatric unit. I have a physical problem." (*Somatization disorder*)	Deficient Knowledge (psychological causes for physical symptoms)
Verbal complaints of pain, with evidence of psychological contributing factors, and excessive use of analgesics (*Pain disorder*)	Chronic Pain
Seeking to be alone; refusal to participate in therapeutic activities (*Pain disorder*)	Social Isolation
Preoccupation with and unrealistic interpretation of bodily signs and sensations (*Hypochondriasis*)	Fear (of having a serious disease)
Transformation of internalized anger into physical complaints and hostility toward others (*Hypochondriasis*)	Chronic Low Self-esteem
Loss or alteration in physical functioning without evidence of organic pathology; "la belle indifference" (*Conversion disorder*)	Disturbed Sensory Perception
Need for assistance to carry out self-care activities such as eating, dressing, maintaining hygiene, and toileting due to alteration in physical functioning (*Conversion disorder*)	Self-Care Deficit
Preoccupation with imagined defect; verbalizations that are out of proportion to any actual physical abnormality that may exist; numerous visits to plastic surgeons or dermatologists seeking relief (*Body dysmorphic disorder*)	Disturbed Body Image
Loss of memory (*Dissociative amnesia*)	Disturbed Thought Processes
Verbalizations of frustration over lack of control and dependence on others (*Dissociative amnesia*)	Powerlessness
Fear of unknown circumstances surrounding emergence from the fugue state (*Dissociative fugue*)	Risk for Other-Directed Violence
Sudden travel away from home with inability to recall previous identity (*Dissociative fugue*)	Ineffective Coping
Unresolved grief; depression; self-blame associated with childhood abuse (*DID*)	Risk for Suicide
Presence of more than one personality within the individual (*DID*)	Disturbed Personal Identity
Alteration in the perception or experience of the self or the environment (*Depersonalization disorder*)	Disturbed Sensory Perception (Visual and Kinesthetic)

depiction of this theory of multiple causation is presented in the Transactional Model of Stress/Adaptation.

Diagnosis/Outcome Identification

Nursing diagnoses are formulated from the data gathered during the assessment phase and with background knowledge regarding predisposing factors to the disorder. Table 31–1 presents a list of client behaviors and the NANDA nursing diagnoses that correspond to those behaviors, which may be used in planning care for clients with somatoform and dissociative disorders.

Outcome Criteria

The following criteria may be used for measurement of outcomes in the care of the client with somatoform and dissociative disorders.

The client:

1. Effectively uses adaptive coping strategies during stressful situations without resorting to physical symptoms (*somatoform and pain disorders*).

2. Verbalizes relief from pain and demonstrates adaptive coping strategies during stressful situations to prevent the onset of pain (*pain disorder*).

3. Interprets bodily sensations rationally; verbalizes understanding of the significance the irrational fear held for him or her; and has decreased the number and frequency of physical complaints (*hypochondriasis*).

4. Is free of physical disability and is able to verbalize understanding of the correlation between the loss of or alteration in function and extreme emotional stress (*conversion disorder*).

5. Verbalizes a realistic perception of his or her appearance and expresses feelings that reflect a positive body image (*body dysmorphic disorder*).

6. Can recall events associated with a traumatic or stressful situation (*dissociative amnesia*).

7. Can recall all events of past life (*dissociative amnesia and dissociative fugue*).

8. Can verbalize the extreme anxiety that precipitated the dissociation (*dissociative disorders*).

9. Can demonstrate more adaptive coping strategies to avert dissociative behaviors in the face of severe anxiety (*dissociative disorders*).

10. Verbalizes understanding of the existence of multiple personalities and the purposes they serve (*dissociative identity disorder*).
11. Is able to maintain a sense of reality during stressful situations (*dissociative disorders*).

Planning/Implementation

The following section presents a group of selected nursing diagnoses, with short- and long-term goals and nursing interventions for each.

Ineffective Coping

Ineffective coping is defined as the "inability to form a valid appraisal of the stressors, inadequate choices of practiced responses, and/or inability to use available resources" (NANDA International [NANDA-I], 2007, p. 59).

Client Goals

Outcome criteria include short- and long-term goals. Timelines are individually determined.

Short-Term Goal

● Within 2 weeks, the client will verbalize understanding of correlation between physical symptoms and psychological problems.

Long-Term Goal

● By time of discharge from treatment, the client will demonstrate ability to cope with stress by means other than preoccupation with physical symptoms.

Interventions

● Monitor the physician's ongoing assessments, laboratory reports, and other data to maintain assurance that the possibility of organic pathology is clearly ruled out. Review findings with the client. Accurate medical assessment is vital for the provision of adequate and appropriate care. Honest explanation may help the client understand the psychological implications.
● Recognize and accept that the physical complaint is real to the client, even though no organic etiology can be identified. Denial of the client's feelings is nontherapeutic and interferes with establishment of a trusting relationship.
● Identify gains that the physical symptoms are providing for the client: increased dependency, attention, and distraction from other problems. Identification of underlying motivation is important in assisting the client with problem resolution.

● Initially, fulfill the client's most urgent dependency needs, but gradually withdraw attention to physical symptoms. Minimize time given in response to physical complaints. Anxiety and maladaptive behaviors will increase if dependency needs are ignored initially. Gradual withdrawal of positive reinforcement will discourage repetition of maladaptive behaviors.
● Explain to the client that any new physical complaints will be referred to the physician and give no further attention to them. Follow up on the physician's assessment of the complaint. The possibility of organic pathology must always be considered. Failure to do so could jeopardize client safety.
● Encourage the client to verbalize fears and anxieties. Explain that attention will be withdrawn if rumination about physical complaints begins. Follow through. Without consistency of limit setting, change will not occur.
● Help the client recognize that physical symptoms often occur because of, or are exacerbated by, specific stressors. Discuss alternative coping responses to these stressors. The client may need help with problem solving. Give positive reinforcement for adaptive coping strategies.
● Have the client keep a diary of appearance, duration, and intensity of physical symptoms. A separate record of situations that the client finds especially stressful should also be kept. Comparison of these records may provide objective data from which to observe the relationship between physical symptoms and stress.
● Help the client identify ways to achieve recognition from others without resorting to physical complaints. Positive recognition from others enhances self-esteem and minimizes the need for attention through maladaptive behaviors.
● Discuss how interpersonal relationships are affected by the client's narcissistic behavior. Explain how this behavior alienates others. The client may not realize how he or she is perceived by others.
● Provide instruction in relaxation techniques and assertiveness skills. These approaches decrease anxiety and increase self-esteem, which facilitate adaptive responses to stressful situations.

Fear (of Having a Serious Disease)

Fear is defined as the "response to a perceived threat that is consciously recognized as a danger" (NANDA-I, 2007, p. 87).

Client Goals

Outcome criteria include short- and long-term goals. Timelines are individually determined.

Short-Term Goal

● The client will verbalize that fears associated with bodily sensations are irrational (within time limit deemed appropriate for specific individual).

Long-Term Goal

● The client interprets bodily sensations correctly.

Interventions

● Monitor the physician's ongoing assessments and laboratory reports. Organic pathology must be clearly ruled out.
● Refer all new physical complaints to the physician. To assume that all physical complaints are hypochondriacal would place the client's safety in jeopardy.
● Assess what function the client's illness is fulfilling for him or her (e.g., unfulfilled needs for dependency, nurturing, caring, attention, or control). This information may provide insight into reasons for maladaptive behavior and provide direction for planning client care.
● Identify times during which the preoccupation with physical symptoms is worse. Determine the extent of correlation of physical complaints with times of increased anxiety. The client is most likely unaware of the psychosocial implications of the physical complaints. Knowledge of the relationship is the first step in the process for creating change.
● Convey empathy. Let the client know that you understand how a specific symptom may conjure up fears of previous life-threatening illness. Unconditional acceptance and empathy promote a therapeutic nurse–client relationship.
● Initially allow the client a limited amount of time (e.g., 10 minutes each hour) to discuss physical symptoms. Because this has been his or her primary method of coping for so long, complete prohibition of this activity would likely raise the client's anxiety level significantly, further exacerbating the hypochondriacal behavior.
● Help the client determine what techniques may be most useful for him or her to implement when fear and anxiety are exacerbated (e.g., relaxation techniques; mental imagery; thought-stopping techniques; physical exercise). All of these techniques are effective in reducing anxiety and may assist the client in the transition from focusing on fear of physical illness to the discussion of honest feelings.
● Gradually increase the limit on amount of time spent each hour in discussing physical symptoms. If the client violates the limits, withdraw attention. Lack of positive reinforcement may help to extinguish the maladaptive behavior.

● Encourage the client to discuss feelings associated with fear of serious illness. Verbalization of feelings in a nonthreatening environment facilitates expression and resolution of disturbing emotional issues. When the client can express feelings directly, there is less need to express them through physical symptoms.
● Role-play the client's plan for dealing with the fear the next time it assumes control and before it becomes disabling through the exacerbation of physical symptoms. Anxiety and fears are minimized when the client has achieved a degree of comfort through practicing a plan for dealing with stressful situations in the future.

Disturbed Sensory Perception

Disturbed sensory perception is defined as a "change in the amount or patterning of incoming stimuli accompanied by a diminished, exaggerated, distorted, or impaired response to such stimuli" (NANDA-I, 2007, p. 195). Table 31–2 presents this nursing diagnosis in care plan format.

Client Goals

Outcome criteria include short- and long-term goals. Timelines are individually determined.

Short-Term Goal

● The client will verbalize understanding of emotional problems as a contributing factor to the alteration in physical functioning (within time limit appropriate for specific individual).

Long-Term Goal

● The client will demonstrate recovery of lost or altered function.

Interventions

● Monitor the physician's ongoing assessments, laboratory reports, and other data to ensure that the possibility of organic pathology is clearly ruled out. Failure to do so may jeopardize the client's safety.
● Identify primary or secondary gains that the physical symptom is providing for the client (e.g., increased dependency, attention, protection from experiencing a stressful event). These are considered to be etiological factors and will be used to assist in problem resolution.
● Do not focus on the disability, and encourage the client to be as independent as possible. Intervene only when the client requires assistance. Positive reinforcement would encourage continued use of the maladaptive response for secondary gains, such as dependency.

Table 31–2	Care Plan for the Client with Conversion Disorder

NURSING DIAGNOSIS: DISTURBED SENSORY PERCEPTION

RELATED TO: Repressed severe anxiety

EVIDENCED BY: Loss or alteration in physical functioning, without evidence of organic pathology; "la belle indifference"

Outcome Criteria	Nursing Interventions	Rationale
Short-Term Goal ● The client will verbalize understanding of emotional problems as a contributing factor to the alteration in physical functioning (within time limit appropriate for specific individual). **Long-Term Goal** ● The client will demonstrate recovery of lost or altered function.	1. Monitor the physician's ongoing assessments, laboratory reports, and other data to ensure that possibility of organic pathology is clearly ruled out. 2. Identify primary or secondary gains that the physical symptom is providing for the client (e.g., increased dependency, attention, protection from experiencing a stressful event). 3. Do not focus on the disability, and encourage the client to be as independent as possible. Intervene only when client requires assistance. 4. Maintain nonjudgmental attitude when providing assistance to the client. The physical symptom is not within the client's conscious control and is very real to him or her. 5. Do not allow the client to use the disability as a manipulative tool to avoid participation in therapeutic activities. Withdraw attention if the client continues to focus on physical limitation. 6. Encourage the client to verbalize fears and anxieties. Help identify physical symptoms as a coping mechanism that is used in times of extreme stress. 7. Help client identify coping mechanisms that he or she could use when faced with stressful situations, rather than retreating from reality with a physical disability. 8. Give positive reinforcement for identification or demonstration of alternative, more adaptive coping strategies.	1. Failure to do so may jeopardize client safety. 2. Primary and secondary gains are etiological factors and may be used to assist in problem resolution. 3. Positive reinforcement would encourage continual use of the maladaptive response for secondary gains, such as dependency. 4. A judgmental attitude interferes with the nurse's ability to provide therapeutic care for the client. 5. Lack of reinforcement may help to extinguish the maladaptive response. 6. Clients with conversion disorder are usually unaware of the psychological implications of their illness. 7. The client needs assistance with problem solving at this severe level of anxiety. 8. Positive reinforcement enhances self-esteem and encourages repetition of desirable behaviors.

● Maintain a nonjudgmental attitude when providing assistance with self-care activities to the client. The physical symptom is not within the client's conscious control and is very real to him or her.

● Do not allow the client to use the disability as a manipulative tool to avoid participating in therapeutic activities. Withdraw attention if the client continues to focus on the physical limitation. Lack of reinforcement may help to extinguish the maladaptive response.

● Encourage the client to verbalize fears and anxieties. Help identify physical symptoms as a coping mechanism that is used in times of extreme stress. Clients with conversion disorder are usually unaware of the psychological implications of their illness.

● Help the client identify coping mechanisms that he or she could use when faced with stressful situations, rather than retreating from reality with a physical disability. The client needs assistance with problem solving at this severe level of anxiety.

● Give positive reinforcement for identification or demonstration of alternative, more adaptive coping strategies.

Disturbed Thought Processes

Disturbed thought processes is defined as a "disruption in cognitive operations and activities" (NANDA-I, 2007, p. 226).

Client Goals

Outcome criteria include short- and long-term goals. Timelines are individually determined.

Short-Term Goal

● The client will verbalize understanding that loss of memory is related to stressful situation and begin discussing stressful situation with nurse or therapist.

Long-Term Goal

● The client will recover deficits in memory and develop more adaptive coping mechanisms to deal with stressful situations.

Interventions

● Obtain as much information as possible about the client from family and significant others if possible. Consider likes, dislikes, important people, activities, music, and pets. A comprehensive baseline assessment is necessary for the development of an effective plan of care.

● Do not flood the client with data regarding his or her past life. Individuals who are exposed to painful information from which the amnesia is providing protection may decompensate even further into a psychotic state.

● Instead, expose the client to stimuli that represent pleasant experiences form the past, such as smells associated with enjoyable activities, beloved pets, and music known to have been pleasurable to the client. As memory begins to return, engage the client in activities that may provide additional stimulation. Recall often occurs during activities such as these that simulate life experiences.

● Encourage the client to discuss situations that have been especially stressful and to explore the feelings associated with those times. Verbalization of feelings in a nonthreatening environment may help the client come to terms with unresolved issues that may be contributing to the dissociative process.

● Identify specific conflicts that remain unresolved and help the client identify possible solutions. Provide instruction regarding more adaptive ways to respond to anxiety. Unless these underlying conflicts are resolved, any improvement in coping behaviors must be viewed as only temporary.

● Provide positive feedback for decisions made. Respect the client's right to make those decisions independently, and refrain from attempting to influence him or her toward those that may seem more logical. Independent choice provides a feeling of control, decreases feelings of powerlessness, and increases self-esteem.

Disturbed Personal Identity

Disturbed personal identity is defined as the "inability to distinguish between self and nonself" (NANDA-I, 2007, p. 110).

Client Goals

Outcome criteria include short- and long-term goals. Timelines are individually determined.

Short-Term Goals

● The client will verbalize understanding of the existence of multiple personalities within the self.

● The client will be able to recognize stressful situations that precipitate transition from one personality to another.

Long-Term Goals

● The client will verbalize understanding of the reason for existence of each personality and the role each plays for the individual.

● The client will enter into and cooperate with long-term therapy, with the ultimate goal being integration into one personality.

Interventions

● The nurse must develop a trusting relationship with the original personality and with each of the subpersonalities. Trust is the basis of a therapeutic relationship. Each of the personalities views itself as a separate entity and initially must be treated as such.

● Help the client understand the existence of the subpersonalities and the need each serves in the personal identity of the individual. The client may initially be unaware of the dissociative response. Knowledge of the needs each personality fulfills is the first step in the integration process and the client's ability to face unresolved issues without dissociation.

● Help the client identify stressful situations that precipitate transition from one personality to another. Carefully observe and record these transitions. Identification of stressors is required to assist the client in responding more adaptively and to eliminate the need for transition to another personality.

- Use nursing interventions necessary to deal with maladaptive behaviors associated with individual subpersonalities. For example, if one personality is suicidal, precautions must be taken to guard against the client's self-harm. If another personality has a tendency toward physical hostility, precautions must be taken to protect others.
- It may be possible to seek assistance from another personality. For example, a strong-willed personality may help to control the behaviors of the "suicidal" personality.
- Help subpersonalities understand that their "being" will not be destroyed, but rather integrated into a unified identity within the individual. Because the subpersonalities function as separate entities, the idea of total elimination generates fear and defensiveness.
- Provide support during disclosure of painful experiences and reassurance when the client becomes discouraged with lengthy treatment.

Concept Care Mapping

The concept map care plan is an innovative approach to planning and organizing nursing care (see Chapter 9). It is a diagrammatic teaching and learning strategy that allows visualization of interrelationships between medical diagnoses, nursing diagnoses, assessment data, and treatments. Examples of concept map care plans for clients with somatoform and dissociative disorders are presented in Figures 31–3 and 31–4.

Evaluation

Reassessment is conducted to determine if the nursing actions have been successful in achieving the objectives of care. Evaluation of the nursing actions for the client with a somatoform disorder may be facilitated by gathering information using the following types of questions:

- Can the client recognize signs and symptoms of escalating anxiety?
- Can the client intervene with adaptive coping strategies to interrupt the escalating anxiety before physical symptoms are exacerbated?
- Can the client verbalize an understanding of the correlation between physical symptoms and times of escalating anxiety?
- Does the client have a plan for dealing with increased stress to prevent exacerbation of physical symptoms?
- Does the client demonstrate a decrease in ruminations about physical symptoms?
- Have fears of serious illness diminished?
- Does the client demonstrate full recovery from previous loss or alteration of physical functioning?
- Does the client verbalize a realistic perception and satisfactory acceptance of personal appearance?

Evaluation of the nursing actions for the client with a dissociative disorder may be facilitated by gathering information using the following types of questions:

- Has the client's memory been restored?
- Can the client connect occurrence of psychological stress to loss of memory?
- Does the client discuss fears and anxieties with members of the staff in an effort toward resolution?
- Can the client discuss the presence of various personalities within the self?
- Can he or she verbalize why these personalities exist?
- Can the client verbalize situations that precipitate transition from one personality to another?
- Can the client maintain a sense of reality during stressful situations?
- Can the client verbalize a correlation between stressful situations and the onset of depersonalization behaviors?
- Can the client demonstrate more adaptive coping strategies for dealing with stress without resorting to dissociation?

TREATMENT MODALITIES

Somatoform Disorders

Individual Psychotherapy

The goal of psychotherapy is to help clients develop healthy and adaptive behaviors, encourage them to move beyond their somatization, and manage their lives more effectively. The focus is on personal and social difficulties that the client is experiencing in daily life as well as the achievement of practical solutions for these difficulties.

Treatment is initiated with a complete physical examination to rule out organic pathology. Once this has been ensured, the physician turns his or her attention to the client's social and personal problems and away from the somatic complaints.

Group Psychotherapy

Group therapy may be helpful for somatoform disorders because it provides a setting where clients can share their experiences of illness, can learn to verbalize thoughts and feelings, and can be confronted by group members and leaders when they reject responsibility for maladaptive behaviors. It has been reported to be the treatment of choice for both somatization disorder and hypochondriasis, in part because it provides the social support and social interaction that these clients need.

Behavior Therapy

Behavior therapy is more likely to be successful in instances when secondary gain is prominent. This may

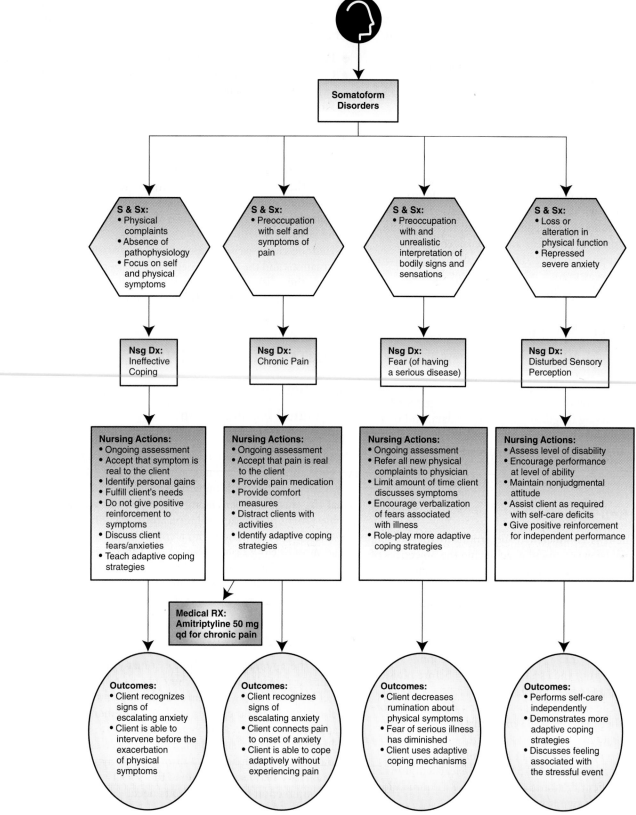

FIGURE 31–3 Concept map care plan for somatoform disorders.

7. In establishing trust with Ellen, the nurse must:

   a. Try to relate to Ellen as though she did not have multiple personalities.
   b. Establish a relationship with each of the personalities separately.
   c. Ignore behaviors that Ellen attributes to Beth.
   d. Explain to Ellen that he or she will work with her only if she maintains the status of the primary personality.

8. The ultimate goal of therapy for Ellen is:

   a. Integration of the personalities into one.
   b. For her to have the ability to switch from one personality to another voluntarily.
   c. For her to select which personality she wants to be her dominant self.
   d. For her to recognize that the various personalities exist.

9. The ultimate goal of therapy will most likely be achieved through:

   a. Crisis intervention and directed association.
   b. Psychotherapy and hypnosis.
   c. Psychoanalysis and free association.
   d. Insight psychotherapy and dextroamphetamines.

10. Which of the following is an appropriate nursing intervention for controlling the behavior of the "suicidal personality," Beth?

   a. When Beth emerges, put the client in restraints.
   b. Keep Ellen in isolation during her hospitalization.
   c. Make a verbal contract with Ellen that Beth will do no harm.
   d. Elicit the help of another, strong-willed personality to help control Beth's behavior.

Test Your **Critical Thinking Skills**

Sam was admitted to the psychiatric unit from the emergency department of a general hospital in the Midwest. The owner of a local bar called the police when Sam suddenly seemed to "lose control. He just went ballistic." The police reported that Sam did not know where he was or how he got there. He kept saying, "My name is John Brown, and I live in Philadelphia." When the police ran an identity check on Sam, they found that he was indeed John Brown from Philadelphia and his wife had reported him missing a month ago. Mrs. Brown explained that about 12 months before his disappearance, her husband, who was a shop foreman at a large manufacturing plant, had been having considerable difficulty at work. He had been passed over for a promotion, and his supervisor had been very critical of his work. Several of his staff had left the company for other jobs, and without enough help, Sam had been unable to meet shop deadlines. Work stress made him very difficult to live with at home. Previously an easygoing, extroverted individual, he became withdrawn and extremely critical of his wife and children. Immediately preceding his disappearance, he had had a violent argument with his 18-year-old son, who called Sam a "loser" and stormed out of the house to stay with some friends. It was the day after this argument that Sam disappeared. The psychiatrist assigns a diagnosis of dissociative fugue.

Answer the following questions related to Sam:

1. Describe the *priority* nursing intervention with Sam as he is admitted to the psychiatric unit.
2. What approach should be taken to help Sam with his problem?
3. What is the long-term goal of therapy for Sam?

REFERENCES

American Psychiatric Association (APA). (2000). *Diagnostic and statistical manual of mental disorders* (4th ed.) Text Revision. Washington, DC: American Psychiatric Association.

Andreasen, N.C., & Black, D.W. (2006). *Introductory textbook of psychiatry* (4th ed.). Washington, DC: American Psychiatric Publishing.

Brunet, A., Holowka, D.W., & Laurence, J.R. (2003). Dissociation. In M.J. Aminoff & R.B. Daroff (Eds.), *Encyclopedia of the neurological sciences*, Vol. 2. New York: Elsevier.

Ford-Martin, P. (2001). Fugue. *Gale encyclopedia of psychology*. Retrieved July 28, 2008 from http://www.findarticles.com/p/articles/mi_g2699/is_0004/ai_2699000474/

Leo, R.J. (2008). Pain disorders. In R.E. Hales, S.C. Yudofsky, & G.O. Gabbard (Eds.), *Textbook of psychiatry* (5th ed.). Washington, DC: American Psychiatric Publishing.

Maldonado, J.R., & Spiegel, D. (2008). Dissociative disorders. In R.E. Hales, S.C. Yudofsky, & G.O. Gabbard (Eds.), *Textbook of psychiatry* (5th ed.). Washington, DC: American Psychiatric Publishing.

NANDA International (NANDA-I). (2007). *Nursing diagnoses: Definitions & classification 2007–2008*. Philadelphia: NANDA-I.

Sadock, B.J., & Sadock, V.A. (2007). *Synopsis of psychiatry: Behavioral sciences/clinical psychiatry* (10th ed.). Philadelphia: Lippincott Williams & Wilkins.

Shahrokh, N.C., & Hales, R.E. (2003). *American psychiatric glossary* (8th ed.). Washington, DC: American Psychiatric Publishing.

Simeon, D., Stein, D.J., & Hollander, E. (1998). Treatment of depersonalization disorder with clomipramine. *Biological Psychiatry, 44*(4), 302–303.

Soares, N., & Grossman, L. (2007, November 28). Somatoform disorder: Conversion. *Emedicine Journal, 2*(9). Retrieved

February 13, 2008 from http://www.emedicine.com/PED/topic2780.htm

Yutzy, S.H. (2003). Somatoform disorders. In R.E. Hales & S.C. Yudofsky (Eds.), *Textbook of clinical psychiatry* (4th ed.). Washington, DC: American Psychiatric Publishing.

CLASSICAL REFERENCES

Freud, S. (1962). The neuro-psychoses of defense. In J. Strachey (Ed.), *Standard edition of the complete psychological works of Sigmund*

Freud, Vol. 3. London: Hogarth Press. (Original work published 1894).

 Internet References

- Additional information about somatoform disorders is located at the following Web sites:
  - http://www.psyweb.com/Mdisord/somatd.html
  - http://www.uib.no/med/avd/med_a/gastro/wilhelms/hypochon.html
  - http://www.emedicine.com/EMERG/topic112.htm
  - http://www.findarticles.com/p/articles/mi_g2601/is_0012/ai_2601001276

- Additional information about dissociative disorders is located at the following Web sites:
  - http://www.human-nature.com/odmh/dissociative.html
  - http://www.nami.org/helpline/dissoc.htm
  - http://www.issd.org/
  - http://www.findarticles.com/cf_dis/g2601/0004/2601000438/p1/article.jhtml
  - http://www.mental-health-matters.com/disorders/
  - http://www.sidran.org/
  - http://www.emedicine.com/med/topic3484.htm

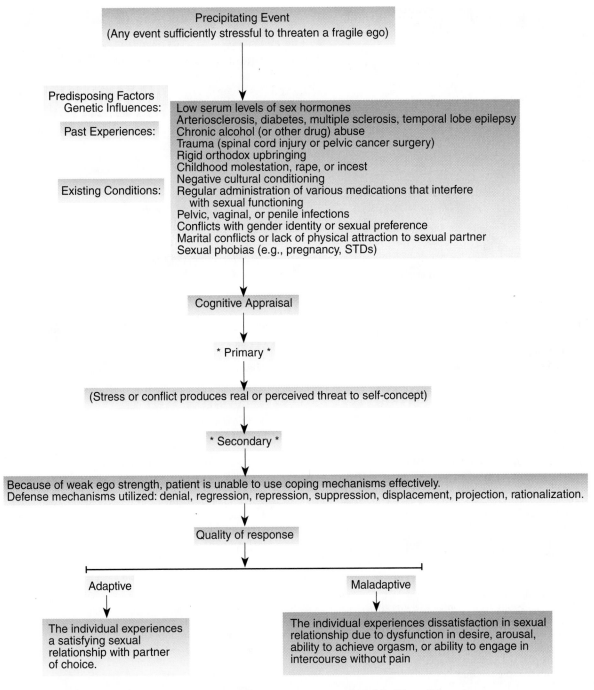

FIGURE 32–2 The dynamics of sexual dysfunction using the Transactional Model of Stress/Adaptation.

but as a guideline from which the nurse may select appropriate topics for gathering information about the client's sexuality. The outline should be individualized according to client needs.

Diagnosis/Outcome Identification

Nursing diagnoses are formulated from the data gathered during the assessment phase and with background knowledge regarding predisposing factors to the disorder. The following nursing diagnoses may be used for the client with sexual disorders:

● Sexual dysfunction related to depression and conflict in relationship or certain biological or psychological contributing factors to the disorder evidenced by loss of sexual desire or ability to perform
● Ineffective sexuality pattern related to conflicts with sexual orientation or variant preferences, evidenced by expressed dissatisfaction with certain sexual behaviors (e.g., voyeurism, transvestitism)

Outcome Criteria

The following criteria may be used for measurement of outcomes in the care of the client with sexual disorders.

BOX 32–1 Sexual History: Content Outline

I. Identify data
  A. Client
    1. Age
    2. Gender
    3. Marital status
  B. Parents
    1. Ages
    2. Dates of death and ages at death
    3. Birthplace
    4. Marital status
    5. Religion
    6. Education
    7. Occupation
    8. Congeniality
    9. Demonstration of affection
    10. Feelings toward parents
  C. Siblings (same information as above)
  D. Marital partner (same information as above)
  E. Children
    1. Ages
    2. Gender
    3. Strengths
    4. Identified problems
II. Childhood sexuality
  A. Family attitudes about sex
    1. Parents' openness about sex
    2. Parents' attitudes about nudity
  B. Learning about sex
    1. Asking parents about sex
    2. Information volunteered by parents
    3. At what age and how did client learn about: pregnancy, birth, intercourse, masturbation, nocturnal emissions, menstruation, homosexuality, STDs
  C. Childhood sex activity
    1. First sight of nude body:
      a. Same gender
      b. Opposite gender
    2. First genital self-stimulation
      a. Age
      b. Feelings
      c. Consequences
    3. First sexual exploration at play with another child
      a. Age (of self and other child)
      b. Gender of other child
      c. Nature of the activity
      d. Feelings and consequences
    4. Sexual activity with older persons
      a. Age (of self and other person)
      b. Gender of other person
      c. Nature of the activity
      d. Client willingness to participate
      e. Feelings and consequences
  D. Did you ever see your parents (or others) having intercourse? Describe your feelings.
  E. Childhood sexual theories or myths:
    1. Thoughts about conception and birth.
    2. Roles of male/female genitals and other body parts in sexuality.
III. Onset of adolescence
  A. In girls:
    1. Information about menstruation:

a. How received: from whom
b. Age received
c. Feelings
    2. Age:
      a. Of first period
      b. When breasts began to develop
      c. At appearance of ancillary and pubic hair
    3. Menstruation
      a. Regularity; discomfort; duration
      b. Feelings about first period
  B. In boys:
    1. Information about puberty:
      a. How received; from whom
      b. Age received
      c. Feelings
    2. Age
      a. Of appearance of ancillary and pubic hair
      b. Change of voice
      c. First orgasm (with or without ejaculation); emotional reaction
IV. Orgastic experiences
  A. Nocturnal emissions (male) or orgasms (female) during sleep.
    1. Frequency
  B. Masturbation
    1. Age begun; ever punished?
    2. Frequency; methods used.
    3. Marital partner's knowledge
    4. Practiced with others? Spouse?
    5. Emotional reactions.
    6. Accompanying fantasies.
  C. Necking and petting ("making out")
    1. Age when begun.
    2. Frequency.
    3. Number of partners.
    4. Types of activity.
  D. Premarital intercourse.
    1. Frequency.
    2. Relationship with and number of partners.
    3. Contraceptives used.
    4. Feelings.
  E. Orgasmic frequency
    1. Past
    2. Present.
V. Feelings about self as masculine/feminine
  A. The male client:
    1. Does he feel masculine?
    2. Accepted by peers?
    3. Sexually adequate?
    4. Feelings/concerns about body:
      a. Size
      b. Appearance
      c. Function
  B. The female client:
    1. Does she feel feminine?
    2. Accepted by peers?
    3. Sexually adequate?
    4. Feelings/concerns about body:
      a. Size
      b. Appearance
      c. Function

REVIEW QUESTIONS

Self-Examination/Learning Exercise

Select the answer that is most appropriate for each of the following questions.

1. Janice, age 24, and her husband are seeking treatment at the sex therapy clinic. They have been married for 3 weeks and have never had sexual intercourse together. Pain and vaginal tightness prevent penile entry. The sexual history reveals Janice was raped when she was 15 years old. The physician would most likely assign which of the following diagnoses to Janice?

   a. Dyspareunia
   b. Vaginismus
   c. Anorgasmia
   d. Sexual aversion disorder

2. The most appropriate nursing diagnosis for Janice would be:

   a. Pain related to vaginal constriction.
   b. Ineffective sexuality pattern related to inability to have vaginal intercourse.
   c. Sexual dysfunction related to history of sexual trauma.
   d. Complicated grieving related to loss of self-esteem because of rape.

3. The first phase of treatment may be initiated by the nurse. It would include which of the following?

   a. Sensate focus exercises
   b. Tense and relaxation exercises
   c. Systematic desensitization
   d. Education about the disorder

4. The second phase of treatment includes which of the following?

   a. Gradual dilation of the vagina
   b. Sensate focus exercises
   c. Hypnotherapy
   d. Administration of minor tranquilizers

5. Statistically, the outcome of therapy for Janice and her husband is likely to:

   a. Be unsuccessful.
   b. Be very successful.
   c. Be of very long duration.
   d. Result in their getting a divorce.

Match each of the paraphilias listed on the left with its correct behavioral description from the column on the right.

_____ 6. Exhibitionism

a. Tom watches his neighbor through her window each night as she undresses for bed. Later he fantasizes about having sex with her.

_____ 7. Transvestic fetishism

b. Frank drives his car up to a strange woman, stops, and asks her for directions. As she is explaining, he reveals his erect penis to her.

_____ 8. Voyeurism

c. Tim, age 17, babysits for his 11-year-old neighbor, Jeff. Six months ago, Tim began fondling Jeff's genitals. They now engage in mutual masturbation each time they are together.

_____ 9. Frotteurism

d. John is 32 years old. He buys women's clothing at the thrift shop. Sometimes he dresses as a woman and goes to a singles' bar. He becomes sexually excited as he fantasizes about men being attracted to him as a women.

_____ 10. Pedophilia

e. Fred rides a crowded subway every day. He stands beside a women he views as very attractive. Just as the subway is about to stop, he places his hand on her breast and rubs his genitals against her buttock. As the door opens, he dashes out and away. Later he fantasizes she is in love with him.

Test Your Critical Thinking Skills

Linda was hospitalized on the psychiatric unit for depression. During her nursing assessment interview, she stated, "According to my husband, I can't do anything right—not even have sex." When asked to explain further, Linda said she and her husband had been married for 17 years. She said that in the beginning, they had experienced a mutually satisfying sexual relationship and "made love" two or three times a week. Their daughter was born after they had been married 2 years, followed 2 years later by the birth of their son. They now have two teenagers (ages 15 and 13) who, by Linda's admission, require a great deal of her time and energy. She says, "I'm too tired for sex. And, besides, the kids might hear. I would be so embarrassed if they did. I walked in on my parents having sex once when I was a teenager, and I thought I would die! And my parents never mentioned it. It was just like it never happened! It was so awful! But sex is just so important to my husband, though, and we haven't had sex in months. We argue all the time about it. I'm afraid it's going to break us up."

Answer the following questions related to Linda:
1. What would be the primary nursing diagnosis for Linda?
2. What interventions might the nurse include in the treatment plan for Linda?
3. What would be a realistic goal for which Linda might strive?

REFERENCES

Administration on Aging. (2007). *A profile of older Americans: 2006.* Washington, DC: U.S. Department of Health and Human Services.

Altman, A., & Hanfling, S. (2003). *Sexuality in midlife and beyond.* Boston: Harvard Health Publications.

American Psychiatric Association (APA). (2000). *Diagnostic and statistical manual of mental disorders* (4th ed.). *Text Revision.* Washington, DC: American Psychiatric Association.

Andreasen, N.C., & Black, D.W. (2006). *Introductory textbook of psychiatry* (4th ed.). Washington, DC: American Psychiatric Publishing.

Bailey, J.M., & Pillard, R.C. (1991). A genetic study of male sexual orientation. *Archives of General Psychiatry, 48*, 1089–1096.

Becker, J.V. & Johnson, B.R. (2008). Gender identity disorders and paraphilias. In R.E. Hales, S.C. Yudofsky, & G.O. Gabbard (Eds.), *Textbook of psychiatry* (5th ed.). Washington, DC: American Psychiatric Publishing.

Becker, J.V. & Stinson, J.D. (2008). Human sexuality and sexual dysfunction. In R.E. Hales, S.C. Yudofsky, & G.O. Gabbard (Eds.), *Textbook of psychiatry* (5th ed.). Washington, DC: American Psychiatric Publishing.

Berman, J., & Berman, L. (2001). *For women only: A revolutionary guide to overcoming sexual dysfunction and reclaiming your sex life.* New York: Henry Holt.

Brosman, S.A., & Leslie, S.W. (2006). Erectile dysfunction. Retrieved June 1, 2007 from http://www.emedicine.com/med/ topic3023.htm

Centers for Disease Control and Prevention (CDC). (2007, March 23). Quadrivalent human papillomavirus vaccine: Recommendations of the Advisory Committee on Immunization Practices. *Morbidity and Mortality Weekly Report, 56*(RR-2), 1–24.

Centers for Disease Control and Prevention (CDC) (2008, June 6). Youth risk behavior surveillance—United States, 2007. *Morbidity and Mortality Weekly Report, 57*(SS-4), 1–131.

Clayton, A.H. (2002). Sexual dysfunction. In S.G. Kornstein & A H. Clayton (Eds.), *Women's mental health.* New York: Guilford.

Cook, L.H. (2003). Nursing care of patients with sexually transmitted diseases. In L.S. Williams & P.D. Hopper (Eds.), *Understanding medical surgical nursing* (2nd ed.). Philadelphia: F.A. Davis.

Dreyfus, E.A. (1998). *Sexuality and sex therapy: When there is sexual dysfunction.* Retrieved on June 1, 2007 from http://www.shpm.com/ articles/sex/sexther2.html

Johnson, R.D. (2003). Homosexuality: Nature or nurture. *AllPsych Journal.* Retrieved June 1, 2007 from http://allpsych.com/journal/homosexuality.html

King, B.M. (2005). *Human sexuality today* (5th ed.). Upper Saddle River, NJ: Pearson Education.

Leiblum, S.R. (1999). Sexual problems and dysfunction: Epidemiology, classification, and risk factors. *The Journal of Gender-Specific Medicine, 2*(5), 41–45.

Masters, W.H., Johnson, V.E., & Kolodny, R.C. (1995). *Human sexuality* (5th ed.). New York: Addison Wesley Longman.

Murray, R.B., & Zentner, J.P. (2001). *Health promotion strategies through the life span* (7th ed.). Upper Saddle River, NJ: Prentice-Hall.

NANDA International (NANDA-I). (2007). *Nursing diagnoses: Definitions & classification 2007–2008.* Philadelphia: NANDA-I.

Nappi, R., Salonia, A., Traish, A.M., van Lunsen, R.H.W., Vardi, Y., Kodiglu, A., & Goldstein, I. (2005). Clinical biologic pathophysiologies of women's sexual dysfunction. *Journal of Sexual Medicine, 2*(1), 4–25.

Noviasky, J.A., Masood, A., & Lo, V. (2004, July 15). Tadalafil for erectile dysfunction. *American Family Physician, 70*(2), 359.

Phillips, N.A. (2000, July 1). Female sexual dysfunction: Evaluation and treatment. *American Family Physician, 62*(1), 127–136, 141–142.

Rhodes, J.C., Kjerulff, K.H., Langenberg, P.W., & Guzinski, G.M. (1999). Hysterectomy and sexual functioning. *Journal of the American Medical Association, 282*(20), 1934–1941.

Robins, L.N., Helzer, J.E., Weissman, M.M., Orvaschel, H., Gruenberg, E., Burke, J.D., & Regier, D.A. (1984). Lifetime prevalence of specific psychiatric disorders in three sites. *Archives of General Psychiatry, 41*, 949–958.

Sadock, B.J., & Sadock, V.A. (2007). *Synopsis of psychiatry: Behavioral sciences/clinical psychiatry* (10th ed.). Philadelphia: Lippincott Williams & Wilkins.

Shenenberger, D., & Knee, T. (2005). Hyperprolactinemia. Retrieved March 26, 2007 from http://www.emedicine.com/med/topic1098.htm

Spear, J. (2001). Changing attitudes towards sex. *Gale Encyclopedia of Psychology* (2nd ed.). Retrieved March 26, 2007 from http://www. findarticles.com/p/articles/mi_g2699/is_0003/ai_2699000313

USA Today. (2003). *Poll shows backlash on gay issues.* Retrieved March 26, 2007 from http://www.usatoday.com/news/washington/2003-07-28-poll_x.htm

Wainright, J.L., Russell, S.T., & Patterson, C.J. (2004). Psychosocial adjustment, school outcomes, and romantic relationships of adolescents with same-sex parents. *Child Development, 75*(6), 1886–1898.

CLASSICAL REFERENCES

Freud, S. (1930). *Three contributions to the theory of sex* (4th ed.). New York: Nervous and Mental Disease Publishing.

Masters, W.H., & Johnson, V.E. (1966). *Human sexual response.* Boston: Little, Brown.

Masters, W.H., & Johnson, V.E. (1970). *Human sexual inadequacy.* Boston: Little, Brown.

@ Internet References

- Additional information about sexual disorders is located at the following Web sites:
  - http://www.sexualhealth.com/
  - http://www.priory.com/sex.htm
  - http://www.emedicine.com/med/topic3439.htm
  - http://www.emedicine.com/med/topic3127.htm

- Additional information about sexually transmitted diseases is located at the following web sites:
  - http://www.cdc.gov/std/
  - http://www.niaid.nih.gov/publications/stds.htm

BOX 33–1   Diagnostic Criteria for Anorexia Nervosa

A. Refusal to maintain body weight at or above a minimally normal weight for age and height (e.g., weight loss leading to maintenance of body weight less than 85% of that expected; or failure to make expected weight gain during period of growth, leading to body weight less than 85% of that expected).
B. Intense fear of gaining weight or becoming fat, even though underweight.
C. Disturbance in the way in which one's body weight or shape is experienced, undue influence of body weight or shape on self-evaluation, or denial of the seriousness of the current low body weight.
D. In postmenarchal females, amenorrhea; i.e., the absence of at least three consecutive menstrual cycles. (A woman is considered to have amenorrhea if her periods occur only following hormone, e.g., estrogen, administration.)
Specify type:
Restricting Type: During the current episode of anorexia nervosa, the person has not regularly engaged in binge-eating or purging behavior (i.e., self-induced vomiting or the misuse of laxatives, diuretics, or enemas).
Binge-Eating/Purging Type: During the current episode of anorexia nervosa, the person has regularly engaged in binge eating or purging behavior (i.e., self-induced vomiting or the misuse of laxatives, diuretics, or enemas).

SOURCE: American Psychiatric Association (2000), with permission.

amount of low-calorie food intake. Compulsive behaviors, such as hand washing, may also be present.

Age at onset is usually early to late adolescence. It is estimated to occur in approximately 1 percent of adolescent females, and is 10 times more common in females than in males (Andreasen & Black, 2006). Psychosexual development is generally delayed.

Feelings of depression and anxiety often accompany this disorder. In fact, some studies have suggested a possible interrelationship between eating disorders and affective disorders. Box 33–1 outlines the *DSM-IV-TR* (APA, 2000) diagnostic criteria for anorexia nervosa.

Background Assessment Data (Bulimia Nervosa)

CORE CONCEPT

Bulimia
Excessive, insatiable appetite.

Bulimia nervosa is an episodic, uncontrolled, compulsive, rapid ingestion of large quantities of food over a short period of time **(binging),** followed by inappropriate compensatory behaviors to rid the body of the excess calories. The food consumed during a binge often has a high caloric content, a sweet taste, and a soft or smooth texture that can be eaten rapidly, sometimes even without being chewed (Sadock & Sadock, 2007). The binging episodes often occur in secret and are usually terminated only by abdominal discomfort, sleep, social interruption, or self-induced vomiting. Although the eating binges may bring pleasure while they are occurring, self-degradation and depressed mood commonly follow.

To rid the body of the excessive calories, the individual may engage in **purging** behaviors (self-induced vomiting, or the misuse of laxatives, diuretics, or enemas) or other inappropriate compensatory behaviors, such as fasting or excessive exercise. There is a persistent overconcern with personal appearance, particularly regarding how they believe others perceive them. Weight fluctuations are common because of the alternating binges and fasts. However, most individuals with bulimia are within a normal weight range—some slightly underweight, some slightly overweight.

Excessive vomiting and laxative or diuretic abuse may lead to problems with dehydration and electrolyte imbalance. Gastric acid in the vomitus also contributes to the erosion of tooth enamel. In rare instances, the individual may experience tears in the gastric or esophageal mucosa.

Some people with this disorder are subject to mood disorders, anxiety disorders, and substance abuse or dependence, most frequently involving amphetamines or alcohol (APA, 2000). Diagnostic criteria for bulimia nervosa are presented in Box 33–2.

Predisposing Factors to Anorexia Nervosa and Bulimia Nervosa

Biological Influences

Genetics. A hereditary predisposition to eating disorders has been hypothesized on the basis of family histories and an apparent association with other disorders for which the likelihood of genetic influences exists. One recent study suggests that genetic factors account for 56 percent of the risk for developing anorexia nervosa (Bulik et al., 2006). Anorexia nervosa is more common among sisters and mothers of those with the disorder than among the general population. Several studies have reported a higher than expected frequency of mood disorders among first-degree biological relatives of people with anorexia nervosa and bulimia nervosa and of substance abuse and dependence in relatives of individuals with bulimia nervosa (APA, 2000).

Neuroendocrine Abnormalities. Some speculation has occurred regarding a primary hypothalamic dysfunction in anorexia nervosa. Studies consistent with this theory have revealed elevated cerebrospinal fluid cortisol levels and a possible impairment of dopaminergic regulation in individuals with anorexia (Halmi, 2008). Additional evidence in the etiological implication of hypothalamic dysfunction is gathered from the fact that many people

---

Box 33 – 2 **Diagnostic Criteria for Bulimia Nervosa**

A. Recurrent episodes of binge eating. An episode of binge eating is characterized by both of the following:
1. Eating, in a discrete period of time (e.g., within any 2-hour period) an amount of food that is definitely larger than most people would eat during a similar period of time and under similar circumstances.
2. A sense of lack of control over eating during the episode (e.g., a feeling that one cannot stop eating or control what or how much one is eating).

B. Recurrent inappropriate compensatory behavior in order to prevent weight gain, such as self-induced vomiting; misuse of laxatives, diuretics, enemas, or other medications; fasting; or excessive exercise.

C. The binge eating and inappropriate compensatory behaviors both occur, on average, at least twice a week for 3 months.

D. Self-evaluation is unduly influenced by body shape and weight.

E. The disturbance does not occur exclusively during episodes of anorexia nervosa.

Specify type:

Purging Type: During the current episode of bulimia nervosa, the person has regularly engaged in self-induced vomiting or the misuse of laxatives, diuretics, or enemas.

Nonpurging Type: During the current episode of bulimia nervosa, the person has used other inappropriate compensatory behaviors, such as fasting or excessive exercise, but has not regularly engaged in self-induced vomiting or the misuse of laxatives, diuretics, or enemas.

SOURCE: American Psychiatric Association (2000), with permission.

---

with anorexia experience amenorrhea before the onset of starvation and significant weight loss.

Neurochemical Influences. Neurochemical influences in bulimia may be associated with the neurotransmitters serotonin and norepinephrine. This hypothesis has been supported by the positive response these individuals have shown to therapy with the selective serotonin reuptake inhibitors (SSRIs). Some studies have found high levels of endogenous opioids in the spinal fluid of clients with anorexia, promoting the speculation that these chemicals may contribute to denial of hunger (Sadock & Sadock, 2007). Some of these individuals have been shown to gain weight when given naloxone, an opioid antagonist.

Psychodynamic Influences

Psychodynamic theories suggest that eating disorders result from very early and profound disturbances in mother–infant interactions. The result is retarded ego development in the child and an unfulfilled sense of separation–individuation. This problem is compounded when the mother responds to the child's physical and emotional needs with food. Manifestations include a disturbance in body identity and a distortion in body image. When events occur that threaten the vulnerable ego, feelings emerge of lack of control over one's body (self). Behaviors associated with food and eating serve to provide feelings of control over one's life.

Family Influences

Conflict Avoidance. In the theory of the family as a system, psychosomatic symptoms, including anorexia nervosa, are reinforced in an effort to avoid spousal conflict. Parents are able to deny marital conflict by defining the sick child as the family problem. In these families, there is an unhealthy involvement between the members (enmeshment); the members strive at all costs to maintain "appearances"; and the parents endeavor to retain the child in the dependent position. Conflict avoidance may be a strong factor in the interpersonal dynamics of some families in which children develop eating disorders.

Elements of Power and Control. The issue of control may become the overriding factor in the family of the client with an eating disorder. These families often consist of a passive father, a domineering mother, and an overly dependent child. A high value is placed on perfectionism in this family, and the child feels he or she must satisfy these standards. Parental criticism promotes an increase in obsessive and perfectionistic behavior on the part of the child, who continues to seek love, approval, and recognition. The child eventually begins to feel helpless and ambivalent toward the parents. In adolescence, these distorted eating patterns may represent a rebellion against the parents, viewed by the child as a means of gaining and remaining in control. The symptoms are often triggered by a stressor that the adolescent perceives as a loss of control in some aspect of his or her life.

Background Assessment Data (Obesity)

Obesity is not classified as a psychiatric disorder in the *DSM-IV-TR*, but because of the strong emotional factors associated with the condition, it may be considered under "Psychological Factors Affecting Medical Condition."

A third category of eating disorder is also being considered by the American Psychiatric Association. Research criteria for binge eating disorder (BED) are included in the *DSM-IV-TR* (see Box 33–3). Obesity is a factor in BED because the individual binges on large amounts of food (as in bulimia nervosa) but does not engage in behaviors to rid the body of the excess calories. The following formula is used to determine extent of obesity in an individual:

$$\text{Body mass index} = \frac{\text{Weight (kg)}}{\text{Height (m)}^2}$$

The BMI range for normal weight is 20 to 24.9. Studies by the National Center for Health Statistics indicate that *overweight* is defined as a BMI of 25.0 to 29.9 (based on U.S. Dietary Guidelines for Americans). Based on criteria of the World Health Organization, *obesity* is defined as a BMI of 30.0 or greater. These guidelines, which were released by the National Heart, Lung, and Blood Institute in July 1998, markedly increased the number of Americans considered to be overweight. The average American woman has

BOX 33 – 3   Research Criteria for Binge-Eating Disorder

A. Recurrent episodes of binge eating. An episode of binge eating is characterized by both of the following:
1. Eating, in a discrete period of time (e.g., within any 2-hour period), an amount of food that is definitely larger than most people would eat in a similar period of time under similar circumstances
2. A sense of lack of control over eating during the episode (e.g., a feeling that one cannot stop eating or control what or how much one is eating)

B. The binge-eating episodes are associated with three (or more) of the following:
1. Eating much more rapidly than normal
2. Eating until feeling uncomfortably full
3. Eating large amounts of food when not feeling physically hungry
4. Eating alone because of being embarrassed by how much one is eating
5. Feeling disgusted with oneself, depressed, or very guilty after overeating

C. Marked distress regarding binge eating is present.

D. The binge eating occurs, on average, at least 2 days a week for 6 months.

Note: The method of determining frequency differs from that used for Bulimia Nervosa; future research should address whether the preferred method of setting a frequency threshold is counting the number of days on which binges occur or counting the number of episodes of binge eating.

E. The binge eating is not associated with the regular use of inappropriate compensatory behaviors (e.g., purging, fasting, excessive exercise) and does not occur exclusively during the course of Anorexia Nervosa or Bulimia Nervosa.

SOURCE: American Psychiatric Association (2000), with permission.

a BMI of 26, and fashion models typically have BMIs of 18 (Priesnitz, 2005). Table 33–1 presents an example of some BMIs based on weight (in pounds) and height (in inches).

Obese people often present with hyperlipidemia, particularly elevated triglyceride and cholesterol levels. They commonly have hyperglycemia and are at risk for developing diabetes mellitus. Osteoarthritis may be evident because of trauma to weight-bearing joints. Work load on the heart and lungs is increased, often leading to symptoms of angina or respiratory insufficiency (National Heart, Lung, and Blood Institute, 2005).

Predisposing Factors to Obesity

Biological Influences

Genetics. Genetics have been implicated in the development of obesity in that 80 percent of offspring of two obese parents are obese (Halmi, 2008). Studies of twins and adoptees reared by normal and overweight parents have also supported this implication of heredity as a predisposing factor to obesity.

Physiological Factors. Lesions in the appetite and satiety centers in the hypothalamus may contribute to overeating and lead to obesity. Hypothyroidism is a problem that interferes with basal metabolism and may lead to weight gain. Weight gain can also occur in response to the decreased insulin production of diabetes mellitus and the increased cortisone production of Cushing's disease.

Lifestyle Factors. On a more basic level, obesity can be viewed as the ingestion of a greater number of calories than are expended. Weight gain occurs when caloric intake exceeds caloric output in terms of basal metabolism and

TABLE 33–1   Body Mass Index (BMI) Chart

BMI	19	20	21	22	23	24	25	26	27	28	29	30	31	32	33	34	35	36	37	38	39	40
Height (inches)											**Body Weight (pounds)**											
58	91	96	100	105	110	115	119	124	129	134	138	143	148	153	158	162	167	172	177	181	186	191
59	94	99	104	109	114	119	124	128	133	138	143	148	153	158	163	168	173	178	183	188	193	198
60	97	102	107	112	118	123	128	133	138	143	148	153	158	163	168	174	179	184	189	194	199	204
61	100	106	111	116	122	127	132	137	143	148	153	158	164	169	174	180	185	190	195	201	206	211
62	104	109	115	120	126	131	136	142	147	153	158	164	169	175	180	186	191	196	202	207	213	218
63	107	113	118	124	130	135	141	146	152	158	163	169	175	180	186	191	197	203	208	214	220	225
64	110	116	122	128	134	140	145	151	157	163	169	174	180	186	192	197	204	209	215	221	227	232
65	114	120	126	132	138	144	150	156	162	168	174	180	186	192	198	204	210	216	222	228	234	240
66	118	124	130	136	142	148	155	161	167	173	179	186	192	198	204	210	216	223	229	235	241	247
67	121	127	134	140	146	153	159	166	172	178	185	191	198	204	211	217	223	230	236	242	249	255
68	125	131	138	144	151	158	164	171	177	184	190	197	203	210	216	223	230	236	243	249	256	262
69	128	135	142	149	155	162	169	176	182	189	196	203	209	216	223	230	236	243	250	257	263	270
70	132	139	146	153	160	167	174	181	188	195	202	209	216	222	229	236	243	250	257	264	271	278
71	136	143	150	157	165	172	179	186	193	200	208	215	222	229	236	243	250	257	265	272	279	286
72	140	147	154	162	169	177	184	191	199	206	213	221	228	235	242	250	258	265	272	279	287	294
73	144	151	159	166	174	182	189	197	204	212	219	227	235	242	250	257	265	272	280	288	295	302
74	148	155	163	171	179	186	194	202	210	218	225	233	241	249	256	264	272	280	287	295	303	311
75	152	160	168	176	184	192	200	208	216	224	232	240	248	256	264	272	279	287	295	303	311	319
76	156	164	172	180	189	197	205	213	221	230	238	246	254	263	271	279	287	295	304	312	320	328

SOURCE: National Heart, Lung, and Blood Institute of the National Institutes of Health (2006).

physical activity. Many overweight individuals lead sedentary lifestyles, making it very difficult to burn off calories.

Psychosocial Influences

The psychoanalytical view of obesity proposes that obese individuals have unresolved dependency needs and are fixed in the oral stage of psychosexual development. The symptoms of obesity are viewed as depressive equivalents, attempts to regain "lost" or frustrated nurturance and caring.

Sadock and Sadock (2007) state:

> Although psychological factors are evidently crucial to the development of obesity, how such psychological factors result in obesity is not known. Overweight persons may suffer from every conceivable psychiatric disorder and come from a variety of disturbed backgrounds. Many obese patients are emotionally disturbed persons who, because of the availability of the overeating mechanism in their environments, have learned to use hyperphagia as a means of coping with psychological problems. Some patients may show signs of serious mental disorder when they attain normal weight because they no longer have that coping mechanism. (p. 742)

Transactional Model of Stress/Adaptation

The etiology of eating disorders is most likely influenced by multiple factors. In Figure 33–1, a graphic depiction of this theory of multiple causation is presented in the Transactional Model of Stress/Adaptation.

Diagnosis/Outcome Identification

Nursing diagnoses are formulated from the data gathered during the assessment phase and with background knowledge regarding predisposing factors to the disorder. Table 33–2 presents a list of client behaviors and the NANDA nursing diagnoses that correspond to those behaviors, which may be used in planning care for clients with eating disorders.

Outcome Criteria

The following criteria may be used for measurement of outcomes in the care of the client with eating disorders:

The client:

1. Has achieved and maintained at least 80 percent of expected body weight.
2. Has vital signs, blood pressure, and laboratory serum studies within normal limits.
3. Verbalizes the importance of adequate nutrition.
4. Verbalizes knowledge regarding consequences of fluid loss caused by self-induced vomiting (or laxative/diuretic abuse) and importance of adequate fluid intake.
5. Verbalizes events that precipitate anxiety and demonstrates techniques for its reduction.
6. Verbalizes ways in which he or she may gain more control of the environment and thereby reduce feelings of helplessness.
7. Expresses interest in the welfare of others and less preoccupation with own appearance.
8. Verbalizes that image of body as "fat" was misperception and demonstrates ability to take control of own life without resorting to maladaptive eating behaviors (anorexia nervosa).
9. Has established a healthy pattern of eating for weight control, and weight loss toward a desired goal is progressing.
10. Verbalizes plans for future maintenance of weight control.

Planning/Implementation

The following section presents a group of selected nursing diagnoses, with short- and long-term goals and nursing interventions for each.

Some institutions use a case management model to coordinate care (see Chapter 9 for more detailed explanation). In case management models, the plan of care may take the form of a critical pathway.

Imbalanced Nutrition: Less than Body Requirements/Deficient Fluid Volume (Risk for or Actual)

Imbalanced nutrition: less than body requirements is defined as "intake of nutrients insufficient to meet metabolic needs" (NANDA International [NANDA-I], 2007, p. 148). *Deficient fluid volume* is defined as "decreased intravascular, interstitial, and/or intracellular fluid" (NANDA-I, 2007, p. 90). Table 33–3 presents this nursing diagnosis in care plan format.

Client Goals

Outcome criteria include short- and long-term goals. Timelines are individually determined.

Short-Term Goals

● The client will gain___ pounds per week (amount to be established by client, nurse, and dietitian).
● The client will drink 125 mL of fluid each hour during waking hours.

Long-Term Goal

● By the time of discharge from treatment, the client will exhibit no signs or symptoms of malnutrition or dehydration.

Interventions

● For the client who is emaciated and is unable or unwilling to maintain an adequate oral intake, the physician may order a liquid diet to be administered via nasogastric

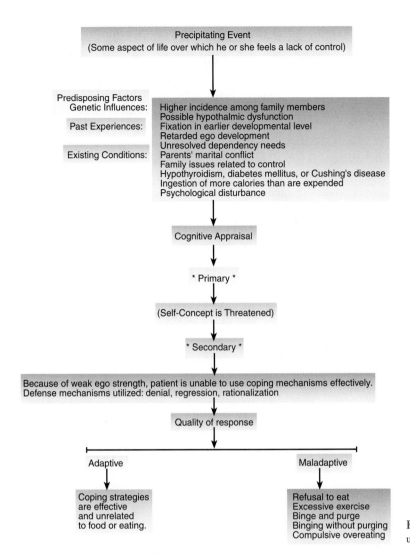

FIGURE 33–1 The dynamics of eating disorders using the Transactional Model of Stress/Adaptation.

TABLE 33–2   Assigning Nursing Diagnoses to Behaviors Commonly Associated with Eating Disorders

Behaviors	Nursing Diagnoses
Refusal to eat; abuse of laxatives, diuretics, and/or diet pills; loss of 15 percent of expected body weight; pale conjunctiva and mucous membranes; poor muscle tone; amenorrhea; poor skin turgor; electrolyte imbalances; hypothermia; bradycardia; hypotension; cardiac irregularities; edema	Imbalanced Nutrition: Less than Body Requirements
Decreased fluid intake; abnormal fluid loss caused by self-induced vomiting; excessive use of laxatives, enemas, or diuretics; electrolyte imbalance; decreased urine output; increased urine concentration; elevated hematocrit; decreased blood pressure; increased pulse rate; dry skin; decreased skin turgor; weakness	Deficient Fluid Volume
Minimizes symptoms; unable to admit impact of disease on life pattern; does not perceive personal relevance of symptoms; does not perceive personal relevance of danger	Ineffective Denial
Compulsive eating; excessive intake in relation to metabolic needs; sedentary lifestyle; weight 20 percent over ideal for height and frame; BMI of 30 or more	Imbalanced Nutrition: More than Body Requirements
Distorted body image; views self as fat, even in the presence of normal body weight or severe emaciation; denies that problem with low body weight exists; difficulty accepting positive reinforcement; self-destructive behavior (self-induced vomiting, abuse of laxatives or diuretics, refusal to eat); lack of eye contact; depressed mood; preoccupation with appearance and how others perceive it	Disturbed Body Image/Low Self-Esteem
Increased tension; increased helplessness; overexcited; apprehensive; fearful; restlessness; poor eye contact; increased difficulty taking oral nourishment; inability to learn	Anxiety (Moderate to Severe)

Table 33–3	Care Plan for Client with Eating Disorders: Anorexia Nervosa and Bulimia Nervosa

NURSING DIAGNOSIS: IMBALANCED NUTRITION: LESS THAN BODY REQUIREMENTS DEFICIENT FLUID VOLUME (RISK FOR OR ACTUAL)

RELATED TO: Refusal to eat/drink; self-induced vomiting; abuse of laxatives/diuretics

EVIDENCED BY: Loss of weight; poor muscle tone and skin turgor; lanugo; bradycardia; hypotension; cardiac arrhythmias; pale, dry mucous membranes

Outcome Criteria	Nursing Interventions	Rationale
Short-Term Goals ● The client will gain___pounds per week (amount to be established by client, nurse, and dietitian) ● The client will drink 125 mL of fluid each hour during waking hours. **Long-Term Goal** ● By the time of discharge from treatment, client will exhibit no signs or symptoms of malnutrition or dehydration.	1. Dietitian will determine number of calories required to provide adequate nutrition and realistic weight gain. 2. Explain to the client that privileges and restrictions will be based on compliance with treatment and direct weight gain. Do not focus on food and eating. 3. Weigh client daily, immediately upon arising and following first voiding. Always use same scale, if possible. Keep strict record of intake and output. Assess skin turgor and integrity regularly. Assess moistness and color of oral mucous membranes. 4. Stay with client during established time for meals (usually 30 min) and for at least 1 hour following meals. 5. If weight loss occurs, use restrictions. Client must understand that if nutritional status deteriorates, tube feedings will be initiated. This is implemented in a matter-of-fact, nonpunitive way. 6. Encourage the client to explore and identify the true feelings and fears that contribute to maladaptive eating behaviors.	1. Adequate calories are required to allow a weight gain of 2-3 pounds per week. 2. The real issues have little to do with food or eating patterns. Focus on the control issues that have precipitated these behaviors. 3. These assessments are important measurements of nutritional status and provide guidelines for treatment. 4. Lengthy mealtimes put excessive focus on food and eating and provide client with attention and reinforcement. The hour following meals may be used to discard food stashed from tray or to engage in self-induced vomiting. 5. Restrictions and limits must be established and carried out consistently to avoid power struggles, to encourage client compliance with therapy, and to ensure client safety. 6. Emotional issues must be resolved if these maladaptive responses are to be eliminated.

tube. Without adequate nutrition, a life-threatening situation exists. Nursing care of the individual receiving tube feedings should be administered according to established hospital procedures.

● For the client who is able and willing to consume an oral diet, the dietitian should determine the appropriate number of calories required to provide adequate nutrition and realistic (according to body structure and height) weight gain.

● Explain the program of behavior modification to client and family. Explain that privileges and restrictions will be based on compliance with treatment and direct weight gain.

● Do not focus on food and eating specifically. Instead, focus on the emotional issues that have precipitated these behaviors.

● Do not discuss food or eating with the client once protocol has been established. Do, however, offer support and positive reinforcement for obvious improvements

in eating behaviors.

● Keep a strict record of intake and output. Weigh the client daily immediately on arising and following first voiding. Always use the same scale, if possible.

● Assess skin turgor and integrity regularly. Assess moistness and color of oral mucous membranes. The condition of the skin and mucous membranes provides valuable data regarding client hydration. Discourage the client from bathing every day if the skin is very dry.

● Sit with the client during mealtimes for support and to observe the amount ingested. A limit (usually 30 minutes) should be imposed on time allotted for meals. Without a time limit, meals can become lengthy, drawn-out sessions, providing the client with attention based on food and eating.

● The client should be observed for at least 1 hour following meals. The client may use this time to discard food that has been stashed from the food tray or to engage in self-induced vomiting. He or she may need to be accompanied to the bathroom if self-induced vomiting is suspected.

● If weight loss occurs, use restrictions. Restrictions and limits must be established and carried out consistently to avoid power struggles and to encourage client compliance with therapy.

● Ensure that the client and family understand that if nutritional status deteriorates, tube feedings will be initiated. This is implemented in a matter-of-fact, nonpunitive way, for the client's safety and protection from a life-threatening condition.

● Encourage the client to explore and identify the true feelings and fears that contribute to maladaptive eating behaviors. Emotional issues must be resolved if these maladaptive responses are to be eliminated.

Ineffective Denial

Ineffective denial is defined as a "conscious or unconscious attempt to disavow the knowledge or meaning of an event to reduce anxiety/fear, but leading to the detriment of health" (NANDA-I, 2007, p. 67).

Client Goals

Outcome criteria include short- and long-term goals. Timelines are individually determined.

Short-Term Goal

● The client will verbalize understanding of the correlation between emotional issues and maladaptive eating behaviors (within time deemed appropriate for individual client).

Long-Term Goal

● By discharge from treatment, the client will demonstrate the ability to discontinue use of maladaptive eating behaviors and to cope with emotional issues in a more adaptive manner.

Interventions

● Establish a trusting relationship with the client by being honest, accepting, and available, and by keeping all promises. Convey unconditional positive regard.

● Acknowledge the client's anger at feelings of loss of control brought about by the established eating regimen associated with the program of behavior modification.

● Avoid arguing or bargaining with the client who is resistant to treatment. State matter-of-factly which behaviors are unacceptable and how privileges will be restricted for noncompliance. It is essential that all staff members are consistent with this intervention.

● Encourage the client to verbalize feelings regarding his or her role within the family and issues related to dependence/independence, the intense need for achievement, and sexuality. Help the client recognize how maladaptive eating behaviors may be related to

these emotional issues. Discuss ways in which he or she can gain control over these problematic areas of life without resorting to maladaptive eating behaviors.

Imbalanced Nutrition: More than Body Requirements

Imbalanced nutrition: more than body requirements is defined as "intake of nutrients that exceeds metabolic needs" (NANDA-I, 2007, p. 149).

Client Goals

Outcome criteria include short- and long-term goals. Timelines are individually determined.

Short-Term Goal

● The client will verbalize understanding of what must be done to lose weight.

Long-Term Goal

● The client will demonstrate a change in eating patterns that results in a steady weight loss.

Interventions

● Encourage the client to keep a diary of food intake. A food diary provides the opportunity for the client to gain a realistic picture of the amount of food ingested and provides a database on which to tailor the dietary program.

● Discuss feelings and emotions associated with eating. This helps to identify when the client is eating to satisfy an emotional need rather than a physiological one.

● With input from the client, formulate an eating plan that includes food from the required food groups with emphasis on low-fat intake. It is helpful to keep the plan as similar to the client's usual eating pattern as possible. The diet must eliminate calories while maintaining adequate nutrition. The client is more likely to stay on the eating plan if he or she is able to participate in its creation and it deviates as little as possible from usual types of foods.

● Identify realistic increment goals for weekly weight loss. Reasonable weight loss (1 to 2 pounds per week) results in more lasting effects. Excessive, rapid weight loss may result in fatigue and irritability and ultimately lead to failure in meeting goals for weight loss. Motivation is more easily sustained by meeting "stair-step" goals.

● Plan a progressive exercise program tailored to individual goals and choice. Exercise may enhance weight loss by burning calories and reducing appetite, increasing energy, toning muscles, and enhancing sense of well-being and accomplishment. Walking is an excellent choice for overweight individuals.

● Discuss the probability of reaching plateaus when weight remains stable for extended periods. The client should know this is likely to happen as changes in metabolism occur. Plateaus cause frustration, and the client may need additional support during these times to remain on the weight-loss program.

● Provide instruction about medications to assist with weight loss if ordered by the physician. Appetite-suppressant drugs (e.g., sibutramine) and others that have weight loss as a side effect (e.g., fluoxetine; topiramate) may be helpful to someone who is severely overweight. They should be used for this purpose for only a short period while the individual attempts to adjust to the new pattern of eating.

Disturbed Body Image/Low Self-Esteem

Disturbed body image is defined as "confusion in mental picture of one's physical self" (NANDA-I, 2007, p. 19). *Low self-esteem* is defined as "negative self-evaluation/feelings about self or self-capabilities" (NANDA-I, 2007, p. 188).

Client Goals (for the Client with Anorexia Nervosa or Bulimia Nervosa)

Outcome criteria include short- and long-term goals. Timelines are individually determined.

Short-Term Goal

● The client will verbally acknowledge misperception of body image as "fat" within specified time (depending on severity and chronicity of condition).

Long-Term Goal

● By the time of discharge from treatment, client will demonstrate an increase in self-esteem as manifested by verbalizing positive aspects of self and exhibiting less preoccupation with own appearance as a more realistic body image is developed.

Client Goals (for the Client with Obesity)

Outcome criteria include short- and long-term goals. Timelines are individually determined.

Short-Term Goal

● The client will begin to accept self based on self-attributes rather than on appearance.

Long-Term Goal

● The client will pursue loss of weight as desired.

Interventions

For the client with anorexia nervosa or bulimia nervosa:

● Help the client to develop a realistic perception of body image and relationship with food. Compare specific measurement of the client's body with the client's perceived calculations. There may be a large discrepancy between the actual body size and the client's perception

of his or her body size. The client needs to recognize that the misperception of body image is unhealthy and that maintaining control through maladaptive eating behaviors is dangerous—even life threatening.

● Promote feelings of control within the environment through participation and independent decision-making. Through positive feedback, help the client learn to accept self as is, including weaknesses as well as strengths. The client must come to understand that he or she is a capable, autonomous individual who can perform outside the family unit and who is not expected to be perfect. Control of his or her life must be achieved in other ways besides dieting and weight loss.

● Help the client realize that perfection is unrealistic, and explore this need with him or her. As the client begins to feel better about self, identifies positive self-attributes, and develops the ability to accept certain personal inadequacies, the need for unrealistic achievement should diminish.

For the client with obesity:

● Assess the client's feelings and attitudes about being obese. Obesity and compulsive eating behaviors may have deep-rooted psychological implications, such as compensation for lack of love and nurturing or a defense against intimacy.

● Ensure that the client has privacy during self-care activities. The obese individual may be sensitive or self-conscious about his or her body.

● Have the client recall coping patterns related to food in family of origin, and explore how these may affect current situation. Parents are role models for their children. Maladaptive eating behaviors are learned within the family system and are supported through positive reinforcement. Food may be substituted by the parent for affection and love, and eating is associated with a feeling of satisfaction, becoming the primary defense.

● Determine the client's motivation for weight loss and set goals. The individual may harbor repressed feelings of hostility, which may be expressed inward on the self. Because of a poor self-concept, the person often has difficulty with relationships. When the motivation is to lose weight for someone else, successful weight loss is less likely to occur.

● Help the client identify positive self-attributes. Focus on strengths and past accomplishments unrelated to physical appearance. It is important that self-esteem not be tied solely to size of the body. The client needs to recognize that obesity need not interfere with positive feelings regarding self-concept and self-worth.

● Refer the client to a support or therapy group. Support groups can provide companionship, increase motivation, decrease loneliness and social ostracism, and give practical solutions to common problems. Group therapy can be helpful in dealing with underlying psychological concerns.

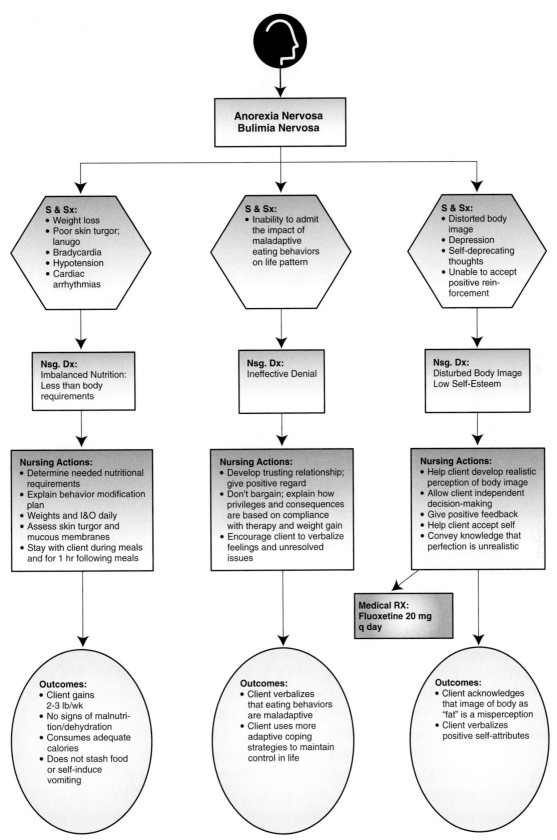

FIGURE 33–2 Concept map care plan for client with anorexia nervosa or bulimia nervosa.

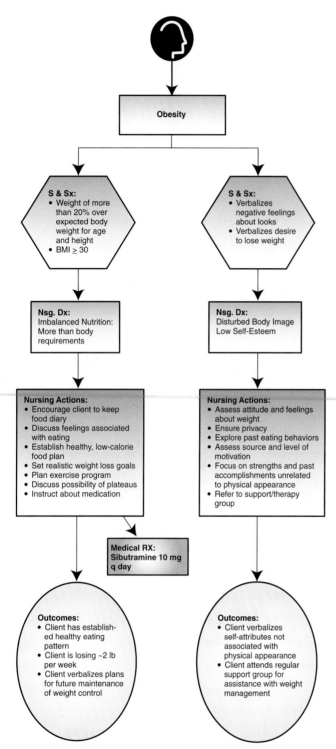

FIGURE 33–3 Concept map care plan for client with obesity.

Concept Care Mapping

The concept map care plan is an innovative approach to planning and organizing nursing care (see Chapter 9). It is a diagrammatic teaching and learning strategy that allows visualization of interrelationships between medical diagnoses, nursing diagnoses, assessment data, and treatments. Examples of concept map care plans for clients with eating disorders are presented in Figures 33–2 and 33–3.

Box 33–4 Topics for Client/Family Education Related to Eating Disorders

Nature of the Illness

1. Symptoms of anorexia nervosa
2. Symptoms of bulimia nervosa
3. What constitutes obesity
4. Causes of eating disorders
5. Effects of the illness or condition on the body

Management of the Illness

1. Principles of nutrition (foods for maintenance of wellness)
2. Ways client may feel in control of life (aside from eating)
3. Importance of expressing fears and feelings, rather than holding them inside.
4. Alternative coping strategies (to maladaptive eating behaviors)
5. For the obese client:
   a. How to plan a reduced-calorie, nutritious diet
   b. How to read food content labels
   c. How to establish a realistic weight loss plan
   d. How to establish a planned program of physical activity
6. Correct administration of prescribed medications (e.g., antidepressants, anorexiants)
7. Indication for and side effects of prescribed medications
8. Relaxation techniques
9. Problem-solving skills

Support Services

1. Weight Watchers International
2. Overeaters Anonymous
3. National Association of Anorexia Nervosa and Associated Disorders (ANAD)
   P.O. Box 7
   Highland Park, IL 60035
   (847) 831-3438
4. The American Anorexia/Bulimia Association, Inc.
   165 W. 46th St., Suite 1108
   New York, NY 10036
   (212) 575-6200

Client/Family Education

The role of client teacher is important in the psychiatric area, as it is in all areas of nursing. A list of topics for client/family education relevant to eating disorders is presented in Box 33–4.

Evaluation

Evaluation of the client with an eating disorder requires a reassessment of the behaviors for which the client sought treatment. Behavioral change will be required on both the part of the client and family members. The following types of questions may provide assistance in gathering data required for evaluating whether the nursing interventions have been effective in achieving the goals of therapy.

For the client with anorexia nervosa or bulimia nervosa:

● Has the client steadily gained 2 to 3 lb per week to at least 80 percent of body weight for age and size?

● Is the client free of signs and symptoms of malnutrition and dehydration?

● Does the client consume adequate calories as determined by the dietitian?

● Have there been any attempts to stash food from the tray to discard later?

● Have there been any attempts to self-induce vomiting?

● Has the client admitted that a problem exists and that eating behaviors are maladaptive?

● Have behaviors aimed at manipulating the environment been discontinued?

● Is the client willing to discuss the real issues concerning family roles, sexuality, dependence/independence, and the need for achievement?

● Does the client understand how he or she has used maladaptive eating behaviors in an effort to achieve a feeling of some control over life events?

● Has the client acknowledged that perception of body image as "fat" is incorrect?

For the client with obesity:

● Has the client shown a steady weight loss since starting the new eating plan?

● Does he or she verbalize a plan to help stay on the new eating plan?

● Does the client verbalize positive self-attributes not associated with body size or appearance?

For the client with anorexia nervosa, bulimia nervosa, or obesity:

● Has the client been able to develop a more realistic perception of body image?

● Has the client acknowledged that past self-expectations may have been unrealistic?

● Does the client accept self as less than perfect?

● Has the client developed adaptive coping strategies to deal with stress without resorting to maladaptive eating behaviors?

TREATMENT MODALITIES

The immediate aim of treatment in eating disorders is to restore the client's nutritional status. Complications of emaciation, dehydration, and electrolyte imbalance can lead to death. Once the physical condition is no longer life-threatening, other treatment modalities may be initiated.

Behavior Modification

Efforts to change the maladaptive eating behaviors of clients with anorexia nervosa and bulimia nervosa have become the widely accepted treatment. The importance of instituting a behavior modification program with these clients is to ensure that the program does not "control" them. Issues of control are central to the etiology of these disorders, and in order for the program to be successful,

the client must perceive that he or she is in control of the treatment.

Successes have been observed when the client with anorexia nervosa is allowed to contract for privileges based on weight gain. The client has input into the care plan and can clearly see what the treatment choices are. The client has control over eating, over the amount of exercise pursued, and, in some instances, even over whether or not to induce vomiting. Goals of therapy, along with the responsibilities of each for goal achievement, are agreed on by client and staff.

Staff and client also agree on a system of rewards and privileges that can be earned by the client, who is given ultimate control. He or she has a choice of whether or not to abide by the contract—a choice of whether or not to gain weight—a choice of whether or not to earn the desired privilege.

This method of treatment gives a great deal of autonomy to the client. It must be understood, however, that

---

IMPLICATIONS OF RESEARCH FOR EVIDENCE-BASED PRACTICE

Long, J.D., & Stevens, K.R. (2004). Using technology to promote self-efficacy for healthy eating in adolescents. *Journal of Nursing Scholarship, 36*(2), 134–139.

Description of the Study: Obesity and overweight have reached epidemic proportions and they are risk factors for the development of chronic disease. The purpose of this study was to test the effects of a classroom and World Wide Web (WWW) educational intervention on self-efficacy for healthy eating. The sample consisted of 63 adolescents in the participant group and 58 in the control group. The age range was between 12 and 16 years. The participant group received the intervention that consisted of 10 hours of classroom and 5 hours of Web-based nutrition education endorsed by the American Cancer Society and the National Cancer Institute. Information is included to encourage healthy eating behaviors that reduce the risk of cancer, obesity, heart disease and diabetes. Participants in the control group received the nutrition education integrated in the health, science, and home economics curriculum. All participants completed six questionnaires to measure dietary knowledge and eating behaviors. Pre- and post-tests were administered to both groups.

Results of the Study: Although no difference was found between groups in food consumption during the month of intervention, the participant group had significantly higher scores related to knowledge of good nutrition and healthy eating behaviors. The study was limited to individual adolescents and did not attempt to initiate change in the home or school environment

Implications for Nursing Practice: Nurses, and especially school nurses, can become actively involved in nutrition education for children and adolescents. The authors report that 9 million young people are overweight—a number that more than doubled in the last 20 years. This has serious implications for nursing to assist in the educational process needed to reverse this unhealthy trend.

IMPLICATIONS OF RESEARCH FOR EVIDENCE-BASED PRACTICE

McIntosh, V.V.W., Jordan, J., Carter, F.A., Luty, S.E., McKenzie, J.M., Bulik, C.M., Frampton, C.M.A., & Joyce, P.R. (2005). Three psychotherapies for anorexia nervosa: A randomized, controlled trial. *American Journal of Psychiatry, 162,* 741–747.

Description of the Study: The objective of this study was to examine the efficacy of three types of therapies in treatment of anorexia nervosa. Fifty-six women (age range: 17 to 40 years) with anorexia nervosa were randomly assigned to one of three treatments. Two were specialized psychotherapies: cognitive behavior therapy (CBT) and interpersonal psychotherapy (IPT). The third (the intervention) included treatment combining clinical management and supportive psychotherapy (called nonspecific supportive clinical management). They participated in 20 therapy sessions over a minimum of 20 weeks. The intervention consisted of education, care, and support, fostering a therapeutic relationship that promotes adherence to treatment. Emphasis was placed on resumption of normal eating and restoration of weight. Information on weight maintenance strategies, energy requirements, and relearning to eat normally were included. Outcomes were measured on a global anorexia nervosa measure using a 4-point ordinal scale:

4 = meets full criteria for the anorexia nervosa spectrum
3 = not full anorexia nervosa, but having a number of features of eating disorders
2 = few features of eating disorders
1 = no significant features of eating disorders

Results of the Study: Fifty-six percent of the participants who received nonspecific supportive clinical management received a score of 1 or 2 on the final outcome measure, compared with 32 percent and 10 percent of those receiving CBT and IPT, respectively. They suggest that IPT may not have been as successful because of the lack of symptom focus and relatively long time taken to decide on the problem area. They hypothesize that the CBT may have been less effective because of the large amount of psychoeducational material and extensive skills acquisition associated with this therapy, and the difficulty of anorexia clients to generate alternatives due to cognitive rigidity. These results were in direct opposition to the original hypothesis generated by the researchers in the beginning of the study.

Implications for Nursing Practice: Nurses in advanced practice are usually trained to provide CBT and IPT. Often, generalist nurses do not have the theoretical background to perform these therapies. The interventions associated with nonspecific supportive clinical management are within the scope of nursing practice, and the results of this study indicate that they are superior to CBT and IPT in the treatment of anorexia nervosa. Nurses could become instrumental in establishing programs based on this type of treatment for individuals with this type of eating disorder.

these behavior modification techniques are helpful for weight restoration only. Concomitant individual and/or family psychotherapy are required to prevent or reduce further morbidity.

Some clinicians incorporate cognitive therapy concepts along with behavior modification techniques. Cognitive therapy helps the client to confront irrational thinking and strive to modify distorted and maladaptive cognitions about body image and eating behaviors. Halmi (2008) states, "Cognitive techniques such as cognitive restructuring and problem solving help the patient deal with distorted and overvalued beliefs about food and thinness and cope with life's stresses" (p. 981).

Individual Therapy

Although individual psychotherapy is not the therapy of choice for eating disorders, it can be helpful when underlying psychological problems are contributing to the maladaptive behaviors. In supportive psychotherapy, the therapist encourages the client to explore unresolved conflicts and to recognize the maladaptive eating behaviors as defense mechanisms used to ease the emotional pain. The goals are to resolve the personal issues and establish more adaptive coping strategies for dealing with stressful situations.

Family Therapy

Kirkpatrick and Caldwell (2001) state:

Eating disorders have a profound effect on families. While these disorders can help bring families together, they always cause some level of distress. Stresses can cause a breakdown of the whole family unit if there isn't some form of intervention. Family therapy aims at finding solutions to help the healing process for everyone in the family. (p. 159)

In many instances, eating disorders may be considered *family* disorders, and resolution cannot be achieved until dynamics within the family have improved. Family therapy deals with education of the members about the disorder's manifestations, possible etiology, and prescribed treatment. Support is given to family members as they deal with feelings of guilt associated with the perception that they may have contributed to the onset of the disorder. Support is also given as they deal with the social stigma of having a family member with emotional problems.

In some instances when the dysfunctional family dynamics are related to conflict avoidance, the family may be noncompliant with therapy, as they attempt to maintain equilibrium by keeping a member in the sick role. When this occurs, it is essential to focus on the functional operations within the family and to help them manage conflict and create change.

Referrals are made to local support groups for families of individuals with eating disorders. Resolution and growth can sometimes be achieved through interaction with others who are experiencing, or have experienced, the numerous problems of living with a family member with an eating disorder.

Psychopharmacology

There are no medications specifically indicated for eating disorders. Various medications have been prescribed for

dysfunctions resulting in diminished activation, minimal pleasure–pain sensibilities, and impaired cognitive functions. These biological etiological factors support the close link between schizotypal personality disorder and schizophrenia and were considered when classifying schizotypal personality disorder with schizophrenia rather than with the personality disorders in the *International Classification of Diseases (ICD-10)* (Skodol & Gunderson, 2008).

The early family dynamics of the individual with schizotypal personality disorder may have been characterized by indifference, impassivity, or formality, leading to a pattern of discomfort with personal affection and closeness. Early on, affective deficits made them unattractive and unrewarding social companions. They were likely shunned, overlooked, rejected, and humiliated by others, resulting in feelings of low self-esteem and a marked distrust of interpersonal relations. Having failed repeatedly to cope with these adversities, they began to withdraw and reduce contact with individuals and situations that evoked sadness and humiliation. Their new inner world provided them with a more significant and potentially rewarding existence than the one experienced in reality.

Antisocial Personality Disorder

Definition and Epidemiological Statistics

Antisocial personality disorder is a pattern of socially irresponsible, exploitative, and guiltless behavior that reflects a disregard for the rights of others (Skodol & Gunderson, 2008). These individuals exploit and manipulate others for personal gain and have a general disregard for the law. They have difficulty sustaining consistent employment and in developing stable relationships. It is one of the oldest and best researched of the personality disorders and has been included in all editions of the *Diagnostic and Statistical Manual of Mental Disorders*. In the United States, prevalence estimates range from 3 percent in men to about 1 percent in women (APA, 2000). The disorder is more common among the lower socioeconomic classes, particularly so among highly mobile residents of impoverished urban areas (Sadock & Sadock, 2007). The *ICD-10* identifies this disorder as *dissocial personality disorder.*

NOTE: The clinical picture, predisposing factors, nursing diagnoses, and interventions for care of clients with antisocial personality disorder are presented later in this chapter.

Borderline Personality Disorder

Definition and Epidemiological Statistics

Borderline personality disorder is characterized by a pattern of intense and chaotic relationships, with affective instability and fluctuating attitudes toward other people. These individuals are impulsive, are directly and indirectly self-destructive, and lack a clear sense of identity. Prevalence estimates of borderline personality range from 2 to 3 percent of the population. It is the most common form of personality disorder (Skodol & Gunderson, 2008). It is more common in women than in men, with female-to-male ratios being estimated as high as 4 to 1 (Finley-Belgrad & Davies, 2006). The *ICD-10* identifies this disorder as *emotionally unstable personality disorder.*

NOTE: The clinical picture, predisposing factors, nursing diagnoses, and interventions for care of clients with borderline personality disorder are presented later in this chapter.

Histrionic Personality Disorder

Definition and Epidemiological Statistics

Histrionic personality disorder is characterized by colorful, dramatic, and extroverted behavior in excitable, emotional people. They have difficulty maintaining longlasting relationships, although they require constant affirmation of approval and acceptance from others. Prevalence of the disorder is thought to be about 2 to 3 percent, and it is more common in women than in men.

Clinical Picture

People with histrionic personality disorder tend to be self-dramatizing, attention seeking, overly gregarious, and seductive. They use manipulative and exhibitionistic behaviors in their demands to be the center of attention. People with histrionic personality disorder often demonstrate, in mild pathological form, what our society tends to foster and admire in its members: to be well liked, successful, popular, extroverted, attractive, and sociable. However, beneath these surface characteristics is a driven quality—an all-consuming need for approval and a desperate striving to be conspicuous and to evoke affection or attract attention at all costs. Failure to evoke the attention and approval they seek often results in feelings of dejection and anxiety.

Individuals with this disorder are highly distractible and flighty by nature. They have difficulty paying attention to detail. They can portray themselves as carefree and sophisticated on the one hand and as inhibited and naive on the other. They tend to be highly suggestible, impressionable, and easily influenced by others. They are strongly dependent.

Interpersonal relationships are fleeting and superficial. The person with histrionic personality disorder, having failed throughout life to develop the richness of inner feelings and lacking resources from which to draw, lacks the ability to provide another with genuinely sustained

Box 34–4 Diagnostic Criteria for Histrionic Personality Disorder

A pervasive pattern of excessive emotionality and attention seeking, beginning by early adulthood and present in a variety of contexts, as indicated by five (or more) of the following:

1. Is uncomfortable in situations in which he or she is not the center of attention.
2. Interaction with others is often characterized by inappropriate sexually seductive or provocative behavior.
3. Displays rapidly shifting and shallow expression of emotions.
4. Consistently uses physical appearance to draw attention to self.
5. Has a style of speech that is excessively impressionistic and lacking in detail.
6. Shows self-dramatization, theatricality, and exaggerated expression of emotion.
7. Is suggestible, i.e., easily influenced by others or circumstances.
8. Considers relationships to be more intimate than they actually are.

SOURCE: American Psychiatric Association (2000), with permission.

affection. Somatic complaints are not uncommon in these individuals, and fleeting episodes of psychosis may occur during periods of extreme stress.

The *DSM-IV-TR* diagnostic criteria for histrionic personality disorder are presented in Box 34–4.

Predisposing Factors

Neurobiological correlates have been proposed in the predisposition to histrionic personality disorder. Coccaro and Siever (2000) relate the characteristics of enhanced sensitivity and reactivity to environmental stimuli to heightened noradrenergic activity in the individual with histrionic personality disorder. They suggested that the trait of impulsivity may be associated with decreased serotonergic activity.

Heredity also may be a factor because the disorder is apparently more common among first-degree biological relatives of people with the disorder than in the general population. Skodol and Gunderson (2008) report on research that suggests that the behavioral characteristics of histrionic personality disorder may be associated with a biogenetically determined temperament. From this perspective, histrionic personality disorder would arise out of "an extreme variation of temperamental disposition."

From a psychosocial perspective, learning experiences may contribute to the development of histrionic personality disorder. The child may have learned that positive reinforcement was contingent on the ability to perform parentally approved and admired behaviors. It is likely that the child rarely received either positive or negative feedback. Parental acceptance and approval came inconsistently and only when the behaviors met parental expectations. Hannig (2007) states:

> The root causes [of histrionic personality disorder] surround an unbonded mother relationship and an abusive paternal relationship. When a child is not the center of a parent's attention, neglect, lack of bonding, and deprivation leaves one starving for attention, approval, praise, and reassurance.

Narcissistic Personality Disorder

Definition and Epidemiological Statistics

Persons with narcissistic personality disorder have an exaggerated sense of self-worth. They lack empathy, and are hypersensitive to the evaluation of others. They believe that they have the inalienable right to receive special consideration and that their desire is sufficient justification for possessing whatever they seek.

This diagnosis appeared for the first time in the third edition of the *Diagnostic and Statistical Manual of Mental Disorders*. However, the concept of **narcissism** has its roots in the 19th century. It was viewed by early psychoanalysts as a normal phase of psychosexual development. The *DSM-IV-TR* (APA, 2000) estimates that the disorder occurs in 2 to 16 percent of the clinical population and in less than 1 percent of the general population. It is diagnosed more often in men than in women.

Clinical Picture

Individuals with narcissistic personality disorder appear to lack humility, being overly self-centered and exploiting others to fulfill their own desires. They often do not conceive of their behavior as being inappropriate or objectionable. Because they view themselves as "superior" beings, they believe they are entitled to special rights and privileges.

Although often grounded in grandiose distortions of reality, their mood is usually optimistic, relaxed, cheerful, and carefree. This mood can easily change, however, because of their fragile self-esteem. If they do not meet self-expectations, do not receive the positive feedback they expect from others, or draw criticism from others, they may respond with rage, shame, humiliation, or dejection. They may turn inward and fantasize rationalizations that convince them of their continued stature and perfection.

The exploitation of others for self-gratification results in impaired interpersonal relationships. In selecting a mate, narcissistic individuals frequently choose a person who will provide them with the praise and positive feedback that they require and who will not ask much from their partner in return.

The *DSM-IV-TR* diagnostic criteria for narcissistic personality disorder are presented in Box 34–5.

Box 34 – 5 Diagnostic Criteria for Narcissistic Personality Disorder

A pervasive pattern of grandiosity (in fantasy or behavior), need for admiration, and lack of empathy, beginning by early adulthood and present in a variety of contexts, as indicated by five (or more) of the following:

1. Has a grandiose sense of self-importance (e.g., exaggerates achievements and talents, expects to be recognized as superior without commensurate achievements).
2. Is preoccupied with fantasies of unlimited success, power, brilliance, beauty, or ideal love.
3. Believes that he or she is "special" and unique and can only be understood by, or should associate with, other special or high-status people (or institutions).
4. Requires excessive admiration.
5. Has a sense of entitlement (i.e., unreasonable expectations of especially favorable treatment or automatic compliance with his or her expectations).
6. Is interpersonally exploitative (i.e., takes advantage of others to achieve his or her own ends).
7. Lacks empathy: Is unwilling to recognize or identify with the feelings and needs of others.
8. Is often envious of others or believes that others are envious of him or her.
9. Shows arrogant, haughty behaviors or attitudes.

SOURCE: American Psychiatric Association (2000), with permission.

Predisposing Factors

Several psychodynamic theories exist regarding the predisposition to narcissistic personality disorder. Skodol and Gunderson (2008) suggest that, as children, these individuals had their fears, failures, or dependency needs responded to with criticism, disdain, or neglect. They grow up with contempt for these behaviors in themselves and others and are unable to view others as sources of comfort and support. They project an image of invulnerability and self-sufficiency that conceals their true sense of emptiness and contributes to their inability to feel deeply.

Mark (2002) suggests that the parents of individuals with narcissistic personality disorder were often narcissistic themselves. The parents were demanding, perfectionistic, and critical, and they placed unrealistic expectations on the child. Children model their parents' behavior, giving way to the adult narcissist. Mark (2002) also suggests that the parents may have subjected the child to physical or emotional abuse or neglect.

Narcissism may also develop from an environment in which parents attempt to live their lives vicariously through their child. They expect the child to achieve the things they did not achieve, possess that which they did not possess, and have life better and easier than they did. The child is not subjected to the requirements and restrictions that may have dominated the parents' lives, and thereby grows up believing he or she is above that which is required for everyone else. Mark (2002) states:

[Some] researchers believe that parents who over-indulge their children or who provide indiscriminate praise and those who do not set limits as to what is appropriate in their children's behavior can also produce adults who will suffer from narcissistic personality disorder. The message here appears to be inconsistency—inconsistency in parenting—the child does not know where to turn or how to behave appropriately; they do not know what is reality and what is fantasy. This of course is a major aspect of the symptoms of narcissistic personality disorder—sufferers tend to shun reality.

Avoidant Personality Disorder

Definition and Epidemiological Statistics

The individual with avoidant personality disorder is extremely sensitive to rejection and because of this may lead a very socially withdrawn life. It is not that he or she is asocial; in fact, there may be a strong desire for companionship. The extreme shyness and fear of rejection, however, create needs for unusually strong guarantees of uncritical acceptance (Sadock & Sadock, 2007). Prevalence of the disorder in the general population is between 0.5 and 1 percent, and it appears to be equally common in men and women (APA, 2000).

Clinical Picture

Individuals with this disorder are awkward and uncomfortable in social situations. From a distance, others may perceive them as timid, withdrawn, or perhaps cold and strange. Those who have closer relationships with them, however, soon learn of their sensitivities, touchiness, evasiveness, and mistrustful qualities.

Their speech is usually slow and constrained, with frequent hesitations, fragmentary thought sequences, and occasional confused and irrelevant digressions. They are often lonely, and express feelings of being unwanted. They view others as critical, betraying, and humiliating. They desire to have close relationships but avoid them because of their fear of being rejected. Depression, anxiety, and anger at oneself for failing to develop social relations are commonly experienced.

The *DSM-IV-TR* diagnostic criteria for avoidant personality disorder are presented in Box 34–6.

Predisposing Factors

It is possible that there is a hereditary influence with avoidant personality disorder because it seems to occur more frequently in certain families (Rettew & Jellinek, 2006). Some infants who exhibit traits of hyperirritability, crankiness, tension, and withdrawal behaviors may possess a temperamental disposition toward an avoidant pattern.

The primary psychosocial predisposing influence to avoidant personality disorder is parental rejection and

Box 34–6 Diagnostic Criteria for Avoidant Personality Disorder

A pervasive pattern of social inhibition, feelings of inadequacy, and hypersensitivity to negative evaluation, beginning by early adulthood and present in a variety of contexts, as indicated by four (or more) of the following:
1. Avoids occupational activities that involve significant interpersonal contact, because of fears of criticism, disapproval, or rejection.
2. Is unwilling to get involved with people unless certain of being liked.
3. Shows restraint within intimate relationships because of the fear of being shamed or ridiculed.
4. Is preoccupied with being criticized or rejected in social situations.
5. Is inhibited in new interpersonal situations because of feelings of inadequacy.
6. Views self as socially inept, personally unappealing, or inferior to others.
7. Is unusually reluctant to take personal risks or to engage in any new activities because they may prove embarrassing.

SOURCE: American Psychiatric Association (2000), with permission.

censure, which is often reinforced by peers (Skodol & Gunderson, 2008). These children are often reared in families in which they are belittled, abandoned, and criticized, such that any natural optimism is extinguished and replaced with feelings of low self-worth and social alienation. They learn to be suspicious and to view the world as hostile and dangerous.

Dependent Personality Disorder

Definition and Epidemiological Statistics

Dependent personality disorder is characterized by "a pervasive and excessive need to be taken care of that leads to submissive and clinging behavior and fears of separation" (APA, 2000). These characteristics are evident in the tendency to allow others to make decisions, to feel helpless when alone, to act submissively, to subordinate needs to others, to tolerate mistreatment by others, to demean oneself to gain acceptance, and to fail to function adequately in situations that require assertive or dominant behavior.

The disorder is relatively common. Sadock and Sadock (2007) discuss the results of one study of personality disorders in which 2.5 percent of the sample were diagnosed with dependent personality disorder. It is more common in women than in men and more common in the youngest children of a family.

Clinical Picture

Individuals with dependent personality disorder have a notable lack of self-confidence that is often apparent in their posture, voice, and mannerisms. They are typically passive and acquiescent to the desires of others. They are overly generous and thoughtful and underplay their own attractiveness and achievements. They may appear to others to "see the world through rose-colored glasses," but when alone, they may feel pessimistic, discouraged, and dejected. Others are not made aware of these feelings; their "suffering" is done in silence.

Individuals with dependent personality disorder assume the passive and submissive role in relationships. They are willing to let others make their important decisions. Should the dependent relationship end, they feel helpless and fearful because they feel incapable of caring for themselves (Skodol & Gunderson, 2008). They may hastily and indiscriminately attempt to establish another relationship with someone they believe can provide them with the nurturance and guidance they need.

They avoid positions of responsibility and become anxious when forced into them. They have feelings of low self-worth and are easily hurt by criticism and disapproval. They will do almost anything, even if it is unpleasant or demeaning, to earn the acceptance of others.

The *DSM-IV-TR* diagnostic criteria for dependent personality disorder are presented in Box 34–7.

Predisposing Factors

An infant may be genetically predisposed to a dependent temperament. Twin studies measuring submissiveness

Box 34–7 Diagnostic Criteria for Dependent Personality Disorder

A pervasive and excessive need to be taken care of that leads to submissive and clinging behavior and fears of separation, beginning by early adulthood and present in a variety of contexts, as indicated by five (or more) of the following:
1. Has difficulty making everyday decisions without an excessive amount of advice and reassurance from others.
2. Needs others to assume responsibility for most major areas of his or her life.
3. Has difficulty expressing disagreement with others because of fear of loss of support or approval. **NOTE:** Do not include realistic fears of retribution.
4. Has difficulty initiating projects or doing things on his or her own (because of a lack of self-confidence in judgment or abilities rather than a lack of motivation or energy).
5. Goes to excessive lengths to obtain nurturance and support from others, to the point of volunteering to do things that are unpleasant.
6. Feels uncomfortable or helpless when alone because of exaggerated fears of being unable to care for him- or herself.
7. Urgently seeks another relationship as a source of care and support when a close relationship ends.
8. Is unrealistically preoccupied with fears of being left to take care of him- or herself.

SOURCE: American Psychiatric Association (2000), with permission.

have shown a higher correlation between identical twins than fraternal twins.

Psychosocially, dependency is fostered in infancy when stimulation and nurturance are experienced exclusively from one source. The infant becomes attached to one source to the exclusion of all others. If this exclusive attachment continues as the child grows, the dependency is nurtured. A problem may arise when parents become overprotective and discourage independent behaviors on the part of the child. Parents who make new experiences unnecessarily easy for the child and refuse to allow him or her to learn by experience encourage their child to give up efforts at achieving autonomy. Dependent behaviors may be subtly rewarded in this environment, and the child may come to fear a loss of love or attachment from the parental figure if independent behaviors are attempted.

Obsessive–Compulsive Personality Disorder

Definition and Epidemiological Statistics

Individuals with obsessive–compulsive personality disorder are very serious and formal and have difficulty expressing emotions. They are overly disciplined, perfectionistic, and preoccupied with rules. They are inflexible about the way in which things must be done and have a devotion to productivity to the exclusion of personal pleasure. An intense fear of making mistakes leads to difficulty with decision-making. The disorder is relatively common and occurs more often in men than in women. Within the family constellation, it appears to be most common in oldest children.

Clinical Picture

Individuals with obsessive–compulsive personality disorder are inflexible and lack spontaneity. They are meticulous and work diligently and patiently at tasks that require accuracy and discipline. They are especially concerned with matters of organization and efficiency and tend to be rigid and unbending about rules and procedures.

Social behavior tends to be polite and formal. They are very "rank conscious," a characteristic that is reflected in their contrasting behaviors with "superiors" as opposed to "inferiors." They tend to be very solicitous to and ingratiating with authority figures. With subordinates, however, the compulsive person can become quite autocratic and condemnatory, often appearing pompous and self-righteous.

People with obsessive–compulsive personality disorder typify the "bureaucratic personality," the so-called company man. They see themselves as conscientious, loyal, dependable, and responsible, and are contemptuous of people whose behavior they consider frivolous and impulsive. Emotional behavior is considered immature and irresponsible.

Although on the surface these individuals appear to be calm and controlled, underneath this exterior lies a great deal of ambivalence, conflict, and hostility. Individuals with this disorder commonly use the defense mechanism of reaction formation. Not daring to expose their true feelings of defiance and anger, they withhold these feelings so strongly that the opposite feelings come forth. The defenses of isolation, intellectualization, rationalization, and undoing also are commonly evident (Skodol & Gunderson, 2008).

The *DSM-IV-TR* diagnostic criteria for obsessive–compulsive personality disorder are presented in Box 34–8.

Predisposing Factors

In the psychoanalytical view, the parenting style in which the individual with obsessive–compulsive personality disorder was reared is one of over-control. These parents expect their children to live up to their imposed standards of conduct and condemn them if they do not. Praise for positive behaviors is bestowed on the child with much less frequency than punishment for undesirable behaviors. In this environment, individuals become experts in learning what they must *not* do to avoid punishment and condemnation rather than what they *can* do

---

BOX 34-8 Diagnostic Criteria for Obsessive–Compulsive Personality Disorder

A pervasive pattern of preoccupation with orderliness, perfectionism, and mental and interpersonal control, at the expense of flexibility, openness, and efficiency, beginning by early adulthood and present in a variety of contexts, as indicated by four (or more) of the following:

1. Is preoccupied with details, rules, lists, order, organization, or schedules to the extent that the major point of the activity is lost.
2. Shows perfectionism that interferes with task completion (e.g., is unable to complete a project because his or her own overly strict standards are not met).
3. Is excessively devoted to work and productivity to the exclusion of leisure activities and friendships (not accounted for by obvious economic necessity).
4. Is overconscientious, scrupulous, and inflexible about matters of morality, ethics, or values (not accounted for by cultural or religious identification).
5. Is unable to discard worn-out or worthless objects even when they have no sentimental value.
6. Is reluctant to delegate tasks or to work with others unless they submit to exactly his or her way of doing things.
7. Adopts a miserly spending style toward both self and others; money is viewed as something to be hoarded for future catastrophes.
8. Shows rigidity and stubbornness.

SOURCE: American Psychiatric Association (2000), with permission.

to achieve attention and praise. They learn to heed rigid restrictions and rules. Positive achievements are expected, taken for granted, and only occasionally acknowledged by their parents, whose comments and judgments are limited to pointing out transgressions and infractions of rules.

Passive–Aggressive Personality Disorder

Definition and Epidemiological Statistics

The *DSM-IV-TR* defines this disorder as a pervasive pattern of negativistic attitudes and passive resistance to demands for adequate performance in social and occupational situations that begins by early adulthood and occurs in a variety of contexts. The name of the disorder is based on the assumption that such people are passively expressing covert aggression. Passive–aggressive disorder has been included in all editions of the *Diagnostic and Statistical Manual of Mental Disorders*, and although no statistics exist that speak to its prevalence, the syndrome appears to be relatively common.

Clinical Picture

Passive–aggressive individuals feel cheated and unappreciated. They believe that life has been unkind to them, and they express envy and resentment over the "easy life" that they perceive others having. When they feel another person has wronged them, they may go to great lengths to seek retribution, or "get even," but always in a subtle and passive manner rather than discussing their feelings with the offending individual. They demonstrate passive resistance and general obstructiveness in response to the expectations of others. As a tactic of interpersonal behavior, passive–aggressive individuals commonly switch among the roles of the martyr, the affronted, the aggrieved, the misunderstood, the contrite, the guilt-ridden, the sickly, and the overworked. In this way, they are able to vent their anger and resentment subtly, while gaining the attention, reassurance, and dependency they crave.

The *DSM-IV-TR* research criteria for passive–aggressive personality disorder are presented in Box 34–9.

Predisposing Factors

Contradictory parental attitudes and behavior are implicated in the predisposition to passive–aggressive personality disorder. In the nuclear family dynamics, at any moment and without provocation, these children may receive the kindness and support they crave or hostility and rejection. Parental responses are inconsistent and unpredictable, and these children internalize the conflicting attitudes toward themselves and others. For

---

> **Box 34–9 Research Criteria for Passive–Aggressive Personality Disorder**
>
> A. A pervasive pattern of negativistic attitudes and passive resistance to demands for adequate performance, beginning by early adulthood and present in a variety of contexts, as indicated by four (or more) of the following:
>   1. Passively resists fulfilling routine social and occupational tasks.
>   2. Complains of being misunderstood and unappreciated by others.
>   3. Is sullen and argumentative.
>   4. Unreasonably criticizes and scorns authority.
>   5. Expresses envy and resentment toward those apparently more fortunate.
>   6. Voices exaggerated and persistent complaints of personal misfortune.
>   7. Alternates between hostile defiance and contrition.
>
> B. Does not occur exclusively during major depressive episodes and is not better accounted for by dysthymic disorder.

SOURCE: American Psychiatric Association (2000), with permission

---

example, they do not know whether to think of themselves as competent or incompetent and are unsure as to whether they love or hate those on whom they depend. Double-bind communication may also be exhibited in these families. Expressions of concern and affection may be verbalized, only to be negated and undone through subtle and devious behavioral manifestations. This *approach–avoidance* pattern is modeled by the children, who then become equally equivocal and ambivalent in their own thinking and actions.

Through this type of environment, children learn to control their anger for fear of provoking parental withdrawal and not receiving love and support—even on an inconsistent basis. Overtly the child appears polite and undemanding; hostility and inefficiency are manifested only covertly and indirectly.

APPLICATION OF THE NURSING PROCESS

Borderline Personality Disorder (Background Assessment Data)

Historically, there have been a group of clients who did not classically conform to the standard categories of neuroses or psychoses. The designation "borderline" was introduced to identify these clients who seemed to fall on the border between the two categories. Other terminology that has been used in an attempt to identify this disorder includes *ambulatory schizophrenia, pseudoneurotic schizophrenia,* and *emotionally unstable personality.* When the term *borderline* was first proposed for inclusion in the third edition of the *DSM,* some psychiatrists feared it

---

Box 34–10 Diagnostic Criteria for Borderline Personality Disorder

A pervasive pattern of instability of interpersonal relationships, self-image, and affects, and marked impulsivity beginning by early adulthood and present in a variety of contexts, as indicated by five (or more) of the following:
1. Frantic efforts to avoid real or imagined abandonment. **NOTE:** Does not include suicidal or self-mutilating behavior covered in criterion 5.
2. A pattern of unstable and intense interpersonal relationships characterized by alternating between extremes of idealization and devaluation.
3. Identity disturbance: markedly and persistently unstable self-image or sense of self.
4. Impulsivity in at least two areas that are potentially self-damaging (e.g., spending, sex, substance abuse, reckless driving, binge eating). **NOTE:** Do not include suicidal or self-mutilating behavior covered in criterion 5.
5. Recurrent suicidal behavior, gestures, or threats, or self-mutilating behavior.
6. Affective instability due to marked reactivity of mood (e.g., intense episodic dysphoria, irritability, or anxiety, usually lasting a few hours and only rarely more than a few days).
7. Chronic feelings of emptiness.
8. Inappropriate, intense anger or difficulty controlling anger (e.g., frequent displays of temper, constant anger, recurrent physical fights).
9. Transient, stress-related paranoid ideation or severe dissociative symptoms.

SOURCE: American Psychiatric Association (2000), with permission.

---

might be used as a "wastebasket" diagnosis for difficult-to-treat clients. However, a specific set of criteria has been established for diagnosing what has been described as "a consistent and stable course of unstable behavior" (Box 34–10).

Clinical Picture

Individuals with borderline personality always seem to be in a state of crisis. Their affect is one of extreme intensity, and their behavior reflects frequent changeability. These changes can occur within days, hours, or even minutes. Often these individuals exhibit a single, dominant affective tone, such as depression, which may give way periodically to anxious agitation or inappropriate outbursts of anger.

Chronic Depression. Depression is so common in clients with this disorder that before the inclusion of borderline personality disorder in the *DSM*, many of these clients were diagnosed as depressed. Depression occurs in response to feelings of abandonment by the mother in early childhood (see "Predisposing Factors"). Underlying the depression is a sense of rage that is sporadically turned inward on the self and externally on the environment. Seldom is the individual aware of the true source of these feelings until well into long-term therapy.

Inability to Be Alone. Because of this chronic fear of abandonment, clients with borderline personality disorder have little tolerance for being alone. They prefer a frantic search for companionship, no matter how unsatisfactory, to sitting with feelings of loneliness, emptiness, and boredom (Sadock & Sadock, 2007).

Patterns of Interaction

Clinging and Distancing. The client with borderline personality disorder commonly exhibits a pattern of interaction with others that is characterized by clinging and distancing behaviors. When clients are clinging to another individual, they may exhibit helpless, dependent, or even childlike behaviors. They overidealize a single individual with whom they want to spend all their time, with whom they express a frequent need to talk, or from whom they seek constant reassurance. Acting-out behaviors, even self-mutilation, may result when they cannot be with this chosen individual. Distancing behaviors are characterized by hostility, anger, and devaluation of others, arising from a feeling of discomfort with closeness. Distancing behaviors also occur in response to separations, confrontations, or attempts to limit certain behaviors. Devaluation of others is manifested by discrediting or undermining their strengths and personal significance.

Splitting. **Splitting** is a primitive ego defense mechanism that is common in people with borderline personality disorder. It arises from their lack of achievement of **object constancy** and is manifested by an inability to integrate and accept both positive and negative feelings. In their view, people—including themselves—and life situations are either all good or all bad. For example, if a caregiver is nurturing and supportive, he or she is lovingly idealized. Should the nurturing relationship be threatened in any way (e.g., the caregiver must move because of his or her job), suddenly the individual is devalued, and the idealized image changes from beneficent caregiver to one of hateful and cruel persecutor.

Manipulation. In their efforts to prevent the separation they so desperately fear, clients with this disorder become masters of manipulation. Virtually any behavior becomes an acceptable means of achieving the desired result: relief from separation anxiety. Playing one individual against another is a common ploy to allay these fears of abandonment.

Self-Destructive Behaviors. Repetitive, self-mutilative behaviors are classic manifestations of borderline personality disorder. Although these acts can be fatal, most commonly they are manipulative gestures designed to elicit a rescue response from significant others. Suicide attempts are quite common and result from feelings of abandonment following separation from a significant other. The endeavor is often attempted, however, incorporating a measure of "safety" into the plan (e.g., swallowing pills in an area where the person will surely be discovered by others; or swallowing pills and making a phone call to report the deed to someone).

Other types of destructive behaviors include cutting, scratching, and burning. Various theories abound regarding why these individuals are able to inflict pain on themselves. One hypothesis suggests they may have higher levels of endorphins in their bodies than most people, thereby increasing their threshold for pain. Another theory relates to the individual's personal identity disturbance. It proposes that since many of the self-mutilating behaviors take place when the individual is in a state of depersonalization and derealization, he or she does not initially feel the pain. The mutilation continues until pain is felt in an attempt to counteract the feelings of unreality. Some clients with borderline personality disorder have reported that ". . . to feel pain is better than to feel nothing." The pain validates their existence.

Impulsivity. Individuals with borderline personality disorder have poor impulse control based on primary process functioning. Impulsive behaviors associated with borderline personality disorder include substance abuse, gambling, promiscuity, reckless driving, and binging and purging (APA, 2000). Many times these acting-out behaviors occur in response to real or perceived feelings of abandonment.

Predisposing Factors to Borderline Personality Disorder

Biological Influences

Biochemical. Cummings and Mega (2003) have suggested a possible serotonergic defect in clients with borderline personality disorder. In positron emission tomography using α-[^{11}C]methyl-L-tryptophan (α-[^{11}C]MTrp), which reflects serotonergic synthesis capability, clients with borderline personality demonstrated significantly decreased α-[^{11}C]MTrp in medial frontal, superior temporal, and striatal regions of the brain. Cummings and Mega (2003) state:

> These functional imaging studies support a medial and orbitofrontal abnormality that may promote the impulsive aggression demonstrated by patients with the borderline personality disorder. (p. 230)

Genetic. The decrease in serotonin also may have genetic implications for borderline personality disorder. Sadock and Sadock (2007) report that depression is common in the family backgrounds of clients with borderline personality disorder. They state:

> These patients have more relatives with mood disorders than do control groups, and persons with borderline personality disorder often have mood disorder as well. (p. 791)

Psychosocial Influences

Childhood Trauma. Studies have shown that many individuals with borderline personality disorder were reared in families with chaotic environments. Finley-Belgrad and Davies (2006) state, "Risk factors [for borderline personality disorder] include family environments characterized by trauma, neglect, and/or separation; exposure to sexual and physical abuse; and serious parental psychopathology such as substance abuse and antisocial personality disorder." Forty to 71 percent of borderline personality disorder clients report having been sexually abused, usually by a non-caregiver (National Institute of Mental Health [NIMH], 2006). In some instances, this disorder has been likened to posttraumatic stress disorder in response to childhood trauma and abuse. Oldham and associates (2006) state:

> Even when full criteria for comorbid PTSD are not present, patients with borderline personality disorder may experience PTSD-like symptoms. For example, symptoms such as intrusion, avoidance, and hyperarousal may emerge during psychotherapy. Awareness of the trauma-related nature of these symptoms can facilitate both psychotherapeutic and pharmacological efforts in symptom relief. (p. 1267)

Developmental Factors

Theory of Object Relations

According to Mahler's theory of object relations (Mahler et al., 1975), the infant passes through six phases from birth to 36 months, when a sense of separateness from the parenting figure is finally established. These phases include the following:

- **Phase 1 (Birth to 1 Month), Autistic Phase.** During this period, the baby spends most of his or her time in a half-waking, half-sleeping state. The main goal is fulfillment of needs for survival and comfort.
- **Phase 2 (1 to 5 Months), Symbiotic Phase.** At this time, there is a type of psychic fusion of mother and child. The child views the self as an extension of the parenting figure, although there is a developing awareness of external sources of need fulfillment.
- **Phase 3 (5 to 10 Months), Differentiation Phase.** The child is beginning to recognize that there is a separateness between the self and the parenting figure.
- **Phase 4 (10 to 16 Months), Practicing Phase.** This phase is characterized by increased locomotor functioning and the ability to explore the environment independently. A sense of separateness of the self is increased.
- **Phase 5 (16 to 24 Months), Rapprochement Phase.** Awareness of separateness of the self becomes acute. This is frightening to the child, who wants to regain some lost closeness but not return to symbiosis. The child wants the mother there as needed for "emotional refueling" and to maintain feelings of security.

● **Phase 6 (24 to 36 Months), On the Way to Object Constancy Phase.** In this phase, the child completes the individuation process and learns to relate to objects in an effective, constant manner. A sense of separateness is established, and the child is able to internalize a sustained image of the loved object or person when out of sight. Separation anxiety is resolved.

The individual with borderline personality disorder becomes fixed in the rapprochement phase of development. This occurs when the child shows increasing separation and autonomy. The mother, who feels secure in the relationship as long as the child is dependent, begins to feel threatened by the child's increasing independence. The mother may indeed be experiencing her own fears of abandonment. In response to separation behaviors, the mother withdraws the emotional support or "refueling" that is so vitally needed during this phase for the child to feel secure. Instead, the mother rewards clinging, dependent behaviors, and punishes (withholding emotional support) independent behaviors. With his or her sense of emotional survival at stake, the child learns to behave in a manner that satisfies the parental wishes. An internal conflict develops within the child, based on fear of abandonment. He or she wants to achieve independence common to this stage of development, but fears that mother will withdraw emotional support as a result. This unresolved fear of abandonment remains with the child into adulthood. Unresolved grief for the nurturing they failed to receive results in internalized rage that manifests itself in the depression so common in people with borderline personality disorder.

Diagnosis/Outcome Identification

Nursing diagnoses are formulated from the data gathered during the assessment phase and with background knowledge regarding predisposing factors to the disorder. Table 34–2 presents a list of client behaviors and the NANDA nursing diagnoses that correspond to these behaviors, which may be used in planning care for clients with borderline personality disorder.

Outcome Criteria

The following criteria may be used for measurement of outcomes in the care of clients with borderline personality disorder.

The client:

1. Has not harmed self.
2. Seeks out staff when desire for self-mutilation is strong.
3. Is able to identify true source of anger.
4. Expresses anger appropriately.
5. Relates to more than one staff member.
6. Completes activities of daily living independently.
7. Does not manipulate one staff member against the other in order to fulfill own desires.

Planning/Implementation

The following section presents a group of selected nursing diagnoses, with short- and long-term goals and nursing interventions for each.

TABLE 34–2 Assigning Nursing Diagnoses to Behaviors Commonly Associated with Borderline Personality Disorder

Behaviors	Nursing Diagnoses
History of self-injurious behavior; history of inability to plan solutions; impulsivity; irresistible urge to damage self; feels threatened with loss of significant relationship	Risk for Self-Mutilation
History of suicide attempts; suicidal ideation; suicidal plan; impulsiveness; childhood abuse; fears of abandonment; internalized rage	Risk for Self-Directed Violence; Risk for Suicide
Body language (e.g., rigid posture, clenching of fists and jaw, hyperactivity, pacing, breathlessness, threatening stances); history of childhood abuse; impulsivity; transient psychotic symptomatology	Risk for Other-Directed Violence
Depression; persistent emotional distress; rumination; separation distress; traumatic distress; verbalizes feeling empty; inappropriate expression of anger	Complicated Grieving
Alternating clinging and distancing behaviors; staff splitting; manipulation	Impaired Social Interaction
Feelings of depersonalization and derealization	Disturbed Personal Identity
Transient psychotic symptoms (disorganized thinking; misinterpretation of the environment); increased tension; decreased perceptual field	Anxiety (severe to panic)
Dependent on others; excessively seeks reassurance; manipulation of others; inability to tolerate being alone	Chronic Low Self-Esteem

Risk for Self-Mutilation/Risk for Self-Directed or Other-Directed Violence

Risk for self-mutilation is defined as "at risk for deliberate self-injurious behavior causing tissue damage with the intent of causing nonfatal injury to attain relief of tension" (NANDA International [NANDA-I], 2007, p. 193). *Risk for self-directed or other-directed violence* is defined as "at risk for behaviors in which an individual demonstrates that he/she can be physically, emotionally, and/or sexually harmful to self or others" (NANDA-I, 2007, pp. 240, 242).

Client Goals

Outcome criteria include short- and long-term goals. Timelines are individually determined.

Short-Term Goals

- The client will seek out staff member if feelings of harming self or others emerge.
- The client will not harm self or others.

Long-Term Goal

- The client will not harm self or others.

Interventions

- Observe the client's behavior frequently. Do this through routine activities and interactions; avoid appearing watchful and suspicious. Close observation is required so that intervention can occur if required to ensure client's (and others') safety.
- Secure a verbal contract from client that he or she will seek out a staff member when the urge for self-mutilation is experienced. Discussing feelings of self-harm with a trusted individual provides some relief to the client. A contract gets the subject out in the open and places some of the responsibility for his or her safety with the client. An attitude of acceptance of the client as a worthwhile individual is conveyed.
- If self-mutilation occurs, care for the client's wounds in a matter-of-fact manner. Do not give positive reinforcement to this behavior by offering sympathy or additional attention. Lack of attention to the maladaptive behavior may decrease repetition of its use.
- Encourage the client to talk about feelings he or she was having just before this behavior occurred. To problem-solve the situation with the client, knowledge of the precipitating factors is important.
- Act as a role model for the appropriate expression of angry feelings, and give positive reinforcement to the client when attempts to conform are made. It is vital that the client expresses angry feelings because suicide and other self-destructive behaviors are often viewed as a result of anger turned inward on the self.
- Remove all dangerous objects from the client's environment so that he or she may not purposefully or inadvertently use them to inflict harm to self or others.

- Try to redirect violent behavior with physical outlets for the client's anxiety (e.g., punching bag, jogging). Physical exercise is a safe and effective way of relieving pent-up tension.
- Have sufficient staff available to indicate a show of strength to the client if it becomes necessary. This conveys to the client evidence of control over the situation and provides some physical security for staff.
- Administer tranquilizing medications as ordered by the physician or obtain an order if necessary. Monitor the client for effectiveness of the medication and for the appearance of adverse side effects. Tranquilizing medications such as anxiolytics or antipsychotics may have a calming effect on the client and may prevent aggressive behaviors.
- Use of mechanical restraints or isolation room may be required if less restrictive interventions are unsuccessful. Follow the policy and procedure prescribed by the institution in executing this intervention. The Joint Commission on Accreditation of Healthcare Organizations (JCAHO) requires that the physician re-evaluate and issue a new order for restraints every 4 hours for adults and every 1 to 2 hours for children and adolescents. JCAHO requires that the client in restraints be observed every 15 minutes to ensure that circulation to extremities is not compromised (check temperature, color, pulses); to assist the client with needs related to nutrition, hydration, and elimination; and to position the client so that comfort is facilitated and aspiration is prevented. Some institutions may require continuous monitoring of restrained clients, particularly those who are highly agitated, and for whom there is a high risk of self- or accidental injury.
- If warranted by high acuity of the situation, staff may need to be assigned on a one-to-one basis. Because of their extreme fear of abandonment, clients with borderline personality disorder should not be left alone at a stressful time as it may cause an acute rise in anxiety and agitation levels.

Complicated Grieving

Complicated grieving is defined as "a disorder that occurs after the death of a significant other [or any other loss of significance to the individual], in which the experience of distress accompanying bereavement fails to follow normative expectations and manifests in functional impairment" (NANDA-I, 2007, p. 98). Table 34–3 presents this nursing diagnosis in care plan format.

Client Goals

Outcome criteria include short- and long-term goals. Timelines are individually determined.

Short-Term Goal

- Within 5 days, the client will discuss with nurse or therapist maladaptive patterns of expressing anger.

IMPLICATIONS OF RESEARCH FOR EVIDENCED-BASED PRACTICE

Zanarini, M.C., & Frankenburg, F.R. (2001). Olanzapine treatment of female borderline personality disorder patients: A double-blind, placebo-controlled pilot study. *Journal of Clinical Psychiatry*, 62(11), 849–854.

Description of the Study: The intent of this study was to compare the efficacy and safety of olanzapine versus placebo in the treatment of women meeting the criteria for borderline personality disorder (BPD). Subjects included 28 women meeting the Revised Diagnostic Interview for Borderlines and the *DSM-IV* criteria for BPD. The subjects were randomly assigned, 19 to olanzapine and 9 to placebo. Treatment duration was 6 months. Outcomes were self-reported on the Symptom Checklist-90, which measured changes in anxiety, depression, paranoia, anger/hostility, and interpersonal sensitivity.

Results of the Study: Olanzapine was associated with a significantly greater rate of improvement over time than placebo in all of the symptom areas studied except depression. Weight gain was modest but higher in the olanzapine group than in the placebo group. No serious movement disorders were noted.

Implications for Nursing Practice: Olanzapine appears to be a safe and effective agent in the treatment of women meeting the criteria for BPD. Nurses who work with individuals who have BPD should be familiar with this medication and understand the nursing implications associated with its administration. The implications of this study are particularly significant for nurses who have prescriptive authority and treat clients with BPD.

Long-Term Goal

● By the time of discharge from treatment, the client will be able to identify the true source of angry feelings, accept ownership of these feelings, and express them in a socially acceptable manner, in an effort to satisfactorily progress through the grieving process.

Interventions

● Convey an accepting attitude—one that creates a non-threatening environment for the client to express feelings. Be honest and keep all promises. An accepting attitude conveys to the client that you believe he or she is a worthwhile person. Trust is enhanced.

● Identify the function that anger, frustration, and rage serve for the client. Allow him or her to express these feelings within reason. Verbalization of feelings in a nonthreatening environment may help the client come to terms with unresolved issues.

● Encourage the client to discharge pent-up anger through participation in large motor activities (e.g., brisk walks, jogging, physical exercises, volleyball, punching bag, exercise bike). Physical exercise provides a safe and effective method for discharging pent-up tension.

● Explore with the client the true source of anger. This is painful therapy that often leads to regression as the client deals with feelings of early abandonment. It seems that sometimes the client must "get worse before he or she can get better." Reconciliation of the feelings associated with this stage is necessary before progression through the grieving process can continue.

● As anger is displaced onto the nurse or therapist, caution must be taken to guard against the negative effects of countertransference (see Chapter 7). These are very difficult clients who have the capacity for eliciting a whole array of negative feelings from the therapist. The existence of negative feelings by the nurse or therapist must be acknowledged, but they must not be allowed to interfere with the therapeutic process.

● Explain the behaviors associated with the normal grieving process. Help the client recognize his or her position in this process. Knowledge of the acceptability of the feelings associated with normal grieving may help to relieve some of the guilt that these responses generate.

● Help the client understand appropriate ways of expressing anger. Give positive reinforcement for behaviors used to express anger appropriately. Act as a role model. It is appropriate to let the client know when he or she has done something that has generated angry feelings in you. Role modeling ways to express anger in an appropriate manner is a powerful learning tool.

● Set limits on acting-out behaviors and explain the consequences of violation of those limits. Be supportive, yet consistent and firm, in caring for this client. The client lacks sufficient self-control to limit maladaptive behaviors, so assistance is required. Without consistency on the part of all staff members working with this client, a positive outcome will not be achieved.

Impaired Social Interaction

Impaired social interaction is defined as "insufficient or excessive quantity or ineffective quality of social exchange" (NANDA-I, 2007, p. 204).

Client Goals

Outcome criteria include short- and long-term goals. Timelines are individually determined.

Short-Term Goal

● Within 5 days, the client will discuss with nurse or therapist behaviors that impede the development of satisfactory interpersonal relationships.

Long-Term Goals

● By the time of discharge from treatment, the client will interact appropriately with others in the therapy setting in both social and therapeutic activities.

● By the time of discharge from treatment, the client will display no evidence of splitting or clinging and distancing behaviors in interpersonal relationships.

Table 34–3	Care Plan for the Client with Borderline Personality Disorder

NURSING DIAGNOSIS: COMPLICATED GRIEVING

RELATED TO: Maternal deprivation during rapprochement phase of development (internalized as a loss, with fixation in anger stage of grieving process)

EVIDENCED BY: Depressed mood, acting-out behaviors

Outcome Criteria	Nursing Interventions	Rationale
Short-Term Goal ● Within 5 days, the client will discuss with nurse or therapist maladaptive patterns of expressing anger. **Long-Term Goal** ● By time of discharge from treatment, the client will be able to identify the true source of angry feelings, accept ownership of these feelings, and express them in a socially acceptable manner, in an effort to satisfactorily progress through the grieving process.	1. Convey an accepting attitude—one that creates a nonthreatening environment for the client to express feelings. Be honest and keep all promises. 2. Identify the function that anger, frustration, and rage serve for the client. Allow him or her to express these feelings within reason. 3. Encourage client to discharge pent-up anger through participation in large motor activities (e.g., brisk walks, jogging, physical exercises, volleyball, punching bag, exercise bike). 4. Explore with client the true source of the anger. This is a painful therapy that often leads to regression as the client deals with the feelings of early abandonment. 5. As anger is displaced onto the nurse or therapist, caution must be taken to guard against the negative effects of countertransference. These are very difficult clients who have the capacity for eliciting a whole array of negative feelings from the therapist. 6. Explain the behaviors associated with the normal grieving process. Help the client recognize his or her position in this process. 7. Help client to understand appropriate ways to express anger. Give positive reinforcement for behaviors used to express anger appropriately. Act as a role model. 8. Set limits on acting-out behaviors and explain consequences of violation of those limits. Be supportive, yet consistent and firm in caring for this client.	1. An accepting attitude conveys to the client that you believe he or she is a worthwhile person. Trust is enhanced. 2. Verbalization of feelings in a nonthreatening environment may help client come to terms with unresolved issues. 3. Physical exercise provides a safe and effective method for discharging pent-up tension. 4. Reconciliation of the feelings associated with this stage is necessary before progression through the grieving process can continue. 5. The existence of negative feelings by the nurse or therapist must be acknowledged, but they must not be allowed to interfere with the therapeutic process. 6. Knowledge of the acceptability of the feelings associated with normal grieving may help to relieve some of the guilt that these responses generate. 7. Positive reinforcement enhances self-esteem and encourages repetition of desirable behaviors. 8. Client lacks sufficient self-control to limit maladaptive behaviors, so assistance is required from staff. Without consistency on the part of all staff members working with this client, however, a positive outcome will not be achieved.

Interventions

● Encourage the client to examine these behaviors (to recognize that they are occurring). He or she may be unaware of splitting or of clinging and distancing pattern of interaction with others. Recognition must take place before change can occur.

● Help the client understand that you will be available, without reinforcing dependent behaviors.

Knowledge of your availability may provide needed security.

● Rotate staff members who work with the client in order to avoid his or her developing a dependence on particular individuals. The client must learn to relate to more than one staff member in an effort to decrease the use of splitting and to diminish fears of abandonment.

● With the client, explore feelings that relate to fears of abandonment and engulfment. Help him or her to understand that clinging and distancing behaviors are engendered by these fears. Exploration of feelings with a trusted individual may help the client come to terms with unresolved issues.

● Help the client understand how these behaviors interfere with satisfactory relationships. He or she may be unaware of how others perceive these behaviors and why they are not acceptable.

● Assist the client to work toward achievement of object constancy. Be available, without promoting dependency. Give positive reinforcement for independent behaviors. The client must resolve fears of abandonment in the process toward developing the ability to establish satisfactory intimate relationships.

CLINICAL PEARL

Recognize when client is playing one staff member against another. Remember that splitting is the primary defense mechanism of these individuals, and the impressions they have of others as either "good" or "bad" are a manifestation of this defense. Do not listen as client tries to degrade other staff members. Suggest that client discuss the problem directly with staff person involved.

Concept Care Mapping

The concept map care plan is an innovative approach to planning and organizing nursing care (see Chapter 9). It is a diagrammatic teaching and learning strategy that allows visualization of interrelationships between medical diagnoses, nursing diagnoses, assessment data, and treatments. An example of a concept map care plan for a client with borderline personality disorder is presented in Figure 34–1.

Evaluation

Reassessment is conducted to determine if the nursing actions have been successful in achieving the objectives of care. Evaluation of the nursing actions for the client with borderline personality disorder may be facilitated by gathering information using the following types of questions:

● Has the client been able to seek out staff when feeling the desire for self-harm?

● Has the client avoided self-harm?

● Can the client correlate times of desire for self-harm to times of elevation in level of anxiety?

● Can the client discuss feelings with staff (particularly feelings of depression and anger)?

● Can the client identify the true source toward which the anger is directed?

● Can the client verbalize understanding of the basis for his or her anger?

● Can the client express anger appropriately?

● Can the client function independently?

● Can the client relate to more than one staff member?

● Can the client verbalize the knowledge that the staff members will return and are not abandoning the client when leaving for the day?

● Can the client separate from the staff in an appropriate manner?

● Can the client delay gratification and refrain from manipulating others in order to fulfill own desires?

● Can the client verbalize resources within the community from whom he or she may seek assistance in times of extreme stress?

Antisocial Personality Disorder (Background Assessment Data)

In the *DSM-I*, antisocial behavior was categorized as a "sociopathic or psychopathic" reaction that was symptomatic of any of several underlying personality disorders. The *DSM-II* represented it as a distinct personality type, a distinction that has been retained in subsequent editions. The *DSM-IV-TR* diagnostic criteria for antisocial personality disorder are presented in Box 34–11.

Individuals with antisocial personality disorder are seldom seen in most clinical settings, and when they are, it is commonly a way to avoid legal consequences. Sometimes they are admitted to the healthcare system by court order for psychological evaluation. Most frequently, however, these individuals may be encountered in prisons, jails, and rehabilitation services.

Clinical Picture

Skodol and Gunderson (2008) describe antisocial personality disorder as a pattern of socially irresponsible, exploitative, and guiltless behavior that reflects a disregard for the rights of others. These individuals exploit and manipulate others for personal gain and have a general disregard for the law. They have difficulty sustaining consistent employment and in developing stable relationships. They appear cold and callous, often intimidating others with their brusque and belligerent manner. They tend to be argumentative and, at times, cruel and malicious. They lack warmth and compassion and are often suspicious of these qualities in others.

Individuals with antisocial personality have a very low tolerance for frustration, act impetuously, and are unable to delay gratification. They are restless and easily bored, often taking chances and seeking thrills, as if they were immune to danger.

When things go their way, individuals with this disorder act cheerful, even gracious and charming. Because of their

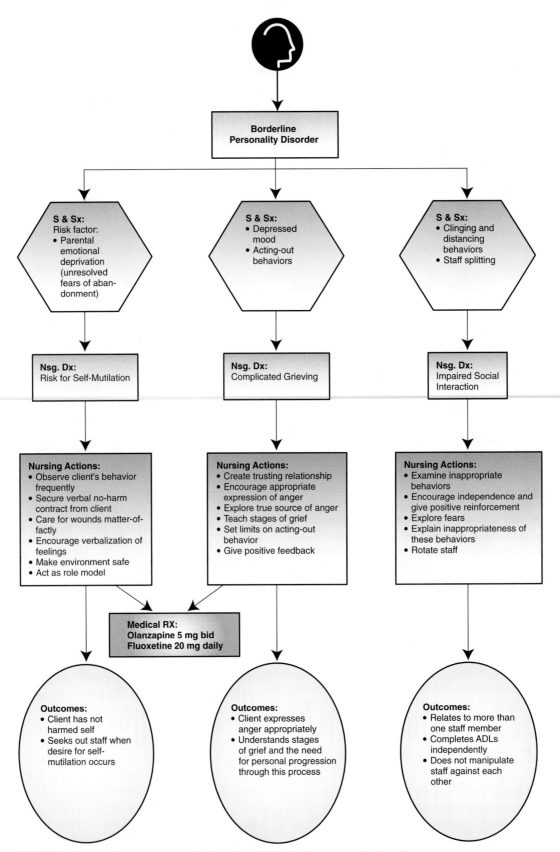

Borderline Personality Disorder

S & Sx:
Risk factor:
• Parental emotional deprivation (unresolved fears of abandonment)

S & Sx:
• Depressed mood
• Acting-out behaviors

S & Sx:
• Clinging and distancing behaviors
• Staff splitting

Nsg. Dx:
Risk for Self-Mutilation

Nsg. Dx:
Complicated Grieving

Nsg. Dx:
Impaired Social Interaction

Nursing Actions:
• Observe client's behavior frequently
• Secure verbal no-harm contract from client
• Care for wounds matter-of-factly
• Encourage verbalization of feelings
• Make environment safe
• Act as role model

Nursing Actions:
• Create trusting relationship
• Encourage appropriate expression of anger
• Explore true source of anger
• Teach stages of grief
• Set limits on acting-out behavior
• Give positive feedback

Nursing Actions:
• Examine inappropriate behaviors
• Encourage independence and give positive reinforcement
• Explore fears
• Explain inappropriateness of these behaviors
• Rotate staff

Medical RX:
Olanzapine 5 mg bid
Fluoxetine 20 mg daily

Outcomes:
• Client has not harmed self
• Seeks out staff when desire for self-mutilation occurs

Outcomes:
• Client expresses anger appropriately
• Understands stages of grief and the need for personal progression through this process

Outcomes:
• Relates to more than one staff member
• Completes ADLs independently
• Does not manipulate staff against each other

FIGURE 34–1 Concept map care plan for client with borderline personality disorder.

Box 34–11 Diagnostic Criteria for Antisocial Personality Disorder

A. There is a pervasive pattern of disregard for and violation of the rights of others occurring since age 15 years, as indicated by three (or more) of the following:
1. Failure to conform to social norms with respect to lawful behaviors as indicated by repeatedly performing acts that are grounds for arrest.
2. Deceitfulness, as indicated by repeated lying, use of aliases, or conning others for personal profit or pleasure.
3. Impulsivity or failure to plan ahead.
4. Irritability and aggressiveness, as indicated by repeated physical fights or assaults.
5. Reckless disregard for safety of self or others.
6. Consistent irresponsibility, as indicated by repeated failure to sustain consistent work behavior or honor financial obligations.
7. Lack of remorse, as indicated by being indifferent to or rationalizing having hurt, mistreated, or stolen from another.

B. Individual is at least 18 years old.
C. There is evidence of conduct disorder with onset before age 15 years.
D. The occurrence of antisocial behavior is not exclusively during the course of schizophrenia or a manic episode.

SOURCE: American Psychiatric Association (2000), with permission.

---

low tolerance for frustration, this pleasant exterior can change very quickly. When what they desire at the moment is challenged, they are likely to become furious and vindictive. Easily provoked to attack, their first inclination is to demean and dominate. They believe that "good guys come in last," and show contempt for the weak and underprivileged. They exploit others to fulfill their own desires, showing no trace of shame or guilt for their behavior.

Individuals with antisocial personalities see themselves as victims, using projection as the primary ego defense mechanism. They do not accept responsibility for the consequences of their behavior. Gorman, Raines, and Sultan (2002) state:

> Manipulative individuals have come to suspect that any person or institution may try to control them, rendering them powerless and vulnerable to attack. (p.168)

In their own minds, this perception justifies their malicious behavior, lest they be the recipient of unjust persecution and hostility from others.

Satisfying interpersonal relationships are not possible because individuals with antisocial personalities have learned to place their trust only in themselves. They have a philosophy that "everyone is out to 'help number one' and that one should stop at nothing to avoid being pushed around" (APA, 2000).

One of the most distinctive characteristics of individuals with antisocial personalities is their tendency to ignore conventional authority and rules. They act as though established social norms and guidelines for self-discipline and cooperative behavior do not apply to

them. They are flagrant in their disrespect for the law and for the rights of others.

Predisposing Factors to Antisocial Personality Disorder

Biological Influences

The *DSM-IV-TR* reports that antisocial personality is more common among first-degree biological relatives of those with the disorder than among the general population (APA, 2000). Twin and adoptive studies have implicated the role of genetics in antisocial personality disorder (Skodol & Gunderson, 2008). These studies of families of individuals with antisocial personality show higher numbers of relatives with antisocial personality or alcoholism than are found in the general population. The studies have also shown that children of parents with antisocial behavior are more likely to be diagnosed with antisocial personality, even when they are separated at birth from their biological parents and reared by individuals without the disorder.

Characteristics associated with temperament in the newborn may be significant in the predisposition to antisocial personality. Parents who bring their children with behavior disorders to clinics often report that the child displayed temper tantrums from infancy and would become furious when awaiting a bottle or a diaper change. As these children mature, they commonly develop a bullying attitude toward other children. Parents report that they are undaunted by punishment and generally quite unmanageable. They are daring and foolhardy in their willingness to chance physical harm and, they seem unaffected by pain.

Fischer and associates (2002) identified attention-deficit hyperactivity disorder and conduct disorder during childhood and adolescence as predisposing factors to antisocial personality disorder.

Although these biogenetic influences may describe some familial pattern to the development of antisocial personality disorder, no basic pathological process has yet been determined as an etiological factor. Bienenfeld (2006) states:

> Low levels of behavioral inhibition may be mediated by serotonergic dysregulation in the septohippocampal system. There may also be developmental or acquired abnormalities in the prefrontal brain systems and reduced autonomic activity in antisocial personality disorder. This may underlie the low arousal, poor fear conditioning, and decision-making deficits described in antisocial personality disorder.

Family Dynamics

Antisocial personality disorder frequently arises from a chaotic home environment. Parental deprivation during the first 5 years of life appears to be a critical predisposing factor in the development of antisocial personality disorder. Separation due to parental delinquency appears to be more highly correlated with the disorder than is parental loss from other causes. The presence or intermittent appearance of inconsistent impulsive parents, not the loss of a consistent parent, is environmentally *most* damaging.

Studies have shown that individuals with antisocial personality disorder often have been severely physically abused in childhood. The abuse contributes to the development of antisocial behavior in several ways. First, it provides a model for behavior. Second, it may result in injury to the child's central nervous system, thereby impairing the child's ability to function appropriately. Finally, it engenders rage in the victimized child, which is then displaced onto others in the environment.

A number of factors associated with disordered family functioning have been implicated in the development of antisocial personality (Hill, 2003; Skodol & Gunderson, 2008; Ramsland, 2007). The following circumstances may influence the predisposition to antisocial personality disorder:

1. Absence of parental discipline
2. Extreme poverty
3. Removal from the home
4. Growing up without parental figures of both sexes
5. Erratic and inconsistent methods of discipline
6. Being "rescued" each time they are in trouble (never having to suffer the consequences of one's own behavior)
7. Maternal deprivation

Diagnosis/Outcome Identification

Nursing diagnoses are formulated from the data gathered during the assessment phase and with background knowledge regarding predisposing factors to the disorder. Table 34–4 presents a list of client behaviors and the NANDA nursing diagnoses that correspond to those behaviors, which may be used in planning care for clients with antisocial personality disorder.

Outcome Criteria

The following criteria may be used for measurement of outcomes in the care of the client with antisocial personality disorder.

The client:

1. Discusses angry feelings with staff and in group sessions.
2. Has not harmed self or others.
3. Can rechannel hostility into socially acceptable behaviors.
4. Follows rules and regulations of the therapy environment.
5. Can verbalize which of his or her behaviors are not acceptable.

IMPLICATIONS OF RESEARCH FOR EVIDENCE-BASED PRACTICE

Dekovic, M., Janssens, J.A.M., & Van As, N.M.C. (2003). Family predictors of antisocial behavior in adolescence. *Family Process, 42*(2), 223–235.

Description of the Study: The objective of this study was to examine the combined and unique ability of different aspects of family functioning to predict involvement in antisocial behavior in a large community (nonclinical) sample of adolescents. The aspects of family functioning that were measured included:

1. *Proximal factors:* parental childrearing behaviors and the quality of the parent-adolescent relationship
2. *Distal factors:* parental characteristics (e.g., depression; parental confidence in his or her competence as a parent)
3. *Contextual factors:* family characteristics (e.g., family cohesion, quality of the marital relationship; involvement between members)
4. *Global factors:* family socioeconomic status; family composition (e.g., single-parent family)

The researchers hypothesized that proximal factors would play a stronger role in future antisocial behavior than the other three variables. The sample included 508 families with an adolescent between 12 and 18 years of age. There were 254 females and 254 males. The parent sample consisted of 969 parents (502 mothers and 467 fathers). Ninety-one percent of the families were intact families, 7 percent of the parents were divorced or separated, and 2 percent were widowed. There was a wide range of socioeconomic and educational backgrounds, although the parents with low educational and occupational levels were slightly underrepresented. Data were gathered in the subjects' homes through a battery of questionnaires administered individually to adolescents, mothers, and fathers.

Results of the Study: Results showed that proximal factors were significant predictors of antisocial behavior, independent of their shared variance with other factors. Also consistent with the hypothesized model, the effects of distal and contextual factors appear to be mostly indirect: after their association with proximal factors was taken into account, these factors were no longer significantly related to antisocial behavior. Global indicators of family functioning (socioeconomic status and family composition) were unrelated to adolescent antisocial behavior. This study showed that supportive parents, parents who use more subtle means of guidance (i.e., supervision rather than punitive strategies) and parents who are consistent in their behavior toward adolescents, have a lower risk that their child would become involved in antisocial behavior. Adolescents who are exposed to coercive and hostile parenting probably adopt this aggressive style of interacting with others. The parent-adolescent relationship that was characterized by elevated levels of conflict and a lack of closeness and acceptance emerged as a risk factor for involvement in antisocial behavior. Parental depression, conflict in the marital dyad, and lack of cohesion between members were also found to influence adolescent antisocial behavior, but less directly than the proximal factors.

Implications for Nursing Practice: Nurses must use this information to design and implement effective parenting programs. Nurses can become actively involved in teaching parents, in inpatient, outpatient, and community education programs. The researchers state, "The findings of this study suggest that, when designing interventions that focus on family factors, in addition to teaching parents adequate child-rearing skills, more attention should be given to finding methods to improve the general *quality* of the parent-adolescent relationship."

TABLE 34-4 **Assigning Nursing Diagnoses to Behaviors Commonly Associated with Antisocial Personality Disorder**

Behaviors	Nursing Diagnoses
Body language (e.g., rigid posture, clenching of fists and jaw, hyperactivity, pacing, breathlessness, threatening stances); cruelty to animals; rage reactions; history of childhood abuse; history of violence against others; impulsivity; substance abuse; negative role-modeling; inability to tolerate frustration	Risk for Other-Directed Violence
Disregard for societal norms and laws; absence of guilty feelings; inability to delay gratification; denial of obvious problems; grandiosity; hostile laughter; projection of blame and responsibility; ridicule of others; superior attitude toward others	Defensive Coping
Manipulation of others to fulfill own desires; inability to form close, personal relationships; frequent lack of success in life events; passive-aggressiveness; overt aggressiveness (hiding feelings of low self-esteem)	Chronic Low Self-Esteem
Inability to form a satisfactory, enduring, intimate relationship with another; dysfunctional interaction with others; use of unsuccessful social interaction behaviors	Impaired Social Interaction
Demonstration of inability to take responsibility for meeting basic health practices; history of lack of health-seeking behavior; demonstrated lack of knowledge regarding basic health practices; lack of expressed interest in improving health behaviors	Ineffective Health Maintenance

6. Shows regard for the rights of others by delaying gratification of own desires when appropriate.
7. Does not manipulate others in an attempt to increase feelings of self-worth.
8. Verbalizes understanding of knowledge required to maintain basic health needs.

Planning/Implementation

The following section presents a group of selected nursing diagnoses, with short- and long-term goals and nursing interventions for each.

Risk for Other-Directed Violence

Risk for other-directed violence is defined as "at risk for behaviors in which an individual demonstrates that he/she can be physically, emotionally, and/or sexually harmful to others" (NANDA-I, 2007, p. 240).

Client Goals

Outcome criteria include short- and long-term goals. Timelines are individually determined.

Short-Term Goals

● Within 3 days, the client will discuss angry feelings and situations that precipitate hostility.
● The client will not harm others.

Long-Term Goal

● The client will not harm others.

Interventions

● Convey an accepting attitude toward this client. Feelings of rejection are undoubtedly familiar to him or her. Work on development of trust. Be honest, keep all promises, and convey the message to the client that it is not *him* or *her*, but the *behavior* that is unacceptable. An attitude of acceptance promotes feelings of self-worth. Trust is the basis of a therapeutic relationship.
● Maintain a low level of stimuli in the client's environment (low lighting, few people, simple decor, low noise level). A stimulating environment may increase agitation and promote aggressive behavior.
● Observe the client's behavior frequently. Do this through routine activities and interactions; avoid appearing watchful and suspicious. Close observation is required so that intervention can occur if needed to ensure the client's (and others') safety.
● Remove all dangerous objects from the client's environment so that he or she may not purposefully or inadvertently use them to inflict harm to self or others.
● Help the client identify the true object of his or her hostility (e.g., "You seem to be upset with . . ."). Because of weak ego development, the client may be misusing the defense mechanism of displacement. Helping him or her recognize this in a nonthreatening manner may help reveal unresolved issues so that they may be confronted.
● Encourage the client to gradually verbalize hostile feelings. Verbalization of feelings in a nonthreatening environment may help client come to terms with unresolved issues.

- Explore with the client alternative ways of handling frustration (e.g., large motor skills that channel hostile energy into socially acceptable behavior). Physically demanding activities help to relieve pent-up tension.
- The staff should maintain and convey a calm attitude toward the client. Anxiety is contagious and can be transferred from staff to client. A calm attitude provides the client with a feeling of safety and security.
- Have sufficient staff available to present a show of strength to the client if necessary. This conveys to the client evidence of control over the situation and provides some physical security for the staff.
- Administer tranquilizing medications as ordered by the physician or obtain an order if necessary. Monitor the client for effectiveness of the medication as well as for appearance of adverse side effects. Antianxiety agents (e.g., lorazepam, chlordiazepoxide, oxazepam) produce a calming effect and may help to allay hostile behaviors. (**NOTE:** Medications are not often prescribed for clients with antisocial personality disorder because of these individuals' strong susceptibility to addictions.)
- If the client is not calmed by "talking down" or by medication, use of mechanical restraints may be necessary. Be sure to have sufficient staff available to assist. Follow protocol established by the institution in executing this intervention. JCAHO requires that the physician re-evaluate and issue a new order for restraints every 4 hours for adults ages 18 years and older. Never use restraints as a punitive measure but rather as a protective measure for a client who is out of control.
- JCAHO requires that the client in restraints be observed every 15 minutes to ensure that circulation to extremities is not compromised (check temperature, color, pulses); to assist the client with needs related to nutrition, hydration, and elimination; and to position the client so that comfort is facilitated and aspiration is prevented. Some institutions may require continuous one-to-one monitoring of restrained clients, particularly those who are highly agitated and for whom there is a high risk of self- or accidental injury.

Defensive Coping

Defensive coping is defined as "repeated projection of falsely positive self-evaluation based on a self-protective pattern that defends against underlying perceived threats to positive self-regard" (NANDA-I, 2007, p. 57).

Client Goals

Outcome criteria include short- and long-term goals. Timelines are individually determined.

Short-Term Goals

- Within 24 hours after admission, the client will verbalize understanding of treatment setting rules and regulations and the consequences for violation of them.

- The client will verbalize personal responsibility for difficulties experienced in interpersonal relationships within (time period reasonable for client).

Long-Term Goals

- By the time of discharge from treatment, the client will be able to cope more adaptively by delaying gratification of own desires and following rules and regulations of the treatment setting.
- By the time of discharge from treatment, the client will demonstrate ability to interact with others without becoming defensive, rationalizing behaviors, or expressing grandiose ideas.

Interventions

- From the onset, the client should be made aware of which behaviors are acceptable and which are not. Explain consequences of violation of the limits. Consequences must involve something of value to the client. All staff must be consistent in enforcing these limits. Consequences should be administered in a matter-of-fact manner immediately following the infraction. Because the client cannot (or will not) impose own limits on maladaptive behaviors, these behaviors must be delineated and enforced by staff. Undesirable consequences may help to decrease repetition of these behaviors.
- Do not attempt to coax or convince the client to do the "right thing." Do not use the words "You should (or shouldn't) . . ."; instead, use the words "You will be expected to . . ." The ideal would be for this client to eventually internalize societal norms, beginning with this step-by-step, "either/or" approach on the unit (*either* you do [don't do] this, *or* this will occur). Explanations must be concise, concrete, and clear, with little or no capacity for misinterpretation.
- Provide positive feedback or reward for acceptable behaviors. Positive reinforcement enhances self-esteem and encourages repetition of desirable behaviors.
- In an attempt to assist the client to delay gratification, begin to increase the length of time requirement for acceptable behavior in order to achieve the reward. For example, 2 hours of acceptable behavior may be exchanged for a phone call; 4 hours of acceptable behavior for 2 hours of television; 1 day of acceptable behavior for a recreational therapy bowling activity; 5 days of acceptable behavior for a weekend pass.
- A milieu unit provides the appropriate environment for the client with antisocial personality. The democratic approach, with specific rules and regulations, community meetings, and group therapy sessions emulates the type of societal situation in which the client must learn to live. Feedback from peers is often more effective than confrontation from an authority figure. The client learns to follow the rules of the

group as a positive step in the progression toward internalizing the rules of society.

● Help the client to gain insight into his or her own behavior. Often, these individuals rationalize to such an extent that they deny that their behavior is inappropriate. (e.g., "The owner of this store has so much money, he'll never miss the little bit I take. He has everything, and I have nothing. It's not fair! I deserve to have some of what he has.") The client must come to understand that certain behaviors will not be tolerated within the society and that severe consequences will be imposed on those individuals who refuse to comply. The client must *want* to become a productive member of society before he or she can be helped.

● Talk about past behaviors with the client. Discuss which behaviors are acceptable by societal norms and which are not. Help the client identify ways in which he or she has exploited others. Encourage client to explore how he or she would feel if the circumstances were reversed. An attempt may be made to enlighten the client to the sensitivity of others by promoting self-awareness in an effort to help the client gain insight into his or her own behavior.

● Throughout the relationship with the client, maintain an attitude of "It is not *you*, but *your behavior*, that is unacceptable." An attitude of acceptance promotes feelings of dignity and self-worth.

Concept Care Mapping

The concept map care plan is an innovative approach to planning and organizing nursing care (see Chapter 9). It is a diagrammatic teaching and learning strategy that allows visualization of interrelationships between medical diagnoses, nursing diagnoses, assessment data, and treatments. An example of a concept map care plan for a client with antisocial personality disorder is presented in Figure 34–2.

Evaluation

Reassessment is conducted to determine if the nursing actions have been successful in achieving the objectives of care. Evaluation of the nursing actions for the client with antisocial personality disorder may be facilitated by gathering information using the following types of questions:

● Does the client recognize when anger is getting out of control?

● Can the client seek out staff instead of expressing anger in an inappropriate manner?

● Can the client use other sources for rechanneling anger (e.g., physical activities)?

● Has harm to others been avoided?

● Can the client follow rules and regulations of the therapeutic milieu with little or no reminding?

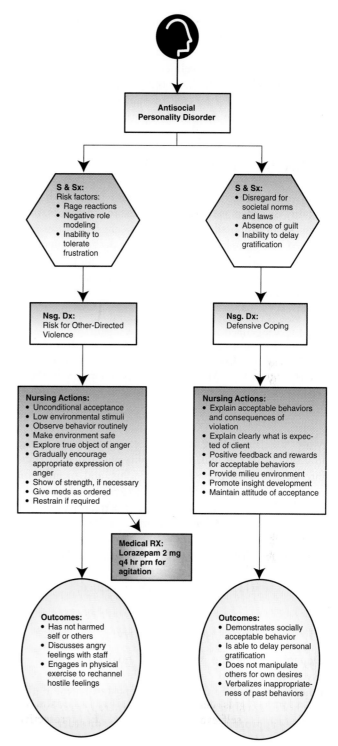

FIGURE 34–2 Concept map care plan for client with antisocial personality disorder.

● Can the client verbalize which behaviors are appropriate and which are not?

● Does the client express a desire to change?

● Can the client delay gratifying own desires in deference to those of others when appropriate?

● Does the client refrain from manipulating others to fulfill own desires?

- Does the client fulfill activities of daily living willingly and independently?
- Can the client verbalize methods of achieving and maintaining optimal wellness?
- Can the client verbalize community resources from which he or she can seek assistance with daily living and healthcare needs when required?

TREATMENT MODALITIES

Few would argue that treatment of individuals with personality disorders is difficult and, in some instances, may even seem impossible. Personality characteristics are learned very early in life and perhaps may even be genetic. It is not surprising, then, that these enduring patterns of behavior may take years to change, if change occurs. Skodol and Gunderson (2008) state:

> Because personality disorders have been thought to consist of deeply ingrained attitudes and behavior patterns that consolidate during development and have endured since early adulthood, they have traditionally been believed to be very resistant to change. Moreover, treatment efforts are further confounded by the degree to which patients with personality disorders do not recognize their maladaptive personality traits as undesirable or in need of change. (p. 831)

Most clinicians believe it best to strive for lessening the inflexibility of the maladaptive traits and reducing their interference with everyday functioning and meaningful relationships. Little research exists to guide the decision of which therapy is most appropriate in the treatment of personality disorders. Selection of intervention is generally based on the area of greatest dysfunction, such as cognition, affect, behavior, or interpersonal relations. Following is a brief description of various types of therapies and the disorders to which they are customarily suited.

Interpersonal Psychotherapy

Depending on the therapeutic goals, interpersonal psychotherapy with personality disorders is brief and time-limited, or it may involve long-term exploratory psychotherapy. Interpersonal psychotherapy may be particularly appropriate because personality disorders largely reflect problems in interpersonal style.

Long-term psychotherapy attempts to understand and modify the maladjusted behaviors, cognition, and affects of clients with personality disorders that dominate their personal lives and relationships. The core element of treatment is the establishment of an empathic therapist–client relationship, based on collaboration and guided discovery in which the therapist functions as a role model for the client.

Interpersonal psychotherapy is suggested for clients with paranoid, schizoid, schizotypal, borderline, dependent, narcissistic, and obsessive-compulsive personality disorders.

Psychoanalytical Psychotherapy

The treatment of choice for individuals with histrionic personality disorder has been psychoanalytical psychotherapy (Skodol & Gunderson, 2008). Treatment focuses on the unconscious motivation for seeking total satisfaction from others and for being unable to commit oneself to a stable, meaningful relationship.

Milieu or Group Therapy

This treatment is especially appropriate for individuals with antisocial personality disorder, who respond more adaptively to support and feedback from peers. In milieu or group therapy, feedback from peers is more effective than in one-to-one interaction with a therapist. Group therapy—particularly homogenous supportive groups that emphasize the development of social skills—may be helpful in overcoming social anxiety and developing interpersonal trust and rapport in clients with avoidant personality disorder (Skodol & Gunderson, 2008). Feminist consciousness-raising groups can be useful in helping dependent clients struggling with social-role stereotypes.

Cognitive/Behavioral Therapy

Behavioral strategies offer reinforcement for positive change. Social skills training and assertiveness training teach alternative ways to deal with frustration. Cognitive strategies help the client recognize and correct inaccurate internal mental schemata. This type of therapy may be useful for clients with obsessive-compulsive, passive-aggressive, antisocial, and avoidant personality disorders.

Psychopharmacology

Psychopharmacology may be helpful in some instances. Although these drugs have no effect in the direct treatment of the disorder itself, some symptomatic relief can be achieved. Antipsychotic medications are helpful in the treatment of psychotic decompensations experienced by clients with paranoid, schizotypal, and borderline personality disorders (Coccaro & Siever, 2000).

A variety of pharmacological interventions have been used with borderline personality disorder. The selective serotonin reuptake inhibitors (SSRIs) and monoamine oxidase inhibitors (MAOIs) have been successful in decreasing impulsivity and self-destructive acts in these clients. The MAOIs are not commonly used, however, because of concerns about violations of dietary restrictions and the higher risk of fatality with overdose

REFERENCES

American Psychiatric Association. (2000). *Diagnostic and statistical manual of mental disorders*. (4th ed.) *Text revision*. Washington, DC: American Psychiatric Association.

Andreasen, N.C., & Black, D.W. (2006). *Introductory textbook of psychiatry*, (4th ed.). Washington, DC: American Psychiatric Publishing.

Bienenfeld, D. (2006). Personality disorders. Retrieved March 29, 2007 from http://www.emedicine.com/med/topic3472.htm

Coccaro, E.F., & Siever, L.J. (2000). The neuropsychopharmacology of personality disorders. *Psychopharmacology: The fourth generation of progress*. The American College of Neuropsychopharmacology. Retrieved March 29, 2007 from http://www.acnp.org/G4/GN401000152/CH148.html

Cummings, J.L., & Mega, M.S. (2003). *Neuropsychiatry and behavioral neuroscience*. New York: Oxford University Press.

Finley-Belgrad, E.A., & Davies, J.A. (2006). Personality disorder: Borderline. Retrieved March 29, 2007 from http://www.emedicine.com/ped/topic270.htm

Fischer, M., Barkley, R.A., Smallish, L., & Fletcher, K. (2002). Young adult follow-up of hyperactive children: Self-reported psychiatric disorders, comorbidity, and the role of childhood conduct problems and teen CD. *Journal of Abnormal Child Psychology, 30*(5), 463–475.

Gorman, L., Raines, M.L., & Sultan, D.F. (2002). *Psychosocial nursing for general patient care* (2nd ed.). Philadelphia: F.A. Davis.

Hannig, P.J. (2007). *Histrionic personality disorder*. Retrieved March 29, 2007 from http://www.nvo.com/psych_help/histrionicpersonality-disorder

Hill, J. (2003). Early identification of individuals at risk for antisocial personality disorder. *British Journal of Psychiatry, 182* (Suppl. 44), s11–s14.

Mark, R. (2002). *How to deal with narcissistic personality disorder*. Retrieved March 29, 2007 from http://wiwi.essortment.com/narcissisticp_rwmn.htm

NANDA International (NANDA-I). (2007). *Nursing diagnoses: Definitions & classification 2007–2008*. Philadelphia: NANDA-I.

National Institute of Mental Health (NIMH). (2006). Borderline personality disorder: Raising questions, finding answers. Retrieved March 30, 2007 from http://www.nimh.nih.gov/publicat/bpd.cfm

Oldham, J.M., Gabbard, G.O., Goin, M.K., Gunderson, J., Soloff, P., Spiegel, D., Stone, M., & Phillips, K.A. (2006). Practice guideline for the treatment of patients with borderline personality disorder. In *The American Psychiatric Association Practice Guidelines for the Treatment of Psychiatric Disorders, Compendium 2006*. Washington, DC: American Psychiatric Publishing.

Ramsland, K. (2007). *Born or made? Theories of psychopathy*. Retrieved March 30, 2007 from http://www.crimelibrary.com/criminal_mind/psychology/psychopath/2.html?sect=4

Rettew, D.C., & Jellinek, M.S. (2006). *Personality disorder: Avoidant personality*. Retrieved March 29, 2007 from http://www.emedicine.com/ped/topic189.htm

Sadock, B.J., & Sadock, V.A. (2007). *Synopsis of psychiatry: Behavioral sciences/clinical psychiatry* (10th ed.). Philadelphia: Lippincott Williams & Wilkins.

Skodol, A.E. & Gunderson, J.G. (2008). Personality disorders. In R.E. Hales, S.C. Yudofsky, & G.O. Gabbard (Eds.), *Textbook of psychiatry* (5th ed.). Washington, DC: American Psychiatric Publishing.

CLASSICAL REFERENCES

Erikson, E. (1963). *Childhood and society* (2nd ed.). New York: WW Norton.

Sullivan, H.S. (1953). *The interpersonal theory of psychiatry*. New York: WW Norton.

Mahler, M., Pine, F., & Bergman, A. (1975). *The psychological birth of the human infant*. New York: Basic Books.

@ Internet References

- Additional information about personality disorders is located at the following Web sites:
  - http://www.mentalhealth.com/dis/p20-pe04.html
  - http://www.mentalhealth.com/dis/p20-pe08.html
  - http://www.mentalhealth.com/dis/p20-pe05.html
  - http://www.mentalhealth.com/dis/p20-pe09.html
  - http://www.mentalhealth.com/dis/p20-pe06.html
  - http://www.mentalhealth.com/dis/p20-pe07.html
  - http://www.mentalhealth.com/dis/p20-pe10.html
  - http://www.mentalhealth.com/dis/p20-pe01.html
  - http://www.mentalhealth.com/dis/p20-pe02.html
  - http://www.mentalhealth.com/dis/p20-pe03.html
  - http://www.mentalhealth.com/p13.html#Per

the occurrence of cancer and autoimmune disorders, provide some evidence for this theory and the proposition that error or mutation occurs at the molecular and cellular level.

Wear-and-Tear Theory

Proponents of this theory believe that the body wears out on a scheduled basis. Free radicals, which are the waste products of metabolism, accumulate and cause damage to important biological structures. Free radicals are molecules with unpaired electrons that exist normally in the body; they also are produced by ionizing radiation, ozone, and chemical toxins. According to this theory, free radicals cause DNA damage, cross-linkage of collagen, and the accumulation of age pigments.

Environmental Theory

According to this theory, factors in the environment (e.g., industrial carcinogens, sunlight, trauma, and infection) bring about changes in the aging process. Although these factors are known to accelerate aging, the impact of the environment is a secondary rather than a primary factor in aging. Science is only beginning to uncover the many environmental factors that affect aging.

Immunity Theory

Immunity theory describes an age-related decline in the immune system. As people age, their ability to defend against foreign organisms decreases, resulting in susceptibility to diseases such as cancer and infection. Along with the diminished immune function, a rise in the body's autoimmune response occurs, leading to the development of autoimmune diseases such as rheumatoid arthritis and allergies to food and environmental agents.

Neuroendocrine Theory

This theory proposes that aging occurs because of a slowing of the secretion of certain hormones that have an impact on reactions regulated by the nervous system. This is most clearly demonstrated in the pituitary gland, thyroid, adrenals, and the glands of reproduction. Although research has given some credence to a predictable biological clock that controls fertility, there is much more to be learned from the study of the neuroendocrine system in relation to a systemic aging process that is controlled by a "clock."

Psychosocial Theories

Psychosocial theories focus on social and psychological changes that accompany advancing age, as opposed to the biological implications of anatomic deterioration. Several theories have attempted to describe how attitudes and behavior in the early phases of life affect people's reactions during the late phase. This work is called the process of "successful aging."

Personality Theory

Personality theories address aspects of psychological growth without delineating specific tasks or expectations of older adults. Murray and Zentner (2001) state, "Evidence supports the general hypothesis that personality characteristics in old age are highly correlated with early life characteristics" (p. 802). In extreme old age, however, people show greater similarity in certain characteristics, probably because of similar declines in biological functioning and societal opportunities.

In a classic study by Reichard, Livson, and Peterson (1962), the personalities of older men were classified into five major categories according to their patterns of adjustment to aging. According to this study:

1. *Mature men* are considered well-balanced persons who maintain close personal relationships. They accept both the strengths and weaknesses of their age, finding little to regret about retirement and approaching most problems in a relaxed or convivial manner without continually having to assess blame.
2. *"Rocking chair" personalities* are found in passive–dependent individuals who are content to lean on others for support, to disengage, and to let most of life's activities pass them by.
3. *Armored men* have well-integrated defense mechanisms, which serve as adequate protection. Rigid and stable, they present a strong silent front and often rely on activity as an expression of their continuing independence.
4. *Angry men* are bitter about life, themselves, and other people. Aggressiveness is common, as is suspicion of others, especially of minorities or women. With little tolerance for ambiguity or frustration, they have always shown some instability in work and their personal lives, and now feel extremely threatened by old age.
5. *Self-haters* are similar to angry men, except that most of their animosity is turned inward on themselves. Seeing themselves as dismal failures, being old only depresses them all the more.

The investigators identified the mature, "rocking chair," and armored categories as characteristic of healthy, adjusted individuals and the angry and self-hater categories as less successful at aging. In all cases, the evidence suggested that the personalities of the subjects, although distinguished by age-specific criteria, had not changed appreciably throughout most of adulthood.

In a more recent study of personality traits, Srivastava and associates (2003) examined the "big five" personality trait dimensions in a large sample to determine how personality changes over the life span. Age range of the subjects was from 21 to 60. The personality traits tested included conscientiousness, agreeableness, neuroticism, openness, and extraversion. They found that conscientiousness (being organized and disciplined) increased throughout the age range studied, with the largest increases during the 20s. Agreeableness (being warm, generous, and helpful) increased most during a person's 30s. Neuroticism (being anxious and emotionally labile) declined with age for women, but did not decline for men. Openness (being receptive to new experiences) showed small declines with age for both men and women. Extraversion (being outwardly expressive and interested in the environment) declined for women but did not change in men. This study contradicts the view that personality traits tend to stop changing in early adulthood. These researchers suggest that personality traits change gradually but systematically throughout the life span.

Developmental Task Theory

Developmental tasks are the activities and challenges that one must accomplish at specific stages in life to achieve successful aging. Erikson (1963) described the primary task of old age as being able to see one's life as having been lived with integrity. In the absence of achieving that sense of having lived well, the older adult is at risk for becoming preoccupied with feelings of regret or despair.

Disengagement Theory

Disengagement theory describes the process of withdrawal by older adults from societal roles and responsibilities. According to the theory, this withdrawal process is predictable, systematic, inevitable, and necessary for the proper functioning of a growing society. Older adults were said to be happy when social contacts diminished and responsibilities were assumed by a younger generation. The benefit to the older adult is thought to be in providing time for reflecting on life's accomplishments and for coming to terms with unfulfilled expectations. The benefit to society is thought to be an orderly transfer of power from old to young.

There have been many critics of this theory, and the postulates have been challenged. For many healthy and productive older individuals, the prospect of a slower pace and fewer responsibilities is undesirable.

Activity Theory

In direct opposition to the disengagement theory is the activity theory of aging, which holds that the way to age successfully is to stay active. Multiple studies have validated the positive relationship between maintaining

meaningful interaction with others and physical and mental well-being.

Sadock and Sadock (2007) suggest that social integration is the prime factor in determining psychosocial adaptation in later life. Social integration refers to how the aging individual is included and takes part in the life and activities of his or her society. This theory holds that the maintenance of activities is important to most people as a basis for deriving and sustaining satisfaction, self-esteem, and health.

Continuity Theory

This theory, also known as the developmental theory, is a follow-up to the disengagement and activity theories. It emphasizes the individual's previously established coping abilities and personal character traits as a basis for predicting how the person will adjust to the changes of aging. Basic lifestyle characteristics are likely to remain stable in old age, barring physical or other types of complications that necessitate change. A person who has enjoyed the company of others and an active social life will continue to enjoy this lifestyle into old age. One who has preferred solitude and a limited number of activities will probably find satisfaction in a continuation of this lifestyle.

Maintenance of internal continuity is motivated by the need for preservation of self-esteem, ego integrity, cognitive function, and social support. As they age, individuals maintain their self-concept by reinterpreting their current experiences so that old values can take on new meanings in keeping with present circumstances. Internal self-concepts and beliefs are not readily vulnerable to environmental change; and external continuity in skills, activities, roles, and relationships can remain remarkably stable into the 70s. Physical illness or death of friends and loved ones may preclude continued social interaction (Sadock & Sadock, 2007).

THE NORMAL AGING PROCESS

Biological Aspects of Aging

Individuals are unique in their physical and psychological aging processes, as influenced by their predisposition or resistance to illness; the effects of their external environment and behaviors; their exposure to trauma, infections, and past diseases; and the health and illness practices they have adopted during their life spans. As the individual ages, there is a quantitative loss of cells and changes in many of the enzymatic activities within cells, resulting in a diminished responsiveness to biological demands made on the body. Age-related changes occur at different rates for different individuals, although in actuality, when growth stops aging begins. This section presents a brief overview of the normal biological changes that occur with the aging process.

Skin

One of the most dramatic changes that occurs in aging is the loss of elastin in the skin. This effect, as well as changes in collagen, causes aged skin to wrinkle and sag. Excessive exposure to sunlight compounds these changes and increases the risk of developing skin cancer.

Fat redistribution results in a loss of the subcutaneous cushion of adipose tissue. Thus, older people lose "insulation" and are more sensitive to extremes of ambient temperature than are younger people (Stanley, Blair, & Beare, 2005). A lower supply of blood vessels to the skin results in a slower rate of healing.

Cardiovascular System

The age-related decline in the cardiovascular system is thought to be the major determinant of decreased tolerance for exercise and loss of conditioning and the overall decline in energy reserve. The aging heart is characterized by modest hypertrophy with reduced ventricular compliance and diminished cardiac output (Murray & Zentner, 2001; Sadock & Sadock, 2007). This results in a decrease in response to work demands and some diminishment of blood flow to the brain, kidneys, liver, and muscles. Heart rate also slows with time. If arteriosclerosis is present, cardiac function is further compromised.

Respiratory System

Thoracic expansion is diminished by an increase in fibrous tissue and loss of elastin. Pulmonary vital capacity decreases, and the amount of residual air increases. Scattered areas of fibrosis in the alveolar septa interfere with exchange of oxygen and carbon dioxide. These changes are accelerated by the use of cigarettes or other inhaled substances. Cough and laryngeal reflexes are reduced, causing decreased ability to defend the airway. Decreased pulmonary blood flow and diffusion ability result in reduced efficiency in responding to sudden respiratory demands.

Musculoskeletal System

Skeletal aging involving the bones, muscles, ligaments, and tendons probably generates the most frequent limitations on activities of daily living experienced by aging individuals. Loss of muscle mass is significant, although this occurs more slowly in men than in women. Demineralization of the bones occurs at a rate of about 1 percent per year throughout the life span in both men and women. However, this increases to approximately 10 percent in women around **menopause**, making them particularly vulnerable to **osteoporosis.**

Individual muscle fibers become thinner and less elastic with age. Muscles become less flexible following disuse. There is diminished storage of muscle glycogen, resulting in loss of energy reserve for increased activity. These changes are accelerated by nutritional deficiencies and inactivity.

Gastrointestinal System

In the oral cavity, the teeth show a reduction in dentine production, shrinkage and fibrosis of root pulp, gingival retraction, and loss of bone density in the alveolar ridges. There is some loss of peristalsis in the stomach and intestines, and gastric acid production decreases. Levels of intrinsic factor may also decrease, resulting in vitamin B_{12} malabsorption in some aging individuals. A significant decrease in absorptive surface area of the small intestine may be associated with some decline in nutrient absorption. Motility slowdown of the large intestine, combined with poor dietary habits, dehydration, lack of exercise, and some medications, may give rise to problems with constipation.

There is a modest decrease in size and weight of the liver resulting in losses in enzyme activity required to deactivate certain medications by the liver. These age-related changes can influence the metabolism and excretion of these medications. These changes, along with the pharmacokinetics of the drug, must be considered when giving medications to aging individuals.

Endocrine System

A decreased level of thyroid hormones causes a lowered basal metabolic rate. Decreased amounts of adrenocorticotropic hormone may result in less efficient stress response.

Impairments in glucose tolerance are evident in aging individuals (Pietraniec-Shannon, 2003). Studies of glucose challenges show that insulin levels are equivalent to or slightly higher than those from younger challenged individuals, although peripheral insulin resistance appears to play a significant role in carbohydrate intolerance. The observed glucose clearance abnormalities and insulin resistance in older people may be related to many factors other than biological aging (e.g., obesity, family history of diabetes) and may be influenced substantially by diet or exercise.

Genitourinary System

Age-related declines in renal function occur because of a steady attrition of nephrons and sclerosis within the glomeruli over time (Stanley, Blair, & Beare, 2005).

Vascular changes affect blood flow to the kidneys and results in reduced glomerular filtration and tubular function (Murray & Zentner, 2001). Elderly people are prone to develop the syndrome of inappropriate antidiuretic hormone secretion, and levels of blood urea nitrogen and creatinine may be elevated slightly. The overall decline in renal functioning has serious implications for physicians in prescribing medications for elderly individuals.

In men, enlargement of the prostate gland is common as aging occurs. Prostatic hypertrophy is associated with an increased risk for urinary retention and may also be a cause of urinary incontinence (Beers & Jones, 2004). Loss of muscle and sphincter control, as well as the use of some medications, may cause urinary incontinence in women. Not only is this problem a cause of social stigma, but also, if left untreated, it increases the risk of urinary tract infection and local skin irritation. Normal changes in the genitalia are discussed in the section on "Sexual Aspects of Aging."

Immune System

Aging results in changes in both cell-mediated and antibody-mediated immune responses. The size of the thymus gland declines continuously from just beyond puberty to about 15 percent of its original size at age 50. The consequences of these changes include a greater susceptibility to infections and a diminished inflammatory response that results in delayed healing. There is also evidence of an increase in various autoantibodies (e.g., rheumatoid factor) as a person ages, increasing the risk of autoimmune disorders (Beers & Jones, 2004).

Because of the overall decrease in efficiency of the immune system, the proliferation of abnormal cells is facilitated in the elderly individual. Cancer is the best example of aberrant cells allowed to proliferate due to the ineffectiveness of the immune system.

Nervous System

With aging, there is an absolute loss of neurons, which correlates with decreases in brain weight of about 10 percent by age 90 (Murray & Zentner, 2001). Gross morphological examination reveals gyral atrophy in the frontal, temporal, and parietal lobes; widening of the sulci; and ventricular enlargement. However, it must be remembered that these changes have been identified in careful study of adults with normal intellectual function.

The brain has enormous reserve, and little cerebral function is lost over time, although greater functional decline is noted in the periphery (Stanley, Blair, & Beare, 2005). There appears to be a disproportionately greater loss of cells in the cerebellum, the locus ceruleus, the substantia nigra, and olfactory bulbs, accounting for some of the more characteristic aging behaviors such as mild gait disturbances, sleep disruptions, and decreased smell and taste perception.

Some of the age-related changes within the nervous system may be due to alterations in neurotransmitter release, uptake, turnover, catabolism, or receptor functions (Beers & Jones, 2004). A great deal of attention is being given to brain biochemistry and in particular to the neurotransmitters acetylcholine, dopamine, norepinephrine, and epinephrine. These biochemical changes may be responsible for the altered responses of many older persons to stressful events and some biological treatments.

Sensory Systems

Vision. Visual acuity begins to decrease in mid-life. Presbyopia (blurred near vision) is the standard marker of aging of the eye. It is caused by a loss of elasticity of the crystalline lens, and results in compromised accommodation.

Cataract development is inevitable if the individual lives long enough for the changes to occur. Cataracts occur when the lens of the eye becomes less resilient (due to compression of fibers) and increasingly opaque (as proteins lump together), ultimately resulting in a loss of visual acuity.

The color in the iris may fade, and the pupil may become irregular in shape. A decrease in production of secretions by the lacrimal glands may cause dryness and result in increased irritation and infection. The pupil may become constricted, requiring an increase in the amount of light needed for reading.

Hearing. Hearing changes significantly with the aging process. Gradually over time, the ear loses its sensitivity to discriminate sounds because of damage to the hair cells of the cochlea. The most dramatic decline appears to be in perception of high-frequency sounds.

Although hearing loss is significant in all aging individuals, the decline is more dramatic in men than in women. Men are twice as likely as women are to have hearing loss (Murray & Zentner, 2001).

Taste and Smell. Taste sensitivity decreases over the life span. Taste discrimination decreases, and bitter taste sensations predominate. Sensitivity to sweet and salty tastes is diminished.

The deterioration of the olfactory bulbs is accompanied by loss of smell acuity. The aromatic component of taste perception diminishes.

Touch and Pain. Organized sensory nerve receptors on the skin continue to decrease throughout the life span; thus, the touch threshold increases with age (Pietraniec-Shannon, 2003). The ability to feel pain also decreases in response to these changes, and the ability to perceive and interpret painful stimuli changes. These changes have critical implications for the elderly in their potential lack of ability to use sensory warnings for escaping serious injury.

Psychological Aspects of Aging

Memory Functioning

Age-related memory deficiencies have been extensively reported in the literature. Although **short-term memory** seems to deteriorate with age, perhaps because of poorer sorting strategies, **long-term memory** does not show similar changes. However, in nearly every instance, well-educated, mentally active people do not exhibit the same decline in memory functioning as their age peers who lack similar opportunities to flex their minds. Nevertheless, with few exceptions, the time required for memory scanning is longer for both recent and remote recall among older people. This can sometimes be attributed to social or health factors (e.g., stress, fatigue, illness), but it can also occur because of certain normal physical changes associated with aging (e.g., decreased blood flow to the brain).

Intellectual Functioning

There appears to be a high degree of regularity in intellectual functioning across the adult age span. Crystallized abilities, or knowledge acquired in the course of the socialization process, tend to remain stable over the adult life span. Fluid abilities, or abilities involved in solving novel problems, tend to decline gradually from young to old adulthood. In other words, intellectual abilities of older people do not decline but do become obsolete. The age of their formal educational experiences is reflected in their intelligence scoring.

Learning Ability

The ability to learn is not diminished by age. Studies, however, have shown that some aspects of learning do change with age. The ordinary slowing of reaction time with age for nearly all tasks or the over-arousal of the central nervous system may account for lower performance levels on tests requiring rapid responses. Under conditions that allow for self-pacing by the participant, differences in accuracy of performance diminish. Ability to learn continues throughout life, although strongly influenced by interests, activity, motivation, health, and experience. Adjustments do need to be made in teaching methodology and time allowed for learning.

Adaptation to the Tasks of Aging

Loss and Grief. Individuals experience losses from the very beginning of life. By the time individuals reach their 60s and 70s, they have experienced numerous losses, and mourning has become a lifelong process. Unfortunately, with the aging process comes a convergence of losses, the timing of which makes it impossible for the aging individual to complete the grief process in response to one loss before another occurs. Because grief is cumulative, this can result in **bereavement overload**, which has been implicated in the predisposition to depression in the elderly.

Attachment to Others. Many studies have confirmed the importance of interpersonal relationships at all stages in the life cycle. Murray and Zentner (2001) state:

> [Social networks] contribute to well-being of the senior by promoting socialization and companionship, elevating morale and life satisfaction, buffering the effects of stressful events, providing a confidant, and facilitating coping skills and mastery. (p. 756)

This need for **attachment** is consistent with the activity theory of aging that correlates the importance of social integration with successful adaptation in later life.

Maintenance of Self-Identity. Self-concept and self-image appear to remain stable over time. Factors that have been shown to favor good psychosocial adjustment in later life are sustained family relationships, maturity of ego defenses, absence of alcoholism, and absence of depressive disorder (Vaillant, 2003). Studies show that the elderly have a strong need for and remarkable capability of retaining a persistent self-concept in the face of the many changes that contribute to instability in later life.

Dealing with Death. Death anxiety among the aging is apparently more of a myth than a reality. Studies have not supported the negative view of death as an overriding psychological factor in the aging process. Various investigators who have worked with dying persons report that it is not death itself, but abandonment, pain, and confusion that are feared. What many desire most is someone to talk with, to show them their life's meaning is not shattered merely because they are about to die (Kübler-Ross, 1969; Murray & Zentner, 2001).

Psychiatric Disorders in Later Life

The later years constitute a time of especially high risk for emotional distress. Sadock and Sadock (2007) state:

> Several psychosocial risk factors predispose older people to mental disorders. These risk factors include loss of social roles, loss of autonomy, the deaths of friends and relatives, declining health, increased isolation, financial constraints, and decreased cognitive functioning. (p. 1353)

Dementia. Dementing disorders are the most common causes of psychopathology in the elderly (Sadock & Sadock, 2007). About half of these disorders are of the Alzheimer's type, which is characterized by an insidious onset and a gradually progressive course of cognitive impairment. No curative treatment is currently available. Symptomatic treatments, including pharmacological interventions, attention to the environment, and family support, can help to maximize the client's level of functioning.

Delirium. Delirium is one of the most common and important forms of psychopathology in later life. A number of factors have been identified that predispose elderly people to delirium, including structural brain disease, reduced capacity for homeostatic regulation, impaired vision and hearing, a high prevalence of chronic disease, reduced resistance to acute stress, and age-related changes in the pharmacokinetic and pharmacodynamics of drugs. Delirium needs to be recognized and the underlying condition treated as soon as possible. A high mortality is associated with this condition.

Depression. Depressive disorders are the most common affective illnesses occurring after the middle years. The incidence of increased depression among elderly people is influenced by the variables of physical illness, functional disability, cognitive impairment, and loss of a spouse (Stanley, Blair, & Beare, 2005). Hypochondriacal symptoms are common in the depressed elderly. Symptomatology often mimics that of dementia, a condition that is referred to as pseudodementia. (See Table 26-3 for a comparison of the symptoms of dementia and pseudodementia.) Suicide is more prevalent in the elderly, with declining health and decreased economic status being considered important influencing factors. Treatment of depression in the elderly individual is with psychotropic medications or electroconvulsive therapy.

Schizophrenia. Schizophrenia and delusional disorders may continue into old age or may manifest themselves for the first time only during senescence (Blazer, 2008). In most instances, individuals who manifest psychotic disorders early in life show a decline in psychopathology as they age. Late-onset schizophrenia (after age 60) is not common, but when it does occur, it often is characterized by delusions or hallucinations of a persecutory nature. The course is chronic, and treatment is with neuroleptics and supportive psychotherapy.

Anxiety Disorders. Most anxiety disorders begin in early to middle adulthood, but some appear for the first time after age 60. Sadock and Sadock (2007) state:

> The fragility of the autonomic nervous system in older persons may account for the development of anxiety after a major stressor. Because of concurrent physical disability, older persons react more severely to posttraumatic stress disorder than younger persons. (p. 1355)

In older adults, symptoms of anxiety and depression often accompany each other, making it difficult to determine which disorder is dominant.

Personality Disorders. Personality disorders are uncommon in the elderly population. The incidence of personality disorders among individuals over age 65 is less than 5 percent. Most elderly people with personality disorder have likely manifested the symptomatology for many years.

Sleep Disorders. Sleep disorders are very common in the aging individual. Sleep disturbances affect 50 percent

Turvey, C.L., Conwell, Y., Jones, M.P., Phillips, C., Simonsick, E., Pearson, J.L., & Wallace, R. (2002). Risk factors for late-life suicide: A prospective, community-based study. *American Journal of Geriatric Psychiatry*, 10(4), 398–406.

Description of the Study: Studies have suggested that a negative or depressive mental outlook, being widowed or divorced, sleeping more than 9 hours per day, and drinking more than three alcoholic beverages per day were risk factors for late-life suicide. The primary aim of this study was to examine the relationship between completed suicide in late life and physical health, disability, and social support. The participants were 14,456 individuals selected from a general population of elderly subjects age 65 and older. Control subjects were a group of 420 individuals who were matched by age and sex. It was a 10-year longitudinal study beginning in 1981. Variables were assessed at baseline, year 3, and year 6, with a 10-year mortality follow-up. Baseline variables included sleep quality, social support, alcohol use, medical illness, physical impairment, cognitive impairment, and depressive symptoms.

Results of the Study: The 10-year mortality follow-up indicated that 75 percent of the control subjects had died, but none had died from suicide. Twenty-one of the 14,456 participants committed suicide within the follow-up period. Twenty of the 21 suicide victims were male. Average age was 78.6 years, with a range from 67 to 90 years. The most common means was gunshot. Other means included hanging, cutting, overdose, drowning, carbon monoxide inhalation, and one participant jumped to his death. In this study, presence of friends or relatives to confide in was negatively associated with suicide. Likewise, regular church attendance was more common in control subjects than the participant sample, indicating an even wider range of community support. Those who committed suicide had reported more depressive symptoms than those who did not, but they did not consume more alcohol (inconsistent with previous studies). Poor sleep quality was positively correlated with suicide in this study, but no specific physical illness was identified as a predisposition. The authors identify the small suicide sample as a limitation of this study.

Implications for Nursing Practice: This study identified depression, poor sleep quality, and limited social support as important variables in the potential for elderly suicide. Sleep disturbance may be an important indicator of depression, whereas limited social support may be a contributing factor. The study provides reinforcement for the U.S. Department of Health and Human Services (USDHHS) recommendation in their *National Strategy for Suicide Prevention: Goals and Objectives for Action* (2001). The USDHHS recommends detection and treatment of depression as a strategy to prevent late-life suicide. The authors state, "Because both depression and social support are amenable to intervention, this study provides further evidence for the possible effectiveness of such strategies to reduce suicides among older adults." Nurses can become actively involved in assessing for these risk factors, as well as planning, implementing, and evaluating the effectiveness of strategies for preventing suicide in the elderly population.

of people age 65 and older who live at home and 66 percent of those who live in long-term care facilities (Stanley, Blair, & Beare, 2005). Some common causes of sleep disturbances among elderly people include age-dependent decreases in the ability to sleep ("sleep decay"); increased prevalence of sleep apnea; depression; dementia; anxiety; pain; impaired mobility; medications; and psychosocial factors such as loneliness, inactivity, and boredom. Sedative-hypnotics, along with nonpharmacological approaches, are often used as sleep aids with the elderly. Changes in aging associated with metabolism and elimination must be considered when maintenance medications are administered for chronic insomnia in the aging client.

Sociocultural Aspects of Aging

Old age brings many important socially induced changes, some of which have the potential for negative effect on both the physical and mental well-being of older persons. In American society, old age is defined arbitrarily as being 65 years or older because that is the age when most people have been able to retire with full Social Security and other pension benefits. Recent legislation has increased the age beyond 65 years for full Social Security benefits. Currently, the age increases yearly (based on year of birth) until 2027, when the age for full benefits will be 67 years for all individuals.

Elderly people in virtually all cultures share some basic needs and interests. There is little doubt that most individuals choose to live the most satisfying life possible until their demise. They want protection from hazards and release from the weariness of everyday tasks. They want to be treated with the respect and dignity that is deserving of individuals who have reached this pinnacle in life; and they want to die with the same respect and dignity.

From the beginning of human culture, the aged have had a special status in society. Even today, in some cultures the aged are the most powerful, the most engaged, and the most respected members of the society. This has not been the case in the modern industrial societies, although trends in the status of the aged differ widely between one industrialized country and another. For example, the status and integration of the aged in Japan have remained relatively high when compared with other industrialized nations, such as the United States. There are subcultures in the U.S., however, in which the elderly are afforded a higher degree of status than they receive in the mainstream population. Examples include Latino Americans, Asian Americans, and African Americans. The aged are awarded a position of honor in cultures that place emphasis on family cohesiveness. In these cultures, the aged are revered for their knowledge and wisdom gained through their years of life experiences (Giger & Davidhizar, 2004).

Many negative stereotypes color the perspective on aging in the United States. Ideas that elderly individuals are always tired or sick, slow and forgetful, isolated and lonely, unproductive, and angry determine the way younger individuals relate to the elderly in this society. Increasing disregard for the elderly has resulted in a type of segregation, as aging individuals voluntarily seek out or are involuntarily placed in special residences for the aged.

Assisted living centers, retirement apartment complexes, and even entire retirement communities intended solely for individuals over age 50, are becoming more and more common. In 2006, about half (51.4 percent) of persons age 65 and older lived in nine states, with the largest numbers in California, Florida, New York, Texas, and Pennsylvania (AoA, 2008). It is important for elderly individuals to feel part of an integrated group, and they are migrating to these areas in an effort to achieve this integration. This phenomenon provides additional corroboration for the activity theory of aging, and the importance of attachment to others.

Employment is another area in which the elderly experience discrimination. Although compulsory retirement has been virtually eliminated, discrimination still exists in hiring and promotion practices. Many employers are not eager to retain or hire older workers. It is difficult to determine how much of the failure to hire and promote results from discrimination based on age alone and how much of it is related to a realistic and fair appraisal of the aged employee's ability and efficiency. It is true that some elderly individuals are no longer capable of doing as good a job as a younger worker; however, there are many who likely can do a *better* job than their younger counterparts, if given the opportunity. Nevertheless, surveys have shown that some employers accept the negative stereotypes about elderly individuals and believe that older workers are hard to please, set in their ways, less productive, frequently absent, and involved in more accidents.

The status of the elderly may improve with time and as their numbers increase with the aging of the "baby boomers." As older individuals gain political power, the benefits and privileges designed for the elderly will increase. There is power in numbers, and the 21st century promises power for people age 65 and older.

Sexual Aspects of Aging

Sexuality and the sexual needs of elderly people are frequently misunderstood, condemned, stereotyped, ridiculed, repressed, and ignored. Americans have grown up in a society that has liberated sexual expression for all other age groups, but still retains certain Victorian standards regarding sexual expression by the elderly. Negative stereotyped notions concerning sexual interest and activity of the elderly are common. Some of these include ideas that older people have no sexual interests or desires; that they are sexually undesirable; or that they are too fragile or too ill to engage in sexual activity. Some people even believe it is disgusting or comical to consider elderly individuals as sexual beings.

These cultural stereotypes undoubtedly play a large part in the misperception many people hold regarding sexuality of the aged, and they may be reinforced by the common tendency of the young to deny the inevitability of aging. With reasonable good health and an interesting and interested partner, there is no inherent reason why individuals should not enjoy an active sexual life well into late adulthood (Altman & Hanfling, 2003).

Physical Changes Associated with Sexuality

Many of the changes in sexuality that occur in later years are related to the physical changes that are taking place at that time of life.

Changes in Women. Menopause may begin anytime during the 40s or early 50s. During this time there is a gradual decline in the functioning of the ovaries and the subsequent production of estrogen, which results in a number of changes. The walls of the vagina become thin and inelastic, the vagina itself shrinks in both width and length, and the amount of vaginal lubrication decreases noticeably. Orgastic uterine contractions may become spastic. All of these changes can result in painful penetration, vaginal burning, pelvic aching, or irritation on urination. In some women, the discomfort may be severe enough to result in an avoidance of intercourse. Paradoxically, these symptoms are more likely to occur with infrequent intercourse of only one time a month or less. Regular and more frequent sexual activity results in a greater capacity for sexual performance (King, 2005). Other symptoms that are associated with menopause in some women include hot flashes, night sweats, sleeplessness, irritability, mood swings, migraine headaches, urinary incontinence, and weight gain.

Some menopausal women elect to take hormone replacement therapy for relief of these changes and symptoms. With estrogen therapy, the symptoms of menopause are minimized or do not occur at all. However, some women choose not to take the hormone because of an increased risk of breast cancer, and when given alone, an increased risk of endometrial cancer. To combat this latter effect, many women also take a second hormone, progesterone. Taken for 7 to 10 days during the month, progesterone decreases the risk of estrogen-induced endometrial cancer. Some physicians prescribe a low dose of progesterone that is taken, along with estrogen, for the entire month. A combination pill, taken in this manner, is also available.

Results of the Women's Health Initiative (WHI), as reported in the *Journal of the American Medical Association*, indicate that the combination pill is associated with an increased risk of cardiovascular disease and breast cancer (Rossouw et al., 2002). Benefits related to colon cancer and osteoporosis were reported; however, investigators stopped this arm of the study and suggested discontinuation of this type of therapy.

Changes in Men. Testosterone production declines gradually over the years, beginning between ages 40 and 60. A major change resulting from this hormone reduction is that erections occur more slowly and require more direct genital stimulation to achieve. There may also be a modest decrease in the firmness of the erection in men older than age 60. The refractory period lengthens with age, increasing the amount of time following orgasm before the man may achieve another erection. The volume of ejaculate gradually decreases, and the force of ejaculation lessens. The testes become somewhat smaller, but most men continue to produce viable sperm well into old age. Prolonged control over ejaculation in middle-aged and elderly men may bring increased sexual satisfaction for both partners.

Sexual Behavior in the Elderly

Coital frequency in early marriage and the overall quantity of sexual activity between age 20 and 40 correlate significantly with frequency patterns of sexual activity during aging (Masters, Johnson, & Kolodny, 1995). Although sexual interest and behavior do appear to decline somewhat with age, studies show that significant numbers of elderly men and women have active and satisfying sex lives well into their 80s. A survey commissioned by the American Association of Retired Persons (AARP) provided some revealing information regarding the sexual attitudes and behavior of senior citizens. Some statistics from the survey are summarized in Table 35–1. The information from this survey clearly indicates that sexual activity can and does continue well past the 70s for healthy active individuals who have regular opportunities for sexual expression. King (2005) states: "For healthy men and women with healthy partners, sexual activity will probably continue throughout life if they had a positive attitude about sex when they were younger."

SPECIAL CONCERNS OF THE ELDERLY POPULATION

Retirement

Statistics reflect that a larger percentage of Americans are living longer and that many of them are retiring earlier. Reasons often given for the increasing pattern of early retirement include health problems, Social Security and other pension benefits, attractive "early out" packages offered by companies, and long-held plans (e.g., turning a hobby into a money-making situation).

TABLE 35–1	Sexuality at Midlife and Beyond: 2004 Update of Attitudes and Behaviors			
	Ages	Men (%)	Women (%)	Both
Have sex at least once a week:	45–59			~ 50 %
	60–74	30	24	
Report very satisfied with physical relationship	All	65	57	
Very satisfied with emotional relationship	All	69	63	
Report sexual activity is important to their overall quality of life	All	65	34	
Believe nonmarital sex is okay	<60	75	70	
	60–69	74	59	
	≥70	63	50	
Describe their partners as physically attractive	45–49	56	59	
	50–59	62	52	
	60–69	58	46	
	≥70	53	49	
Report always or usually having an orgasm with sexual intercourse	45–49	92	84	
	50–59	96	71	
	60–69	91	63	
	≥70	85	55	
Report being impotent	45–49	2		
	50–59	6		
	60–69	11		
	≥70	32		
Report having sought treatment for a sex problem from a professional	All	27	10	
Report having used medicine, hormones, or other treatments to improve sexual functioning	45–49	16	5	
	50–59	20	9	
	60–69	26	9	
	≥70	25	3	
What would most improve your sex life?	45–59			Less stress; more free time; resolve partner issues
	≥60			Better health for self/partner; finding a partner

SOURCE: Adapted from American Association of Retired Persons (AARP), 2005.

Even eliminating the mandatory retirement age and the possibility of delaying the age of eligibility for Social Security benefits from 65 to 67 by the year 2027 is not expected to have a significant effect on the trend toward earlier retirement.

Sadock and Sadock (2007) report that of those people who voluntarily retire, most reenter the work force within 2 years. The reasons they give for doing this include negative reactions to being retired, feelings of being unproductive, economic hardship, and loneliness.

About 5.5 million older Americans were in the labor force (working or actively seeking work) in 2006. These included 3.1 million men and 2.4 million women, and constituted 3.5 percent of the U.S. labor force (AoA, 2008).

Retirement has both social and economical implications for elderly individuals. The role is fraught with a great deal of ambiguity and is one that requires many adaptations on the part of those involved.

Social Implications

Retirement is often anticipated as an achievement in principle, but met with a great deal of ambiguity when it actually occurs. Our society places a great deal of importance on productivity, making as much money as possible, and doing it at as young an age as possible. These types of values contribute to the ambiguity associated with retirement. Although leisure has been acknowledged as a legitimate reward for workers, leisure during retirement historically has lacked the same social value. Adjustment to this life cycle event becomes more difficult in the face of societal values that are in direct conflict with the new lifestyle.

Historically, many women have derived a good deal of their self-esteem from their families—birthing them, rearing them, and being a "good mother." Likewise, many men have achieved self-esteem through work-related activities—creativity, productivity, and earning money. With the termination of these activities may come a loss of self-worth, resulting in depression in some individuals who are unable to adapt satisfactorily. Murray and Zentner (2001) list four developmental tasks related to successful adaptation in retirement:

● Remaining actively involved and having a sense of belonging unrelated to work
● Reevaluating life satisfaction related to family and social relations and spiritual life rather than to work

- Reevaluating the world's outlook, keeping a view of the world that is coherent and meaningful and a view that one's own world is meaningful
- Maintaining a sense of health, integrating mind and body to avoid complaints or illness when work is no longer the focus (p. 811)

American society often identifies an individual by his or her occupation. This is reflected in the conversation of people who are meeting each other for the first time. Undoubtedly, most everyone has either asked or been asked at some point in time, "What do you do?" or "Where do you work?" Occupation determines status, and retirement represents a significant change in status. The basic ambiguity of retirement occurs in an individual's or society's definition of this change. Is it undertaken voluntarily or involuntarily? Is it desirable or undesirable? Is one's status made better or worse by the change?

In looking at the trend of the past two decades, we may presume that retirement is becoming, and will continue to become, more accepted by societal standards. With more and more individuals retiring earlier and living longer, the growing number of aging people will spend a significantly longer time in retirement. At present, retirement has become more of an institutionalized expectation and there appears to be increasing acceptance of it as a social status.

Economical Implications

Because retirement is generally associated with 20 to 40 percent reduction in personal income, the standard of living after retirement may be adversely affected. Most older adults derive postretirement income from a combination of Social Security benefits, public and private pensions, and income from savings or investments.

In 2006, the median income in households containing families headed by persons 65 or older was $39,649 and 3.4 million elderly people were below the poverty level (AoA, 2008). The rate of those living in poverty was higher among women than men and higher among African Americans and Latino Americans than whites.

The Social Security Act of 1935 promised assistance with financial security for the elderly. Since then, the original legislation has been modified, yet the basic philosophy remains intact. Its effectiveness, however, is now being questioned. Faced with deficits, the program is forced to pay benefits to those currently retired from both the reserve funds and monies being collected at present. There is genuine concern about future generations, when there may be no reserve funds from which to draw. Because many of the programs that benefit older adults depend on contributions from the younger population, the growing ratio of older Americans to younger people may affect society's ability to supply the goods and services necessary to meet this expanding demand.

Medicare and **Medicaid** were established by the government to provide medical care benefits for elderly and indigent Americans. Medicaid funds are matched by the states, and coverage varies significantly from state to state. Medicare covers only a percentage of healthcare costs; therefore, to reduce risk related to out-of-pocket expenditures, many older adults purchase private "medigap" policies designed to cover charges in excess of those approved by Medicare.

The magnitude of retirement earnings depends almost entirely on pre-retirement income. The poor will remain poor and the wealthy are unlikely to lower their status during retirement; however, for many in the middle classes, the relatively fixed income sources may be inadequate, possibly forcing them to face financial hardship for the first time in their lives.

Long-Term Care

Stanley, Blair, and Beare (2005) state, "The concept of long-term care covers a broad spectrum of comprehensive health care that addresses both illness and wellness and the support services necessary to provide the physical, social, spiritual, and economic needs of persons with chronic illnesses, including disabilities" (p. 94). Long-term care facilities are defined by the level of care they provide. They may be skilled nursing facilities, intermediate care facilities, or a combination of the two. Some institutions provide convalescent care for individuals recovering from acute illness or injury, some provide long-term care for individuals with chronic illness or disabilities, and still others provide both types of assistance.

Most elderly individuals prefer to remain in their own homes or in the homes of family members for as long as this can meet their needs without deterioration of family or social patterns. Many elderly individuals are placed in institutions as a last resort only after heroic efforts have been made to keep them in their own or a relative's home. The increasing emphasis on home health care has extended the period of independence for aging individuals.

Fewer than 5 percent of the population aged 65 and older live in nursing homes. The percentage increases dramatically with age, ranging from 1.3 percent for persons aged 65 to 74, 4.4 percent for persons aged 75 to 84, to 15.4 percent for persons aged 85 and older (AoA, 2008). A profile of the "typical" elderly nursing home resident is about 80 years of age, white, female, widowed, with multiple chronic health conditions.

Risk Factors for Institutionalization

In determining who in our society will need long-term care, several factors have been identified that appear to place people at risk. The following risk factors are taken into consideration to predict potential need for services and to estimate future costs.

Age. Because people grow older in very different ways, and the range of differences becomes greater with the passage of time, age is becoming a less relevant characteristic than it was historically. However, because of the high prevalence of chronic health conditions and disabilities, as well as the greater chance of diminishing social supports associated with advancing age, the 65-and-older population is often viewed as an important long-term care target group.

Health. Level of functioning, as determined by ability to perform various behaviors or activities—such as bathing, eating, mobility, meal preparation, handling finances, judgment, and memory—is a measurable risk factor. The need for ongoing assistance from another person is critical in determining the need for long-term care.

Mental Health Status. Mental health problems are risk factors in assessing need for long-term care. Many of the symptoms associated with certain mental disorders (especially the dementias) such as memory loss, impaired judgment, impaired intellect, and disorientation would render the individual incapable of meeting the demands of daily living independently.

Socioeconomic and Demographic Factors. Low income generally is associated with greater physical and mental health problems among the elderly. Because many elderly individuals have limited finances, they are less able to purchase care resources available outside of institutions (e.g., home healthcare), although Medicare and Medicaid now contribute a limited amount to this type of noninstitutionalized care.

Women are at greater risk of being institutionalized than men, not because they are less healthy but because they tend to live longer and, thus, reach the age at which more functional and cognitive impairments occur. They are also more likely to be widowed. Whites have a higher rate of institutionalization than nonwhites. This may be related to cultural and financial influences.

Marital Status, Living Arrangements, and the Informal Support Network. Individuals who are married and live with a spouse are the least likely of all disabled people to be institutionalized. Those who live alone without resources for home care and with few or no relatives living nearby to provide informal care are at higher risk for institutionalization.

Attitudinal Factors

Many people dread the thought of even visiting a nursing home, let alone moving to one or placing a relative in one. The media picture and subsequent reputation of nursing homes has not been positive. Stories of substandard care and patient abuse have scarred the industry, making it difficult for those facilities that are clean, well-managed, and provide innovative, quality care to their residents to rise above the stigma.

State and national licensing boards perform periodic inspections to ensure that standards set forth by the federal government are being met. These standards address quality of patient care as well as adequacy of the nursing home facility. Yet, many elderly individuals and their families perceive nursing homes as a place to go to die, and the fact that many of these institutions are poorly equipped, understaffed, and disorganized keeps this societal perception alive. There are, however, many excellent nursing homes that strive to go beyond the minimum federal regulations for Medicaid and Medicare reimbursement. In addition to medical, nursing, rehabilitation, and dental services, social and recreational services are provided to increase the quality of life for elderly people living in nursing homes. These activities include playing cards, bingo, and other games; parties; church activities; books; television; movies; and arts, crafts, and other classes. Some nursing homes provide occupational and professional counseling. These facilities strive to enhance opportunities for improving quality of life and for becoming "places to live," rather than "places to die."

Elder Abuse

Abuse of elderly individuals, which at times has been referred to in the media as "**granny-bashing**," is a serious form of family violence. Sadock and Sadock (2007) estimate that 10 percent of individuals older than age 65 are the victims of abuse or neglect. The abuser is often a relative who lives with the elderly person and may be the assigned caregiver. Typical caregivers who are likely to be abusers of the elderly were described by Murray and Zentner (2001) as being under economic stress, substance abusers, themselves the victims of previous family violence, and exhausted and frustrated by the caregiver role. Identified risk factors for victims of abuse included being a white female age 70 and older, being mentally or physically impaired, being unable to meet daily self-care needs, and having care needs that exceeded the caretaker's ability.

Abuse of elderly individuals may be psychological, physical, or financial. Neglect may be intentional or unintentional. Psychological abuse includes yelling, insulting, harsh commands, threats, silence, and social isolation. Physical abuse is described as striking, shoving, beating, or restraint. Financial abuse refers to misuse or theft of finances, property, or material possessions. Neglect implies failure to fulfill the physical needs of an individual who cannot do so independently. Unintentional neglect is inadvertent, whereas intentional neglect is deliberate. In addition, elderly individuals may be the victims of sexual abuse, which is sexual intimacy between two persons that occurs without the consent of one of the persons involved. Another type of abuse, which has been called "**granny-dumping**" by the media, involves abandoning elderly

BOX 35 – 1 Examples of Elder Abuse

Physical Abuse

Striking, hitting, beating
Shoving
Bruising
Cutting
Restraining

Psychological Abuse

Yelling
Insulting, name-calling
Harsh commands
Threats
Ignoring, silence, social isolation
Withholding of affection

Neglect (intentional or unintentional)

Withholding food and water
Inadequate heating
Unclean clothes and bedding
Lack of needed medication
Lack of eyeglasses, hearing aids, false teeth

Financial Abuse or Exploitation

Misuse of the elderly person's income by the caregiver
Forcing the elderly person to sign over financial affairs to
  another person against his or her will or without sufficient knowledge about the transaction

Sexual Abuse

Sexual molestation; rape
Any type of sexual intimacy against the elderly person's will

SOURCES: Stanley, Blair, & Beare (2005); Sadock & Sadock (2007);
and Murray & Zentner (2001).

individuals at emergency departments, nursing homes, or other facilities—literally leaving them in the hands of others when the strain of caregiving becomes intolerable. Types of elder abuse are summarized in Box 35–1.

Elder victims often minimize the abuse or deny that it has occurred. The elderly person may be unwilling to disclose information because of fear of retaliation, embarrassment about the existence of abuse in the family, protectiveness toward a family member, or unwillingness to institute legal action. Adding to this unwillingness to report is the fact that infirm elders are often isolated so their mistreatment is less likely to be noticed by those who might be alert to symptoms of abuse. For these reasons, detection of abuse in the elderly is difficult at best.

Factors that Contribute to Abuse

A number of contributing factors have been implicated in the abuse of elderly individuals.

Longer Life. The 65-and-older age group has become the fastest growing segment of the population. Within this segment, the number of elderly older than age 75 has increased most rapidly. This trend is expected to continue well into the 21st century. The 75 and older age group is the one most likely to be physically or mentally impaired, requiring assistance and care from family members. This group also is the most vulnerable to abuse from caregivers.

Dependency. Dependency appears to be the most common precondition in domestic abuse. Changes associated with normal aging or induced by chronic illness often result in loss of self-sufficiency in the elderly person, requiring that they become dependent on another for assistance with daily functioning. Long life may also consume finances to the point that the elderly individual becomes financially dependent on another as well. This dependence increases the elderly person's vulnerability to abuse.

Stress. The stress inherent in the caregiver role is a factor in most abuse cases. Some clinicians believe that elder abuse results from individual or family psychopathology. Others suggest that even psychologically healthy family members can become abusive as the result of the exhaustion and acute stress caused by overwhelming caregiving responsibilities. This is compounded in an age group that has been dubbed the "sandwich generation"—those individuals who elected to delay childbearing so that they are now at a point in their lives when they are "sandwiched" between providing care for their children and providing care for their aging parents.

Learned Violence. Children who have been abused or witnessed abusive and violent parents are more likely to evolve into abusive adults. Stanley, Blair, and Beare (2005) state:

Violence is a learned behavior that is passed down from generation to generation in some families because violence has been modeled as an acceptable coping behavior, with no substantial penalties for the behavior. This model suggests that a child who grows up in a violent family will also become violent. Some believe that elder mistreatment may be related to retribution on the part of an adult offspring who was abused as a child. (p. 290)

Identifying Elder Abuse

Because so many elderly individuals are reluctant to report personal abuse, healthcare workers need to be able to detect signs of mistreatment when they are in a position to do so. Box 35–1 listed a number of *types* of elder abuse. The following *manifestations* of the various categories of abuse have been identified (Murray & Zentner, 2001; Stanley, Blair, & Beare, 2005):

● Indicators of psychological abuse include a broad range of behaviors such as the symptoms associated with depression, withdrawal, anxiety, sleep disorders, and increased confusion or agitation.

- Indicators of physical abuse may include bruises, welts, lacerations, burns, punctures, evidence of hair pulling, and skeletal dislocations and fractures.
- Neglect may be manifested as consistent hunger, poor hygiene, inappropriate dress, consistent lack of supervision, consistent fatigue or listlessness, unattended physical problems or medical needs, or abandonment.
- Sexual abuse may be suspected when the elderly person is presented with pain or itching in the genital area, bruising or bleeding in external genitalia, vaginal, or anal areas, or unexplained sexually transmitted disease.
- Financial abuse may be occurring when there is an obvious disparity between assets and satisfactory living conditions or when the elderly person complains of a sudden lack of sufficient funds for daily living expenses.

Healthcare workers often feel intimidated when confronted with cases of elder abuse. In these instances, referral to an individual experienced in management of victims of such abuse may be the most effective approach to evaluation and intervention. Healthcare workers are responsible for reporting any suspicions of elder abuse. An investigation is then conducted by regulatory agencies, whose job it is to determine if the suspicions are corroborated. Every effort must be made to ensure the client's safety, but it is important to remember that a competent elderly person has the right to choose his or her healthcare options. As inappropriate as it may seem, some elderly individuals choose to return to the abusive situation. In this instance, he or she should be provided with names and phone numbers to call for assistance if needed. A follow-up visit by an adult protective service representative should be conducted.

Increased efforts need to be made to ensure that healthcare providers have comprehensive training in the detection of and intervention in elder abuse. More research is needed to increase knowledge and understanding of the phenomenon of elder abuse and ultimately to effect more sophisticated strategies for prevention, intervention, and treatment.

Suicide

Although persons older than age 65 comprise only 12.4 percent of the population, they represent a disproportionately high percentage of individuals who commit suicide. Of all suicides, 16 percent are committed by this age group (American Association of Suicidology [AAS], 2006). The group especially at risk appears to be white men. Predisposing factors include loneliness, financial problems, physical illness, loss, and depression (Sadock & Sadock, 2007).

Although the rate of suicide among the elderly remains high, the numbers of suicides among this age group dropped steadily from 1930 to 1980. Investigators who study these trends surmise that this decline was due

to increases in services for older people and an understanding of their problems in society. Then from 1980 to 1986, the number of suicides among people age 65 and older increased by 25 percent, which suggests that other factors are contributing to the problem. However, since 1987, there has been a gradual decline in the number of elderly suicides.

It has been suggested that increased social isolation may be a contributing factor to suicide among the elderly. The number of elderly individuals who are divorced, widowed, or otherwise living alone has increased. Men seem especially vulnerable after the loss of a spouse, with a relative risk three times that of married men (O'Connell et al., 2004).

The National Institute of Mental Health [NIMH] (2006) suggests that major depression is a significant predictor of suicide in older adults. Unfortunately, it is widely under-recognized and under-treated by the medical community. The NIMH (2006) states:

> Several studies have found that many older adults who die by suicide—up to 75 percent—have visited a primary care physician within a month of their suicide. These findings point to the urgency of enhancing both the detection and the adequate treatment of depression as a means of reducing suicide risk among older persons.

Many elderly individuals express symptoms associated with depression that are never recognized as such. Any sign of helplessness or hopelessness should elicit a supportive intervening response. Stanley, Blair, and Beare (2005) suggest that, in assessing suicide intention, while using concern and compassion, direct questions such as the following should be asked:

- Have you thought life is not worth living?
- Have you considered harming yourself?
- Do you have a plan for hurting yourself?
- Have you ever acted on that plan?
- Have you ever attempted suicide?

Components of intervention with a suicidal elderly person should include demonstrations of genuine concern, interest, and caring; indications of empathy for their fears and concerns; and help in identifying, clarifying, and formulating a plan of action to deal with the unresolved issue. If the elderly person's behavior seems particularly lethal, additional family or staff coverage and contact should be arranged to prevent isolation.

APPLICATION OF THE NURSING PROCESS

Assessment

Assessment of the elderly individual may follow the same framework used for all adults, but with consideration of the possible biological, psychological, sociocultural, and sexual changes that occur in the normal aging process described previously in this chapter. In no other area of nursing is it more important for nurses to practice holistic nursing than with the elderly. Older adults are likely to have multiple physical problems that contribute to problems in other areas of their lives. Obviously, these components cannot be addressed as separate entities. Nursing the elderly is a multifaceted, challenging process because of the multiple changes occurring at this time in the life cycle and the way in which each change affects every aspect of the individual.

Several considerations are unique to assessment of the elderly. Assessment of the older person's thought processes is a primary responsibility. Knowledge about the presence and extent of disorientation or confusion will influence the way in which the nurse approaches elder care.

Information about sensory capabilities is also extremely important. Because hearing loss is common, the nurse should lower the pitch and loudness of his or her voice when addressing the older person. Looking directly into the face of the older person when talking facilitates communication. Questions that require a declarative sentence in response should be asked; in this way, the nurse is able to assess the client's ability to use words correctly. Visual acuity can be determined by assessing adaptation to the dark, color matching, and the perception of color contrast. Knowledge about these aspects of sensory functioning is essential in the development of an effective care plan.

The nurse should be familiar with the normal physical changes associated with the aging process. Examples of some of these changes include:

● Less effective response to changes in environmental temperature, resulting in hypothermia.
● Decreases in oxygen use and the amount of blood pumped by the heart, resulting in cerebral anoxia or hypoxia.
● Skeletal muscle wasting and weakness, resulting in difficulty in physical mobility.
● Limited cough and laryngeal reflexes, resulting in risk of aspiration.
● Demineralization of bones, resulting in spontaneous fracturing.
● Decrease in gastrointestinal motility, resulting in constipation.
● Decrease in the ability to interpret painful stimuli, resulting in risk of injury.

Common psychosocial changes associated with aging include:

● Prolonged and exaggerated grief, resulting in depression.
● Physical changes, resulting in disturbed body image.
● Changes in status, resulting in loss of self-worth.

This list is by no means exhaustive. The nurse should consider many other alterations in his or her assessment of the client. Knowledge of the client's functional capabilities is essential for determining the physiological, psychological, and sociological needs of the elderly individual. Age alone does not preclude the occurrence of all these changes. The aging process progresses at a wide range of variance, and each client must be assessed as a unique individual.

Diagnosis/Outcome Identification

Virtually any nursing diagnosis may be applicable to the aging client, depending on individual needs for assistance. Based on normal changes that occur in the elderly, the following nursing diagnoses may be considered:

Physiologically Related Diagnoses

● Risk for trauma related to confusion, disorientation, muscular weakness, spontaneous fractures, falls.
● Hypothermia related to loss of adipose tissue under the skin, evidenced by increased sensitivity to cold and body temperature below 98.6 degrees.
● Decreased cardiac output related to decreased myocardial efficiency secondary to age-related changes, evidenced by decreased tolerance for activity and decline in energy reserve.
● Ineffective breathing pattern related to increase in fibrous tissue and loss of elasticity in lung tissue, evidenced by dyspnea and activity intolerance.
● Risk for aspiration related to diminished cough and laryngeal reflexes.
● Impaired physical mobility related to muscular wasting and weakness, evidenced by need for assistance in ambulation.
● Imbalanced nutrition, less than body requirements, related to inefficient absorption from gastrointestinal tract, difficulty chewing and swallowing, anorexia, difficulty in feeding self, evidenced by wasting syndrome, anemia, weight loss.
● Constipation related to decreased motility; inadequate diet; insufficient activity or exercise, evidenced by decreased bowel sounds; hard, formed stools; or straining at stool.
● Stress urinary incontinence related to degenerative changes in pelvic muscles and structural supports associated with increased age, evidenced by reported or observed dribbling with increased abdominal pressure or urinary frequency.
● Urinary retention related to prostatic enlargement, evidenced by bladder distention, frequent voiding of small amounts, dribbling, or overflow incontinence.
● Disturbed sensory perception related to age-related alterations in sensory transmission, evidenced by

- The elderly population represents a disproportionately high percentage of individuals who commit suicide.
- Dementing disorders are the most frequent causes of psychopathology in the elderly. Sleep disorders are very common.
- The need for sexual expression by the elderly is often misunderstood within our society. Although many physical changes occur at this time of life that alter an individual's sexuality, if he or she has reasonably good health and a willing partner, sexual activity can continue well past the 70s for most people.
- Retirement has both social and economical implications for elderly individuals. Society often equates an individual's status with occupation, and loss of employment may result in the need for adjustment in the standard of living because retirement income may be reduced by 20 to 40 percent of pre-retirement earnings.
- Less than 5 percent of the population aged 65 and older live in nursing homes. A profile of the typical elderly nursing home resident is a white woman about 78 years old, widowed, with multiple chronic health conditions. Much stigma is attached to what some still call "rest homes" or "old age homes," and many elderly people still equate them with a place "to go to die."
- The strain of the caregiver role has become a major dilemma in our society. Elder abuse is sometimes inflicted by caregivers for whom the role has become overwhelming and intolerable. There is an intense need to find assistance for these people, who must provide care for their loved ones on a 24-hour basis. Home health care, respite care, support groups, and financial assistance are needed to ease the burden of this role strain.
- Caring for elderly individuals requires a special kind of inner strength and compassion. The poem that follows conveys a vital message for nurses.

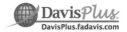

DavisPlus
DavisPlus.fadavis.com   **For additional clinical tools and study aids, visit DavisPlus.**

What Do You See, Nurse?

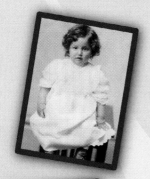

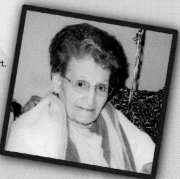

What do you see, nurse, what do you see?
    What are you thinking when you look at me?
A crabbed old woman, not very wise.
    Uncertain of habit, with faraway eyes.
Who dribbles her food and makes no reply
    When you say in a loud voice, "I do wish you'd try."
Who seems not to notice the things that you do
    And forever is losing a stocking or shoe.
Who unresisting or not, lets you do as you will
    With bathing and feeding, the long day to fill.
Is that what you're thinking, is that what you see?
    Then open your eyes, you're not looking at me.
I'll tell you who I am as I sit there so still.
    As I move at your bidding, as I eat at your will.
I'm a small child of ten with a father and a mother,
    Brothers and sisters who love one another.

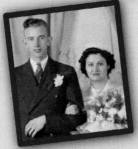

A young girl at sixteen with wings on her feet
    Dreaming that soon now a lover she'll meet.
A bride soon at twenty—my heart gives a leap
    Remembering the vows that I promised to keep.
At twenty-five, now, I have young of my own
    Who need me to build a secure happy home.
A woman of thirty, my young now grow fast
    Bound to each other with ties that should last.

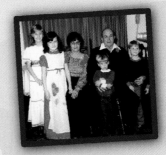

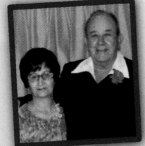

At forty my young will now soon be gone,
    But my man stays beside me to see I don't mourn.
At fifty once more babies play round my knee.
    Again we know children, my loved one and me.

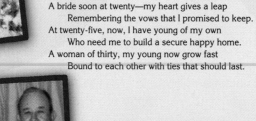

Dark days are upon me, my husband is dead.
    I look at the future, I shudder with dread.
For my young are all busy rearing young of their own.
    And I think of the years and the love I have known.

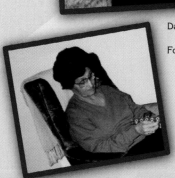

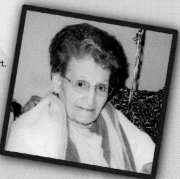

I'm an old woman now and nature is cruel.
    Tis her jest to make old age look like a fool.
The body it crumbles, grace and vigor depart.
    There is now just a stone where I once had a heart.
But inside this old carcass a young girl still dwells.
    And now and again my battered heart swells.

I remember the joys, I remember the pain.
    And I'm loving and living life all over again.
I think of the years all too few—gone so fast.
    And accept the stark fact that nothing can last.
So open your eyes, nurse, open and see.
    Not a crabbed old woman—look closer—SEE ME.

Author Unknown

REVIEW QUESTIONS

Self-Examination/Learning Exercise

Select the answer that is most appropriate for each of the following questions.

Situation: Stanley, a 72-year-old widower, was brought to the hospital by his son, who reports that Stanley has become increasingly withdrawn. He has periods of confusion and forgetfulness, but most of the time his thought processes are intact. He eats very little and has lost some weight. His wife died 5 years ago and the son reports, "He did very well. He didn't even cry." Stanley attended the funeral of his best friend 1 month ago, after which these symptoms began. Stanley has been admitted for testing and evaluation.

1. In her admission assessment, the nurse notices an open sore on Stanley's arm. When she questions him about it he says, "I scraped it on the fence 2 weeks ago. It's smaller than it was." How might the nurse analyze these data?

   a. Stanley was trying to commit suicide.
   b. The delay in healing may indicate that Stanley has developed skin cancer.
   c. A diminished inflammatory response in the elderly increases healing time.
   d. Age-related skin changes and distribution of adipose tissue delay healing in the elderly.

2. Stanley is deaf on his right side. Which is the most appropriate nursing intervention for communicating with Stanley?

   a. Speak loudly into his left ear.
   b. Speak to him from a position on his left side.
   c. Speak face-to-face in a high-pitched voice.
   d. Speak face-to-face in a low-pitched voice.

3. Why is it important to have the nurse check the temperature of the water before Stanley takes a shower?

   a. Stanley may catch cold if the water temperature is too low.
   b. Stanley may burn himself because of a higher pain threshold.
   c. Stanley has difficulty discriminating between hot and cold.
   d. The water must be exactly 98.6°F.

4. From the information provided in the situation, which would be the priority nursing diagnosis for Stanley?

   a. Complicated grieving
   b. Imbalanced nutrition: less than body requirements
   c. Social isolation
   d. Risk for injury

5. The physician diagnoses Stanley with major depression. A suicide assessment is conducted. Why is Stanley at high risk for suicide?

   a. All depressed people are at high risk for suicide.
   b. Stanley is in the age group in which the highest percentage of suicides occur.
   c. Stanley is a white man, recently bereaved, living alone.
   d. His son reports that Stanley owns a gun.

6. Which of the following would be a *priority* nursing intervention with Stanley?

   a. Take blood pressure once each shift.
   b. Ensure that Stanley attends group activities.
   c. Encourage Stanley to eat all of the food on his food tray.
   d. Encourage Stanley to talk about his wife's death.

7. In group exercise, Stanley becomes tired and short of breath very quickly. This is most likely due to:

   a. Age-related changes in the cardiovascular system.
   b. Stanley's sedentary lifestyle.

    c. The effects of pathological depression.

    d. Medication the physician has prescribed for depression.

8. Stanley says to the nurse, "I'm all alone now. My wife is gone. My best friend is gone. My son is busy with his work and family. I might as well just go, too." Which is the best response by the nurse?

    a. "Are you thinking that you want to die, Stanley?"

    b. "You have lots to live for, Stanley."

    c. "Cheer up, Stanley. You have so much to be thankful for."

    d. "Tell me about your family, Stanley."

9. Stanley says to the nurse, "I don't want to go to that crafts class. I'm too old to learn anything." Based on knowledge of the aging process, which of the following is a true statement?

    a. Memory functioning in the elderly most likely reflects loss of long-term memories of remote events.

    b. Intellectual functioning declines with advancing age.

    c. Learning ability remains intact, but time required for learning increases with age.

    d. Cognitive functioning is rarely affected in aging individuals.

10. According to the literature, which of the following is most important for Stanley to maintain a healthy, adaptive old age?

    a. To remain socially interactive

    b. To disengage slowly in preparation of the last stage of life

    c. To move in with his son and family

    d. To maintain total independence and accept no help from anyone

Test Your Critical Thinking Skills

Mrs. M., age 76, is seeing her primary physician for her regular 6-month physical exam. Mrs. M's husband died 2 years ago, at which time she sold her home in Kansas and came to live in California with her only child, a daughter. The daughter is married and has 3 children (one in college and two teenagers at home). The daughter reports that her mother is becoming increasingly withdrawn, stays in her room, and eats very little. She has lost 13 pounds since her last 6-month visit. The primary physician refers Mrs. M. to a psychiatrist who hospitalizes her for evaluation. He diagnoses Mrs. M. with Major Depression.

Mrs. M. tells the nurse, "I didn't want to leave my home, but my daughter insisted. I would have been all right. I miss my friends and my church. Back home I drove my car everywhere. But there's too much traffic out here. They sold my car and I have to depend on my daughter or grandkids to take me places.

I hate being so dependent! I miss my husband so much. I just sit and think about him and our past life all the time. I don't have any interest in meeting new people. I want to go home!!"

Mrs. M. admits to having some thoughts of dying, although she denies feeling suicidal. She denies having a plan or means for taking her life. "I really don't want to die, but I just can't see much reason for living. My daughter and her family are so busy with their own lives. They don't need me—or even have time for me!"

Answer the following questions about Mrs. M:

1. What would be the *primary* nursing diagnosis for Mrs. M.?
2. Formulate a short-term goal for Mrs. M.
3. From the assessment data, identify the major problem that may be a long-term focus of care for Mrs. M.

REFERENCES

American Association of Retired Persons (AARP). (2005). *Sexuality at Midlife and Beyond: 2004 Update of Attitudes and Behaviors.* Retrieved April 5, 2007 from http://www.aarp.org/research/family/lifestyles/2004_sexuality.html

Administration on Aging (AoA). (2008). *A profile of older Americans: 2007.* Washington, DC: U.S. Department of Health and Human Services.

Altman, A., & Hanfling, S. (2003). *Sexuality in midlife and beyond.* Boston, MA: Harvard Health Publications.

American Geriatrics Society. (2005). Summary of Geriatric and Chronic Care Management Act of 2005 (S. 40/H.R. 467). Retrieved April 5, 2007 from http://www.americangeriatrics.org/policy/summ_gerchroniccaremgmt05PF.shtml

American Association of Suicidology (AAS). (2006). *Elderly suicide fact sheet.* Retrieved on July 7, 2007 from http://www.suicidology.org

Beers, M.H., & Jones, T.V. (Eds.). (2004). *The Merck manual of health & aging.* Whitehouse Station, NJ: Merck Research Laboratories.

Blazer, D. (2008).Treatment of seniors. In R.E. Hales, S.C. Yudofsky, & G.O. Gabbard (Eds.), *Textbook of psychiatry* (5th ed.). Washington, DC: American Psychiatric Publishing.

Giger, J.N., & Davidhizar, R.E. (2004). *Transcultural nursing: Assessment and intervention* (4th ed.). St. Louis: C.V. Mosby.

King, B.M. (2005). *Human sexuality today* (5th ed.). Upper Saddle River, NJ: Pearson Prentice-Hall.

Masters, W.H., Johnson, V.E., & Kolodny, R.C. (1995). *Human sexuality* (5th ed.). New York: Addison-Wesley Longman.

Murray, R.B., & Zentner, J.P. (2001). *Health promotion strategies through the life span* (7th ed.). Upper Saddle River, NJ: Prentice-Hall.

National Center for Health Statistics (NCHS). (2007). *Health, United States, 2007.* U.S. Department of Health and Human Services, Centers for Disease Control and Prevention. DHHS Publication No. 2007–1232.

National Center for Health Statistics (NCHS). (2006). *Older Americans Update 2006: Key indicators of well-being.* Federal Interagency Forum on Aging-Related Statistics. Washington, DC: U.S. Government Printing Office.

National Institute of Mental Health [NIMH]. (2006). *Older adults: Depression and suicide facts.* Retrieved April 5, 2007 from http://www.nimh.nih.gov/publicat/elderlydepsuicide.cfm

O'Connell, H., Chin, A.V., Cunningham, C., & Lawlor, B.A. (2004). Recent developments: Suicide in older people. *British Medical Journal, 329,* 895–899.

Pietraniec-Shannon, M. (2003). Nursing care of elderly patients. In L.S. Williams & P.D. Hopper (Eds.), *Understanding medical-surgical nursing* (2nd ed.). Philadelphia: F.A. Davis.

Roberts, C.M. (1991). *How did I get here so fast?* New York: Warner Books.

Rogers-Seidl, F.F. (1997). *Geriatric nursing care plans* (2nd ed.). St. Louis: Mosby Year Book.

Rossouw, J.E., Anderson, G.L., Prentice, R.L., LaCroix, A.Z., Kooperberg, C., Stefanick, M.L., Jackson, R.D., Beresford, S.A.A., Howard, B.V., Johnson, K.C., Kotchen, J.M., & Ockene, J. (2002, July 17). Risks and benefits of estrogen plus progestin in healthy postmenopausal women: Principal results from the Women's Health Initiative randomized controlled trial. *Journal of the American Medical Association, 288*(3), 321–333, 366–368.

Sadock, B.J., & Sadock, V.A. (2007). *Synopsis of psychiatry: Behavioral sciences/clinical psychiatry* (10th ed.). Philadelphia: Lippincott Williams & Wilkins.

Srivastava, S., John, O.P., Gosling, S.D., & Potter, J. (2003). Development of personality in early and middle adulthood: Set like plaster or persistent change? *Journal of Personality and Social Psychology, 84*(5), 1041–1053.

Stanley, M., Blair, K.A., & Beare, P.G. (2005). *Gerontological nursing: Promoting successful aging with older adults* (3rd ed.). Philadelphia: F.A. Davis.

Vaillant, G.E. (2003). *Aging Well: Surprising guideposts to a happier life from the landmark Harvard study of adult development.* New York: Little, Brown, & Company.

CLASSICAL REFERENCES

Erikson, E.H. (1963). *Childhood and society* (2nd ed.). New York: W.W. Norton.

Kübler-Ross, E. (1969). *On death and dying.* New York: Macmillan.

Reichard, S., Livson, F., & Peterson, P.G. (1962). *Aging and personality.* New York: John Wiley & Sons.

 ## Internet References

● Additional sources related to aging are located at the following Web sites:
  - http://www.4woman.org/Menopause
  - http://www.aarp.org/
  - http://www.oaktrees.org/elder/
  - http://www.acjnet.org/docs/eldabpfv.html
  - http://www.ssa.gov/
  - http://www.nih.gov/nia/
  - http://www.medicare.gov/
  - http://www.seniorlaw.com/
  - http://www.growthhouse.org/cesp.html
  - http://www.agenet.com/
  - http://www.aoa.dhhs.gov/
  - http://www.nsclc.org/

36
CHAPTER

Victims of Abuse
or Neglect

CHAPTER OUTLINE

OBJECTIVES

HISTORICAL PERSPECTIVES

PREDISPOSING FACTORS

APPLICATION OF THE NURSING PROCESS

TREATMENT MODALITIES

SUMMARY AND KEY POINTS

REVIEW QUESTIONS

KEY TERMS

acquaintance rape
child sexual abuse
compounded rape
    reaction
controlled response
    pattern
cycle of battering
date rape
emotional abuse
emotional neglect

expressed response
    pattern
marital rape
physical neglect
safe house or shelter
sexual exploitation of a
    child
silent rape reaction
statutory rape

CORE CONCEPTS

abuse
battering
incest
neglect
rape

OBJECTIVES

After reading this chapter, the student will be able to:

1. Discuss historical perspectives associated with intimate partner abuse, child abuse, and sexual assault.
2. Describe epidemiological statistics associated with intimate partner abuse, child abuse, and sexual assault.
3. Discuss characteristics of victims and victimizers.
4. Identify predisposing factors to abusive behaviors.
5. Describe physical and psychological effects on the victims of intimate

partner abuse, child abuse, and sexual assault.
6. Identify nursing diagnoses, goals of care, and appropriate nursing interventions for care of victims of intimate partner abuse, child abuse, and sexual assault.
7. Evaluate nursing care of victims of intimate partner abuse, child abuse, and sexual assault.
8. Discuss various modalities relevant to treatment of victims of abuse.

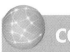

CORE CONCEPT

Abuse
The maltreatment of one person by another.

Abuse is on the rise in this society. Books, newspapers, movies, and television inundate their readers and viewers with stories of "man's inhumanity to man" (no gender bias intended).

Nearly 5.3 million intimate partner victimizations occur each year among United States women ages 18 and older, and 3.2 million occur among men (Centers for Disease Control and Prevention [CDC], 2006). More injuries are attributed to intimate partner violence than to all rapes, muggings, and automobile accidents combined.

Rape is vastly underreported in the United States. Because many of these attacks occurring daily go unreported and unrecognized, sexual assault can be considered a silent-violent epidemic in the United States today.

An increase in the incidence of child abuse and related fatalities has also been documented. In 2005, an estimated 3.3 million cases of possible child abuse or neglect were reported to child protective services, and about 30 percent of these cases were substantiated (U.S. Department of Health and Human Services [USDHHS], 2007). An estimated 1,460 children died from causes related to abuse or neglect in 2005.

Abuse affects all populations equally. It occurs among all races, religions, economic classes, ages, and educational backgrounds. The phenomenon is cyclical in that many abusers were themselves victims of abuse as children.

This chapter discusses intimate partner violence, child abuse (including neglect), and sexual assault. Elder abuse is discussed in Chapter 35. Factors that predispose individuals to commit acts of abuse against others, as well as the physical and psychological effects on the victims, are examined.

Nursing of individuals who have experienced abusive behavior from others is presented within the context of the nursing process. Various treatment modalities are described.

HISTORICAL PERSPECTIVES

Family violence is not a new problem; in fact, it is probably as old as humankind and has been documented as far back as Biblical times. In the United States, spouse and child abuse arrived with the Puritans; however, it was not until 1973 that public outrage initiated an active movement against the practice. Child abuse became a mandatory reportable occurrence in the United States in 1968. Responsibility for the protection of elders from abuse rests primarily with the states. In 1987, Congress passed

amendments to the Older Americans Act of 1965 that provide for state Area Agencies on Aging to assess the need for elder abuse prevention services. These events have made it possible for individuals who once felt powerless to stop the abuse against them, to come forward and seek advice, support, and protection.

Historically, violence against female partners (whether in a married or an unmarried intimate relationship) has not been considered a social problem but rather a fact of life. Some individuals have been socialized within their cultural context to accept violence against women in relationships (American Nurses Association [ANA], 1998).

From Roman times until the beginning of the 20th century, women were considered the personal property of men. Very early on in Roman times, women were purchased as brides, and their status, as well as that of their children, was closely akin to that of slaves. Violent beatings and even death occurred if women acted contrary to their husband's wishes or to the social code of the time.

Women historically have been socialized to view themselves as sexual objects. In early Biblical times, women were expected to subjugate themselves to the will of men, and those who refused were often severely punished. Rape is largely a crime against women, although men and children also fall victim to this heinous act. Rape is the extreme manifestation of the domination of one individual over another. Rape is viewed as a ritual of power.

During the Puritan era, "spare the rod and spoil the child" was a theme supported by the Bible. Children were considered the property of their parents and could be treated accordingly. Harsh treatment by parents was justified by the belief that severe physical punishment was necessary to maintain discipline, transmit educational decisions, and expel evil spirits. Change began in the mid-19th and early 20th centuries with the child welfare movement and the passage of laws for the protection of children.

Historical examination reveals an inclination toward violence among human beings from very early in civilization. Little has changed, for violence permeates every aspect of today's society, the victims of which are inundating the health care system. Aside from the individual physical, psychological, and social devastation that violence incurs, there are economic implications as well. The World Health Organization (WHO) reports that in the United States alone, costs related to interpersonal violence reach 3.3 percent of the gross domestic product (WHO, 2005).

PREDISPOSING FACTORS

What predisposes individuals to be abusive? Although no one really knows for sure, several theories have been espoused. A brief discussion of ideas associated with biological, psychological, and sociocultural views is presented here.

Biological Theories

Neurophysiological Influences

Various components of the neurological system in both humans and animals have been implicated in both the facilitation and inhibition of aggressive impulses. Areas of the brain that may be involved include the temporal lobe, the limbic system, and the amygdaloid nucleus (Tardiff, 2003).

Biochemical Influences

Studies show that various neurotransmitters—in particular norepinephrine, dopamine, and serotonin—may play a role in the facilitation and inhibition of aggressive impulses (Hollander, Berlin, & Stein, 2008). This theory is consistent with the "fight or flight" arousal described by Selye (1956) in his theory of the response to stress, which was described in Chapter 1. An explanation of these biochemical influences on violent behavior is presented in Figure 36–1.

Genetic Influences

Various genetic components related to aggressive behavior have been investigated. Some studies have linked increased aggressiveness with selective inbreeding in mice, suggesting the possibility of a direct genetic link. Another genetic characteristic that was once thought to have some implication for aggressive behavior was the genetic karyotype XYY. The XYY syndrome has been found to contribute to aggressive behavior in a small percentage of cases (Sadock & Sadock, 2007). The evidence linking this chromosomal aberration to aggressive and deviant behavior has not yet been firmly established.

Disorders of the Brain

Organic brain syndromes associated with various cerebral disorders have been implicated in the predisposition to aggressive and violent behavior (Sadock & Sadock, 2007; Cummings & Mega, 2003; Tardiff, 2003). Brain tumors, particularly in the areas of the limbic system and the temporal lobes; trauma to the brain, resulting in cerebral changes; and diseases, such as encephalitis (or medications that may effect this syndrome) and epilepsy, particularly temporal lobe epilepsy, have all been implicated.

Psychological Theories

Psychodynamic Theory

The psychodynamic theorists imply that unmet needs for satisfaction and security result in an underdeveloped ego and a weak superego. It is thought that when frustration occurs, aggression and violence supply this individual with a dose of power and prestige that boosts the self-image and validates a significance to his or her life that is lacking. The immature ego cannot prevent dominant id behaviors from occurring, and the weak superego is unable to produce feelings of guilt.

Learning Theory

Children learn to behave by imitating their role models, which are usually their parents. Models are more likely to be imitated when they are perceived as prestigious or influential, or when the behavior is followed by positive reinforcement. Children may have an idealistic perception of their parents during the very early developmental stages but, as they mature, may begin to imitate the behavior patterns of their teachers, friends, and others. Individuals who were abused as children or whose parents disciplined with physical punishment are more likely to behave in an abusive manner as adults (Tardiff, 2003).

Adults and children alike model many of their behaviors after individuals they observe on television and in movies. Unfortunately, modeling can result in maladaptive as well as adaptive behavior, particularly when children view heroes triumphing over villains by using violence. It is also possible that individuals who have a biological predisposition toward aggressive behavior may be more susceptible to negative role modeling.

Sociocultural Theories

Societal Influences

Although they agree that perhaps some biological and psychological aspects are influential, social scientists believe that aggressive behavior is primarily a product of one's culture and social structure.

American society essentially was founded on a general acceptance of violence as a means of solving problems. The concept of relative deprivation has been shown to have a profound effect on collective violence within a society. Kennedy and associates (1998) have stated:

> Studies have shown that poverty and income are powerful predictors of homicide and violent crime. The effect of the growing gap between the rich and poor is mediated through an undermining of social cohesion, or social capital, and decreased social capital is in turn associated with increased firearm homicide and violent crime. (p. 7)

Indeed, the United States was populated by the violent actions of one group of people over another. Since that time, much has been said and written, and laws have been passed, regarding the civil rights of all people. However, to this day many people would agree that the

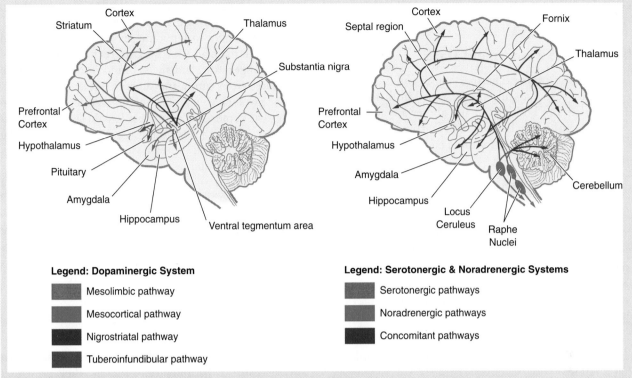

FIGURE 36–1 Neurobiology of violence.

Neurotransmitters

Neurotransmitters that have been implicated in the etiology of aggression and violence include decreases in serotonin, and increases in norepinephrine and dopamine (Hollander, Berlin, & Stein, 2008; Tardiff, 2003).

Associated Areas of the Brain

- Limbic structures: Emotional alterations
- Prefrontal & frontal cortices: Modulation of social judgment
- Amygdala: Anxiety, rage, fear
- Hypothalamus: Stimulates sympathetic nervous system in "fight-or-flight" response
- Hippocampus: Learning and memory

Medications Used to Modulate Aggression

1. Studies have suggested that selective serotonin reuptake inhibitors (SSRIs) may reduce irritability and aggression consistent with the hypothesis of reduced serotonergic activity in aggression.
2. Mood stabilizers that dampen limbic irritability may be important in reducing the susceptibility to react to provocation or threatening stimuli by overactivation of limbic system structures such as the amygdala (Siever, 2002). Carbamazepine (Tegretol), diphenylhydantoin (Dilantin), and divalproex sodium (Depakote) have yielded positive results. Lithium has also been used effectively in violent individuals (Tardiff, 2003).
3. Anti-adrenergic agents such as ß-blockers (e.g., propranolol) have been shown to reduce aggression in some individuals, presumably by dampening excessive noradrenergic activity (Siever, 2002).
4. In their ability to modulate excessive dopaminergic activity, antipsychotics—both typical and atypical—have been helpful in the control of aggression and violence, particularly in individuals with co-morbid psychosis.

statement "All men are created equal" is hypocritical in our society.

Societal influences may also contribute to violence when individuals realize that their needs and desires are not being met relative to other people (Tardiff, 2003). When poor and oppressed people find that they have limited access through legitimate channels, they are more likely to resort to delinquent behaviors in an effort to obtain desired ends. This lack of opportunity and subsequent delinquency may even contribute to a subculture of violence within a society.

APPLICATION OF THE NURSING PROCESS

Background Assessment Data

Data related to intimate partner abuse, child abuse and neglect, and sexual assault are presented in this section. Characteristics of both victim and abuser are addressed. This information may be used as background knowledge in designing plans of care for these clients.

Intimate Partner Abuse

CORE CONCEPT

Battering
A pattern of coercive control founded on and supported by physical and/or sexual violence or threat of violence of an intimate partner.

The National Coalition Against Domestic Violence (2007) states:

> Battering is a pattern of behavior used to establish power and control over another person through fear and intimidation, often including the threat or use of violence. Battering happens when one person believes they are entitled to control another.

The American Medical Association (2007) defines domestic violence as:

> An ongoing, debilitating experience of physical, psychological, and/or sexual abuse in the home, associated with increased isolation from the outside world and limited personal freedom and accessibility to resources . (p. 7)

Physical abuse between domestic partners may be known as spouse abuse, domestic or family violence, wife or husband battering, or intimate partner or relationship abuse. United States Bureau of Justice statistics for 2004 (2007) reflected the following: (1) approximately 85 percent of victims of intimate violence were women, (2) women ages 20 to 34 experienced the highest per capita rates of intimate violence, (3) intimate partners committed 3 percent of the nonfatal violence against men. In the same study, approximately 64 percent of women and 54 percent of men reported the victimizations to the police. The most common reason for not reporting among women was "fear of reprisal." Among men, the most common reason for not reporting was because it was a "private or personal matter."

Profile of the Victim

Battered women represent all age, racial, religious, cultural, educational, and socioeconomic groups. They may be married or single, housewives or business executives. Many women who are battered have low self-esteem, commonly adhere to feminine sex-role stereotypes, and often accept the blame for the batterer's actions. Feelings of guilt, anger, fear, and shame are common. They may be isolated from family and support systems.

Some women who are in violent relationships grew up in abusive homes and may have left those homes, even gotten married, at a very young age in order to escape the abuse. The battered woman views her relationship as male dominant, and as the battering continues, her ability to see the options available to her and to make decisions concerning her life (and possibly those of her children) decreases. The phenomenon of *learned helplessness* may be applied to the woman's progressing inability to act on her own behalf. Learned helplessness occurs when an individual comes to understand that regardless of his or her behavior, the outcome is unpredictable and usually undesirable.

Profile of the Victimizer

Men who batter usually are characterized as persons with low self-esteem. Pathologically jealous, they present a "dual personality," one to the partner and one to the rest of the world (Meskill & Conner, 2003). They are often under a great deal of stress, but have limited ability to cope with the stress. The typical abuser is very possessive and perceives his spouse as a possession. He becomes threatened when she shows any sign of independence or attempts to share herself and her time with others. Small children are often ignored by the abuser; however, they may also become the targets of abuse as they grow older, particularly if they attempt to protect their mother from abuse. The abuser also may use threats of taking the children away as a tactic of emotional abuse.

The abusing man typically wages a continuous campaign of degradation against his female partner. He insults and humiliates her and everything she does at every opportunity. He strives to keep her isolated from others and totally dependent on him. He demands to know where she is at every moment, and when she tells him he challenges her honesty. He achieves power and control through intimidation.

The Cycle of Battering

In her classic studies of battered women and their relationships, Walker (1979) identified a cycle of predictable behaviors that are repeated over time. The behaviors can be divided into three distinct phases that vary in time and intensity both within the same relationship and among different couples. Figure 36–2 depicts a graphic representation of the **cycle of battering.**

Phase I. The Tension-Building Phase. During this phase, the woman senses that the man's tolerance for

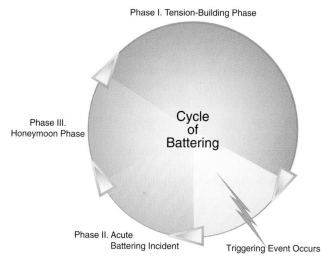

FIGURE 36–2 The cycle of battering.

frustration is declining. He becomes angry with little provocation but, after lashing out at her, may be quick to apologize. The woman may become very nurturing and compliant, anticipating his every whim in an effort to prevent his anger from escalating. She may just try to stay out of his way.

Minor battering incidents may occur during this phase, and in a desperate effort to avoid more serious confrontations, the woman accepts the abuse as legitimately directed toward her. She denies her anger and rationalizes his behavior (e.g., "I need to do better;" "He's under so much stress at work;" "It's the alcohol. If only he didn't drink"). She assumes the guilt for the abuse, even reasoning that perhaps she *did* deserve the abuse, just as her aggressor suggests.

The minor battering incidents continue, and the tension mounts as the woman waits for the impending explosion. The abuser begins to fear that his partner will leave him. His jealousy and possessiveness increase, and he uses threats and brutality to keep her in his captivity. Battering incidents become more intense, after which the woman becomes less and less psychologically capable of restoring equilibrium. She withdraws from him, which he misinterprets as rejection, further escalating his anger toward her. Phase I may last from a few weeks to many months or even years.

Phase II. The Acute Battering Incident. This phase is the most violent and the shortest, usually lasting up to 24 hours. It most often begins with the batterer justifying his behavior to himself. By the end of the incident, however, he cannot understand what has happened, only that in his rage he has lost control over his behavior.

This incident may begin with the batterer wanting to "just teach her a lesson." In some instances, the woman may intentionally provoke the behavior. Having come to a point in phase I in which the tension is unbearable, long-term battered women know that once the acute phase is behind them, things will be better.

During phase II, women feel their only option is to find a safe place to hide from the batterer. The beating is severe, and many women can describe the violence in great detail, almost as if dissociation from their bodies had occurred. The batterer generally minimizes the severity of the abuse. Help is usually sought only in the event of severe injury or if the woman fears for her life or those of her children.

Phase III. Calm, Loving, Respite ("Honeymoon") Phase. In this phase, the batterer becomes extremely loving, kind, and contrite. He promises that the abuse will never recur and begs her forgiveness. He is afraid she will leave him and uses every bit of charm he can muster to ensure this does not happen. He believes he now can control his behavior, and because now he has "taught her a lesson," he believes she will not "act up" again.

He plays on her feelings of guilt, and she desperately wants to believe him. She wants to believe that he *can* change, and that she will no longer have to suffer abuse. During this phase the woman relives her original dream of ideal love and chooses to believe that *this* is what her partner is *really* like.

This loving phase becomes the focus of the woman's perception of the relationship. She bases her reason for remaining in the relationship on this "magical" ideal phase and hopes against hope that the previous phases will not be repeated. This hope is evident even in those women who have lived through a number of horrendous cycles.

Although phase III usually lasts somewhere between the lengths of time associated with phases I and II, it can be so short as to almost pass undetected. In most instances, the cycle soon begins again with renewed tensions and minor battering incidents. In an effort to "steal" a few precious moments of the phase III kind of loving, the battered woman becomes a collaborator in her own abusive lifestyle. Victim and batterer become locked together in an intense, symbiotic relationship.

Why Does She Stay?

Probably the most common response that battered women give for staying is that they fear for their life and/or the lives of their children. As the battering progresses, the man gains power and control through intimidation and instilling fear with threats such as, "I'll kill you and the kids if you try to leave." Challenged by these threats, and compounded by her low self-esteem and sense of powerlessness, the woman sees no way out. In fact, she may try to leave only to return when confronted by her partner and the psychological power he holds over her.

Women have been known to stay in an abusive relationship for many reasons, some of which include the following (Family Violence Law Center, 2003; National Coalition Against Domestic Violence, 2007):

● *For the children*: She may fear losing custody of the children if she leaves.

● *For financial reasons*: She may have no financial resources, access to the resources, or job skills.
● *Fear of retaliation*: Her partner may have told her that if she leaves he will find her and kill her and the children.
● *Lack of a support network*: She may be under pressure from family members to stay in the marriage and try to work things out.
● *Religious reasons*: She may have religious beliefs against divorce. Some clergy strive only to help save the marriage at all costs (rather than to focus on stopping the violence).
● *Hopefulness*: She remembers good times and love in the relationship and has hope that her partner will change his behavior and they can have good times again.

IMPLICATIONS OF RESEARCH FOR EVIDENCE-BASED PRACTICE

Sachs, B., Hall, L.A., Lutenbacher, M., & Rayens, M.K. (1999). Potential for abusive parenting by rural mothers with low-birth-weight children. *Image: Journal of Nursing Scholarship*, 31(1), 21–25.

Description of the Study: The purpose of this study was to describe factors influencing the potential for abusive parenting by rural mothers of low-birth-weight (LBW) children. The convenience sample in this study included 48 mothers of LBW children, ranging in age from 18 to 39 years, all living in a rural area of the state, and all living with their LBW infant at the time of the study. Average length of the children's hospitalization after birth was 6 weeks, and the average age at time of the study was 9 months. In-home interviews were conducted using structured questionnaires to assess the mothers' everyday stressors, depressive symptoms, functional social support, quality of family relationships, and child abuse potential.

Results of the Study: According to the questionnaires used for measurement, 54 percent of the mothers indicated a high level of depressive symptoms and 63 percent indicated a high potential for physical child abuse. No significant differences were noted in depressive symptoms and potential for child abuse by birth weight, health status of the child, or time since hospital discharge. Mothers with high child abuse potential reported more everyday stressors and depressive symptoms, less functional social support, and poorer family functioning. Because in this study everyday stressors and the two social support systems (functional social support and quality of family relationships) were examined as predictors of depressive symptoms, it is suggested that everyday stressors exerts both a direct and an indirect effect on mothers' potential for child abuse. The strongest predictor of child abuse potential was mothers' depressive symptoms.

Implications for Nursing Practice: The researchers conclude that rural mothers of LBW children are at risk for abusive parenting. This study demonstrated the adverse effects of everyday stressors, minimal social resources, and depressive symptoms on mothers' potential for abusive parenting. Nurses should provide attention to the mental health of mothers living in isolated, rural areas. Information should be made available to these mothers regarding community resources that offer social support and childcare assistance. Nurses could establish and conduct educational programs to improve parenting skills and promote more positive child health outcomes.

Child Abuse

Erik Erikson (1963) stated, "The worst sin is the mutilation of a child's spirit." Children are vulnerable and relatively powerless, and the effects of maltreatment are infinitely deep and long lasting. Child maltreatment typically includes physical or emotional injury, physical or emotional neglect, or sexual acts inflicted upon a child by a caregiver. The Child Abuse Prevention and Treatment Act (CAPTA), as amended and reauthorized in 2003, identifies a minimum set of acts or behaviors that characterize maltreatment (Child Welfare Information Gateway [CWIG], 2006a). States may use these as foundations on which to establish state legislation.

Physical Abuse

Physical abuse of a child includes "any physical injury as a result of punching, beating, kicking, biting, burning, shaking, throwing, stabbing, choking, hitting (with a hand, stick, strap, or other object), burning, or otherwise harming a child" (CWIG, 2006a). Maltreatment is considered whether or not the caretaker intended to cause harm, or even if the injury resulted from over-discipline or physical punishment. The most obvious way to detect it is by outward physical signs. However, behavioral indicators also may be evident.

Signs of Physical Abuse. Indicators of physical abuse may include any of the following (CWIG, 2006b). The child:

● Has unexplained burns, bites, bruises, broken bones, or black eyes.
● Has fading bruises or other marks noticeable after an absence from school.
● Seems frightened of the parents and protests or cries when it is time to go home.
● Shrinks at the approach of adults
● Reports injury by a parent or another adult caregiver.

Physical abuse may be suspected when the parent or other adult caregiver (CWIG, 2006b):

● Offers conflicting, unconvincing, or no explanation for the child's injury.
● Describes the child as "evil," or in some other very negative way.
● Uses harsh physical discipline with the child.
● Has a history of abuse as a child.

Emotional Abuse

Emotional abuse involves a pattern of behavior on the part of the parent or caretaker that results in serious impairment of the child's social, emotional, or intellectual functioning. Examples of emotional injury include belittling or rejecting the child, ignoring the child, blaming the child for things over which he or she has no control, isolating the child from normal social experiences, and using harsh and inconsistent discipline. Behavioral indicators of emotional injury may include (CWIG, 2006b):

- Shows extremes in behavior, such as overly compliant or demanding behavior, extreme passivity, or aggression.
- Is either inappropriately adult (e.g., parenting other children) or inappropriately infantile (e.g., frequently rocking or head-banging)
- Is delayed in physical or emotional development
- Has attempted suicide
- Reports a lack of attachment to the parent

Emotional abuse may be suspected when the parent or other adult caregiver (CWIG, 2006b):

- Constantly blames, belittles, or berates the child.
- Is unconcerned about the child and refuses to consider offers of help for the child's problems.
- Overtly rejects the child.

Physical and Emotional Neglect

CORE CONCEPT

Neglect
Physical neglect of a child includes refusal of or delay in seeking health care, abandonment, expulsion from the home or refusal to allow a runaway to return home, and inadequate supervision.

Emotional neglect refers to a chronic failure by the parent or caretaker to provide the child with the hope, love, and support necessary for the development of a sound, healthy personality.

Indicators of Neglect. The possibility of neglect may be considered when the child (CWIG, 2006b):

- Is frequently absent from school.
- Begs or steals food or money.
- Lacks needed medical or dental care, immunizations, or glasses.
- Is consistently dirty and has severe body odor.
- Lacks sufficient clothing for the weather.
- Abuses alcohol or other drugs.
- States that there is no one at home to provide care.

The possibility of neglect may be considered when the parent or other adult caregiver (CWIG, 2006b):

- Appears to be indifferent to the child.
- Seems apathetic or depressed.
- Behaves irrationally or in a bizarre manner.
- Is abusing alcohol or other drugs.

Sexual Abuse of a Child

Various definitions of **child sexual abuse** are available in the literature. CAPTA defines sexual abuse as:

Employment, use, persuasion, inducement, enticement, or coercion of any child to engage in, or assist any other person to engage in, any sexually explicit conduct or any simulation of such conduct for the purpose of producing any visual depiction of such conduct; or the rape, and in cases of caretaker or inter-familial relationships, statutory rape, molestation, prostitution, or other form of sexual exploitation of children, or incest with children. (CWIG, 2006a)

Included in the definition is **sexual exploitation of a child,** in which a child is induced or coerced into engaging in sexually explicit conduct for the purpose of promoting any performance, and child sexual abuse, in which a child is being used for the sexual pleasure of an adult (parent or caretaker) or any other person.

CORE CONCEPT

Incest
The occurrence of sexual contacts or interaction between, or sexual exploitation of, close relatives, or between participants who are related to each other by a kinship bond that is regarded as a prohibition to sexual relations (e.g., caretakers, stepparents, stepsiblings) (Sadock & Sadock, 2007).

Indicators of Sexual Abuse. Child abuse may be considered a possibility when the child (NCCAN, 2003):

- Has difficulty walking or sitting.
- Suddenly refuses to change for gym or to participate in physical activities.
- Reports nightmares or bedwetting.
- Experiences a sudden change in appetite.
- Demonstrates bizarre, sophisticated, or unusual sexual knowledge or behavior.
- Becomes pregnant or contracts a venereal disease, particularly if younger than age 14.
- Runs away.
- Reports sexual abuse by a parent or another adult caregiver.

Sexual abuse may be considered a possibility when the parent or other adult caregiver (CWIG, 2006b):

- Is unduly protective of the child or severely limits the child's contact with other children, especially of the opposite sex.
- Is secretive and isolated.
- Is jealous or controlling with family members.

Characteristics of the Abuser

A number of factors have been associated with adults who abuse or neglect their children. Sadock and Sadock (2007) report that 90 percent of parents who abuse their children were severely physically abused by their own mothers or fathers. Murray and Zentner (2001) identify the following as additional characteristics that may be associated with abusive parents:

- Experiencing a stressful life situation (e.g., unemployment; poverty)
- Having few, if any, support systems; commonly isolated from others
- Lacking understanding of child development or care needs
- Lacking adaptive coping strategies; angers easily; has difficulty trusting others
- Expecting the child to be perfect; may exaggerate any mild difference the child manifests from the "usual"

The Incestuous Relationship

A great deal of attention has been given to the study of father-daughter incest. In these cases there is usually an impaired sexual relationship between the parents. Communication between the parents is ineffective, which prevents them from correcting their problems. Typically, the father is domineering, impulsive, and physically abusing; whereas the mother is passive and submissive, and denigrates her role as wife and mother. She is often aware of, or at least strongly suspects, the incestuous behavior between the father and daughter but may believe in or fear her husband's absolute authority over the family. She may deny that her daughter is being harmed and may actually be grateful that her husband's sexual demands are being met by someone other than herself.

Onset of the incestuous relationship typically occurs when the daughter is 8 to 10 years of age and commonly begins with genital touching and fondling. In the beginning, the child may accept the sexual advances from her father as signs of affection. As the incestuous behavior continues and progresses, the daughter usually becomes more bewildered, confused, and frightened, never knowing whether her father will be paternal or sexual in his interactions with her (Sadock & Sadock, 2007).

The relationship may become a love-hate situation on the part of the daughter. She continues to strive for the ideal father-daughter relationship but is fearful and hateful of the sexual demands he places on her. The mother may be alternately caring and competitive as she witnesses her husband's possessiveness and affections directed toward her daughter. Out of fear that his daughter may expose their relationship, the father may attempt to interfere with her normal peer relationships (Sadock & Sadock, 2007).

It has been suggested that some fathers who participate in incestuous relationships may have unconscious homosexual tendencies and have difficulty achieving a stable heterosexual orientation. On the other hand, some men have frequent sex with their wives and several of their own children but are unwilling to seek sexual partners outside the nuclear family because of a need to maintain the public facade of a stable and competent patriarch. Although the oldest daughter in a family is most vulnerable to becoming a participant in father–daughter incest, some fathers form sequential relationships with several daughters. If incest has been reported with one daughter, it should be suspected with all of the other daughters (Murray & Zentner, 2001).

The Adult Survivor of Incest

Several common characteristics have been identified in adults who have experienced incest as children. Basic to these characteristics is a fundamental lack of trust resulting from an unsatisfactory parent–child relationship, which causes low self-esteem and a poor sense of identity. Children of incest often feel trapped, for they have been admonished not to talk about the experience and may be afraid, or even fear for their lives, if they are exposed. If they do muster the courage to report the incest, particularly to the mother, they frequently are not believed. This is confusing to the child, who is then left with a sense of self-doubt and the inability to trust his or her own feelings. The child develops feelings of guilt with the realization over the years that the parents are using him or her in an attempt to solve their own problems.

Childhood sexual abuse is likely to distort the development of a normal association of pleasure with sexual activity (Reeves, 2003). Peer relationships are often delayed, altered, inhibited, or perverted. In some instances, individuals who were sexually abused as children completely retreat from sexual activity and avoid all close interpersonal relationships throughout life. Other adult manifestations of childhood sexual abuse in women include diminished libido, vaginismus, nymphomania, and promiscuity. In male survivors of childhood sexual abuse, impotence, premature ejaculation, exhibitionism, and compulsive sexual conquests may occur. Lerner (2005) suggests that adult survivors of incest are at risk for experiencing symptoms of posttraumatic stress disorder, sexual dysfunction, somatization disorders, compulsive sexual behaviors, depression, anxiety, eating disorders, substance use disorders, and intolerance of or constant search for intimacy.

The conflicts associated with pain (either physical or emotional) and sexual pleasure experienced by children who are sexually abused are commonly manifested symbolically in adult relationships. Women who were abused as children commonly enter into relationships with men who abuse them physically, sexually, or emotionally (Bensley, VanEenwyk, & Wynkoop, 2003).

Adult survivors of incest who decide to come forward with their stories usually are estranged from nuclear family members. They are blamed by family members for disclosing the "family secret" and often accused of overreacting to the incest. Frequently the estrangement becomes permanent when family members continue to deny the behavior and the individual is accused of lying. In recent years, a number of celebrities have come forward with stories of their childhood sexual abuse. Some have chosen to make the disclosure only after the death of their parents. Revelation of these past activities can be one way of contributing to the healing process for which incest survivors so desperately strive.

Sexual Assault

CORE CONCEPT

Rape
The expression of power and dominance by means of sexual violence, most commonly by men over women, although men may also be rape victims.

Sexual assault is viewed as any type of sexual act in which an individual is threatened or coerced, or forced to submit against his or her will. Rape, a type of sexual assault, occurs over a broad spectrum of experiences ranging from the surprise attack by a stranger to insistence on sexual intercourse by an acquaintance or spouse. Regardless of the defining source, one common theme always emerges: Rape is an act of aggression, not one of passion.

Acquaintance rape (called **date rape** if the encounter is a social engagement agreed to by the victim) is a term applied to situations in which the rapist is acquainted with the victim. They may be out on a first date, may have been dating for a number of months, or merely may be acquaintances or schoolmates. College campuses are the location for a staggering number of these types of rapes, a great many of which go unreported. An increasing number of colleges and universities are establishing programs for rape prevention and counseling for victims of rape.

Marital rape, which has been recognized only in recent years as a legal category, is the case in which a spouse may be held liable for sexual abuse directed at a marital partner against that person's will. Historically, with societal acceptance of the concept of women as marital property, the legal definition of rape held an exemption within the marriage relationship. In 1993, marital rape became a crime in all 50 states, under at least one section of the sexual offenses code. In 17 states and the District of Columbia, there are no exemptions from rape prosecution granted to husbands. However, in 33 states, there are still some exemptions given to husbands from rape prosecution.

Statutory rape is defined as unlawful intercourse between a person who is over the age of consent and a person who is under the age of consent. The legal age of consent varies from state to state, ranging from age 14 to 18 (King, 2005). An adult who has intercourse with a person who is under the age of consent can be arrested for statutory rape, although the interaction may have occurred between consenting individuals.

Profile of the Victimizer

Older profiles of the individual who rapes were described by Abrahamsen (1960) and Macdonald (1971), who identified the rapist's childhood as "mother-dominated" and the mother as "seductive but rejecting." The behavior of the mother toward the son was described as overbearing, with seductive undertones. Mother and son shared little secrets, and she rescued him when his delinquent acts created problems with others. However, she was quick to withdraw her love and attention when he went against her wishes, a rejection that was powerful and unyielding. She was domineering and possessive of the son, a dominance that often continued into his adult life. Macdonald (1971) stated:

> The seductive mother arouses overwhelming anxiety in her son with great anger, which may be expressed directly toward her but more often is displaced onto other women. When this seductive behavior is combined with parental encouragement of assaultive behavior, the setting is provided for personality development in the child which may result in sadistic, homicidal sexual attacks on women in adolescence or adult life.

Many rapists report growing up in abusive homes (McCormack, 2002). Even when the parental brutality is discharged by the father, the anger may be directed toward the mother who did not protect her child from physical assault. More recent feminist theories suggest that the rapist displaces this anger on the rape victim because he cannot directly express it toward other men (Sadock & Sadock, 2007). Another feminist view suggests that rape is most common in societies that encourage aggressiveness in males, have distinct gender roles, and in which men regard women's roles as inferior (King, 2005).

Statistics show that the greatest number of rapists are between the ages of 25 and 44. Of rapists, 51 percent are white, 47 percent are African-American, and the remaining 2 percent come from all other races (Sadock & Sadock, 2007). Many are either married or cohabiting at the time of their offenses. For those with previous criminal activity, the majority of their convictions are for crimes against property rather than against people. Most rapists do not have histories of mental illness.

The Victim

Rape can occur at any age. Although victims have been reported as young as 15 months old and as old as 82 years, the high-risk age group appears to be 20 to 34 years (U.S. Bureau of Justice, 2007). Of rape victims, 70 to 75 percent are single women, and the attack frequently occurs in or close to the victim's own neighborhood.

Scully (1994), in a study of a prison sample of rapists, found that in "stranger rapes," victims were not chosen for any reason having to do with appearance or behavior, but simply because the individual happened to be in a certain place at a certain time. Scully states:

> The most striking and consistent factor in all the stranger rapes, whether committed by a lone assailant or a group, is the unfortunate fact that the victim was "just there" in a location unlikely to draw the attention of a passerby. Almost every one of these men said exactly the same thing, "It could have been any woman," and a few added that because it was dark, they could not even see what their victim looked like very well. (p. 175)

In her study, Scully found that 62 percent of the rapists used a weapon, most frequently a knife. Most suggested that they used the weapon to terrorize and subdue the victim but not to inflict serious injury. The presence of a weapon (real or perceived) appears to be the principal measure of the degree to which a woman resists her attacker.

Rape victims who present themselves for care shortly after the crime has occurred likely may be experiencing an overwhelming sense of violation and helplessness that began with the powerlessness and intimidation experienced during the rape. Burgess (2007) identified two emotional patterns of response that may occur within hours after a rape and with which health care workers may be confronted in the emergency department or rape crisis center. In the **expressed response pattern**, the victim expresses feelings of fear, anger, and anxiety through such behaviors as crying, sobbing, smiling, restlessness, and tension. In the **controlled response pattern**, the feelings are masked or hidden, and a calm, composed, or subdued affect is seen.

The following manifestations may be evident in the days and weeks after the attack (Burgess, 2007):

- Contusions and abrasions about various parts of the body
- Headaches, fatigue, sleep pattern disturbances
- Stomach pains, nausea and vomiting
- Vaginal discharge and itching, burning upon urination, rectal bleeding and pain
- Rage, humiliation, embarrassment, desire for revenge, and self-blame
- Fear of physical violence and death

The long-term effects of sexual assault depend largely on the individual's ego strength, social support system, and the way he or she was treated as a victim (Burgess, 2007). Various long-term effects include increased restlessness, dreams and nightmares, and phobias (particularly those having to do with sexual interaction). Some women report that it takes years to get over the experience; they describe a sense of vulnerability and a loss of control over their own lives during this period. They feel defiled and unable to wash themselves clean, and some women are unable to remain living alone in their home or apartment.

Some victims develop a **compounded rape reaction**, in which additional symptoms such as depression and sui-

cide, substance abuse, and even psychotic behaviors may be noted (Burgess, 2007). Another variation has been called the **silent rape reaction**, in which the victim tells no one about the assault. Anxiety is suppressed and the emotional burden may become overwhelming. The unresolved sexual trauma may not be revealed until the woman is forced to face another sexual crisis in her life that reactivates the previously unresolved feelings.

Diagnosis/Outcome Identification

Nursing diagnoses are formulated from the data gathered during the assessment phase and with background knowledge regarding predisposing factors to the situation. Some common nursing diagnoses for victims of abuse include:

- Rape-trauma syndrome related to sexual assault evidenced by verbalizations of the attack; bruises and lacerations over areas of body; severe anxiety.
- Powerlessness related to cycle of battering evidenced by verbalizations of abuse; bruises and lacerations over areas of body; fear for her safety and that of her children; verbalizations of no way to get out of the relationship.
- Delayed growth and development related to abusive family situation evidenced by sudden onset of enuresis, thumb sucking, nightmares, inability to perform self-care activities appropriate for age.

Outcome Criteria

The following criteria may be used to measure outcomes in the care of abuse victims:

The client who has been sexually assaulted:
- Is no longer experiencing panic anxiety.
- Demonstrates a degree of trust in the primary nurse.
- Has received immediate attention to physical injuries.
- Has initiated behaviors consistent with the grief response.

The client who has been physically battered:
- Has received immediate attention to physical injuries.
- Verbalizes assurance of his or her immediate safety.
- Discusses life situation with primary nurse.
- Can verbalize choices from which he or she may receive assistance.

The child who has been abused:
- Has received immediate attention to physical injuries.
- Demonstrates trust in primary nurse by discussing abuse through the use of play therapy.
- Is demonstrating a decrease in regressive behaviors.

Planning/Implementation

Table 36–1 provides a plan of care for the client who has been a victim of abuse. Nursing diagnoses are presented,

Table 36–1 Care Plan for Victims of Abuse

NURSING DIAGNOSIS: RAPE-TRAUMA SYNDROME

RELATED TO: Sexual assault

EVIDENCED BY: Verbalizations of the attack; bruises and lacerations over areas of body; severe anxiety

Outcome Criteria	Nursing Interventions	Rationale
Short-Term Goal: ● Client's physical wounds will heal without complication. **Long-Term Goal:** ● Client will begin a healthy grief resolution, initiating the process of physical and psychological healing (time to be individually determined).	1. It is important to communicate the following to the victim of sexual assault: ● You are safe here. ● I'm sorry that it happened. ● I'm glad you survived. ● It's not your fault. No one deserves to be treated this way. ● You did the best that you could. 2. Explain every assessment procedure that will be conducted and why it is being conducted. Ensure that data collection is conducted in a caring, nonjudgmental manner. 3. Ensure that the client has adequate privacy for all immediate post-crisis interventions. Try to have as few people as possible providing the immediate care or collecting immediate evidence. 4. Encourage the client to give an account of the assault. Listen, but do not probe. 5. Discuss with the client whom to call for support or assistance. Provide information about referrals for aftercare.	1. The woman who has been sexually assaulted fears for her life and must be reassured of her safety. She may also be overwhelmed with self-doubt and self-blame, and these statements instill trust and validate self-worth. 2. This may serve to decrease fear/anxiety and increase trust. 3. The post-trauma client is extremely vulnerable. Additional people in the environment increase this feeling of vulnerability and serve to escalate anxiety. 4. Nonjudgmental listening provides an avenue for catharsis that the client needs to begin healing. A detailed account may be required for legal follow-up, and a caring nurse, as client advocate, may help to lessen the trauma of evidence collection. 5. Because of severe anxiety and fear, the client may need assistance from others during this immediate post-crisis period. Provide referral information in writing for later reference (e.g., psychotherapist, mental health clinic, community advocacy group).

NURSING DIAGNOSIS: POWERLESSNESS

RELATED TO: Cycle of battering

EVIDENCED BY: Verbalizations of abuse; bruises and lacerations over areas of body; fear for own safety and that of children; verbalizations of no way to get out of the relationship

Outcome Criteria	Nursing Interventions	Rationale
Short-Term Goal: ● Client will recognize and verbalize choices available, thereby perceiving some control over life situation. **Long-Term Goal:** ● Client will exhibit control over life situation by making decision about what to do regarding living with cycle of abuse.	1. In collaboration with physician, ensure that all physical wounds, fractures, and burns receive immediate attention. Take photographs if the victim will permit. 2. Take the woman to a private area to do the interview.	1. Client safety is a nursing priority. Photographs may be called in as evidence if charges are filed. 2. If the client is accompanied by the man who did the battering, she is not likely to be truthful about her injuries.

Continued on following page

Table 36–1 *(Continued)*

3. If she has come alone or with her children, assure her of her safety. Encourage her to discuss the battering incident. Ask questions about whether this has happened before, whether the abuser takes drugs, whether the woman has a safe place to go, and whether she is interested in pressing charges.

4. Ensure that "rescue" efforts are not attempted by the nurse. Offer support, but remember that the final decision must be made by the client.

5. Stress to the victim the importance of safety. She must be made aware of the variety of resources that are available to her. These may include crisis hot lines, community groups for women who have been abused, shelters, counseling services, and information regarding the victim's rights in the civil and criminal justice system. Following a discussion of these available resources, the woman may choose for herself. If her decision is to return to the marriage and home, this choice also must be respected.

3. Some women will attempt to keep secret how their injuries occurred in an effort to protect the partner or because they are fearful that the partner will kill them if they tell.

4. Making her own decision will give the client a sense of control over her life situation. Imposing judgments and giving advice are nontherapeutic.

5. Knowledge of available choices decreases the victim's sense of powerlessness, but true empowerment comes only when she chooses to use that knowledge for her own benefit.

NURSING DIAGNOSIS: DELAYED GROWTH AND DEVELOPMENT

RELATED TO: Abusive family situation

EVIDENCED BY: Sudden onset of enuresis, thumb sucking, nightmares, inability to perform self-care activities appropriate for age.

Outcome Criteria	Nursing Interventions	Rationale
Short-Term Goal: • Client will develop trusting relationship with nurse and report how evident injuries were sustained. **Long-Term Goal:** • Client will demonstrate behaviors consistent with age-appropriate growth and development.	1. Perform complete physical assessment of the child. Take particular note of bruises (in various stages of healing), lacerations, and client complaints of pain in specific areas. Do not overlook or discount the possibility of sexual abuse. Assess for nonverbal signs of abuse: aggressive conduct, excessive fears, extreme hyperactivity, apathy, withdrawal, age-inappropriate behaviors.	1. An accurate and thorough physical assessment is required to provide appropriate care for the client.
	2. Conduct an in-depth interview with the parent or adult who accompanies the child. Consider: If the injury is being reported as an accident, is the explanation reasonable? Is the injury consistent with the explanation? Is the injury consistent with the child's developmental capabilities?	2. Fear of imprisonment or loss of child custody may place the abusive parent on the defensive. Discrepancies may be evident in the description of the incident, and lying to cover up involvement is a common defense that may be detectable in an in-depth interview.
	3. Use games or play therapy to gain child's trust. Use these techniques to assist in describing his or her side of the story.	3. Establishing a trusting relationship with an abused child is extremely difficult. He or she may not even want to be touched. These types of play activities can provide a nonthreatening environment that may enhance the child's attempt to discuss these painful issues.

Outcome Criteria	Nursing Interventions	Rationale
	4. Determine whether the nature of the injuries warrants reporting to authorities. Specific state statutes must enter into the decision of whether to report suspected child abuse. Individual state statutes regarding what constitutes child abuse and neglect may be found at http://www.childwelfare.gov/systemwide/laws_policies/search/index.cfm	4. A report is commonly made if there is reason to suspect that a child has been injured as a result of physical, mental, emotional, or sexual abuse. "Reason to suspect" exists when there is evidence of a discrepancy or inconsistency in explaining a child's injury. Most states require that the following individuals report cases of suspected child abuse: all health care workers, all mental health therapists, teachers, child-care providers, firefighters, emergency medical personnel, and law enforcement personnel. Reports are made to the Department of Health and Human Services or a law enforcement agency.

along with outcome criteria, appropriate nursing interventions, and rationales for each.

Concept Care Mapping

The concept map care plan is an innovative approach to planning and organizing nursing care (see Chapter 9). It is a diagrammatic teaching and learning strategy that allows visualization of interrelationships between medical diagnoses, nursing diagnoses, assessment data, and treatments. An example of a concept map care plan for a client who is the victim of abuse is presented in Figure 36–3.

Evaluation

Evaluation of nursing actions to assist victims of abuse must be considered on both a short- and a long-term basis.

Short-term evaluation may be facilitated by gathering information using the following types of questions:

● Has the individual been reassured of his or her safety?
● Is this evidenced by a decrease in panic anxiety?
● Have wounds been properly cared for and provision made for follow-up care?
● Have emotional needs been attended to?
● Has trust been established with at least one person to whom the client feels comfortable relating the abusive incident?
● Have available support systems been identified and notified?
● Have options for immediate circumstances been presented?

Long-term evaluation may be conducted by health care workers who have contact with the individual long after the immediate crisis has passed.

● Is the individual able to conduct activities of daily living satisfactorily?
● Have physical wounds healed properly?
● Is the client appropriately progressing through the behaviors of grieving?
● Is the client free of sleep disturbances (nightmares, insomnia); psychosomatic symptoms (headaches, stomach pains, nausea/vomiting); regressive behaviors (enuresis, thumb sucking, phobias); and psychosexual disturbances?
● Is the individual free from problems with interpersonal relationships?
● Has the individual considered the alternatives for change in his or her personal life?
● Has a decision been made relative to the choices available?
● Is he or she satisfied with the decision that has been made?

TREATMENT MODALITIES

Crisis Intervention

The focus of the initial interview and follow-up with the client who has been sexually assaulted is on the rape incident alone. Problems identified but unassociated with the rape are not dealt with at this time. The goal of crisis intervention is to help victims return to their previous lifestyle as quickly as possible.

The client should be involved in the intervention from the beginning. This promotes a sense of competency, control, and decision-making. Because an overwhelming sense of powerlessness accompanies the rape experience, active involvement by the victim is both a validation of personal worth and the beginning of the recovery process. Crisis intervention is time limited—usually 6 to

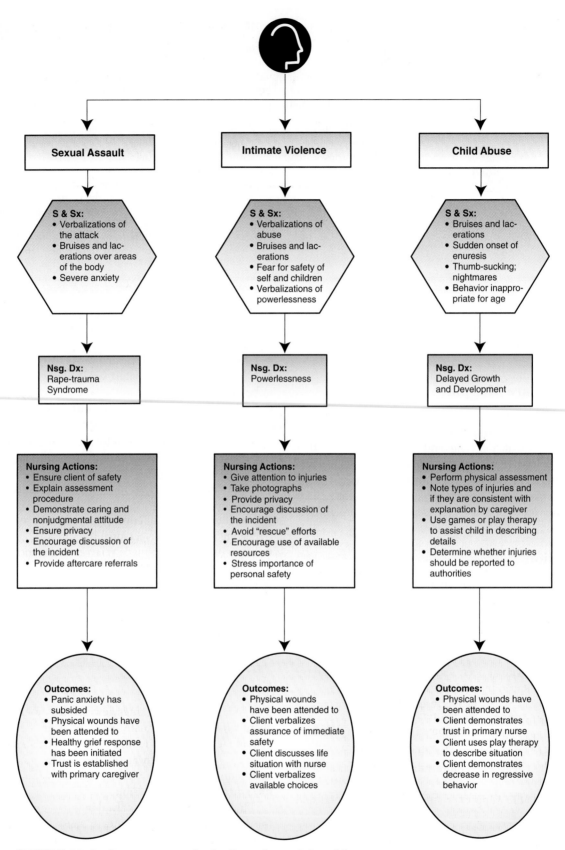

FIGURE 36–3 Concept map care plan for clients who are victims of abuse.

REFERENCES

American Medical Association (AMA). (2007). *Diagnostic and treatment guidelines on domestic violence.* Retrieved July 9, 2007 from http://www.ama-assn.org/ama/pub/category/3548.html

American Nurses Association (ANA). (1998). *Culturally competent assessment for family violence.* Washington, DC: American Nurses Publishing.

Bensley, L., VanEenwyk, J., & Wynkoop, K.S. (2003). Childhood family violence history and women's risk for intimate partner violence and poor health. *American Journal of Preventive Medicine, 25*(1), 38–44.

Burgess, A. (2007). Rape violence. *Nurse Spectrum/Nurseweek CE: Course 60025.* Retrieved July 8, 2007 from http://www.nurse.com/CE/60025

Centers for Disease Control and Prevention (CDC). (2006). *Intimate partner violence: Fact sheet.* Retrieved July 8, 2007 from http://www.cdc.gov/ncipc/factsheets/ipvfacts.htm

Child Welfare Information Gateway (CWIG). (2006a). *What is child abuse and neglect?* Retrieved July 8, 2007 from http://www.childwelfare.gov/pubs/factsheets/whatiscan.cfm

Child Welfare Information Gateway (CWIG). (2006b). *Recognizing child abuse and neglect: Signs and symptoms.* Retrieved July 8, 2007 from http://www.childwelfare.gov/pubs/factsheets/signs.cfm

Cummings, J.L., & Mega, M.S. (2003). *Neuropsychiatry and behavioral neuroscience.* New York: Oxford University Press.

Family Violence Law Center. (2003). *Why do women stay in violent relationships?* Retrieved April 1, 2007 from http://www.fvlc.org

Hollander, E., Berlin, H.A., & Stein, D.J. (2008). Impulse-control disorders not elsewhere classified. In R.E. Hales, S.C. Yudofsky, & G.O. Gabbard (Eds.), *Textbook of psychiatry* (5th ed.). Washington, DC: American Psychiatric Publishing.

Kennedy, B.P., Kawachi, I., Prothrow, S.D., Lochner, K., & Gupta, V. (1998). Social capital, income inequality, and firearm violent crime. *Social Science and Medicine, 47*(1), 7–17.

King, B.M. (2005). *Human sexuality today* (5th ed.). Upper Saddle River, NJ: Pearson Education.

Lerner, M. (2005). *Adult manifestations of childhood sexual abuse.* New York: The American Academy of Experts in Traumatic Stress.

McCormack, J. (2002, May). Sexual offenders' perceptions of their early interpersonal relationships: An attachment perspective. *Journal of Sex Research, 39*(2), 85–93.

Meskill, J., & Conner, M. (2003). *Understanding and dealing with domestic violence against women.* Retrieved March 31, 2007 from http://www.oregoncounseling.org/

Murray, R.B., & Zentner, J.P. (2001). *Health promotion strategies through the life span* (7th ed.). Upper Saddle River, NJ: Prentice-Hall.

National Coalition Against Domestic Violence. (2007). *What is battering?* Retrieved March 31, 2007 from http://www.ncadv.org/learn/TheProblem_100.html

Reeves, C.R. (2003). *Childhood: It should not hurt.* Huntersville, NC: LTI Publishing.

Sadock, B.J., & Sadock, V.A. (2007). *Synopsis of psychiatry: Behavioral sciences/clinical psychiatry* (10th ed.). Philadelphia: Lippincott Williams & Wilkins.

Scully, D. (1994). *Understanding sexual violence: A study of convicted rapists.* New York: Routledge.

Siever, L.J. (2002, August). Neurobiology of impulsive-aggressive personality disordered patients. *Psychiatric Times, 19*(8): Online.

Tardiff, K.J. (2003). Violence. In R.E. Hales & S.C. Yudofsky (Eds.), *Textbook of clinical psychiatry* (4th ed.). Washington, DC: American Psychiatric Publishing.

United States Bureau of Justice. (2007). *Intimate partner violence in the U.S.* Retrieved July 8, 2007 from http://www.ojp.gov/bjs

United States Department of Health and Human Services (USDHHS). (2007). *Child Maltreatment 2005.* Retrieved July 8, 2007 from http://www.acf.dhhs.gov/programs/cb/pubs/cm05/summary.htm

World Health Organization (WHO). (2005). The economic dimensions of interpersonal violence. Geneva, Switzerland: WHO.

CLASSICAL REFERENCES

Abrahamsen D. (1960). *The psychology of crime.* New York: John Wiley & Sons.

Erikson, E.H. (1963). *Childhood and society* (2nd ed.). New York: W.W. Norton.

Macdonald, J.M. (1971). *Rape: Offenders and their victims.* Springfield, IL: Charles C Thomas.

Selye, H. (1956). *The stress of life.* New York: McGraw-Hill.

Walker, L.E. (1979). *The battered woman.* New York: Harper & Row.

@ Internet References

● Additional information related to child abuse is located at the following Web sites:
  • http://www.childwelfare.gov
  • http://endabuse.org/
  • http://www.child-abuse.com
  • http://www.nlm.nih.gov/medlineplus/childabuse.html

● Additional information related to sexual assault is located at the following Web sites:
  • http://www.vaw.umn.edu/
  • http://www.nlm.nih.gov/medlineplus/rape.html

● Additional information related to domestic violence is located at the following Web sites:
  • http://www.ndvh.org/
  • http://home.cybergrrl.com/dv/book/toc.html
  • http://crisis-support.org/
  • http://www.ama-assn.org/ama/pub/category/3242.html

37
CHAPTER

Community Mental Health Nursing

CHAPTER OUTLINE

KEY TERMS

case management
case manager
deinstitutionalization
diagnostically related
    groups (DRGs)

managed care
mobile outreach units
prospective payment
shelters
store-front clinics

CORE CONCEPTS

community
primary prevention
secondary prevention
tertiary prevention

OBJECTIVES

After reading this chapter, the student will be able to:

1. Discuss the changing focus of care in the field of mental health.
2. Define the concepts of care associated with the model of public health:
   a. Primary prevention
   b. Secondary prevention
   c. Tertiary prevention
3. Differentiate between the roles of basic level and advanced practice psychiatric/mental health registered nurses.
4. Define the concepts of case management and identify the role of case management in community mental health nursing.
5. Discuss primary prevention of mental illness within the community.
6. Identify populations at risk for mental illness within the community.
7. Discuss nursing intervention in primary prevention of mental illness within the community.

8. Discuss secondary prevention of mental illness within the community.
9. Describe treatment alternatives related to secondary prevention within the community.
10. Discuss tertiary prevention of mental illness within the community as it relates to the seriously mentally ill and homeless mentally ill.
11. Relate historical and epidemiological factors associated with caring for the seriously mentally ill and homeless mentally ill within the community.
12. Identify treatment alternatives for care of the seriously mentally ill and homeless mentally ill within the community.
13. Apply steps of the nursing process to care of the seriously mentally ill and homeless mentally ill within the community.

The retiree may be faced with these questions: Can I face loss of job satisfaction? Will I feel the separation from people close to me at work? If I need continued employment on a part-time basis to supplement Social Security payments, will the old organization provide it, or must I adjust to a new job? Shall I remain in my present home or seek a different one because of easier maintenance or reduced cost of upkeep? Might a different climate be better, and if so, will I miss my relatives and neighbors? (p. 812)

Support can also be provided in a group environment. Support groups of individuals undergoing the same types of experiences can be extremely helpful. Nurses can form and lead these types of groups to assist retiring individuals through this critical period. These groups can also serve to provide information about available resources that offer assistance to individuals in or nearing retirement, such as information concerning Medicare, Social Security, and Medicaid; information related to organizations that specialize in hiring retirees; and information regarding ways to use newly acquired free time constructively.

Situational Crises

Situational crises are acute responses that occur as a result of an external circumstantial stressor. The number and types of situational stressors are limitless and may be real or exist only in the perception of the individual. Some types of situational crises that put individuals at risk for mental illness include the following.

Poverty. A number of studies have identified poverty as a direct correlation to emotional illness. This may have to do with the direct consequences of poverty, such as inadequate and crowded living conditions, nutritional deficiencies, medical neglect, unemployment, or being homeless.

High Rate of Life Change Events. Miller and Rahe (1997) found that frequent changes in life patterns due to a large number of significant events occurring in close proximity tend to decrease a person's ability to deal with stress, and physical or emotional illness may be the result. These include life change events such as death of a loved one, divorce, being fired from a job, a change in living conditions, a change in place of employment or residence, physical illness, or a change in body image caused by the loss of a body part or function.

Environmental Conditions. Environmental conditions can create situational crises. Tornados, floods, hurricanes, and earthquakes have wreaked devastation on thousands of individuals and families in recent years.

Trauma. Individuals who have encountered traumatic experiences must be considered at risk for emotional illness. These include traumatic experiences usually considered outside the range of usual human experience, such as participating in military combat, being a victim of violent personal assault, undergoing torture, being taken hostage or kidnapped, or being the victim of a natural or manmade disaster (APA, 2000).

Nursing intervention at the primary level of prevention with individuals experiencing situational crises is aimed at maintaining the highest possible level of functioning while offering support and assistance with problem solving during the crisis period. Interventions for nursing of clients in crisis include the following:

● Use a reality-oriented approach. The focus of the problem is on the here and now.
● Remain with the individual who is experiencing panic anxiety.
● Establish a rapid working relationship by showing unconditional acceptance, by active listening, and by attending to immediate needs.
● Discourage lengthy explanations or rationalizations of the situation; promote an atmosphere for verbalization of true feelings.
● Set firm limits on aggressive, destructive behaviors. At high levels of anxiety, behavior is likely to be impulsive and regressive. Establish at the outset what is acceptable and what is not, and maintain consistency.
● Clarify the problem that the individual is facing. The nurse does this by describing his or her perception of the problem and comparing it with the individual's perception of the problem.
● Help the individual determine what he or she believes precipitated the crisis.
● Acknowledge feelings of anger, guilt, helplessness, and powerlessness, while taking care not to provide positive feedback for these feelings.
● Guide the individual through a problem-solving process by which he or she may move in the direction of positive life change:
  ● Help the individual confront the source of the problem that is creating the crisis response.
  ● Encourage the individual to discuss changes he or she would like to make. Jointly determine whether desired changes are realistic.
  ● Encourage exploration of feelings about aspects that cannot be changed, and explore alternative ways of coping more adaptively in these situations.
  ● Discuss alternative strategies for creating changes that are realistically possible.
  ● Weigh benefits and consequences of each alternative.
  ● Assist the individual to select alternative coping strategies that will help alleviate future crises.
● Identify external support systems and new social networks from whom the individual may seek assistance in times of stress.

Nursing at the level of primary prevention focuses largely on education of the consumer to prevent initiation or exacerbation of mental illness. An example of just one type of teaching plan for use in primary prevention situations is presented in Table 37–1.

TABLE 37–1	Client Education for Primary Prevention: Drugs of Abuse

Class of Drugs	Effects	Symptoms of Overdose	Trade Names	Common Names	Effects on the Body (Chronic or High-Dose Use)
CNS Depressants					
Alcohol	Relaxation, loss of inhibitions, lack of concentration, drowsiness, slurred speech, sleep	Nausea, vomiting; shallow respirations; cold, clammy skin; weak, rapid pulse; coma; possible death.	Ethyl alcohol, beer, gin, rum, vodka, bourbon, whiskey, liqueurs, wine, brandy, sherry, champagne.	Booze, alcohol, liquor, drinks, cocktails, high-balls, nightcaps, moonshine, white lightning, firewater.	Peripheral nerve damage, skeletal muscle wasting, encephalopathy, psychosis, cardiomyopathy, gastritis, esophagitis, pancreatitis, hepatitis, cirrhosis of the liver, leukopenia, thrombocytopenia, sexual dysfunction.
Other (barbiturates and non-barbiturates)	Same as alcohol.	Anxiety, fever, agitation, hallucinations, disorientation, tremors, delirium, convulsions, possible death.	Seconal Nembutal Amytal Valium Librium Chloral hydrate Miltown	Red birds Yellow birds Blue birds Blues/yellows Green & whites Mickies Downers	Decreased REM sleep, respiratory depression, hypotension, possible kidney or liver damage, sexual dysfunction.
CNS Stimulants					
Amphetamines and related drugs	Hyperactivity, agitation, euphoria, insomnia, loss of appetite.	Cardiac arrhythmias, headache, convulsions, hypertension, rapid heart rate, coma, possible death.	Dexedrine, Didrex, Tenuate, Preludin, Ritalin, Plegine, Ionamin, Sanorex	Uppers, pep pills, wakeups, bennies, eye-openers, speed, black beauties, sweet A's	Aggressive, compulsive behavior; paranoia; hallucinations; hypertension.
Cocaine	Euphoria, hyperactivity, restlessness, talkativeness, increased pulse, dilated pupils.	Hallucinations, convulsions, pulmonary edema, respiratory failure, coma, cardiac arrest, possible death.	Cocaine hydrochloride	Coke, flake, snow, dust, happy dust, gold dust, girl, cecil, C, toot, blow, crack	Pulmonary hemorrhage; myocardial infarction; ventricular fibrillation.
Opioids	Euphoria, lethargy, drowsiness, lack of motivation.	Shallow breathing, slowed pulse, clammy skin, pulmonary edema, respiratory arrest, convulsions, coma, possible death.	Heroin Morphine Codeine Dilaudid Demerol Methadone Percodan Talwin Opium	Snow, stuff, H, Harry, horse M, morph, Miss Emma Schoolboy Lords Doctors Dollies Perkies T's Big O, black stuff	Respiratory depression, constipation, fecal impaction, hypotension, decreased libido, retarded ejaculation, impotence, orgasm failure.
Hallucinogens	Visual hallucinations, disorientation, confusion, paranoid delusions, euphoria, anxiety, panic, increased pulse.	Agitation, extreme hyperactivity, violence, hallucinations, psychosis, convulsions, possible death.	LSD PCP Mescaline DMT STP	Acid, cube, big D Angel dust, Hog, crystal Mesc Businessman's trip Serenity and peace	Panic reaction, acute psychosis, flashbacks.
Cannabinols	Relaxation, talkativeness, lowered inhibitions, euphoria, mood swings.	Fatigue, paranoia, delusions, hallucinations, possible psychosis.	Cannabis Hashish	Marijuana, pot, grass, joint, Mary Jane, MJ Hash, rope, Sweet Lucy	Tachycardia, orthostatic hypotension, chronic bronchitis, problems with infertility, amotivational syndrome.

BOX 37 – 1   Secondary Prevention Case Study: Parenthood

The identified patient was a petite, doll-like 4-year-old girl named Tanya. She was the older of two children in a Latino American family. The other child was a boy named Joseph, aged 2. The mother was 5 months pregnant with their third child. The family had been referred to the nurse after Tanya was placed in foster care following a report to the Department of Health and Human Services by her nursery school teacher that the child had marks on her body suspicious of child abuse.

The parents, Paulo and Annette, were in their mid-20s. Paulo had lost his job at an aircraft plant 3 months ago and had been unable to find work since. Annette brought in a few dollars from cleaning houses for other people, but the family was struggling to survive.

Paulo and Annette were angry at having to see the nurse. After all, "Parents have the right to discipline their children." The nurse did not focus on the *intent* of the behavior, but instead looked at factors in the family's life that could be viewed as stressors. This family had multiple stressors: poverty, the father's unemployment, the age and spacing of the children, the mother's chronic fatigue from work at home and in other people's homes, and finally, having a child removed from the home against the parents' wishes.

During therapy with this family, the nurse discussed the behaviors associated with various developmental levels. She also discussed possible deviations from these norms and when they should be reported to the physician. The nurse and the family discussed Tanya's behavior, and how it compared with the norms.

The parents also discussed their own childhoods. They were able to relate some of the same types of behaviors that they observed in Tanya. But they both admitted that they came from families whose main method of discipline was physical punishment. Annette had been the oldest child in her large family and had been expected to "keep the younger ones in line." When she had not done so, she was punished with her father's belt. She expressed anger toward her father, although she had never been allowed to express it at the time.

Paulo's father had died when he was a small boy, and Paulo had been expected to be the "man of the family." From the time he was very young, he worked at odd jobs to bring money into the home. Because of this, he had little time for the usual activities of childhood and adolescence. He held much resentment toward the young men who "had everything and never had to work for it."

Paulo and Annette had high expectations for Tanya. In effect, they expected her to behave in a manner well beyond her developmental level. These expectations were based on the reflections of their own childhoods. They were uncomfortable with the spontaneity and playfulness of childhood because they had had little personal experience with these behaviors. When Tanya balked and expressed the verbal assertions common to early childhood, Paulo and Annette interpreted these behaviors as defiance toward them and retaliated with anger in the manner in which they had been parented.

With the parents, the nurse explored feelings and behaviors from their past so that they were able to understand the correlation to their current behaviors. They learned to negotiate ways to deal with Tanya's age-appropriate behaviors. In combined therapy with Tanya, they learned how to relate to her childishness, and even how to enjoy playing with both of their children.

The parents ceased blaming each other for the family's problems. Annette had spent a good deal of her time deprecating Paulo for his lack of support of his family, and Paulo blamed Annette for being "unable to control her daughter." Communication patterns were clarified, and life in the family became more peaceful.

Without a need to "prove himself" to his wife, Paulo's efforts to find employment met with success because he no longer felt the need to turn down jobs that he believed his wife would perceive to be beneath his capabilities. Annette no longer works outside the home, and both she and Paulo participate in the parenting chores. Tanya and her siblings continue to demonstrate age-appropriate developmental progression.

Historical and Epidemiological Aspects

In 1955, more than half a million individuals resided in public mental hospitals. More recent statistics indicate that approximately 100,000 persons with mental illness inhabit these institutions on a long-term basis (Sadock & Sadock, 2003).

Deinstitutionalization of persons with serious mental illness began in the 1960s as national policy change and with a strong belief in the individual's right to freedom. Other considerations included the deplorable conditions of some of the state asylums, the introduction of neuroleptic medications, and the cost-effectiveness of caring for these individuals in the community setting.

Deinstitutionalization began to occur rapidly and without sufficient planning for the needs of these individuals as they reentered the community. Those who were fortunate enough to have support systems to provide assistance with living arrangements and sheltered employment experiences most often received the outpatient treatment they required. Those without adequate support, however,

either managed to survive on a meager existence or were forced to join the ranks of the homeless. Some ended up in nursing homes meant to provide care for individuals with physical disabilities.

Certain segments of our population with severe and persistent mental illness have been left untreated: the elderly, the "working poor," the homeless, and those individuals previously covered by funds that have been cut by various social reforms. These circumstances have promoted in individuals with severe and persistent mental illness a greater number of crisis-oriented emergency department visits and hospital admissions, and repeated confrontations with law enforcement officials.

In 2002, President George W. Bush established the New Freedom Commission on Mental Health. This commission was charged with the task of conducting a comprehensive study of the United States mental health service delivery system. They were to identify unmet needs and barriers to services and recommend steps for improvement in services and support for individuals with serious mental illness. In July 2003, the commission presented its final report to the President (President's New Freedom Commission on Mental Health, 2003). The Commission identified the following five barriers:

1. **Fragmentation and gaps in care for children.** About 7 to 9 percent of all children (ages 9 to 17) have a serious emotional disturbance (SED). The Commission found that services for children are even more fragmented than those for adults, with more uncoordinated funding and differing eligibility requirements. Only a fraction of children with SED appear to have access to school-based or school-linked mental health services. Children with SED who are identified for special education services have higher levels of absenteeism, higher drop-out rates, and lower levels of academic achievement than students with other disabilities.

2. **Fragmentation and gaps in care for adults with serious mental illness.** The Commission expressed concern that so many adults with serious mental illness are homeless, dependent on alcohol or drugs, unemployed, and go without treatment. According to the World Health Organization (WHO), neuropsychiatric conditions account for 13 percent of the total Disability Adjusted Life Years (DALYs) lost due to all disease and injuries in the world, and are expected to increase by 15 percent by the year 2020 (WHO, 2004). The Commission identifies public attitudes and the stigma associated with mental illness as a major barrier to treatment. Stigma is often internalized by individuals with mental illness, leading to hopelessness, lower self-esteem, and isolation. Stigma deprives these individuals of the support they need to recover.

3. **High unemployment and disability for people with serious mental illness.** Undetected, untreated, and poorly treated mental disorders interrupt careers, leading many individuals into lives of disability, poverty, and long-term dependence. The Commission found a 90 percent unemployment rate among adults with serious mental illness—the worst level of employment of any group of people with disabilities. Some surveys have shown that many individuals with serious mental illness *want* to work, and could, with modest assistance. However, the largest "program" of assistance the United States has for people with mental illness is disability payments. Sadly, societal stigma is also reflected in employment discrimination against people with mental illness.

4. **Older adults with mental illnesses are not receiving care.** The Commission reports that about 5 to 10 percent of older adults have major depression, yet most are not properly recognized and treated. The report states:

> Older people are reluctant to get care from specialists. They feel more comfortable going to their primary

care physician. Still, they are often more sensitive to the stigma of mental illness, and do not readily bring up their sadness and despair. If they acknowledge problems, they are more likely than young people to describe physical symptoms. Primary care doctors may see their suffering as "natural" aging, or treat their reported physical distress instead of the underlying mental disorder. What is often missed is the deep impact of depression on older people's capacity to function in ways that are seemingly effortless for others.

5. **Mental health and suicide prevention are not yet national priorities.** The fact that the United States has failed to prioritize mental health puts many lives at stake. Families struggle to maintain equilibrium while communities strain (and often fail) to provide needed assistance for adults and children who suffer from mental illness. Over 30,000 lives are lost annually to suicide. About 90 percent of those who take their life have a mental disorder. Many individuals who commit suicide have not had the care in the months before their death that would help them to affirm life. Both the American Psychiatric Association and the National Mental Health Association have called on the U.S. Congress to pass parity legislation. Lack of equal access to insurance coverage is conspicuous evidence of the low priority placed on mental health treatment.

The Commission outlined the following goals and recommendations for mental health reform:

Goal 1. Americans will understand that mental health is essential to overall health.
Commission recommendations:
- Advance and implement a national campaign to reduce the stigma of seeking care and a national strategy for suicide prevention.
- Address mental health with the same urgency as physical health.

Goal 2. Mental health care will be consumer and family driven.
Commission recommendations:
- Develop an individualized plan of care for every adult with a serious mental illness and child with a serious emotional disturbance.
- Involve consumers and families fully in orienting the mental health system toward recovery.
- Align relevant Federal programs to improve access and accountability for mental health services.
- Create a Comprehensive State Mental Health Plan.
- Protect and enhance the rights of people with mental illness.

Goal 3. Disparities in mental health services will be eliminated.
Commission recommendations:
- Improve access to quality care that is culturally competent.

● Improve access to quality care in rural and geographically remote areas.

Goal 4. Early mental health screening, assessment, and referral to services will be common practice.
Commission recommendations:
● Promote the mental health of young children.
● Improve and expand school mental health programs.
● Screen for co-occurring mental and substance use disorders and link with integrated treatment strategies.
● Screen for mental disorders in primary health care, across the life span, and connect to treatment and supports.

Goal 5. Excellent mental health care will be delivered and research will be accelerated.
Commission recommendations:
● Accelerate research to promote recovery and resilience, and ultimately to cure and prevent mental illnesses.
● Advance evidence-based practices using dissemination and demonstration projects, and create a public-private partnership to guide their implementation.
● Improve and expand the workforce providing evidence-based mental health services and supports.
● Develop the knowledge base in four understudied areas: mental health disparities, long-term effects of medications, trauma, and acute care.

Goal 6. Technology will be used to access mental health care and information.
Commission recommendations:
● Use health technology and telehealth to improve access and coordination of mental health care, especially for Americans in remote areas or in underserved populations.
● Develop and implement integrated electronic health record and personal health information systems.

If these proposals became reality, it would surely mean improvement in the care of individuals with severe and persistent mental illness. Many nurse leaders see this period of health care reform as an opportunity for nurses to expand their roles and assume key positions in education, prevention, assessment, and referral. Nurses are, and will continue to be, in key positions to assist individuals with severe and persistent mental illness to remain as independent as possible, to manage their illness within the community setting, and to strive to minimize the number of hospitalizations required.

Treatment Alternatives

Community Mental Health Centers. The goal of community mental health centers in caring for individuals with severe and persistent mental illness is to improve coping ability and prevent exacerbation of acute symptoms. A major obstacle in meeting this goal has been the lack of advocacy or sponsorship for clients who require services from a variety of sources. This has placed responsibility for health care on an individual with mental illness who is often barely able to cope with everyday life. Case management has become a recommended method of treatment for individuals with severe and persistent mental illness.

The ANA (1992) has endorsed case management as an effective method of providing care for clients in the community who require long-term assistance, and nurses as uniquely qualified case managers:

> Nurses bring broad-based and unique skills and knowledge to case management. The role of the nurse as a coordinator of care has been integral to defining nursing practice for decades. The coordination of services and care is the primary function of case managers. This role is a logical extension of the nursing role. (p. 14)

Bower (1992) identified five core components and nursing role functions that blend with the steps of the nursing process to form a framework for nursing case management. The core components include:

● **Interaction.** The nurse must develop a trusting relationship with the client, family members, and other service providers. During an initial screening process the nurse determines if the client is eligible for case management according to preestablished guidelines and, if not, refers the client for appropriate assistance elsewhere.
● **Assessment: Establishment of a Database.** The nurse conducts a comprehensive assessment of the client's physical health status, functional capability, mental status, personal and community support systems, financial resources, and environmental conditions. The data are then analyzed and appropriate nursing diagnoses formulated.
● **Planning.** A service care plan is devised with client participation. The plan should include mutually agreed-on goals, specific actions directed toward goal achievement, and selection of essential resources and services through collaboration among health care professionals, the client, and the family or significant others.
● **Implementation.** In this phase, the client receives the needed services from the appropriate providers. In some instances the nursing case manager is also a provider of care, whereas in others, he or she is only the coordinator of care.
● **Evaluation.** The case manager continuously monitors and evaluates the client's responses to interventions

BOX 37–2 Nursing Case Management in the Community Mental Health Center: A Case Study

Michael, 73 years old with a history of multiple psychiatric admissions, has lived in various adult foster homes and boarding houses for the past 10 years. He was originally diagnosed as having schizophrenia, but he was recently rediagnosed as having bipolar disorder, mania. His symptoms are well controlled with lithium 300 mg three times a day, which is prescribed by the outpatient psychiatrist.

The nurse practitioner/case manager in the outpatient clinic coordinates Michael's care, advocates for his needs, and counsels him regarding his health problems. She orders routine blood tests to assess his lithium levels. When Michael experienced visual disturbances, she referred him for an emergency eye evaluation. He was found to have a retinal detachment and was sent to a local VA hospital for emergency surgery. After his eye surgery, the nurse practitioner arranged transportation to his follow-up visits with the eye doctor and instructed him about his eye care and instillation of his eye drops. Michael did not like putting eye drops in his eye and tended to neglect doing it. Because he also had glaucoma and required ongoing treatment with pilocarpine and timolol maleate eye drops twice daily, he needed a great deal of education and reassurance to continue using the eye drops.

In addition to routine quarterly visits for ongoing case management, the nurse practitioner also performs his annual health assessment consisting of history, review of systems, mental status exam, and physical assessment. During Michael's last physical exam, the nurse practitioner detected a thyroid mass and referred him for a complete evaluation including thyroid function tests, a thyroid scan, and evaluation by a surgeon and an endocrinologist. She discussed his thyroid problem with the surgeon and the endocrinologist, and they determined that Michael would best benefit from thyroid replacement (i.e., levothyroxine sodium 0.1 mg daily).

Because Michael eats all of his meals in restaurants, the nurse was concerned about his diet. A brief diet review revealed that his diet was low in vitamin C. He was then instructed in which foods and juices he should include in his daily menu. The nurse practitioner discussed ways that Michael could get the best nutrition for the least cost.

Michael currently is living in a boarding house and is totally responsible for taking his own medication, attending to his activities of daily living, and managing his own money. He has very limited income and depends on donations for many of his clothing needs.

Despite his age, he is quite active and alert. He attends many VA-sponsored social activities and does daily volunteer work at the VA, such as pushing wheelchairs, running errands, and escorting other veterans to clinic appointments. His nurse case manager arranged for him to receive free lunches as a reward for some of his volunteer activities.

Nursing case management has helped this elderly gentleman with severe and persistent psychiatric illness and many years of hospitalization to live independently within the community setting.

SOURCE: From Pittman (1989), with permission.

and progress toward preestablished goals. Regular contact is maintained with client, family or significant others, and direct service providers. Ongoing care coordination continues until outcomes have been achieved. The client may then be discharged or assigned to inactive status, as appropriate.

A case study of nursing case management within a community mental health center is presented in Box 37–2.

Assertive Community Treatment (ACT). The National Alliance for the Mentally Ill (NAMI) defines ACT as a service-delivery model that provides comprehensive, locally based treatment to people with serious and persistent mental illnesses (NAMI, 2007). ACT is a type of case-management program that provides highly individualized services directly to consumers. It is a team approach, and includes members from psychiatry, social work, nursing, substance abuse, and vocational rehabilitation. The ACT team provides these services 24 hours a day, seven days a week, 365 days a year.

NAMI (2007) identifies the primary goals of ACT as follows:

● To lessen or eliminate the debilitating symptoms of mental illness each individual client experiences

● To minimize or prevent recurrent acute episodes of the illness

● To meet basic needs and enhance quality of life

● To improve functioning in adult social and employment roles

● To enhance an individual's ability to live independently in his or her own community

● To lessen the family's burden of providing care

The ACT team provides treatment, rehabilitation, and support services to individuals with severe and persistent mental illness who are unable on their own to receive treatment from a traditional model of case management. The team is usually able to provide most services with minimal referrals to other mental health programs or providers. Services are provided within community settings, such as a person's home, local restaurants, parks, nearby stores, and any other place that the individual requires assistance with living skills.

Studies have shown that ACT clients spend significantly less time in hospitals and more time in independent living situations, have less time unemployed, earn more income from competitive employment, experience more positive social relationships, express greater satisfaction with life, and are less symptomatic (NAMI, 2007). Only about half of the states currently have ACT programs established or under pilot testing. NAMI (2007) states:

Despite the documented treatment success of ACT, only a fraction of those with the greatest needs have access to this uniquely effective program. In the United States, adults with severe and persistent mental illnesses constitute one-half to one percent of the adult population. It is estimated that 10 to 20 percent of this group could be helped by the ACT model if it were available.

Day/Evening Treatment/Partial Hospitalization Programs.
Day or evening treatment programs (also called partial hospitalization) are designed to prevent institutionalization or to ease the transition from inpatient hospitalization to community living. Various types of treatment are offered. Many include therapeutic community (milieu) activities; individual, group, and family therapies; psychoeducation; alcohol and drug education; crisis intervention; therapeutic recreational activities; and occupational therapy. Many programs offer medication administration and monitoring as part of their care. Some programs have established medication clinics for individuals on long-term psychopharmacological therapy. These clinics may include educational classes and support groups for individuals with similar conditions and treatments.

Partial hospitalization programs generally offer a comprehensive treatment plan formulated by an interdisciplinary team of psychiatrists, psychologists, nurses, occupational and recreational therapists, and social workers. Nurses take a leading role in the administration of partial hospitalization programs. They lead groups, provide crisis intervention, conduct individual counseling, act as role models, and make necessary referrals for specialized treatment. Use of the nursing process provides continual evaluation of the program, and modifications can be made as necessary.

Partial hospitalization programs have proven to be an effective method of preventing hospitalization for many individuals with severe and persistent mental illness. They are a way of transitioning these individuals from the acute care setting back into the mainstream of the community. For some individuals who have been deinstitutionalized, they provide structure, support, opportunities for socialization, and an improvement in their overall quality of life.

Community Residential Facilities.
Community residential facilities for persons with severe and persistent mental illness are known by many names: group homes, halfway houses, foster homes, boarding homes, sheltered care facilities, transitional housing, independent living programs, social-rehabilitation residences, and others. These facilities differ by the purpose for which they exist and the activities that they offer.

Some of these facilities provide food, shelter, housekeeping, and minimal supervision and assistance with activities of daily living. Others may also include a variety of therapies and serve as a transition between hospital and independent living. In addition to the basics, services might include individual and group counseling, medical care, job training or employment assistance, and leisure-time activities.

A wide variety of personnel staff these facilities. Some facilities have live-in professionals who are available at all times, some have professional staff who are on call for intervention during crisis situations, and some are staffed by volunteers and individuals with little knowledge or background for understanding and treating persons with severe and persistent mental illness.

The concept of transitional housing for individuals with serious mental illness is sound and has proved in many instances to be a successful means of therapeutic support and intervention for maintaining them within the community. However, without guidance and planning, transition to the community can be futile. These individuals may be ridiculed and rejected by the community. They may be targets of unscrupulous individuals who take advantage of their inability to care for themselves satisfactorily. These behaviors may increase maladaptive responses to the demands of community living and exacerbate the mental illness. A period of structured reorientation to the community in a living situation that is supervised and monitored by professionals is more likely to result in a successful transition for the individual with severe and persistent mental illness.

Psychiatric Home Health Care.
For the individual with serious mental illness who no longer lives in a structured, supervised setting, home health care may be the element that helps to keep him or her living independently. To receive home health care, individuals must validate their homebound status for the prospective payer (Medicare, Medicaid, most insurance companies, and Veteran's Administration [VA] benefits). An acute psychiatric diagnosis is not enough to qualify for the service. The client must show that he or she is unable to leave the home without considerable difficulty or the assistance of another person. The plan of treatment and subsequent charting must explain why the client's psychiatric disorder keeps him or her at home and justify the need for home services.

Homebound clients most often have diagnoses of depression, dementia, anxiety disorders, bipolar affective disorder, and schizophrenia. Many elderly clients are homebound because of medical conditions that impair mobility and necessitate home care.

Nurses who provide psychiatric home care must have an in-depth knowledge of psychopathology, psychopharmacology, and how medical and physical problems can be influenced by psychiatric impairments. These nurses must be highly adept at performing biopsychosocial assessments. They must be sensitive to changes in behavior that signal that the client is decompensating psychiatrically or medically so that early intervention may be implemented.

Another important job of the psychiatric home health nurse is monitoring compliance with the regimen of psychotropic medications. Some clients who are receiving injectable medications remain on home health care only until they can be placed on oral medications. Those clients receiving oral medications require close monitoring for compliance and assistance with the uncomfortable side effects of some of these drugs. Medication noncompliance is responsible for approximately two thirds of psychiatric hospital readmissions. Home health nurses can assist clients with this problem by helping them to see the relationship between control of their psychiatric symptoms and compliance with their medication regimen.

Client populations that benefit from psychiatric home health nursing include:

1. **Elderly Clients.** These individuals may not have a psychiatric diagnosis, but they may be experiencing emotional difficulties that have arisen from medical, sociocultural, or developmental factors. Depressed mood and social isolation are common.
2. **Persons with Severe and Persistent Mental Illness.** These individuals have a history of psychiatric illness and hospitalization. They require long-term medications and continual supportive care. Common diagnoses include recurrent major depression, schizophrenia, and bipolar disorder.
3. **Individuals in Acute Crisis Situations.** These individuals are in need of crisis intervention and and/or short-term psychotherapy.

The American Nurses Association (ANA) (1999) defines home health nursing as:

> . . . the practice of nursing applied to a client with a health condition in the client's place of residence. Clients and their designated caregivers are the focus of home health nursing practice. The goal of care is to initiate, manage, and evaluate the resources needed to promote the client's optimal level of well-being and function. (p. 3)

Medicare requires that psychiatric home nursing care be provided by "psychiatrically trained nurses," which they define as, ". . . nurses who have special training and/or experience beyond the standard curriculum required for a registered nurse" (Centers for Medicare & Medicaid Services [CMS], 2005).

The guidelines that cover psychiatric nursing services are not well defined by CMS. This has presented some reimbursement problems for psychiatric nurses in the past. The CMS statement regarding psychiatric nursing services is presented in Box 37–3.

Preparation for psychiatric home health nursing, in addition to the registered nurse licensure, should include several years of psychiatric inpatient treatment experience. It is also recommended that the nurse have medical-surgical nursing experience, because of common client physical comorbidity and the holistic nursing perspective. Additional training and experience in psychotherapy is viewed as an asset. However, psychotherapy is not the

---

> **BOX 37–3 CMS Guidelines for Psychiatric Home Nursing Care**
>
> **Psychiatric Evaluation, Therapy, and Teaching**
>
> The evaluation, psychotherapy, and teaching needed by a patient suffering from a diagnosed psychiatric disorder that requires active treatment by a psychiatrically trained nurse and the costs of the psychiatric nurse's services may be covered as a skilled nursing service. Psychiatrically trained nurses are nurses who have special training and/or experience beyond the standard curriculum required for a registered nurse. The services of the psychiatric nurse are to be provided under a plan of care established and reviewed by a physician.

SOURCE: Centers for Medicare and Medicaid Services (2005).

primary focus of psychiatric home nursing care. In fact, most reimbursement sources do not pay for exclusively insight-oriented therapy. Crisis intervention, client education, and hands-on care are common interventions in psychiatric home nursing care.

The psychiatric home health nurse provides comprehensive nursing care, incorporating interventions for physical and psychosocial problems into the treatment plan. The interventions are based on the client's mental and physical health status, cultural influences, and available resources. The nurse is accountable to the client at all times during the therapeutic relationship. Nursing interventions are carried out with appropriate knowledge and skill, and referrals are made when the need is outside the scope of nursing practice. Continued collaboration with other members of the health care team (e.g., psychiatrist, social worker, psychologist, occupational therapist, and/or physical therapist) is essential for maintaining continuity of care.

A case study of psychiatric home health care and the nursing process is presented in Box 37–4. A plan of care for Mrs. C. (the client in the case study) is presented in Table 37–2. Nursing diagnoses are presented, along with outcome criteria, appropriate nursing interventions, and rationale for each.

Care for the Caregivers. Another aspect of psychiatric home health care is to provide support and assistance to primary caregivers. When family is the provider of care on a 7-day-a-week, 24-hour-a-day schedule for a loved one with a severe and persistent mental disorder, it can be very exhausting and very frustrating. A care plan for primary caregivers is presented in Table 37–3.

The Homeless Population

Historical and Epidemiological Aspects

In 1992, Dr. Richard Lamb, a recognized expert in the field of severe and persistent mental illness, wrote:

> Alec Guinness, in his memorable role as a British Army colonel in *Bridge on the River Kwai*, exclaims at the end of the

required by the forensic nurse is the ability to assess patterned injury by differentiating marks such as defense wounds, grab marks, and fingernail marks. Clinical forensic nurses focus on observation of the communication and interaction patterns of suspected abuse victims and perpetrators. Many nurses come to forensic nursing from acute-care settings of emergency room nursing, critical care nursing, and perioperative nursing.

In the coroner's office, death notification entails stabilization of the family situation and grief support, skills that are basic to nursing practice. Expert skills in physical assessment, clinical history taking and interviewing, and use of technology have helped advance this nursing role.

Because of their awareness of the effects of violence in society and their ability to assess situations in which potential for violence exists, clinical forensic nurses are often called upon for consultation. By identifying risk factors and cues for violence in health care and workplace settings, these nurses can assist in the development of strategies, policies, and protocols to manage risk and reduce violence and injury. They also assist in the debriefing or resolution of violent events in a workplace or community.

The Sexual Assault Nurse Examiner (SANE)

The **sexual assault nurse examiner (SANE)** is a clinical forensic registered nurse who has received specialized training to provide care to the sexual assault victim. The SANE performs physical and psychosocial examination and collection of physical evidence, therapeutic interactions to minimize the trauma and initiate healing, coordination of referral and collaboration with community-based agencies involved in the rehabilitation of victims, and the judicial processing of sexual assault. The first programs training SANEs were developed in the United States in the late 1970s. SANEs may now earn national certification through the IAFN Forensic Nursing Certification Board and the Center for Nursing Education and Testing.

Forensic Psychiatric Nursing Specialty

Forensic psychiatric nurses integrate psychiatric/mental health nursing philosophy and practice with knowledge of the criminal justice system and assessment of the sociocultural influences on the individual client, the family, and the community, to provide comprehensive psychiatric and mental health nursing. Forensic psychiatric nurses work with mentally ill offenders and with victims of crime. They help victims cope with their emotional wounds and assist in the assessment and care of perpetrators. They focus on identification and change of behaviors that link criminal offenses or reactions to them. These nurses assist perpetrators and victims of crime in dealing with the courts and other aspects of the criminal justice system, minimizing further victimization and promoting functional abilities.

Functional applications of forensic psychiatric nursing include assessment of inmates for physical fitness, criminal responsibility, disposition, and early release. Forensic psychiatric nurses also provide mental health treatment for convicted offenders and those who are not found criminally responsible. In the criminal justice system, forensic psychiatric nurses deal with destructive, aggressive, and socially unacceptable behavior. These nurses provide interventions that encourage individuals to exercise self-control, foster individual change in behavior, and, in the process, protect other members of society and property.

There has been an increase in the involvement of forensic psychiatric nurses (especially those prepared for advanced practice) in the assessment and treatment of forensic psychiatric patients. These practitioners are involved in the development and refining of clinical roles in forensic psychiatric nursing and are in a position to promote intervention strategies that increase the likelihood of rehabilitation and reintegration of the forensic client into society.

Correctional/Institutional Nursing Specialty

Correctional/institutional nurses work in secure settings, providing treatment, rehabilitation and health promotion to clients who have been charged with or convicted of crimes. Settings include jails, state and federal prisons, and halfway houses. Prior to the 1960s, most nurses gave little thought to working in the correctional system, even though jails and correctional facilities have always been a part of the community at large. There is a growing awareness of the potential for the correctional population as a target of successful health interventions. Some nurses have created private practices or consultation services in which they identify the health needs and arrange for the care of people detained in custody. This service is provided separate from acute care, which is located in a secured hospital or infirmary section of the institution. Such services are just emerging as health care alternatives and will serve as the model from which community based care, aimed at decreasing recidivism among those incarcerated, will develop. To guide professional nursing practice, the ANA has published the 2007 edition of *Corrections Nursing: Scope and Standards of Practice*.

Nurses in General Practice

In addition to nurses in specialty practice, nurses in general practice find forensic nursing knowledge of growing importance. Forensic applications in the acute care setting emphasize the use of forensic knowledge and awareness of criminal justice implications for assessment, documentation of care, and reporting of information to police or other law enforcement agencies. Nurses who work in emergency departments and in critical care units are often in positions to preserve evidence of what might be a criminal offense. Victims of automobile accidents or apparent accidental overdoses are not always what they appear to be. Knowledge of what to look for and how to collect evidence, in addition to knowing whom to call and when, can be valuable in finding out what really happened in such cases. Clients often come into acute care settings with what are first thought to be injuries that are the result of an accident. However, preservation of evidence such as stomach contents, clothing residue, or marks on the skin surface can provide a very different picture—one of injury caused by a self-inflicted wound or violence perpetrated by another.

This chapter focuses on two specialties in forensic nursing: the clinical forensic nurse specialist in trauma care settings and the psychiatric forensic nurse in correctional facilities.

APPLICATION OF THE NURSING PROCESS IN CLINICAL FORENSIC NURSING IN TRAUMA CARE

Assessment

Lynch, Roach, and Sadler (2006) state, "Forensic nurse specialists are specifically trained to deal with cases of sexual assault, child abuse, acute psychiatric emergencies, and death investigation" (p. 603). All traumatic injuries in which liability is suspected are considered within the scope of forensic nursing. Reports to legal agencies are required to ensure follow-up investigation; however, the protection of clients' rights remains a nursing priority.

McPeck (2002) reports on the performance of forensic nurses in the aftermath of the September 11, 2001 attack on New York City and Washington, DC. He states:

> [Forensic nurses] worked as mortuary assistants to collect and process biological and evidentiary remains of the victims, many of whom are still missing and probably never will be found. The forensic nurses provided clinical care and support for about 2,000 police officers, firefighters, and emergency workers who were at Ground Zero at any one time. Forensic nurses are trained to intervene in crises and offer that kind of mental support. (p. 25)

With the rise of violence in our society reaching epidemic proportions, the role of the clinical forensic nurse in the care of trauma clients in the emergency department is expanding. The forensic clinical nurse specialist may be the ideal liaison between legal and medical agencies.

Lynch (2006) identifies several areas of assessment in which the clinical forensic nurse specialist may become involved. Some of these include the preservation of evidence, investigation of wound characteristics, and deaths in the emergency department.

Preservation of Evidence

Intentional traumas in the emergency department may be crime related or self-inflicted. Crime-related evidence is essential and must be safeguarded in a manner consistent with the investigation. Brown (2007) identifies common types of evidence as clothing, bullets, gunshot powder on the skin, bloodstains, hairs, fibers, grass, and any other type of debris that is found on the individual, such as fragments of glass, paint, and wood. Often this type of evidence is destroyed in the clinical setting when health care personnel are unaware of its potential value in an investigation. It is important that this type of evidence be saved and documented in all medical or accident instances that have legal implications.

Investigation of Wound Characteristics

When clients present to the emergency department with wounds from undiagnosed trauma, it is important for the clinical forensic nurse specialist to make a detailed documentation of the injuries. Failure to do so may interfere with the administration of justice should legal implications later arise. The following categories of medicolegal injuries are identified (Brown, 2007; Lynch, 2006):

● Sharp force injuries: includes stab wounds and other wounds resulting from penetration with a sharp object.
● Blunt force injuries: includes cuts and bruises resulting from the impact of a blunt object against the body.
● Dicing injuries: multiple, minute cuts and abrasions caused by contact with shattered glass (e.g., often occur in motor vehicle accidents)
● Patterned injuries: specific injuries that reflect the pattern of the weapon used to inflict the injury.
● Bite mark injuries: a type of patterned injury inflicted by human or animal.
● Defense wounds: injuries that reflect the victim's attempt to defend himself or herself from attack.
● Hesitation wounds: usually superficial, sharp force wounds; often found perpendicular to the lower part of the body and may reflect self-inflicted wounds.
● Fast-force injuries: usually gunshot wounds; may reflect various patterns of injury.

Nurses managing the client's care in the emergency department must be able to make assessments about the type of wound, the weapon involved, and an estimate of the length of time between the injury and presentation for treatment.

Deaths in the Emergency Department

When deaths occur in the emergency department as a result of abuse or accident, evidence must be retained, the death must be reported to legal authorities, and an investigation is conducted. It is therefore essential that the nurse carefully document the appearance, condition, and behavior of the victim upon arrival at the hospital. The information gathered from the client and family (or others accompanying the client) may serve to facilitate the postmortem investigation and may be used during criminal justice proceedings.

The critical factor is to be able to determine if the cause of death is natural or unnatural. A death is deemed *natural* if it occurs because of a congenital anomaly or a disease process that interferes with vital organ functioning (Lynch, 2006). In the emergency department, most deaths are sudden and unexpected. Those that are considered natural most commonly involve the cardiovascular, respiratory, and central nervous systems. Deaths that are considered *unnatural* include those from trauma, from self-inflicted acts, or from injuries inflicted by another. Legal authorities must be notified of all deaths related to unnatural circumstances.

Nursing Diagnosis

Clinical forensic nurse specialists in the trauma care setting analyze the information gathered during assessment of the client to formulate nursing diagnoses. Common nursing diagnoses relevant to forensic clients in the emergency department include:

● Impaired tissue integrity
● Risk for post-trauma syndrome
● Fear
● Anxiety
● Risk for self-mutilation
● Risk for suicide
● Risk for complicated grieving

Planning/Implementation

Preservation of Evidence

When a trauma victim is admitted to the emergency department, the most obvious priority intervention is medical stabilization. This priority must be balanced against the need to protect rapidly deteriorating physical evidence that can determine if a crime has occurred.

Wounds must be examined to speculate about the type of weapon used and to estimate age of the wound. Clothing must be checked for blood, semen, gunshot residue, or trace materials such as hair, fibers, and other debris. Clothing that is removed from a victim should not be shaken, so any evidence that may be adhering to it is not lost. Each separate item of clothing should be carefully placed in a paper bag, sealed, dated, timed, and signed. Plastic bags should never be used because of the tendency for condensation to occur. This promotes the growth of mold and the decay of biological tissue, which results in contamination of the evidence (Brown, 2007; Lynch, 2006).

When the trauma is sexual assault, a SANE may be called to the emergency department. SANEs usually work on-call, and because most sexual assault victims are women, female nurses are employed as SANEs. Male victims of sexual assault also most often prefer to work with a female SANE, because the perpetrators are usually men and because of the subsequent mistrust of men following the attack.

Ledray (2001) suggests the following essential components of a forensic examination of the sexual assault survivor in the emergency department:

Treatment and Documentation of Injuries

Emergency department (ED) staff typically performs the initial assessments when a sexual assault victim arrives. Vital signs and treatment of serious injuries often occur before the arrival of the SANE. Unless the injuries are life threatening, the forensic examination should occur before medical treatment is administered so as not to destroy physical evidence that is needed to establish that a sexual crime has occurred.

It is often expected that a sexual assault survivor must exhibit cuts and bruises in the genital or nongenital area. It has been estimated that there are no visible physical injuries in 40 to 60 percent of sexual assaults (American Medical Association [AMA], 1999). Absence of physical trauma does not necessarily mean that no force was used and that consent was given. This, however, is the case often used by defense attorneys in court. The AMA (1999) suggests the use of a traumagram—a diagram of a nude figure on which the locations of visible injuries are made. A written description of the color, size, and location of each wound, abrasion, and laceration is then documented. With the client's permission, photographs of the wounds should be taken for accurate documentation.

The nurse may use a **colposcope** to examine for tears and abrasions inside the vaginal area. A colposcope is an instrument that contains a magnifying lens and to which a 35 mm camera can be attached.

Some states have legally mandated procedures, and some acute care settings also have established protocols, for gathering evidence in cases of sexual assault. In some instances, "rape kits" are available for collecting specimens and lab samples in a competent manner that is consistent with legal requirements and that will not interfere with the victim's option to pursue criminal charges. In addition to the vaginal examination, oral and rectal examinations may be conducted. Fingernail scrapings and body, head, and pubic hair samples should also be collected. Client hair samples are important to be able to differentiate from those of the assailant. As previously stated, all evidence should be sealed in paper, *not* plastic, bags to prevent the possible growth of mildew from accumulation of moisture inside the plastic container, and subsequent contamination of the evidence.

Some states may require a urine specimen to test for pregnancy or screen for drugs. It is best, if possible, to wait until the initial internal examination is complete before collecting the urine sample. However, the AMA (1999) states, "Patients needing to urinate before the internal examination should be allowed to do so, with a notation being made in the medical record."

Maintaining the Proper Chain of Evidence

Ledray (2001) states, "Maintaining a proper chain-of-evidence is as important as collecting the proper evidence." Unless the proper chain-of-evidence has been maintained, it cannot be used successfully in a court of law to convict an assailant. The AMA (1999) states,

> To preserve the chain of evidence and the freshness of the samples, check to ensure that they are properly labeled, sealed, refrigerated when necessary, and kept under observation or properly locked until rendered to the proper legal authority. (p. 13)

Treatment and Evaluation of Sexually Transmitted Diseases (STDs)

The AMA (1999) recommends counseling about, and prophylaxis for, STDs to sexual assault victims. Conducted within 72 hours of the attack, several tests and interventions are available. Prophylactic antibiotics may be given to prevent chlamydia, gonorrhea, trichomoniasis, and bacterial vaginosis according to guidelines from the Centers for Disease Control (CDC) (AMA, 1999). They also recommend post-exposure prophylaxis using hepatitis B immunoglobulin. Information also should be provided describing symptoms of STDs for which there are no preventive measures. Because incubation periods vary, the importance of follow-up testing must be emphasized.

There is no proven prophylactic intervention for human HIV infection, and this is a growing concern of sexual assault victims. Even though the CDC reports that the risk for acquiring HIV infection through sexual assault is low in most cases, some states mandate testing for HIV as part of the sexual assault protocol. The AMA (1999) states, "Baseline testing can diagnose or rule out preexisting HIV infection, but repeated testing after 6 months and again in 1 year is recommended, particularly when the assailant is known to be HIV positive or the serostatus is unknown" (p. 15).

Pregnancy Risk Evaluation and Prevention

It is important that sexual assault victims receive information related to risks and interventions for prevention of conception as a result of the assault. Evaluation of pregnancy risk is based on the client's ability to relay accurate information about the occurrence of her last menses so that an estimate can be made of time of ovulation. Prophylactic regimens are 97 to 98 percent effective if started within 24 hours of the sexual attack and are generally only recommended within 72 hours (Ledray, 2001). If the client chooses, a regimen of ethinyl estradiol and norgestrel (Ovral) can be administered. Two tablets are taken at the time of treatment and two tablets are taken 12 hours later. An antiemetic, such as trimethobenzamide (Tigan), may be given to prevent nausea and vomiting, the most common side effects of the medication.

Crisis Intervention and Arrangements for Follow-Up Counseling

In the hours immediately following the sexual assault, the rape victim experiences an overwhelming sense of violation and helplessness that began with the powerlessness and intimidation experienced during the rape. Burgess (2007) has identified two emotional response patterns that may occur within hours after a rape and that health care workers may encounter in the emergency department or rape crisis center. In the *expressed response pattern*, the victim expresses feelings of fear, anger, and anxiety through such behaviors as crying, sobbing, smiling, restlessness, and tension. In the *controlled response pattern*, the feelings are masked or hidden, and a calm, composed, or subdued affect is seen. Brown (2007) suggests that helping the victim to regain a sense of control—that is, helping her to make decisions about what she wants to do—can be an effective method of enhancing recovery. Brown (2007) states:

> Lack of control during a rape or sexual assault creates special needs in victims. These women need to feel in control [of everything that happens in the ED]. Any hint of lack of control can trigger an uncooperative, difficult, or anxious response, and they may be lost to follow-up. Providing as much control as possible for these women in clinical situations within safety guidelines may greatly increase their comfort level.

This is also an important time to ensure that the victim understands that she is not to blame for what has happened. She may be blaming herself and feeling guilty for certain behaviors, such as drinking or walking alone late at night, that may have placed her in a vulnerable position. It is important to communicate the following to the victim of sexual assault:

- You are safe here.
- I'm sorry that it happened.
- I'm glad you survived.
- It's not your fault. No one deserves to be treated this way.
- You did the best that you could.

Before she leaves the emergency department, the individual should be advised about the importance of returning for follow-up counseling. She should be given the names of individuals to call for support. Often a survivor will not follow up with aftercare because she is too ashamed or is fearful of having to relive the nightmare of the attack by sharing the information in group or individual counseling. For this reason, it may be important for the nurse to get permission from the individual to allow a counselor to call her to make a follow-up appointment.

Deaths in the Emergency Department

The emergency department becomes the scene of legal investigation when death occurs in the trauma care setting. Evidence is preserved and the body is protected until the investigation has been completed. Hufft and Peternelj-Taylor (2003) state:

> When investigating a death scene, the clinical forensic nurse interviews witnesses, takes charge of the body, examines the body, photographs the body, secures physical evidence, arranges body transport, and gathers records. The coroner is usually in charge of death investigation. Nurses working in this capacity initiate or assist with death investigation under selected circumstances of homicide, violence, suicide, and suspicious circumstances that indicate a violation of criminal law (e.g., presence of illegal drugs, a body found in water, a fire, explosion). (p. 421)

Anatomical Gifts

When a sudden and unexpected death occurs in the trauma care setting, the clinical forensic nurse may become involved in organ/tissue donation. Some states now require that a request for organ/tissue donation be made of the family when a death occurs under certain circumstances. This is a very painful period for family members, and nurses may feel it is an inappropriate time to present the information associated with an anatomical request. However, most nurses employed in trauma care recognize that organ/tissue recovery for transplantation is a requisite component of their work. Shafer (2006) states:

> The forensic nurse examiner (FNE) can serve as a bridge between families of the bereaved and the medical examiner. Time spent with grieving families, helping them to cope with the events surrounding the death of their loved one, is certainly a role in which the FNE, as a nurse, would excel. Organ and tissue donation are often the only comfort that a family gains in an otherwise tragic situation. The FNE works closely with the organ recovery coordinator by coordinating information in donation situations, and she or he works jointly with other healthcare professionals by assisting families in moving forward through their loss. (p. 232)

Evaluation

Evaluation of the clinical forensic nursing process in the trauma care setting involves ongoing measurement of the diagnostic criteria aimed at resolution of identified real or potential problems. The following types of questions may provide assistance in the evaluation process.

1. Have the physical and psychological needs of the survivors who present themselves to the emergency department been met?
2. Has the evidence in potential criminal investigations been handled such that it can be used in a credible manner?
3. Has the sexual assault survivor received information related to choices pertaining to STDs, pregnancy, and follow-up counseling?
4. In the instance of sudden and unexpected death in the emergency department, have the needs of the grieving family been met?

5. Have the importance of anatomical donations been communicated?

The role of the clinical forensic nurse in trauma care continues to expand. With the level of societal violence at epidemic proportions, clinical forensic nurses potentially may intervene in the examination of victims of all types of abuse situations. The clinical forensic nurse specialist must also strive to be proactive, beginning with educating emergency department staff in the philosophy and interventions of clinical forensic nursing practice. Within the community, proactive responsibilities may include providing information about environmental hazards and issues that may affect public health and safety. Effectiveness of these changes provides measurement for ongoing evaluation.

APPLICATION OF THE NURSING PROCESS IN FORENSIC PSYCHIATRIC NURSING IN CORRECTIONAL FACILITIES

Assessment

Notwithstanding the positive intentions of deinstitutionalization, some negative consequences may have ensued. Raphael (2000) states:

> To the extent that the untreated mentally ill commit crimes and receive prison sentences at a relatively high rate, "deinstitutionalization" of the mentally ill from state and county hospitals may increase prison populations. Indeed, the pronounced increase in the U.S. prison population over the past three decades occurred concurrently with unprecedented declines in the numbers of committed mentally ill. [Trends in continual declines in the mental hospital population] appear to support the contention that deinstitutionalization has shifted the burden of providing services for the mentally ill onto the criminal justice system—i.e., jails and prisons have become de facto mental institutions. (pp. 1-2)

It was believed that deinstitutionalization increased the freedom of mentally ill individuals in accordance with the principle of "least restrictive alternative." Because of inadequate community-based services, however, many of these individuals drifted into poverty and homelessness, increasing their vulnerability to criminalization. Because the bizarre behavior of mentally ill individuals living on the street is sometimes offensive to community standards, law enforcement officials have the authority to protect the welfare of the public and the safety of the individual by initiating emergency hospitalization. Legal criteria for commitment are so stringent in most cases, however, that arrest becomes an easier way of getting the mentally ill person off the street if a criminal statute has been violated. According to the Bureau of Justice, more than half of all prison and jail inmates have some form of mental health problem (James & Glaze, 2006). Some of these individuals are incarcerated as a result of the increasingly popular "guilty but mentally ill" verdict. With this verdict, the individual is deemed mentally ill, yet is held criminally responsible for his actions. He or she is incarcerated and receives special treatment, if needed, but no different from that available for and needed by any prisoner.

The U.S. Department of Justice has reported that U.S. prisons and jails held more than 2 million inmates in 2006 (Sabol, Minton, & Harrison, 2007). The report stated that 43.9 percent of the national jail population was white, 38.6 percent were African American, 15.6 percent were Hispanic, and 1.9 percent were American Indians, Alaska Natives, Asians, Pacific Islanders, or of two or more races. Men accounted for 87 percent of the total.

Care of the mentally-ill offender population is a highly specialized area of nursing practice. The rationale of imprisonment for criminal behavior has been identified as:

● Retribution to society
● Deterrence of future crimes
● Rehabilitation and repentance
● Protection of society

If an institution bases its orientation on retribution and deterrence of criminal activity, the prison will reflect a punishment-oriented atmosphere. If rehabilitation and repentance are accepted as a basis for change, mental health programs that encourage reflection and insight may be a part of the correctional setting. Because at times these basic objectives may seem incompatible with each other, nurses who work in correctional facilities may struggle with a cognitive dissonance founded in their basic nursing value system.

IMPLICATIONS OF RESEARCH FOR EVIDENCE-BASED PRACTICE

Yurkovich, E. & Smyer, T. (2000, June). Health maintenance behaviors of individuals with severe and persistent mental illness in a state prison. *Journal of Psychosocial Nursing and Mental Health Services, 38(6),* 20–31.

Description of the Study: The purpose of this study was to define health and health-seeking behaviors of incarcerated individuals experiencing severe and persistent mental illness (SPMI) in a state prison. The researchers conducted a comparative analysis of these findings to two studies that explored the same questions with individuals experiencing SPMI and attending two different community treatment centers. The researchers also examined strategies used by inmates with SPMI to prevent loss of control and maintain health in the prison environment. Information was gathered by in-depth interview using a semi-structured interview guide, participant observation, and review of inmates' charts. Nineteen

prisoners with SPMI participated. Age range was 21 to 56 and educational level ranged from 4 to 18 years. Fifteen prisoners had committed crimes against person and 4 had committed crimes against property. Criminal activity was related to substance abuse in 15 of the cases. All interviews were conducted in a room set aside for the researchers in the prison infirmary.

Results of the Study: Individuals in the community are able to define their environment through use of healthcare providers and the trusted informal system of peers, friends, and relatives. Individuals with SPMI in the corrections facility do not have this connection. Negative response from other inmates to the behavior of inmates with SPMI reduces their ability to seek an appropriate level of assistance and maintain a healthy status. Some comparisons from the study are as follows:

Variable	Community-Based Individuals	Inmates with SPMI
Relationships	Maintains a balance within family	Maintains relationships based on purpose (e.g., to provide protection or prevent abuse)
Feelings	Controls negative feelings and prevents destructive outcome when feeling angry (e.g., leave hostile environment)	Control of negative feelings by self-imposed solitude, lock down, or withdrawal from socialization areas
Attitude	Builds self-esteem through purpose or goal completion	Lack of opportunity for building self esteem
Functional Behaviors	Performs ADLs and participates in treatment center activities	Lacks opportunities to perform and participate

The prisoners demonstrated a need for education about their illnesses and medications. They demonstrated little insight into how stress and poor physical health affected their mental illness.

Implications for Nursing Practice: The authors state, "This study communicates a message from prisoners with

SPMI that tells health care providers how they struggle to maintain a healthy status within a toxic environment and what they need to support this process. Nurses within a correctional setting have a responsibility to assist individuals with SPMI to interpret their environment, define role behaviors, and determine how to maintain wellness within the prison system."

Assessing Mental Health Needs of the Incarcerated

Is the provision of mental health care within the custodial environment possible? Or are clinical care concerns incompatible with security issues? What special knowledge and skills must a psychiatric nurse possess to be successful in caring for the mentally ill offender?

Psychiatric diagnoses commonly identified in incarcerated individuals include schizophrenia, bipolar disorder, major depression, substance use disorders, personality disorders, and many have dual diagnoses (Yurkovich & Smyer, 2000). Common psychiatric behaviors include hallucinations, suspiciousness, thought disorders, anger/agitation, and impulsivity. Denial of problems is a common behavior among this population. Use of substances and medication noncompliance are common obstacles to rehabilitation. Substance abuse has been shown to have a strong correlation with recidivism among the prison population. Many individuals report that they were under the influence of illegal substances at the time of their criminal actions, and dual diagnoses are common. Detoxification frequency occurs in jails and prisons, and some deaths have occurred from the withdrawal syndrome because of inadequate treatment during this process.

Metzner and Dvoskin (2004) point out that there is a fundamental difference between prisons and jails. They define local jails, which are usually administered by city or county officials, as "facilities that hold inmates beyond arraignment, generally for 48 hours, but less than a year." In contrast, prisons, which are run by state or federal administrations, are correctional facilities that house individuals convicted of major crimes or felonies and who are serving sentences that are usually in excess of a year. A large portion of offenders who are mentally ill, particularly the acutely psychotic, never reach the prison system. Frequent arrests for minor offenses may lead to numerous jail incarcerations, a sense of loss of control, and a continual state of crisis. The National Center on Institutions and Alternatives (2007) reports that the suicide rate in county jails is several times greater than that of the general population, while the suicide rate in prisons remains slightly higher than in the community.

Special Concerns

Overcrowding and Violence

Numerous studies have shown that crowding affects the level of violence in prisons. The prison system is not capable of handling the burden of large numbers of prisoners for which it has become responsible, and many of the infractions by prisoners are violent in nature. The growing number of prisoners is thought to be related to the increasing war on drugs, longer mandatory sentencing, and the "three strikes and you're out" laws. As this population continues to grow, the solution seems to be to continue to construct larger and larger complexes to house the growing numbers of inmates. The unfortunate truth lies in the fact that violent behavior often proves to be resourceful for the individuals who use it in prison.

Inmate violence directed toward prison staff is also a common occurrence. Light (1991) reported the most frequently cited motives as: inmate resistance to officer's commands, protest of unjust treatment, resistance to searches and attempt to remove contraband, and staff intervention in fights between inmates. Actual or implied verbal threats and swearing are the common everyday language of most offender clients. Nurses who work in correctional facilities must be able to adjust to the commonality of physical and verbal aggression if they are to prevail in this chosen area of specialization.

Sexual Assault

On September 4, 2003, President George W. Bush signed into law the Prison Rape Elimination Act of 2003. This legislation requires the Bureau of Justice Statistics (BJS) to develop new national data collections on the incidence and prevalence of sexual violence within correctional facilities (Beck & Harrison, 2006). Currently, it is estimated that at least 13 percent of inmates in the United States have been sexually assaulted in prison, with many of them suffering repeated assaults (Cornell University Law School, 2007). The majority of these assaults go unreported because the consequences of "ratting" on fellow prisoners are often far more serious than the rape itself.

Rape in prison is viewed as an act of dominance and power, rather than one that is sexually motivated, and the majority of both victims and victimizers are heterosexuals. The typical victim is a young person convicted of a nonviolent crime. They are most likely to be first-time offenders who are small, weak, shy, and inexperienced with prison life. In some instances, sexual assault is used as a means of punishment and social control when the victim is believed to have violated certain unwritten prison codes. Gang rape is not uncommon, and severe physical injury is often the result if the victim attempts to defend himself.

HIV Infection in the Prison Population

The AIDS rate is more than three times higher in state and federal prisons than in the general U.S. population (Kantor, 2006). In addition to sexual conduct, other means of HIV transmission among inmates include fights that result in lacerations, bites, or bleeding. Body piercing and tattooing are popular in prison, and clean instruments for these activities are not available. Intravenous drug use results in sharing of unsterilized injection equipment.

HIV has placed an enormous financial burden on a prison system that was already financially distressed. Some terminally ill prisoners with advanced HIV disease are being granted early compassionate release to family or hospice care and with access to community health services (Kantor, 2006).

The most recent approach to prevention of HIV transmission has shifted from segregation to education. Education of the prison population about HIV is difficult because as many as 50 percent of American prisoners are functionally illiterate, and many do not speak English (Kantor, 2006). Educational programs to meet the communication needs of this special population would be required.

Female Offenders

Women comprise approximately 13 percent of the total population in prisons and jails (Sabol, Minton, & Harrison, 2007). As a minority group, they appear to be discriminated against within the prison system. Their facilities are usually more isolated, making it more difficult for family visits. In some instances, separate institutions do not exist, making it necessary to house male and female offenders in co-correctional facilities. Men are given a greater number of opportunities regarding education and vocational training services. McClellan (2002) states:

> My first study of women prisoners uncovered striking disparity: women prisoners were cited more often for disciplinary infractions than were men. Rules scrupulously enforced in women's institutions were routinely ignored in men's. Although their infractions were less serious in nature, women were punished more severely than men. Operating under the same set of court-mandated formal rules, prisons display two gender-differentiated systems of surveillance and control.

Many women are single mothers who are unable to make adequate provision for their children while they serve their time in prison and who often lose custody of their children to the state. Prison health care is mostly inadequate, and the unique health needs of women often go unmet. Many of these women had very little before they were incarcerated, and have come to expect that little is what they deserve. Many report long histories of sexual and emotional abuse throughout their lives. Depression and acting-out behaviors are common in women's prisons.

Nursing Diagnosis

Forensic psychiatric nurse specialists in correctional facilities analyze the information gathered during assessment of the client to formulate nursing diagnoses. Common nursing diagnoses relevant to forensic clients in correctional facilities include:

● Defensive coping
● Complicated grieving
● Anxiety/Fear
● Disturbed thought processes
● Powerlessness
● Low self-esteem
● Risk for self-mutilation
● Risk for self-directed or other-directed violence
● Ineffective coping
● Ineffective sexuality pattern
● Risk for infection

Planning/Implementation

Psychiatric nurses who work in correctional facilities must be armed with extraordinary psychosocial skills and the knowledge to apply them in the most appropriate manner.

Development of a Therapeutic Relationship

Incarcerated individuals have difficulty trusting anyone associated with authority, including nurses. For most of these individuals, this likely relates back to very early stages of development and lack of nurturing.

Aside from the added difficulty of dealing with this special population, development of a therapeutic relationship in the correctional facility encompasses the same phases of interaction as it does with other clients. Chapter 7 of this text discusses the dynamics of this process at length.

Preinteraction Phase

During this phase, the nurse must examine his or her feelings, fears, and anxieties about working with prisoners, and in particular violent offenders—perhaps murderers, rapists, or pedophiles. This is the phase in which the nurse must determine whether he or she is able to separate the *person* from the *behavior* and provide the unconditional positive regard that Rogers (1951) believed identified each individual as a worthwhile and unique human being.

Orientation (Introductory) Phase

This is the phase in which the nurse works to establish trust with the client. This is a lengthy and intense process with the prisoner population. The characteristics that have been identified as significant to the development of a therapeutic nurse-client relationship—rapport, trust, and genuineness—are commonly met with suspicion on the part of the offender. Empathy may be used as a tool for manipulating the nurse. It is therefore imperative that limits be established and enforced by all of the nursing staff. Testing of limits is commonplace, so consequences for violation must be consistently administered. Splitting treatment team members against each other is a common ploy among inmates (Schafer, 1999).

Touch and self-disclosure, two elements used in the establishment of trust with clients, are most commonly unacceptable with the prisoner population. A handshake may be appropriate, but any other form of touch between nurse and inmate of the opposite gender is usually restricted in most settings. Self-disclosure is commonly used to convey empathy and to promote trust by helping the client view the nurse as an ordinary human being. With the prisoner population, however, the client may seek personal information about the nurse in an effort to maintain control of the relationship. Nurses must maintain awareness of the situation and ensure that personal boundaries are not being violated.

Communication within the correctional facility may prove to be a challenge for the nurse. Slang terminology is commonplace and changes rapidly. Some of these terms are presented in Box 38–1.

Working Phase

Nursing skills are implemented during the working phase of the relationship, and promoting behavioral

---

Box 38–1   Glossary of Prison Slang

Ad-Seg. Administrative segregation. A prisoner placed on ad-seg is being investigated and will go into isolation (the "hole") until the investigation is complete.

Beef. Criminal charges. As, "I caught a burglary beef this time around." Also used to mean a problem. "I have a beef with that guy."

Big Yard. The main recreation yard.

Bit. Prison sentence, usually relatively short. "I got a three-year bit." (opposite of *jolt*)

Bitch, bitched (v). To be sentenced as a "habitual offender."

Blocks. Cellhouses.

Books. Administratively controlled account ledger that lists each prisoner's account balance.

Bone Yard. The visiting trailers, used for overnight visits of wives and/or families.

Bum Beef. A false accusation. Also, a wrongful conviction.

Catch a Ride. To ask a friend with drugs to get you high. "Hey man, can I catch a ride?"

The Chain. The bus transports that bring prisoners to prison. One is shackled and chained when transported. As, "I've been riding the chain," or "I just got in on the chain," or "Is there anyone we know on the chain?"

Check-In. Someone who has submitted to pressure, intimidation, debts, etc., and no longer feels secure in population and "checks in" to a protective custody (PC) unit.

Chi-Mo. Child molester, "chester," "baby-raper," "short-eyes," (as "he has short-eyes," meaning he goes after young kids). The worst of the *rapo* class in the eyes of *convicts*.

Convict. Guys who count in prison; loyal to the code; aren't stool pigeons; their word is good (opposite of *inmate*).

C.U.S. Custody unit supervisor/cellhouse supervisor.

De-Seg. Disciplinary segregation. When a person is on de-seg, he is in isolation (the "hole") for an infraction.

Ding. A disrespectful term for a mentally ill prisoner.

Dry Snitching. To inform on someone indirectly by talking loud or performing suspicious actions when officers are in the area.

Dummy Up; Get on the Dummy. To shut up, to pipe down, to be quiet, especially about one's knowledge of a crime.

E.P.R.D. Earliest possible release date.

Fish. A new arrival, a first-timer, a bumpkin, not wise to prison life.

Gate Money. Money the state gives a prisoner upon his release.

Gate Time. At most prisons they yell "gate time," meaning one can get in or out of their cell. See *lock-up*.

Hacks/Hogs/Pigs/Snouts/Screws/Cops/Bulls. The guards; called "Corrections Officers" by themselves and *inmates*.

Heat Wave. Being under constant suspicion, thereby bringing attention to those around you.

Hit It. Go away, leave, get lost

Hold Your Mud. Not tell, even under pressure of punishment.

The Hole. An isolation ("segregation") cell, used as punishment for offenses.

House. Cell.

Hustle. A professional criminal's avocation. Also refers to any scheme to obtain money or drugs while in prison.

I.K. Inmate kitchen.

I.M.U. Intensive Management Unit. Administration's name for "segregation" or "the hole."

Inmate. Derogatory term for prisoners. Used by guards, administrators, other inmates, or new arrivals who don't know the language yet. Opposite of *convict*.

Jacket. Prison file containing all information on a prisoner. "He's a child molester; it's in his jacket." Also reputation. Prisoners can put false jackets on other prisoners to discredit them.

Jolt. A long sentence. ("I got a life jolt.") Opposite of *bit*.

Jumping-Out. Turning to crime. "I've been jumping out since I was a kid."

Keister. To hide something in the anal cavity.

Lag. A *convict*, as in, "He's an old lag, been at it all his life."

Lifer or "All Day." Anyone doing a life sentence. A life *jolt*.

Lock-Down. When prisoners are confined to their cells.

Lock-Up. Free movement period for prisoners. See also *gate time*.

Lop. Same as *inmate*.

Mule. A person who smuggles drugs into the institution.

On the Leg. A prisoner who is always chatting with and befriending guards.

Paper. A small quantity of drugs packaged for selling.

P.C. Protective custody. Also as in "He's a PC case," meaning weak or untrustworthy.

Point/Outfit. Syringe.

Pruno. Homemade wine.

Punk. Derogatory term meaning homosexual or weak individual.

Rapo. Anyone with a sex crime—generally looked down on by *convicts*.

Rat/Snitch/Stool Pigeon. n., informant. v., to inform.

Stand Point. Watch for "the man" (guard)

Tag/Write-Up. Infraction of institution rules.

The Bag/Sack. Dope.

Tom or George. Meaning "no good"(Tom) or "okay"(George). Used in conversation to indicate if someone or something is okay or not.

Turned Out. To be forced into homosexual acts, or to turn someone out to do things for you; to use someone for your own needs.

White Money. Currency within the institution.

Yard-In/Yard-Out. Closing of the recreation yard (yard-in). Recreation yard opens (yard-out).

change is the primary goal. This is extremely difficult with offenders who commonly deny problems and resist change. Transference and countertransference issues (see Chapter 7) are more common in working with this population than with other psychiatric clients. Issues are discussed in the treatment team meetings, and ongoing modifications are made as required. Following are some of the interventions associated with psychiatric forensic nursing in correctional institutions.

Counseling and Supportive Psychotherapy. Nurses may work with inmates who are experiencing feelings of powerlessness and grief. Women who have left children behind may fear the permanent loss of custody or of never seeing them again. Helping these individuals work through a period of mourning is an important nursing intervention.

Nurses may also counsel victims of sexual assault. Victims of sexual assault in prison often experience the symptoms associated with rape-trauma syndrome. Feelings of helplessness and vulnerability, coupled with shame, humiliation, and embarrassment are characteristic. Internalized rage can become paralytic. Perception of gender identity may even be compromised.

These individuals often become withdrawn and isolated and are at high risk for suicide. The nurse can recognize these symptoms and intervene as required. All unusual behavior should be shared with the treatment team. Interventions for treating specific behaviors (such as depression and suicide, psychotic behaviors, and antisocial behaviors) are located in Units 3 and 4 of this text.

Crisis Intervention. Behaviors such as aggression, self-mutilation, suicide attempts, acute psychotic episodes, and post-trauma responses, require that the nurse be proficient in crisis intervention. Feelings of helplessness and loss of control are pervasive in the prison population. The chaotic, overburdened prison system lacks the resources to provide the kind of services needed to prevent the continual state of crisis these conditions engender. Suicide risk is higher in jails and prisons than it is in the community. Noncompliance with prison rules, feelings of hopelessness, psychopathology, substance abuse, and overcrowded conditions all contribute to the potential for violence. Threatening behaviors must be reported immediately to all members of the treatment team. A strong foundation in crisis intervention theory and techniques is mandatory for nurses who work in correctional institutions.

Education. Opportunities for teaching abound in the correctional facility. As was mentioned previously, however, because of the level of education of many incarcerated individuals, and because many of them speak little English, the teaching plan must be highly individualized. Many have no desire or motivation to learn and resist cooperating with these efforts. Important educational endeavors with these clients include:

● **Health Teaching.** Most criminals are not in good physical condition when they reach prison. They have lived rough lives of smoking, poor diets, substance abuse, and minimal health care. This is an opportunity for nurses to provide information about ways to achieve optimum wellness.

● **HIV/AIDS Education.** Kantor (2006) states:

> All persons entering prison must be informed in clear, simple terms, *and in their own language*, about how to avoid transmission of HIV and other communicable diseases. Educational programs can reduce fears about HIV and its transmission among staff members and inmates. Individual counseling, peer counseling, support groups, and special programs for women, designed by and for prisoners, have been successful in a number of institutions and seem to be the best educational tools.

Some correctional institutions now provide condoms to inmates, but this remains a point of controversy between legal and public health officials.

● **Stress Management.** Nurses can present information and demonstration of stress management techniques. They can help individuals practice reduction of anxiety without resorting to medications or substances.

● **Substance Abuse.** The Federal Bureau of Prisons (2007) has established a comprehensive substance abuse treatment strategy in an effort to change inmates' criminal and drug-using behaviors. This strategy begins with drug abuse education and ends with a strong community transition component. The individuals receive information about alcohol and drugs and the physical, social, and psychological impact of abusing these substances. Since its inception, this program has proved highly successful in decreasing recidivism and relapse rates among its participants.

Nurses can participate in substance abuse treatment programs by providing client education (e.g., the effects of substances on the body; the consequences of sharing needles). They can also form support groups for individuals who abuse substances if one does not exist in the institution. A large percentage of the prison population has a history of substance abuse, and many correlate the commission of their crimes with substance use. This is an important area of need for nursing intervention in the correctional system.

Termination Phase

Ideally, the termination phase of the nurse-client relationship ensures therapeutic closure. This is not always possible in the correctional environment. Prisoners are transferred from one institution to another, and from one part of an institution to another, for a variety of reasons, not the least of which are safety and security of self or others. When possible, it is important for nurses to initiate termination with clients so that at least some semblance of closure can be achieved and a review of goal attainment can be accomplished. Community facilities for mentally ill ex-offenders are few, and recidivism is rampant. Johnson (2007) states:

> The majority of mentally ill offenders need the basic elements of case management. Psychiatric nurses in correctional settings often act as case managers, beginning prerelease

planning upon the initial contact with inmates. Continuation of any treatment and medication from jail and transition to the community-based treatment in a swift manner is critical to success. Unfortunately resources in this area are often lacking. Many inmates may not have predetermined release dates, thereby leading to releases at all hours of the day and night. Prerelease planning and coordination with community-based programs are necessary to promote continuity of care and recidivism. Nurses are vital members of the interdisciplinary team and play significant roles in the assessment, planning, implementation, and evaluation of the case management plan to best meet the needs of patients.

Evaluation

Evaluation of the psychiatric forensic nursing process in the correctional environment involves ongoing measurement of the diagnostic criteria aimed at resolution of identified real or potential problems. The following types of questions may provide assistance in the evaluation process.

● Has a degree of trust been established in the nurse-client relationship?
● Has violence by the offender to self or others been prevented?
● If victimization has occurred, has appropriate care and support been provided to the survivor?
● Have limits been set on inappropriate behaviors, and has consistency of consequences for violation of the limits been administered by all staff?
● Have educational programs been established to provide information about health and wellness, HIV/AIDS, stress management, and substance abuse?

Evaluation is an ongoing process and must be assumed by the entire treatment team. Modification of the treatment plan as required is part of the ongoing evaluation process, and positive change within the system is the ultimate outcome. Nurses who work in correctional facilities are "pioneers" within the nursing profession. To share the knowledge gleaned from this specialty area is an important part of the nursing process.

SUMMARY AND KEY POINTS

● Forensic nursing, which is a growing area within the profession, is composed of a variety of areas of expertise.
● Forensic nurses take care of both victims and perpetrators of crime in a variety of settings, including primary care facilities, hospitals, and correctional institutions.
● The International Association of Forensic Nurses, founded in 1992, now has more than 2500 members.
● Forensic nursing specialties include clinical forensic nursing, the sexual assault nurse examiner, forensic psychiatric nursing, and correctional/institutional nursing.
● Nurses in general practice also find forensic nursing knowledge of importance in their practices, particularly in emergency departments and intensive care units.
● Forensic nurses in trauma care are involved with preservation of evidence, investigation of wound characteristics, and management of responsibilities associated with deaths that occur in the emergency department, including assisting with requests for anatomical gifts.
● Forensic psychiatric nurses in correctional facilities involves care of the mentally ill offender population, as well as the emotional needs of all incarcerated individuals.
● Interventions for the forensic psychiatric nurse include establishment of a therapeutic relationship; providing counseling and supportive psychotherapy; intervening in crises; and providing education concerning health and wellness issues, HIV/AIDS, stress management, and substance abuse.
● The number of educational offerings pertaining to forensic nursing is growing. Some content is taught in traditional nursing courses, whereas some colleges and universities are establishing forensic nursing courses as electives.
● Forensic nursing is fertile ground for nursing research, and the complex nature of the specialty lends itself well to those nurses who seek a challenge within the profession.

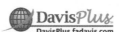

DavisPlus
DavisPlus.fadavis.com

For additional clinical tools and study aids, visit DavisPlus.

REVIEW QUESTIONS

Self-Examination/Learning Exercise

Identify whether each of the following questions is true or false.

1. All traumatic injuries in which liability is suspected are considered within the scope of forensic nursing.

    a._____true   b._____false

2. Clinical forensic nursing in the trauma department encompasses preservation of evidence, investigation of wound characteristics, and sudden deaths in the emergency department (ED).

    a._____true   b._____false

3. Legal authorities must be notified of all deaths, natural or unnatural, that occur in the ED.

    a._____true   b._____false

4. When a trauma victim is admitted to the ED, the most obvious priority intervention is preservation of evidence.

    a._____true   b._____false

5. When clothing is removed, it should be shaken to remove any possible evidence that may be adhering to it.

    a._____true   b._____false

6. Rape victims can be treated prophylactically for sexually transmitted diseases.

    a._____true   b._____false

7. The most common psychiatric behavior that has been identified among mentally ill offenders is thought disorder.

    a._____true   b._____false

8. The AIDS rate is higher in state and federal prisons than in the general population.

    a._____true   b._____false

9. Male offenders receive more educational opportunities in prison than female offenders.

    a._____true   b._____false

10. Correctional institutions are federally mandated to provide condoms to inmates to prevent the transmission of HIV.

    a._____true   b._____false

Test Your **Critical Thinking Skills**

Kim is a 27-year-old woman who recently moved from a small town in Texas to work in the city of Dallas as a reporter for one of the major newspapers. She is 5'6" tall and weighs 115 lb. To keep in shape she likes to jog, which she did regularly in her hometown. She doesn't know anyone in Dallas and has been lonely for her family since arriving. But she has moved into a small apartment in a quiet neighborhood and hopes to meet young people soon though her work and church.

On the first Saturday morning after she moved into her new apartment, Kim decided to get up early and go jogging. It was still dark out, but Kim was not afraid. She had been jogging alone in the dark many times in her hometown. She donned her jogging clothes and headed down the quiet street toward a nearby park. As she entered the park, an individual came out from a dense clump of bushes, put a knife to her throat, and ordered her

to the ground. She was raped and beaten unconscious. She remained in that condition until sunrise when she was found by another jogger who called emergency services, and Kim was taken to the nearest emergency department. Upon regaining consciousness, Kim was hysterical, but a sexual assault nurse examiner (SANE) was called to the scene, and Kim was assigned to a quiet area of the hospital, where the post-rape examination was initiated.

Answer the following questions related to Kim:

1. What are the initial nursing interventions for Kim?
2. What treatments must the nurse ensure that Kim is aware are available for her?
3. What nursing diagnosis would the nurse expect to focus on with Kim in follow-up care?

gives another person legal power to make decisions regarding health care when an individual is no longer capable of making such decisions. Some states have adopted forms that combine the intent of the durable power of attorney for health care (i.e., to have a proxy) and the intent of the living will (i.e., to state choices for end-of-life medical treatment).

Doctors usually follow clearly stated directives. It is important that the physician be informed that an advanced directive exists and what the specific wishes of the client are. In most states, health care professionals are legally bound to honor the client's wishes (Norlander, 2001). In 1990, the U.S. Congress passed legislation requiring that all health care facilities that receive Medicare or Medicaid funds advise clients of their rights to refuse treatment and to make advance directives available to clients on admission (Aiken, 2004). Aiken (2004) states:

Every state has enacted legislation that allows individuals to execute living wills or durable power of attorney for health care. These directives are binding on health care providers. Historically, there were problems between states that had no such legislation and states that did because some states would not accept advance directives from other states. (p. 263)

Catalano (2006) points out that unless a natural death act has been enacted into law by a state, the living will has no mechanism of legal enforcement. These laws have been called "pull the plug" statues and have various names in different states, such as "Removal of Life Support Systems Act" (Connecticut), "Natural Death Act" (Washington), "Declaration of Death Act" (New Jersey), and "Medical Treatment Decision Act" (Arizona) (Mantel, 2007). Catalano (2006) states:

In some states, a living will is considered only advisory and the physician has the right to comply with the living will or treat the client as the physician deems most appropriate. There is no protection for nurses or other health care practitioners against criminal or civil liability in the execution of living wills in states without a natural death act. (p. 149)

Norlander (2001) suggests the following reasons why advance directives sometimes are not honored:

● The advance directive is not available at the time treatment decisions need to be made. This is especially true in emergency situations.
● The advance directive is not clear. Statements such as "no heroic measures" can be interpreted in many different ways.
● The health care proxy is unsure of the client's wishes.

Advance directives allow the client to be in control of decisions at the end of life. It is also a way to spare family and loved ones the burden of making choices without knowing what is most important to the person who is dying.

SUMMARY AND KEY POINTS

● Loss is the experience of separation from something of personal importance.
● Loss is anything that is perceived as such by the individual.
● Loss of any concept of value to an individual can trigger the grief response.
● Elisabeth Kübler-Ross identified five stages that individuals pass through on their way to resolution of a loss. These include denial, anger, bargaining, depression, and acceptance.
● John Bowlby described similar stages that he identified in the following manner: stage I, numbness or protest; stage II, disequilibrium; stage III, disorganization and despair; and stage IV, reorganization.
● George Engel's stages include shock and disbelief, developing awareness, restitution, resolution of the loss, and recovery.
● J. William Worden, a more contemporary clinician, has proposed that bereaved individuals must accomplish a set of tasks in order to complete the grief process. These four tasks include accepting the reality of the loss, working through the pain of grief, adjusting to an environment that has changed because of the loss, and emotionally relocating the lost entity and moving on with life.
● The length of the grief process is highly individual, and it can last for a number of years without being maladaptive.
● The acute stage of the grief process usually lasts a couple of months, but resolution usually lasts much longer.
● Kübler-Ross suggests that a calendar year of experiencing significant events and anniversaries without the lost entity may be required.
● Anticipatory grieving is the experiencing of the feelings and emotions associated with the normal grief process in response to anticipation of the loss.
● Anticipatory grieving is thought to facilitate the grief process when the actual loss occurs.
● Three types of pathological grief reactions have been described. These include the following:
  ● Delayed or inhibited grief in which there is absence of evidence of grief when it ordinarily would be expected.
  ● Distorted or exaggerated grief response in which the individual remains fixed in the anger stage of the grief process and all of the symptoms associated with normal grieving are exaggerated.
  ● Chronic or prolonged grieving in which the individual is unable to let go of grieving behaviors after a extended period of time and in which behaviors are evident that indicate the bereaved individual is not accepting that the loss has occurred.
● Several authors have identified one crucial difference between normal and maladaptive grieving: the loss of self-esteem.

● Feelings of worthlessness are indicative of depression rather than uncomplicated bereavement.
● Very young children do not understand death, but often react to the emotions of adults by becoming more irritable and crying more. They often believe death is reversible.
● School-age children understand the finality of death. Grief behaviors may reflect regression or aggression, school phobias, or sometimes a withdrawal into the self.
● Adolescents are usually able to view death on an adult level. Grieving behaviors may include withdrawal or acting out. Although they understand that their own death is inevitable, the concept is so far-reaching as to be imperceptible.
● By the time a person reaches the 60s or 70s, he or she has experienced numerous losses. Because grief is cumulative, this can result in bereavement overload. Depression is a common response.

● Nurses must be aware of the death rituals and grief behaviors common to various cultures. Some of these rituals associated with African Americans, Asian Americans, Filipino Americans, Jewish Americans, Mexican Americans, and Native Americans were presented in this chapter.
● Hospice is a program that provides palliative and supportive care to meet the special needs of people who are dying and their families.
● The term advance directives refers to either a living will or a durable power of attorney for health care. Advance directives allow clients to be in control of decisions at the end of life, and spare family and loved ones the burden of making choices without knowing what is most important to the person who is dying.

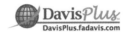 **DavisPlus**
DavisPlus.fadavis.com

For additional clinical tools and study aids, visit DavisPlus.

REVIEW QUESTIONS

Self-Examination/Learning Exercise

Select the answer that is most appropriate for each of the following questions.

1. Which of the following is most likely to initiate a grief response in an individual?

   a. Death of the pet dog
   b. Being told by her doctor that she has begun menopause
   c. Failing an exam
   d. A only
   e. All of the above

2. Nancy, who is dying of cancer, says to the nurse, "I just want to see my new grandbaby. If only God will let me live until she is born. Then I'll be ready to go." This is an example of which of Kübler-Ross's stages of grief?

   a. Denial
   b. Anger
   c. Bargaining
   d. Acceptance

3. Gloria, a recent widow, states, "I'm going to have to learn to pay all the bills. Hank always did that. I don't know if I can handle all of that." This is an example of which of the tasks described by Worden?

   a. Task I. Accepting the reality of the loss
   b. Task II. Working through the pain of grief
   c. Task III. Adjusting to an environment that has changed because of the loss
   d. Task IV. Emotionally relocating the lost entity and moving on with life

4. Engel identifies which of the following as successful resolution of the grief process?

   a. When the bereaved person can talk about the loss without crying
   b. When the bereaved person no longer talks about the lost entity
   c. When the bereaved person puts all remembrances of the loss out of sight
   d. When the bereaved person can discuss both positive and negative aspects about what has been lost.

5. Which of the following is thought to facilitate the grief process?

   a. The ability to grieve in anticipation of the loss
   b. The ability to grieve alone without interference from others
   c. Having recently grieved for another loss
   d. Taking personal responsibility for the loss

6. When Frank's wife of 34 years dies, he is very stoic, handles all the funeral arrangements, doesn't cry or appear sad, and comforts all of the other family members in their grief. Two years later, when Frank's best friend dies, Frank has sleep disturbances, difficulty concentrating, loss of weight, and difficulty performing on his job. This is an example of which of the following maladaptive responses to loss?

   a. Delayed grieving
   b. Distorted grieving
   c. Prolonged grieving
   d. Exaggerated grieving

7. A major difference between normal and maladaptive grieving has been identified by which of the following?

   a. There are no feelings of depression in normal grieving.
   b. There is no loss of self-esteem in normal grieving.
   c. Normal grieving lasts no longer than 1 year.
   d. In normal grief the person does not show anger toward the loss.

8. Which grief reaction can the nurse anticipate in a 10-year-old child?

    a. Statements that the deceased person will soon return
    b. Regressive behaviors, such as loss of bladder control
    c. A preoccupation with the loss
    d. Thinking that they may have done something to cause the death

9. Which of the following is a correct statement when attempting to distinguish normal grief from clinical depression?

    a. In clinical depression, anhedonia is prevalent.
    b. In normal grieving, the person has generalized feelings of guilt.
    c. The person who is clinically depressed relates feelings of depression to a specific loss.
    d. In normal grieving, there is a persistent state of dysphoria.

10. Which of the following is *not* true regarding grieving by an adolescent?

    a. Adolescents may not show their true feelings about the death.
    b. Adolescents tend to have an immortal attitude.
    c. Adolescents do not perceive death as inevitable.
    d. Adolescents may exhibit acting out behaviors as part of their grief.

REFERENCES

Aiken, T.D. (2004). *Legal, ethical, and political issues in nursing* (2nd ed.). Philadelphia: F.A. Davis.

Asante, M.K. (2007). *Contours of the African American culture.* Retrieved April 8, 2007 from http://africawithin.com/asante/contours.htm

Bateman, A.L. (1999). Understanding the process of grieving and loss: A critical social thinking perspective. *Journal of the American Psychiatric Nurses Association, 5*(5), 139–147.

Catalano, J.T. (2006). *Nursing Now! Today's issues, tomorrow's trends* (4th ed.). Philadelphia: F.A. Davis.

Eisendrath, S.J., & Lichtmacher, J.E. (2005). Psychiatric disorders. In L.M. Tierney, S.J. McPhee, & M.A. Papadakis (Eds.), *Current medical diagnosis and treatment* (44th ed.). New York: McGraw-Hill.

Glanville, C.L. (2003). People of African-American heritage. In L.D. Purnell & B.J. Paulanka (Eds.), *Transcultural health care* (2nd ed.). Philadelphia: F.A. Davis.

Halstead, H.L. (2005). Spirituality in older adults. In M. Stanley, K.A. Blair, & P.G. Beare (Eds.), *Gerontological nursing: A health promotion/protection approach* (3rd ed.). Philadelphia: F. A. Davis.

Kaplan, H.I., Sadock, B.J., & Grebb, J.A. (1994). *Synopsis of psychiatry: Behavioral sciences, clinical psychiatry* (7th ed.). Baltimore: Williams & Wilkins.

Mantel, D.L. (2007). Laws on death and dying. *Advance for long-term care management.* Retrieved July 15, 2007 from http://long-term-care.advanceweb.com

Murray, R.B., & Zentner, J.P. (2001). *Health promotion strategies through the life span* (7th ed.). Upper Saddle River, NJ: Prentice Hall.

National Hospice and Palliative Care Organization (NHPCO). (2000). *Standards of Practice for hospice programs.* Alexandria, VA: NHPCO.

Norlander, L. (2001). *To comfort always: A nurse's guide to end of life care.* Washington, DC: American Nurses Publishing.

Nowak, T.T. (2003). Vietnamese-Americans. In L.D. Purnell & B.J. Paulanka (Eds.), *Transcultural health care: A culturally competent approach* (2nd ed.). Philadelphia: F.A. Davis.

Pacquiao, D.F. (2003). People of Filipino Heritage. In L.D. Purnell & B.J. Paulanka (Eds.), *Transcultural health care: A culturally competent approach.* Philadelphia: F.A. Davis.

Periyakoil, V.J. (2005). *Is it grief or depression?* (2nd ed.). End-of-Life/Palliative Education Resource Center. Retrieved April 7, 2007 from http://www.eperc.mcw.edu

Purnell, L.D., & Paulanka, B.J. (2003). *Transcultural health care: A culturally competent approach* (2nd ed.). Philadelphia: F.A. Davis.

Purnell, L.D., & Paulanka, B.J. (2005). *Guide to culturally competent health care.* Philadelphia: F.A. Davis.

Sadock, B.J., & Sadock, V.A. (2003). *Synopsis of psychiatry: Behavioral sciences/clinical psychiatry* (9th ed.). Philadelphia: Lippincott Williams & Wilkins

Selekman, J. (2003). People of Jewish heritage. In L.D. Purnell & B.J. Paulanka (Eds.), *Transcultural health care: A culturally competent approach.* Philadelphia: F.A. Davis.

Still, O., & Hodgins, D. (2003). Navajo Indians. In L.D. Purnell & B.J. Paulanka (Eds.), *Transcultural health care: A culturally competent approach* (2nd ed.). Philadelphia: F.A. Davis.

Wang, Y. (2003). People of Chinese heritage. In L.D. Purnell & B.J. Paulanka (Eds.), *Transcultural health care* (2nd ed.). Philadelphia: F.A. Davis.

Worden, J.W. (2002). *Grief counseling and grief therapy: A handbook for the mental health practitioner* (3rd ed.). New York: Springer.

Zoucha, R., & Purnell, L.D. (2003). People of Mexican heritage. In L.D. Purnell & B.J. Paulanka (Eds.), *Transcultural health care: A culturally competent approach.* Philadelphia: F.A. Davis.

CLASSICAL REFERENCES

Bowlby, J. (1961). Processes of mourning. *International Journal of Psychoanalysis, 42,* 22.

Engel, G. (1964). Grief and grieving. *American Journal of Nursing, 64,* 93.

Kübler-Ross, E. (1969). *On death and dying.* New York: Macmillan.

@ Internet References

● Additional references related to bereavement are located at the following Web sites:

• http://www.journeyofhearts.org
• http://www.nhpco.org
• http://www.aarp.org/griefandloss/

• http://www.hospicefoundation.org
• http://www.bereavement.org
• http://www.caringinfo.org/
• http://www.aahpm.org
• http://www.hpna.org

Answers to Chapter Review Questions

CHAPTER 1. THE CONCEPT OF STRESS ADAPTATION

1. b   2. d   3. a   4. b
5. 1. c 2. d 3. b 4. a
6. 1. d 2. a 3. e 4. b 5. c

CHAPTER 2. MENTAL HEALTH/MENTAL ILLNESS: HISTORICAL AND THEORETICAL CONCEPTS

1. c   2. d   3. b   4. a   5. b   6. d   7. c
8. d   9. c   10. b
11. compensation = b   12. denial = h
13. displacement = a   14. identification = m
15. intellectualization = n   16. introjection = c
17. isolation = k   18. projection = e
19. rationalization = i   20. reaction formation = f
21. regression = d   22. repression = o
23. sublimation = g   24. suppression = j
25. undoing = l

CHAPTER 3. THEORETICAL MODELS OF PERSONALITY DEVELOPMENT

1. b   2. c   3. d   4. b   5. b   6. b   7. a
8. c   9. a   10. b

CHAPTER 4. CONCEPTS OF PSYCHOBIOLOGY

1. c   2. e   3. f   4. b   5. d   6. g   7. a
8. c   9. b   10. a   11. a   12. b   13. d

CHAPTER 5. ETHICAL AND LEGAL ISSUES IN PSYCHIATRIC/MENTAL HEALTH NURSING

1. c   2. a   3. e   4. d   5. b   6. d   7. b
8. e   9. a   10. c

CHAPTER 6. CULTURAL AND SPIRITUAL CONCEPTS RELEVANT TO PSYCHIATRIC/MENTAL HEALTH NURSING

1. c   2. d   3. a   4. d   5. b   6. c   7. c
8. b   9. b   10. a   11. a   12. d

CHAPTER 7. RELATIONSHIP DEVELOPMENT

1. a. The stranger
   b. The resource person
   c. The teacher
   d. The leader
   e. The surrogate
   f. The counselor
2. The counselor
3. It is through establishment of a satisfactory nurse-client relationship that individuals learn to generalize the ability to achieve satisfactory interpersonal relationships to other aspects of their lives.
4. Most often, the goal is directed at learning and growth promotion, in an effort to bring about some type of change in the client's life. This is accomplished through use of the problem-solving model.
5. The therapeutic use of self.
6. 1. d 2. a 3. e 4. b 5. c
7. 1. c 2. a 3. d 4. b
8. c   9. a   10. e

CHAPTER 8. THERAPEUTIC COMMUNICATION

1. In the transactional model of communication, both persons are participating simultaneously. They are mutually perceiving each other, simultaneously listening to each other, and mutually and simultaneously engaged in the process of creating meaning in a relationship.
2. a. One's value system.
   b. Internalized attitudes and beliefs.
   c. Culture and/or religion.
   d. Social status.

e. Gender

f. Background knowledge and experience.

g. Age or developmental level.

h. Type of environment in which the communication takes place.

3. Territoriality is the innate tendency to own space. People "mark" space as their own and feel more comfortable in these spaces. Territoriality affects communication in that an interaction can be more successful if it takes place on "neutral" ground rather than in a space "owned" by one or the other of the communicants.

4. Density refers to the number of people within a given environmental space. It may affect communication in that some studies indicate that a correlation exists between prolonged high density situations and certain behaviors, such as aggression, stress, criminal activity, hostility toward others, and a deterioration of mental and physical health.

5. a. Intimate distance (0–18 inches)—kissing or hugging someone.

b. Personal distance (18–40 inches)—close conversations with friends or colleagues

c. Social distance (4–12 feet)—conversations with strangers or acquaintances (e.g., at a cocktail party).

d. Public distance (>12 feet)—speaking in public.

6. a. Physical appearance and dress (e.g., young men who have hair down past their shoulders may convey a message of rebellion against the establishment).

b. Body movement and posture (e.g., a person with hands on hips standing straight and tall in front of someone seated who must look up to them is conveying a message of power over the seated individual.)

c. Touch (e.g., laying one's hand on the shoulder of another may convey a message of friendship and caring).

d. Facial expressions (e.g., wrinkling up of the nose, raising the upper lip, or raising one side of the upper lip conveys a message of disgust for a situation.).

e. Eye behavior (e.g., direct eye contact, accompanied by a smile and nodding of the head, conveys interest in what the other person is saying).

f. Vocal cues or paralanguage (e.g., a normally soft-spoken individual whose pitch and rate of speaking increases may be perceived as being anxious or tense).

7. S—Sit squarely facing the client.

O—Observe an open posture.

L—Lean forward toward the client.

E—Establish eye contact.

R—Relax.

8. a. Nontherapeutic technique: Disagreeing.

b. The correct answer. Therapeutic technique: Voicing doubt.

9. a. The correct answer. Therapeutic technique: Giving recognition.

b. Nontherapeutic technique: Complimenting—a judgment on the part of the nurse.

10. a. Nontherapeutic: Giving reassurance.

b. Nontherapeutic: Giving disapproval.

c. Nontherapeutic: Introducing an unrelated topic.

d. Nontherapeutic: Indicating an external source of power.

e. The correct answer: Therapeutic technique: Exploring.

11. a. Nontherapeutic: Requesting an explanation.

b. Nontherapeutic: Belittling feelings expressed.

c. Nontherapeutic: Rejecting.

d. The correct answer: Therapeutic technique: Formulating a plan of action.

12. Therapeutic response: "Do you think you should tell him?" Technique: Reflecting.

Nontherapeutic response: "Yes, you must tell your husband about your affair with your boss." Technique: Giving advice.

13. a. The correct answer. Therapeutic technique: Reflecting.

b. Nontherapeutic: Requesting an explanation.

c. Nontherapeutic: Indicating an external source of power.

d. Nontherapeutic: Giving advice.

e. Nontherapeutic: Defending.

f. Nontherapeutic: Making stereotyped comments.

CHAPTER 9. THE NURSING PROCESS IN PSYCHIATRIC/MENTAL HEALTH NURSING

1. Assessment, diagnosis, outcome identification, planning, implementation, evaluation.

2. a. Implementation

b. Diagnosis

c. Evaluation

d. Assessment

e. Planning

f. Outcome identification

3. Nursing diagnoses:

a. Imbalanced nutrition, less than body requirements

b. Social isolation

c. Low self-esteem

Outcomes:

a. Client will gain 2 lb/wk in next 3 weeks

b. Client will voluntarily spend time with peers and staff in group activities on the unit within 7 days.

c. Client will verbalize positive aspects about herself (excluding any references to eating or body image) within 2 weeks.

4. Problem-oriented recording (SOAPIE); Focus Charting®; PIE charting.

CHAPTER 10. THERAPEUTIC GROUPS

1. A group is a collection of individuals whose association is founded upon shared commonalities of interest, values, norms, and/or purpose.

2. a. Teaching group.

Laissez-faire leader.

b. Supportive/therapeutic group.

Democratic leader.

c. Task group.

Autocratic leader.

3. b	4. i	5. k	6. h	7. e	8. j	9. a
10. d	11. f	12. g	13. c	14. e	15. h	16. f
17. d	18. a	19. c	20. g	21. b		

CHAPTER 11. INTERVENTION WITH FAMILIES

1. e	2. a	3. f	4. c	5. b	6. d	7. b
8. c	9. a	10. b				

CHAPTER 12. MILIEU THERAPY—THE THERAPEUTIC COMMUNITY

1. A scientific structuring of the environment in order to effect behavioral changes and to improve the psychological health and functioning of the individual.
2. The goal of milieu therapy/therapeutic community is for the client to learn adaptive coping, interaction, and relationship skills that can be generalized to other aspects of his or her life.

3. c 4. b 5. a 6. d 7. f 8. h 9. b
10. i 11. g 12. j 13. a 14. e 15. c 16. k
17. m 18. l 19. d

CHAPTER 13. CRISIS INTERVENTION

1. c 2. d 3. a 4. b 5. c 6. a 7. d
8. b 9. b 10. d 11. c

CHAPTER 14. RELAXATION THERAPY

3a. (1) Anxiety (moderate to severe) related to lack of self-confidence and fear of making errors
(2) Pain (migraine headaches) related to repressed severe anxiety
(3) Insomnia related to anxiety

3b. Some outcome criteria for Linda might be:
(1) Client will be able to perform duties on the job while maintaining anxiety at a manageable level by practicing deep breathing exercises.
(2) Client will verbalize a reduction in headache pain following progressive relaxation techniques.
(3) Client is able to fall asleep within 30 minutes of retiring by listening to soft music and performing mental imagery exercises.

3c. The deep breathing exercises would be especially good for Linda because she could perform them as many times as she needed to during the working day to relieve her anxiety. With practice, progressive relaxation techniques and mental imagery could also provide relief from anxiety attacks for Linda. Any of these relaxation techniques may be beneficial at bedtime to help induce relaxation and sleep. Biofeedback may provide assistance for relief from migraine headaches. Physical exercise, either in the early morning or late afternoon after work, may provide Linda with renewed energy and combat chronic fatigue. It also relieves pent-up tension.

CHAPTER 15. ASSERTIVENESS TRAINING

1. a. AS 2. a. AG 3. a. NA
   b. PA   b. NA   b. AS
   c. NA   c. PA   c. PA
   d. AG   d. AS   d. AG
4. a. PA 5. a. AS 6. a. NA
   b. AG   b. NA   b. AS
   c. AS   c. PA   c. AG
   d. NA   d. AG   d. PA
7. a. AS 8. a. PA 9. a. AG
   b. PA   b. NA   b. NA
   c. AG   c. AG   c. AS
   d. NA   d. AS   d. PA
10. a. AS
    b. NA
    c. AG
    d. PA

CHAPTER 16. PROMOTING SELF-ESTEEM

1. b 2. a 3. d 4. c 5. a 6. b 7. c
8. e 9. d 10. a

CHAPTER 17. ANGER/AGGRESSION MANAGEMENT

1. Past history of violence; diagnosis of alcohol abuse/intoxication; current behaviors: abusive and threatening.
2. b. This is considered a long-term goal because John must have time to practice and learn this behavior.
3. c. Immediate and ongoing.
4. c 5. a
6. Observe at least every 15 minutes; check circulation (temperature, color, pulses); assist with needs related to nutrition, hydration, and elimination; position for comfort and to prevent aspiration.
7. c 8. a, b, c 9. c 10. b

CHAPTER 18. THE SUICIDAL CLIENT

1. b 2. a 3. c 4. a 5. d 6. c 7. c
8. b 9. d 10. b

CHAPTER 19. BEHAVIOR THERAPY

1. a 2. a 3. b 4. c 5. a 6. b 7. d
8. f, b, d, a, e, c

CHAPTER 20. COGNITIVE THERAPY

1. b 2. d 3. a 4. c 5. c 6. a 7. d
8. a 9. b 10. c

CHAPTER 21. PSYCHOPHARMACOLOGY

1. a 2. c 3. d 4. b 5. c 6. b 7. a
8. b 9. d 10. b

CHAPTER 22. ELECTROCONVULSIVE THERAPY

1. c 2. b 3. a 4. c 5. d 6. a 7. c
8. d 9. b 10. c

CHAPTER 23. COMPLEMENTARY THERAPIES

1. c   2. e   3. f   4. b   5. g   6. a   7. d
8. c   9. d   10. a   11. b

CHAPTER 24. CLIENT EDUCATION

1. a   2. c   3. d   4. c   5. a   6. b   7. c
8. d   9. a   10. b

CHAPTER 25. DISORDERS USUALLY FIRST DIAGNOSED IN INFANCY, CHILDHOOD, OR ADOLESCENCE

1. b   2. c   3. a   4. b   5. b   6. d   7. c
8. d   9. a   10. b

CHAPTER 26. DELIRIUM, DEMENTIA, AND AMNESTIC DISORDERS

1. c   2. b   3. a   4. b   5. d   6. c   7. c
8. a   9. b   10. c and e

CHAPTER 27. SUBSTANCE-RELATED DISORDERS

1. a   2. c   3. b   4. b   5. a   6. c   7. a
8. b   9. d   10. a

CHAPTER 28. SCHIZOPHRENIA AND OTHER PSYCHOTIC DISORDERS

1. b   2. b   3. c   4. d   5. d   6. a   7. c
8. b   9. c   10. d

CHAPTER 29. MOOD DISORDERS

1. c   2. b   3. a   4. d   5. c   6. b   7. c
8. a   9. c   10. b

CHAPTER 30. ANXIETY DISORDERS

1. d   2. c   3. d   4. a   5. b   6. c   7. b
8. c   9. a   10. d

CHAPTER 31. SOMATOFORM AND DISSOCIATIVE DISORDERS

1. a   2. b   3. d   4. b   5. c   6. d   7. b
8. a   9. b   10. d

CHAPTER 32. ISSUES RELATED TO HUMAN SEXUALITY

1. b   2. c   3. d   4. a   5. b   6. b   7. d
8. a   9. e   10. c

CHAPTER 33. EATING DISORDERS

1. c   2. a   3. b   4. b   5. c   6. b
7. c   8. b   9. c   10. a

CHAPTER 34. PERSONALITY DISORDERS

1. d   2. a   3. b   4. d   5. a   6. b   7. c
8. c   9. d   10. b

CHAPTER 35. THE AGING INDIVIDUAL

1. c   2. d   3. b   4. a   5. c   6. d   7. a
8. a   9. c   10. a

CHAPTER 36. VICTIMS OF ABUSE OR NEGLECT

1. b   2. c   3. a   4. d   5. b   6. d   7. a
8. b   9. b   10. d

CHAPTER 37. COMMUNITY MENTAL HEALTH NURSING

1. a   2. b   3. a   4. c   5. d   6. b   7. c
8. d   9. a   10. b

CHAPTER 38. FORENSIC NURSING

1. a   2. a   3. b   4. b   5. b   6. a   7. b
8. a   9. a   10. b

CHAPTER 39. THE BEREAVED INDIVIDUAL

1. e   2. c   3. c   4. d   5. a   6. a   7. b
8. c   9. a   10. c

.59 Parasomnia type

.59 Mixed type

— Substance-Induced Sleep Disorder (*refer to Substance-Related Disorders for substance-specific codes*)

IMPULSE CONTROL DISORDERS NOT ELSEWHERE CLASSIFIED

312.34 Intermittent Explosive Disorder

312.32 Kleptomania

312.33 Pyromania

312.31 Pathological Gambling

312.39 Trichotillomania

312.30 Impulse Control Disorder NOS

ADJUSTMENT DISORDERS

309.xx Adjustment Disorder

.0 With Depressed Mood

.24 With Anxiety

.28 With Mixed Anxiety and Depressed Mood

.3 With Disturbance of Conduct

.4 With Mixed Disturbance of Emotions and Conduct

.9 Unspecified

PERSONALITY DISORDERS

NOTE: *These are coded on Axis II.*

301.0 Paranoid Personality Disorder

301.20 Schizoid Personality Disorder

301.22 Schizotypal Personality Disorder

301.7 Antisocial Personality Disorder

301.83 Borderline Personality Disorder

301.50 Histrionic Personality Disorder

301.81 Narcissistic Personality Disorder

301.82 Avoidant Personality Disorder

301.6 Dependent Personality Disorder

301.4 Obsessive-Compulsive Personality Disorder

301.9 Personality Disorder NOS

OTHER CONDITIONS THAT MAY BE A FOCUS OF CLINICAL ATTENTION

Psychological Factors Affecting Medical Condition

316 *Choose name based on nature of factors:*
Mental Disorder Affecting Medical Condition
Psychological Symptoms Affecting Medical Condition
Personality Traits or Coping Style Affecting Medical Condition
Maladaptive Health Behaviors Affecting Medical Condition
Stress-Related Physiological Response Affecting Medical Condition
Other or Unspecified Psychological Factors Affecting Medical Condition

Medication-Induced Movement Disorders

332.1 Neuroleptic-Induced Parkinsonism

333.92 Neuroleptic Malignant Syndrome

333.7 Neuroleptic-Induced Acute Dystonia

333.99 Neuroleptic-Induced Acute Akathisia

333.82 Neuroleptic-Induced Tardive Dyskinesia

333.1 Medication-Induced Postural Tremor

333.90 Medication-Induced Movement Disorder NOS

Other Medication-Induced Disorder

995.2 Adverse Effects of Medication NOS

Relational Problems

V61.9 Relational Problem Related to a Mental Disorder or General Medical Condition

V61.20 Parent-Child Relational Problem

V61.10 Partner Relational Problem

V61.8 Sibling Relational Problem

V62.81 Relational Problem NOS

Problems Related to Abuse or Neglect

V61.21 Physical Abuse of Child

V61.21 Sexual Abuse of Child

V61.21 Neglect of Child

— — Physical Abuse of Adult

V61.12 (if by partner)

V62.83 (if by person other than partner)

— — Sexual Abuse of Adult

V61.12 (if by partner)

V62.83 (if by person other than partner)

Additional Conditions That May Be a Focus of Clinical Attention

V15.81 Noncompliance with Treatment

V65.2 Malingering

V71.01 Adult Antisocial Behavior

V71.02 Childhood or Adolescent Antisocial Behavior

V62.89 Borderline Intellectual Functioning (coded on Axis II)

780.9 Age-Related Cognitive Decline

V62.82 Bereavement

V62.3   Academic Problem
V62.2   Occupational Problem
313.82   Identity Problem
V62.89   Religious or Spiritual Problem
V62.4   Acculturation Problem
V62.89   Phase of Life Problem

ADDITIONAL CODES

300.9   Unspecified Mental Disorder (nonpsychotic)
V71.09   No Diagnosis or Condition on Axis I
799.9   Diagnosis or Condition Deferred on Axis I
V71.09   No Diagnosis on Axis II
799.9   Diagnosis Deferred on Axis II

NANDA Nursing Diagnoses: Taxonomy II

DOMAINS, CLASSES, AND DIAGNOSES

Domain 1: Health Promotion

Class 1: Health Awareness

Class 2: Health Management

Approved Diagnoses

Effective therapeutic regimen management
Ineffective therapeutic regimen management
Ineffective family therapeutic regimen management
Ineffective community therapeutic regimen
  management
Health-seeking behaviors (specify)
Ineffective health maintenance
Impaired home maintenance
Readiness for enhanced therapeutic regimen
  management
Readiness for enhanced nutrition
Readiness for enhanced immunization status

Domain 2: Nutrition

Class 1: Ingestion

Approved Diagnoses

Ineffective infant feeding pattern
Impaired swallowing
Imbalanced nutrition: Less than body requirements
Imbalanced nutrition: More than body requirements
Risk for imbalanced nutrition: More than body
  requirements

Class 2: Digestion

Class 3: Absorption

Class 4: Metabolism

Approved Diagnoses

Risk for impaired liver function
Risk for unstable blood glucose level

Class 5: Hydration

Approved Diagnoses

Deficient fluid volume
Risk for deficient fluid volume
Excess fluid volume
Risk for imbalanced fluid volume
Readiness for enhanced fluid balance

Domain 3: Elimination and Exchange

Class 1: Urinary Function

Approved Diagnoses

Impaired urinary elimination
Urinary retention
Total urinary incontinence
Functional urinary incontinence
Stress urinary incontinence
Urge urinary incontinence
Reflex urinary incontinence
Risk for urge urinary incontinence
Readiness for enhanced urinary elimination
Overflow urinary incontinence

Class 2: Gastrointestinal Function

Approved Diagnoses

Bowel incontinence
Diarrhea
Constipation
Risk for constipation
Perceived constipation

Class 3: Integumentary Function

Class 4: Respiratory Function

Approved Diagnoses

Impaired gas exchange

Domain 4: Activity/Rest

Class 1: Sleep/Rest

Approved Diagnoses
Insomnia
Sleep deprivation
Readiness for enhanced sleep

Class 2: Activity/Exercise

Approved Diagnoses
Risk for disuse syndrome
Impaired physical mobility
Impaired bed mobility
Impaired wheelchair mobility
Impaired transfer ability
Impaired walking
Deficient diversional activity
Delayed surgical recovery
Sedentary lifestyle

Class 3: Energy Balance

Approved Diagnoses
Energy field disturbance
Fatigue

Class 4: Cardiovascular/Pulmonary Responses

Approved Diagnoses
Decreased cardiac output
Impaired spontaneous ventilation
Ineffective breathing pattern
Activity intolerance
Risk for activity intolerance
Dysfunctional ventilatory weaning response
Ineffective tissue perfusion (specify type: renal, cerebral, cardiopulmonary, gastrointestinal, peripheral)

Class 5: Self-Care

Approved Diagnoses
Dressing/grooming self-care deficit
Bathing/hygiene self-care deficit
Feeding self-care deficit
Toileting self-care deficit
Readiness for enhanced self-care

Domain 5: Perception/Cognition

Class 1: Attention

Approved Diagnoses
Unilateral neglect

Class 2: Orientation

Approved Diagnoses
Impaired environmental interpretation syndrome
Wandering

Class 3: Sensation/Perception

Approved Diagnoses
Disturbed sensory perception (specify: visual, auditory, kinesthetic, gustatory, tactile)

Class 4: Cognition

Approved Diagnoses
Deficient knowledge (specify)
Readiness for enhanced knowledge (specify)
Acute confusion
Chronic confusion
Impaired memory
Disturbed thought processes
Readiness for enhanced decision making
Risk for acute confusion

Class 5: Communication

Approved Diagnoses
Impaired verbal communication
Readiness for enhanced communication

Domain 6: Self-Perception

Class 1: Self-Concept

Approved Diagnoses
Disturbed personal identity
Powerlessness
Risk for powerlessness
Hopelessness
Risk for loneliness
Readiness for enhanced self-concept
Readiness for enhanced power
Risk for compromised human dignity
Readiness for enhanced hope

Class 2: Self-Esteem

Approved Diagnoses
Chronic low self-esteem
Situational low self-esteem
Risk for situational low self-esteem

Class 3: Body Image

Approved Diagnoses
Disturbed body image

Domain 7: Role Relationships

Class 1: Caregiving Roles

Approved Diagnoses

Caregiver role strain
Risk for caregiver role strain
Impaired parenting
Risk for impaired parenting
Readiness for enhanced parenting

Class 2: Family Relationships

Approved Diagnoses

Interrupted family processes
Readiness for enhanced family processes
Dysfunctional family processes: Alcoholism
Risk for impaired parent/infant/child attachment

Class 3: Role Performance

Approved Diagnoses

Effective breastfeeding
Ineffective breastfeeding
Interrupted breastfeeding
Ineffective role performance
Parental role conflict
Impaired social interaction

Domain 8: Sexuality

Class 1: Sexual Identity

Class 2: Sexual Function

Approved Diagnoses

Sexual dysfunction
Ineffective sexuality pattern

Class 3: Reproduction

Domain 9: Coping/Stress Tolerance

Class 1: Post-Trauma Responses

Approved Diagnoses

Relocation stress syndrome
Risk for relocation stress syndrome
Rape-trauma syndrome
Rape-trauma syndrome: Silent reaction
Rape-trauma syndrome: Compound reaction
Post-trauma syndrome
Risk for post-trauma syndrome

Class 2: Coping Responses

Approved Diagnoses

Fear
Anxiety
Death anxiety
Chronic sorrow
Ineffective denial
Ineffective coping
Grieving
Complicated grieving
Risk for complicated grieving
Disabled family coping
Compromised family coping
Defensive coping
Ineffective community coping
Readiness for enhanced coping (individual)
Readiness for enhanced family coping
Readiness for enhanced community coping
Stress overload
Risk-prone health behavior

Class 3: Neurobehavioral Stress

Approved Diagnoses

Autonomic dysreflexia
Risk for autonomic dysreflexia
Disorganized infant behavior
Risk for disorganized infant behavior
Readiness for enhanced organized infant behavior
Decreased intracranial adaptive capacity

Domain 10: Life Principles

Class 1: Values

Approved Diagnoses

Readiness for enhanced hope

Class 2: Beliefs

Approved Diagnoses

Readiness for enhanced spiritual well-being
Readiness for enhanced hope

Class 3: Value/Belief/Action Congruence

Approved Diagnoses

Spiritual distress
Risk for spiritual distress
Decisional conflict (specify)
Noncompliance (specify)
Risk for impaired religiosity
Impaired religiosity

Readiness for enhanced religiosity
Moral distress
Readiness for enhanced decision making

Domain 11: Safety/Protection

Class 1: Infection

Approved Diagnoses
Risk for infection
Readiness for enhanced immunization status

Class 2: Physical Injury

Approved Diagnoses
Impaired oral mucous membrane
Risk for injury
Risk for perioperative positioning injury
Risk for falls
Risk for trauma
Impaired skin integrity
Risk for impaired skin integrity
Impaired tissue integrity
Impaired dentition
Risk for suffocation
Risk for aspiration
Ineffective airway clearance
Risk for peripheral neurovascular dysfunction
Ineffective protection
Risk for sudden infant death syndrome

Class 3: Violence

Approved Diagnoses
Risk for self-mutilation
Self-mutilation
Risk for other-directed violence
Risk for self-directed violence
Risk for suicide

Class 4: Environmental Hazards

Approved Diagnoses
Risk for poisoning
Risk for contamination
Contamination

Class 5: Defensive Processes

Approved Diagnoses
Latex allergy response
Risk for latex allergy response
Readiness for enhanced immunization status

Class 6: Thermoregulation

Approved Diagnoses
Risk for imbalanced body temperature
Ineffective thermoregulation
Hypothermia
Hyperthermia

Domain 12: Comfort

Class 1: Physical Comfort

Approved Diagnoses
Acute pain
Chronic pain
Nausea
Readiness for enhanced comfort

Class 2: Environmental Comfort

Approved Diagnoses
Readiness for enhanced comfort

Class 3: Social Comfort

Approved Diagnoses
Social isolation

Domain 13: Growth/Development

Class 1: Growth

Approved Diagnoses
Delayed growth and development
Risk for disproportionate growth
Adult failure to thrive

Class 2: Development

Approved Diagnoses
Delayed growth and development
Risk for delayed development

SOURCE: *NANDA Nursing Diagnoses: Definitions & Classification 2007-2008.* (2007). Philadelphia: NANDA International. With permission.

Assigning Nursing Diagnoses to Client Behaviors

Following is a list of client behaviors and the NANDA nursing diagnoses that correspond to the behaviors and that may be used in planning care for the client exhibiting the specific behavioral symptoms.

BEHAVIORS	NANDA NURSING DIAGNOSES
Aggression; hostility	Risk for injury; Risk for other-directed violence
Anorexia or refusal to eat	Imbalanced nutrition: Less than body requirements
Anxious behavior	Anxiety (Specify level)
Confusion; memory loss	Confusion, acute/chronic; Disturbed thought processes
Delusions	Disturbed thought processes
Denial of problems	Ineffective denial
Depressed mood or anger turned inward	Complicated grieving
Detoxification; withdrawal from substances	Risk for injury
Difficulty accepting new diagnosis or recent change in health status	Risk-prone health behavior
Difficulty making important life decision	Decisional conflict (specify)
Difficulty sleeping	Insomnia
Difficulty with interpersonal relationships	Impaired social interaction
Disruption in capability to perform usual responsibilities	Ineffective role performance
Dissociative behaviors (depersonalization; derealization)	Disturbed sensory perception (kinesthetic)
Expresses feelings of disgust about body or body part	Disturbed body image
Expresses anger at God	Spiritual distress
Expresses lack of control over personal situation	Powerlessness
Fails to follow prescribed therapy	Ineffective therapeutic regimen management; Noncompliance
Flashbacks, nightmares, obsession with traumatic experience	Post-trauma syndrome
Hallucinations	Disturbed sensory perception (auditory; visual)
Highly critical of self or others	Low self-esteem (chronic; situational)
HIV positive; altered immunity	Ineffective protection
Inability to meet basic needs	Self-care deficit (feeding; bathing/hygiene; dressing/grooming; toileting)
Loose associations or flight of ideas	Impaired verbal communication
Loss of a valued entity, recently experienced	Risk for complicated grieving
Manic hyperactivity	Risk for injury
Manipulative behavior	Ineffective coping
Multiple personalities; gender identity disturbance	Disturbed personal identity
Orgasm, problems with; lack of sexual desire	Sexual dysfunction
Overeating, compulsive	Risk for imbalanced nutrition: More than body requirements

Phobias	Fear
Physical symptoms as coping behavior	Ineffective coping
Potential or anticipated loss of significant entity	Grieving
Projection of blame; rationalization of failures; denial of personal responsibility	Defensive coping
Ritualistic behaviors	Anxiety (severe); ineffective coping
Seductive remarks; inappropriate sexual behaviors	Impaired social interaction
Self-inflicted injuries (non-life-threatening)	Self-mutilation; Risk for self-mutilation
Sexual behaviors (difficulty, limitations, or changes in; reported dissatisfaction)	Ineffective sexuality pattern
Stress from caring for chronically ill person	Caregiver role strain
Stress from locating to new environment	Relocation stress syndrome
Substance use as a coping behavior	Ineffective coping
Substance use (denies use is a problem)	Ineffective denial
Suicidal gestures/threats; suicidal ideation	Risk for suicide; Risk for self-directed violence
Suspiciousness	Disturbed thought processes; ineffective coping
Vomiting, excessive, self-induced	Risk for deficient fluid volume
Withdrawn behavior	Social isolation

Controlled Drug Categories and Pregnancy Categories

DEA CONTROLLED SUBSTANCES SCHEDULES

Classes or schedules are determined by the Drug Enforcement Agency (DEA), an arm of the United States Justice Department, and are based on the potential for abuse and dependence liability (physical and psychological) of the medication. Some states may have stricter prescription regulations. Physicians, dentists, podiatrists, and veterinarians may prescribe controlled substances. Nurse practitioners and physician's assistants may prescribe controlled substances with certain limitations.

Schedule I (C-I)

Potential for abuse is so high as to be unacceptable. May be used for research with appropriate limitations. Examples are LSD and heroin.

Schedule II (C-II)

High potential for abuse and extreme liability for physical and psychological dependence (amphetamines, opioid analgesics, dronabinol, certain barbiturates). Outpatient prescriptions must be in writing. In emergencies, telephone orders may be acceptable if a written prescription is provided within 72 hours. No refills are allowed.

Schedule III (C-III)

Intermediate potential for abuse (less than C-II) and intermediate liability for physical and psychological dependence (certain nonbarbiturate sedatives, certain nonamphetamine CNS stimulants, and limited dosages of certain opioid analgesics). Outpatient prescriptions can be refilled 5 times within 6 months from date of issue if authorized by prescriber. Telephone orders are acceptable.

Schedule IV (C-IV)

Less abuse potential than Schedule III with minimal liability for physical or psychological dependence (certain sedative/hypnotics, certain antianxiety agents, some barbiturates, benzodiazepines, chloral hydrate, pentazocine, and propoxyphene). Outpatient prescriptions can be refilled 6 times within 6 months from date of issue if authorized by prescriber. Telephone orders are acceptable.

Schedule V (C-V)

Minimal abuse potential. Number of outpatient refills determined by prescriber. Some products (cough suppressants with small amounts of codeine, antidiarrheals containing paregoric) may be available without prescription to patients at least 18 years of age.

FDA PREGNANCY CATEGORIES

Category A	Adequate, well-controlled studies in pregnant women have not shown an increased risk of fetal abnormalities.
Category B	Animal studies have revealed no evidence of harm to the fetus, however, there are no adequate and well-controlled studies in pregnant women. OR Animal studies have shown an adverse effect, but adequate and well-controlled studies in pregnant women have failed to demonstrate a risk to the fetus.
Category C	Animal studies have shown an adverse effect and there are no adequate and well-controlled studies in pregnant women. OR No animal studies have been conducted and there are no adequate and well-controlled studies in pregnant women.
Category D	Studies, adequate well-controlled or observational, in pregnant women have demonstrated a risk to the fetus. However, the benefits of therapy may outweigh the potential risk.
Category X	Studies, adequate well-controlled or observational, in animals or pregnant women have demonstrated positive evidence of fetal abnormalities. The use of the product is contraindicated in women who are or may become pregnant.

SOURCE: From Deglin, J.H., & Vallerand, A.H. (2007). *Davis's Drug Guide for Nurses* (10th ed.). Philadelphia: F.D. Davis. With permission.

Sample Teaching Guides

These teaching guides also appear in the Student Workbook (CD-ROM) that accomanies this textbook. They may be printed and used with clients who require this type of instruction.

BENZODIAZEPINES

Patient Medication Instruction Sheet

Patient Name_____ **Drug Prescribed**_____

Directions for Use_____

Examples and Uses of this Medicine:
Benzodiazepines are used to treat moderate to severe anxiety: alprazolam [Xanax], chlordiazepoxide [Librium], clonazepam [Klonopin], clorazepate [Tranxene], diazepam [Valium], lorazepam [Ativan], and oxazepam [Serax]. Some are used to treat insomnia (sleeplessness): flurazepam [Dalmane], temazepam [Restoril], and triazolam [Halcion]. Some are used for muscle spasms and to treat seizure disorders.

Before Using this Medicine, Be Sure to Tell Your Doctor if You:

- Are allergic to any medicine
- Have glaucoma
- Are pregnant, plan to be, or are breastfeeding
- Are taking any other medications

Side Effects of this Medicine:
REPORT THE FOLLOWING SIDE EFFECTS TO YOUR DOCTOR IMMEDIATELY:

- Mental confusion or depression
- Hallucinations (seeing, hearing, or feeling things not there)
- Skin rash or itching
- Sore throat and fever
- Unusual excitement, nervousness, irritability, or trouble sleeping

SIDE EFFECTS THAT MAY OCCUR BUT NOT REQUIRE A DOCTOR'S ATTENTION UNLESS THEY PERSIST LONGER THAN A FEW DAYS:

- Blurred vision, or other changes in vision
- Clumsiness, dizziness, lightheadedness, or slurred speech
- Constipation, diarrhea, nausea, vomiting, or stomach pain
- Difficulty in urination
- Drowsiness, headache, or unusual tiredness or weakness

Other Instructions While Taking this Medication:

- Take this medicine only as your doctor has directed. Do not take more of it or do not take it more often than prescribed. If large doses are taken for a prolonged period of time, it may become habit-forming.
- If you are taking this medicine several times a day and you forget a dose, if it is within an hour or so of the missed dose, go ahead and take it. Otherwise, wait and take the next dose at regular time. Do not double up on a dose if you forget one. Just keep taking the prescribed dosage.
- Do not stop taking the drug abruptly. Can produce serious withdrawal symptoms, such as depression, insomnia, anxiety, abdominal and muscle cramps, tremors, vomiting, sweating, convulsions, delirium. Discuss with the doctor before stopping this medication.
- Do not consume other CNS depressants (including alcohol) while taking this medication.
- Do not take nonprescription medication without approval from physician.
- Rise slowly from the sitting or lying position to prevent a sudden drop in blood pressure.

BUSPIRONE (BuSpar)

Patient Medication Instruction Sheet

Patient Name_____

Directions for Use_____

Uses of this Medicine:
BuSpar is used in the treatment of anxiety disorders. It is also sometimes used to treat the symptoms of premenstrual syndrome.

Before Using this Medicine, Be Sure to Tell Your Doctor if You:

- Are allergic to any medicine
- Are pregnant, plan to be, or are breastfeeding
- Are taking any other medications

Side Effects of this Medicine:
REPORT THE FOLLOWING SIDE EFFECTS TO YOUR DOCTOR IMMEDIATELY:

- Mental confusion or depression
- Hallucinations (seeing, hearing, or feeling things not there)
- Skin rash or itching
- Unusual excitement, nervousness, irritability, or trouble sleeping
- Persistent headache
- Involuntary movements of the head or neck muscles

SIDE EFFECTS THAT MAY OCCUR BUT NOT REQUIRE A DOCTOR'S ATTENTION UNLESS THEY PERSIST LONGER THAN A FEW DAYS:

- Dizziness; lightheadedness
- Drowsiness
- Nausea
- Fatigue
- Headache that subsides

Other Instructions While Taking this Medication:

- Take this medicine only as your doctor has directed. Do not take more of it or do not take it more often than prescribed.
- If you are taking this medicine several times a day and you forget a dose, if it is within an hour or so of the missed dose, go ahead and take it. Otherwise, wait and take the next dose at regular time. Do not double up on a dose if you forget one. Just keep taking the prescribed dosage.
- Do not consume other CNS depressants (including alcohol) while taking this medication.
- Do not take nonprescription medication without approval from physician.
- Rise slowly from the sitting or lying position to prevent a sudden drop in blood pressure.

TRICYCLIC ANTIDEPRESSANTS

Patient Medication Instruction Sheet

Patient Name_____ **Drug Prescribed**_____

Directions for Use_____

Examples and Uses of this Medicine:
Tricyclic antidepressants are used to treat symptoms of depression: amitriptyline [Elavil], amoxapine [Asendin], desipramine [Norpramin], doxepin [Sinequan], imipramine [Tofranil], nortriptyline [Aventyl], protriptyline [Vivactil], and trimipramine [Surmontil]. Doxepin is used to treat depression with anxiety. Clomipramine [Anafranil] is used to treat obsessive–compulsive disorder. Imipramine is also used to treat enuresis (bedwetting) in children.

Before Using this Medicine, Be Sure to Tell Your Doctor if You:

- Are allergic to any medicine
- Have glaucoma
- Have a history of heart problems or high blood pressure
- Are pregnant, plan to be, or are breastfeeding
- Are taking any other medications
- Have a history of seizures

Side Effects of this Medicine:
REPORT THE FOLLOWING SIDE EFFECTS TO YOUR DOCTOR IMMEDIATELY:

- Seizures
- Difficulty urinating
- Irregular heartbeat or chest pain
- Hallucinations
- Skin rash
- Sore throat and fever
- Unusual amount of restlessness and excitement
- Confusion; disorientation

SIDE EFFECTS THAT MAY OCCUR BUT MAY NOT REQUIRE A DOCTOR'S ATTENTION:

- Drowsiness
- Dry mouth
- Nausea
- Sensitivity to the sun (may burn easily)
- Headache
- Constipation

Other Instructions While Taking this Medication:

- Continue to take the medication even though you still have symptoms. It may take as long as 4 weeks before you start feeling better.
- Use caution when driving or operating dangerous machinery. Drowsiness and dizziness can occur. If these side effects don't go away or get worse, report them to the doctor.
- Do not stop taking the drug abruptly. To do so might produce withdrawal symptoms, such as nausea, vertigo, insomnia, headache, malaise, and nightmares. Tell the doctor when you want to stop taking it.
- Use sunscreens and wear protective clothing when spending time outdoors.
- Rise slowly from a sitting or lying position to prevent a sudden drop in blood pressure.
- Take frequent sips of water, chew sugarless gum, or suck on hard candy if dry mouth is a problem.
- You may take this medication with food if nausea is a problem.
- Do not drink alcohol while taking this medication.
- Do not consume other medications (including over-the-counter medications) without the physician's approval while taking this medication. Many medications contain

substances that, in combination with tricyclic antidepressants, could be dangerous.

SELECTIVE SEROTONIN REUPTAKE INHIBITORS (SSRIs)

Patient Medication Instruction Sheet

Patient Name_____ Drug Prescribed_____

Directions for Use_____

Examples and Uses of this Medicine:

SSRIs are used to treat symptoms of depression: citalopram [Celexa], escitalopram [Lexapro], fluoxetine [Prozac], paroxetine [Paxil], and sertraline [Zoloft]. Some are used to treat obsessive–compulsive disorder: fluvoxamine [Luvox], fluoxetine [Prozac], paroxetine [Paxil], and sertraline [Zoloft]. Also bulimia nervosa: fluoxetine [Prozac]; panic disorder and premenstrual dysphoric disorder: fluoxetine [Prozac; Serafem], sertraline [Zoloft] and paroxetine [Paxil]; posttraumatic stress disorder: paroxetine [Paxil] and sertraline [Zoloft], generalized anxiety disorder: escitalopram [Lexapro] and paroxetine [Paxil], and social anxiety disorder: paroxetine [Paxil] and sertraline [Zoloft].

Before Using this Medicine, Be Sure to Tell Your Doctor if You:

- Are allergic to any medicine
- Are pregnant, plan to be, or are breastfeeding
- Are taking any other medications
- Have diabetes

Side Effects of this Medicine:
REPORT THE FOLLOWING SIDE EFFECTS TO YOUR DOCTOR IMMEDIATELY:

- Skin rash
- Fever
- Unusual excitement, nervousness, irritability, or trouble sleeping
- Loss of appetite and weight loss
- Seizures
- Difficulty breathing
- Increased sensitivity to sunburn

SIDE EFFECTS THAT MAY OCCUR BUT MAY NOT REQUIRE A DOCTOR'S ATTENTION:

- Drowsiness
- Dizziness
- Nausea
- Headache
- Impotence or loss of sexual desire (this should be reported to physician if it is troubling to the patient)

Other Instructions While Taking this Medication:

- Continue to take the medication even though you still have symptoms. It may take as long as 4 weeks before you start feeling better.
- Use caution when driving or operating dangerous machinery. Drowsiness and dizziness can occur. If these side effects don't go away or get worse, report them to the doctor.
- Use sunscreens and wear protective clothing when spending time outdoors.
- Rise slowly from a sitting or lying position to prevent a sudden drop in blood pressure.
- Take frequent sips of water, chew sugarless gum, or suck on hard candy if dry mouth is a problem.
- You may take this medication with food if nausea is a problem.
- Avoid drinking alcohol while taking this medication.
- Do not consume other medications (including over-the-counter medications) without the physician's approval while taking this medication. Many medications contain substances that, in combination with SSRI antidepressants, could be dangerous.

MONOAMINE OXIDASE INHIBITORS (MAOIS)

Patient Medication Instruction Sheet

Patient Name_____ Drug Prescribed_____

Directions for Use_____

Examples and Uses of this Medicine:
MAOIs are used to treat the symptoms of depression: isocarboxazid [Marplan], phenelzine [Nardil], tranylcypromine [Parnate], selegiline transdermal system [Emsam].

Before Using this Medicine, Be Sure to Tell Your Doctor if You:

- Are allergic to any medicine
- Have a history of liver or kidney disease
- Have been diagnosed with pheochromocytoma
- Have a history of severe or frequent headaches
- Are pregnant, plan to be, or are breastfeeding
- Have a history of hypertension
- Have a history of heart disease
- Are taking (or have taken in the last 2 weeks) *any* other medication

Side Effects of this Medicine:
REPORT THE FOLLOWING SIDE EFFECTS TO YOUR DOCTOR IMMEDIATELY:

- Severe, pounding headache
- Rapid or pounding heartbeat
- Stiff or sore neck
- Chest pain

- Nausea and vomiting
- Seizures

THE FOLLOWING SIDE EFFECTS SHOULD ALSO BE REPORTED TO THE DOCTOR:

- Dark urine
- Yellowing of eyes or skin
- Hallucinations
- Fainting
- Hyperexcitability
- Confusion
- Fever
- Skin rash
- Disorientation

SIDE EFFECTS THAT MAY OCCUR BUT MAY NOT REQUIRE A DOCTOR'S ATTENTION:

- Constipation
- Diarrhea (unless severe and persistent)
- Dizziness
- Dry Mouth
- Fatigue
- Drowsiness
- Nausea
- Decreased sexual ability

Other Instructions While Taking this Medication:

- Continue to take the medication even though you still have symptoms. It may take as long as 4 weeks before you start feeling better.
- Use caution when driving or operating dangerous machinery. Drowsiness and dizziness can occur.
- Do not stop taking the drug abruptly. To do so might produce withdrawal symptoms, such as nausea, vertigo, insomnia, headache, malaise, and nightmares. Tell the doctor when you want to stop taking it.
- Rise slowly from a sitting or lying position to prevent a sudden drop in blood pressure.
- Take frequent sips of water, chew sugarless gum, or suck on hard candy if dry mouth is a problem.
- You may take this medication with food if nausea is a problem. Do not drink alcohol.
- Do not consume other medications (including over-the-counter medications) without the physician's approval while taking this medication. Many medications contain substances that, in combination with MAOI antidepressants, could be dangerous.
- Do not consume the following foods or medications while taking MAOIs (or for 2 weeks after you stop taking them): aged cheese, raisins, red wine (especially Chianti), beer, chocolate, colas, coffee, tea, sour cream, beef/chicken livers, game meat, canned figs, soy sauce, meat tenderizer (MSG), pickled herring, smoked/processed meats (lunchmeats, sausage, pepperoni), yogurt, yeast products, broad beans, sauerkraut, cold remedies, diet pills, or nasal decongestants. To do so could cause a life-threatening condition.

- Be sure to tell any doctor or dentist that you see that you are taking this medication.
- Follow package directions carefully when applying the selegiline transdermal patch.

HETEROCYCLIC ANTIDEPRESSANTS

Patient Medication Instruction Sheet

Patient Name_____ **Drug Prescribed**_____

Directions for Use_____

Examples and Uses of this Medicine:

Heterocyclic antidepressants are used to treat symptoms of depression: maprotiline [Ludiomil], mirtazapine [Remeron], trazodone [Desyrel], bupropion [Wellbutrin], and nefazodone. Maprotiline is also used to treat anxiety associated with depression. Trazodone is also used to treat insomnia and panic disorder. Bupropion has been shown to be effective in treatment of neuropathic pain, to enhance weight loss, in the treatment of attention deficit hyperactivity disorder, and as a smoking deterrent (Zyban).

Before Using this Medicine, Be Sure to Tell Your Doctor if You:

- Are allergic to any medicine
- Have an eating disorder
- Have a history of heart problems
- Are pregnant, plan to be, or are breastfeeding
- Are taking any other medications
- Have a history of seizures or high blood pressure

Side Effects of this Medicine:
REPORT THE FOLLOWING SIDE EFFECTS TO YOUR DOCTOR IMMEDIATELY:

- Seizures
- Fever, chills
- Sore throat
- Prolonged erection (trazodone)
- Unusual amount of restlessness and excitement
- Irregular heartbeat or chest pain
- Hallucinations
- Skin rash
- Jaundice, anorexia, GI complaints, malaise (signs of liver dysfunction [nefazodone])

SIDE EFFECTS THAT MAY OCCUR BUT NOT REQUIRE A DOCTOR'S ATTENTION UNLESS THEY PERSIST LONGER THAN A FEW DAYS:

- Drowsiness
- Dizziness
- Dry mouth
- Constipation
- Headache
- Nausea

Other Instructions While Taking this Medication:

- Continue to take the medication even though you still have symptoms. It may take as long as 4 weeks before you start feeling better.
- Use caution when driving or operating dangerous machinery. Drowsiness and dizziness can occur. If these side effects don't go away or get worse, report them to the doctor.
- Do not stop taking the drug abruptly. To do so might produce withdrawal symptoms, such as nausea, vertigo, insomnia, headache, malaise, and nightmares. Tell the doctor when you want to stop taking it.
- Rise slowly from a sitting or lying position to prevent a sudden drop in blood pressure.
- Take frequent sips of water, chew sugarless gum, or suck on hard candy if dry mouth is a problem.
- You may take this medication with food if nausea is a problem.
- Do not drink alcohol while taking this medication.
- Do not consume other medications (including over-the-counter medications) without the physician's approval while taking this medication. Many medications contain substances that, in combination with heterocyclic antidepressants, could be dangerous.

SEROTONIN–NOREPINEPHRINE REUPTAKE INHIBITORS (SNRIS)

Patient Medication Instruction Sheet

Patient Name_____ **Drug Prescribed**_____

Directions for Use_____

Examples and Uses of this Medicine:
SNRIs are used to treat symptoms of depression: venlafaxine [Effexor] and duloxetine [Cymbalta]. Venlafaxine is also used to treat generalized anxiety disorder and social anxiety disorder. It has also been effective in treatment of hot flashes, premenstrual dysphoric disorder, and posttraumatic stress disorder. Duloxetine is also used to treat diabetic peripheral neuropathic pain.

Before Using this Medicine, Be Sure to Tell Your Doctor if You:

- Are allergic to any medicine
- Have glaucoma
- Have a history of seizures
- Are pregnant, plan to be, or are breastfeeding
- Are taking any other medications
- Have a history of heart disease

Side Effects of this Medicine:
REPORT THE FOLLOWING SIDE EFFECTS TO YOUR DOCTOR IMMEDIATELY:

- Skin rash
- Seizures

- Unusual amount of restlessness or excitement
- Irregular heartbeat or chest pain

SIDE EFFECTS THAT MAY OCCUR BUT NOT REQUIRE A DOCTOR'S ATTENTION UNLESS THEY PERSIST LONGER THAN A FEW DAYS:

- Dizziness
- Headache
- Constipation
- Dry mouth
- Drowsiness
- Insomnia
- Sexual dysfunction (should be reported to the physician if it is troubling to the patient)
- Nausea

Other Instructions While Taking this Medication:

- Continue to take the medication even though you still have symptoms. It may take as long as 4 weeks before you start feeling better.
- Use caution when driving or operating dangerous machinery. Drowsiness and dizziness can occur. If these side effects don't go away or get worse, report them to the doctor.
- Do not stop taking the drug abruptly. To do so might produce withdrawal symptoms, such as nausea, vertigo, insomnia, headache, malaise, and nightmares. Tell the doctor when you want to stop taking it.
- Rise slowly from a sitting or lying position to prevent a sudden drop in blood pressure.
- Take frequent sips of water, chew sugarless gum, or suck on hard candy if dry mouth is a problem.
- You may take this medication with food if nausea is a problem.
- Do not drink alcohol while taking this medication.
- Do not consume other medications (including over-the-counter medications) without the physician's approval while taking this medication. Many medications contain substances that, in combination with SNRI antidepressants, could be dangerous.

LITHIUM

Patient Medication Instruction Sheet

Patient Name_____

Directions for Use_____

Uses of this Medicine:
Lithium is used for treatment of manic episodes associated with bipolar disorder. Taking lithium regularly also prevents manic episodes or causes fewer, less serious manic episodes in a person with bipolar disorder.

Before Using this Medicine, Be Sure to Tell Your Doctor if You:

- Are allergic to any medicine
- Have heart, kidney, or thyroid disease

- Are pregnant, plan to be, or are breastfeeding
- Are taking any other medication, particularly diuretics, haloperidol, NSAIDs, fluoxetine, or carbamazepine

Side Effects of this Medicine:
REPORT THE FOLLOWING SIDE EFFECTS TO YOUR DOCTOR IMMEDIATELY:

- Lack of coordination
- Persistent nausea and vomiting
- Slurred speech
- Blurred vision
- Ringing in the ears
- Jerking of arms and legs
- Severe diarrhea
- Confusion

SIDE EFFECTS THAT MAY OCCUR BUT MAY NOT REQUIRE A DOCTOR'S ATTENTION UNLESS THEY PERSIST:

- Mild hand tremors
- GI upset; nausea
- Diarrhea
- Dizziness
- Dry mouth

Other Instructions While Taking this Medication:

- Take this medicine exactly as it is prescribed. Do not take more of it or more often than it is prescribed. Sometimes it takes several weeks of taking this medication before you begin to feel better. At some point, you doctor may make an adjustment in the dosage.
- Do not drive or operate dangerous machinery until your response to the medication is adjusted. Drowsiness or dizziness can occur.
- Do not stop taking the medication even if you are feeling fine and don't think you need it. Symptoms of mania can occur.
- Take this medication with food or milk to lessen stomach upset, unless otherwise directed by your doctor.
- Use a normal amount of salt in your food. Drink 8-10 glasses of water each day. Avoid drinks that contain caffeine (that have a diuretic effect). Have blood tests taken to check lithium level every month, or as advised by physician.
- Avoid consuming alcoholic beverages and nonprescription medications without approval from physician.
- Use extra care in hot weather and during activities that cause you to sweat heavily, such as hot baths, saunas, or exercising. The loss of too much water and salt from your body can lead to serious side effects from this medicine.
- Be sure to get enough salt and water in the diet during times of sickness that can deplete the body of water, such as high fever, nausea and vomiting, and diarrhea.
- Carry card at all times identifying the name of medications being taken.

ANTIPSYCHOTICS (CONVENTIONAL)

Patient Medication Instruction Sheet

Patient Name_____ Drug Prescribed_____

Directions for Use_____

Examples:

- Chlorpromazine (Thorazine)
- Perphenazine (Trilafon)
- Thioridazine
- Thiothixene (Navane)
- Fluphenazine (Prolixin)
- Prochlorperazine (Compazine)
- Trifluoperazine (Stelazine)
- Loxapine (Loxitane)
- Molindone (Moban)
- Haloperidol (Haldol)
- Pimozide (Orap)

Uses of this Medicine:
Used in the management of schizophrenia and other psychotic disorders. Chlorpromazine [Thorazine] is also used in bipolar mania. Selected agents are used to treat nausea and vomiting: chlorpromazine [Thorazine], perphenazine, haloperidol [Haldol], and prochlorperazine [Compazine]; pediatric behavior problems: chlorpromazine [Thorazine] and haloperidol [Haldol]; intractable hiccoughs: chlorpromazine [Thorazine] and haloperidol [Haldol]; and Tourette's disorder: haloperidol [Haldol] and pimozide [Orap].

Before Using this Medicine, Be Sure to Tell Your Doctor if You:

- Are allergic to any medicine
- Have history of seizures
- Have liver or heart disease
- Have any blood disorders
- Are pregnant, plan to be, or are breastfeeding
- Are taking any other medications (either prescription or over-the-counter)
- Have any other medical problem

Side Effects of this Medicine:
REPORT THE FOLLOWING SIDE EFFECTS TO YOUR DOCTOR IMMEDIATELY:

- Difficulty urinating
- Shuffling walk
- Yellow eyes and skin
- Wormlike movements of the tongue
- Fainting
- Skin rash
- Sore throat
- Seizures
- Fever
- Muscle spasms or stiffness
- Excitement or restlessness
- Jerky movements of head, face, or neck

- Unusual bleeding; easy bruising
- Unusually fast heartbeat

SIDE EFFECTS THAT MAY OCCUR BUT MAY NOT REQUIRE A DOCTOR'S ATTENTION:

- Dry mouth
- Nausea
- Weight gain
- Blurred vision
- Decreased sweating
- Dizziness
- Constipation
- Increased sensitivity to sun burn
- Drowsiness

Other Instructions While Taking this Medication:

- Use caution when driving or operating dangerous machinery. Drowsiness and dizziness can occur.
- Do not stop taking the drug abruptly after long-term use. To do so might produce withdrawal symptoms, such as nausea, vomiting, gastritis, headache, tachycardia, insomnia, tremulousness.
- Use sunscreens and wear protective clothing when spending time outdoors. Skin is more susceptible to sunburn, which can occur in as little as 30 minutes.
- Rise slowly from a sitting or lying position to prevent a sudden drop in blood pressure.
- Take frequent sips of water, chew sugarless gum, or suck on hard candy, if experiencing a problem with dry mouth.
- Dress warmly in cold weather and avoid extended exposure to very high or low temperatures. Body temperature is harder to maintain with this medication.
- Do not drink alcohol while on antipsychotic therapy. These drugs potentiate each other's effects.
- Do not consume other medications (including over-the-counter products) without physician's approval. Many medications contain substances that interact with antipsychotics in a way that may be harmful.
- Continue to take medication, even if feeling well and as though it is not needed. Symptoms may return if medication is discontinued.
- Some of these medications may turn the urine pink to red or reddish brown. This is harmless.

ANTIPSYCHOTICS (Atypical)

Patient Medication Instruction Sheet

Patient Name_____ Drug Prescribed_____

Directions for Use_____

Examples:

- Risperidone (Risperdal)
- Clozapine (Clozaril)
- Olanzapine (Zyprexa)
- Quetiapine (Seroquel)
- Ziprasidone (Geodon)
- Aripiprazole (Abilify)
- Paliperidone (Invega)

Uses of this Medicine:

Used in the management of schizophrenia and other psychotic disorders. Selected agents are used to treat bipolar mania: ziprasidone [Geodon], olanzapine [Zyprexa], quetiapine [Seroquel], risperidone [Risperdal], and aripiprazole [Abilify].

Before Using this Medicine, Be Sure to Tell Your Doctor if You:

- Are allergic to any medicine
- Have history of seizures
- Have any blood disorders
- Have liver or heart disease
- Are pregnant, plan to be, or are breastfeeding
- Are taking any other medications (either prescription or over-the-counter)
- Have any other medical problem

Side Effects of this Medicine:
REPORT THE FOLLOWING SIDE EFFECTS TO YOUR DOCTOR IMMEDIATELY:

- Difficulty urinating
- Shuffling walk
- Yellow eyes and skin
- Wormlike movements of the tongue
- Fainting
- Skin rash
- Sore throat
- Seizures
- Fever
- Muscle spasms or stiffness
- Excitement or restlessness
- Jerky movements of head, face, or neck
- Unusual bleeding; easy bruising
- Unusually fast heartbeat

SIDE EFFECTS THAT MAY OCCUR BUT MAY NOT REQUIRE A DOCTOR'S ATTENTION:

- Dry mouth
- Nausea
- Weight gain
- Blurred vision
- Decreased sweating
- Dizziness
- Constipation
- Increased sensitivity to sun burn
- Drowsiness

Other Instructions While Taking this Medication:

- Use caution when driving or operating dangerous machinery. Drowsiness and dizziness can occur.

- Do not stop taking the drug abruptly after long-term use. To do so might produce withdrawal symptoms, such as nausea, vomiting, gastritis, headache, tachycardia, insomnia, tremulousness.
- Use sunscreens and wear protective clothing when spending time outdoors. Skin is more susceptible to sunburn, which can occur in as little as 30 minutes.
- Rise slowly from a sitting or lying position to prevent a sudden drop in blood pressure.
- Take frequent sips of water, chew sugarless gum, or suck on hard candy, if you have dry mouth.
- Dress warmly in cold weather and avoid extended exposure to very high or low temperatures. Body temperature is harder to maintain with this medication.
- Do not drink alcohol while on antipsychotic therapy. These drugs potentiate each other's effects.
- Do not consume other medications (including over-the-counter products) without physician's approval. Many medications contain substances that interact with antipsychotics in a way that may be harmful.
- Continue to take medication, even if feeling well and as though it is not needed. Symptoms may return if medication is discontinued.
- Report weekly (if receiving clozapine therapy) to have blood levels drawn and to obtain a weekly supply of the drug.

AGENTS FOR ATTENTION-DEFICIT/ HYPERACTIVITY DISORDER (ADHD)

Patient Medication Instruction Sheet

Patient Name_____ **Drug Prescribed**_____

Directions for Use_____

Examples and Uses of this Medicine:
These medications are used in the treatment of Attention-Deficit/Hyperactivity Disorder (ADHD) in children and adults: dextroamphetamine sulfate [Dexedrine], methamphetamine [Desoxyn], lisdexamphetamine [Vyvanse], dextroamphetamine/amphetamine mixture [Adderall], dexmethylphenidate [Focalin], methylphenidate [Ritalin and others], and atomoxetine [Strattera]. The antidepressant bupropion [Wellbutrin] is also used to treat ADHD.

Before Using this Medicine, Be Sure to Tell Your Doctor if You:

- Are allergic to any medicine
- Have glaucoma
- Have a history of tics or Tourette's disorder
- Have a history of heart disease
- Have a history of hyperthyroidism
- Have any other medical problem
- Are pregnant, plan to be, or are breastfeeding
- Are taking any other medications

- Have arteriosclerosis
- Have high blood pressure
- Have taken an MAOI within 14 days

Side Effects of this Medicine:
REPORT THE FOLLOWING SIDE EFFECTS TO YOUR DOCTOR IMMEDIATELY:

- Insomnia
- Rapid, pounding heartbeat
- Restlessness or agitation
- Severe, persistent headache
- Skin rash

SIDE EFFECTS THAT MAY OCCUR BUT MAY NOT REQUIRE A DOCTOR'S ATTENTION:

- Dry mouth
- Dizziness
- Constipation
- Anorexia
- Nausea
- Headache

Other Instructions While Taking this Medication:

- Use caution in driving or operating dangerous machinery. Dizziness can occur.
- Do not stop taking the drug abruptly. To do so can cause fatigue and mental depression. Tell the physician if you wish to discontinue this medication.
- Take medication no later than 6 hours before bedtime to prevent insomnia.
- Do not take other medications (including over-the-counter drugs) without physician's approval. Many medications contain substances that, in combination with CNS stimulants, can be harmful.
- Diabetic clients should monitor blood sugar two or three times a day or as instructed by the physician. Be aware of need for possible alteration in insulin requirements because of changes in food intake, weight, and activity.
- Avoid consumption of large amounts of caffeinated products (coffee, tea, colas, chocolate). They may increase restlessness and stimulation.
- Carry a card or other identification at all times describing medications being taken.

MOOD STABILIZING AGENTS (Anticonvulsants)

Patient Medication Instruction Sheet

Patient Name_____ **Drug Prescribed**_____

Directions for Use_____

Examples and Uses of this Medicine:
These medications are used in the treatment of seizure disorders and bipolar disorder: carbamazepine [Tegretol],

clonazepam [Klonopin], valproic acid [Depakote], lamotrigine [Lamictal], gabapentin [Neurontin], and topiramate [Topamax]. Selected agents are used for migraine prophylaxis: valproic acid, gabapentin, topiramate; in panic disorder: clonazepam; and in resistant schizophrenia: carbamazepine, valproic acid.

Before Using this Medicine, Be Sure to Tell Your Doctor if You:

- Are allergic to any medicine
- Have glaucoma
- Have a history of kidney disease
- Have a history of heart disease
- Have a history of liver disease
- Are pregnant, plan to be, or are breastfeeding
- Are taking any other medications
- Have taken an MAOI within 14 days
- Have high blood pressure
- Have any other medical problem

Side Effects of this Medicine:
REPORT THE FOLLOWING SIDE EFFECTS TO YOUR DOCTOR IMMEDIATELY:

- Easy bruising
- Unusual bleeding
- Pale stools or dark urine
- Diminished vision or eye pain (with topiramate)
- Suspected pregnancy
- Skin rash
- Yellow skin or eyes
- Sore throat or fever
- Abdominal pain
- Severe nausea and vomiting

SIDE EFFECTS THAT MAY OCCUR BUT MAY NOT REQUIRE A DOCTOR'S ATTENTION:

- Drowsiness
- Dizziness
- Constipation
- Headache
- Nausea
- Blurred vision
- Impaired concentration
- Increased sensitivity to the sun

Other Instructions While Taking This Medication:

- Use caution in driving or operating dangerous machinery. Dizziness can occur.
- Do not stop taking the drug abruptly. To do so may cause serious adverse reactions. Tell the physician if you wish to discontinue this medicine.
- Use sunblock lotion and protective clothing to protect from sunburn.
- Women taking oral contraceptives may need to choose another form of birth control, as their effectiveness is compromised with carbamazepine or topiramate.

- Do not take alcohol or other CNS depressants while you are taking this medication.
- Do not take other medications (including over-the-counter drugs) without physician's approval.
- Take medication as prescribed by physician. Do not take larger dose or more frequently than prescribed.
- Carry identification describing medication regimen.

DEPRESSION

What Is Depression?

It is normal to feel "blue" sometimes. In fact, feelings of sadness or disappointment are quite common, particularly in response to a loss, a failure, or even a change. Depression is different than just feeling "blue" or unhappy. The severity of the feelings, how long they last, and the presense of the other symptoms are some of the factors that separate normal sadness from depression. Depression is more common in women that it is in men, and the probability increases with age.

What Are the Symptoms of Depression?

(From the National Institute of Mental Health)

- Persistent sad, anxious or "empty" feeling
- Loss of interest or pleasure in ordinary activities, including sex
- Decreased energy, fatigue, feeling "slowed down"
- Sleep problems (insomnia, oversleeping, early-morning waking)
- Eating problems (loss of appetite or weight, weight gain)
- Difficulty concentrating, remembering, or making decisions
- Recurring aches and pains that don't respond to treatment
- Irritability
- Excessive crying
- Feelings of hopelessness or pessimism
- Feelings of guilt, worthlessness, or helplessness
- Thoughts of death or suicide; a suicide attempt

What Causes Depression?

The causes of depression are not fully known. It is most likely caused by a combination of factors.

Genetic. A lot of research has been done to determine if depression is hereditary. Although no direct mode of hereditary transmission has been discovered, it has been found that depression does run in families. You are more likely to get depressed if a close biological relative has or has had the illness.

Biological. Eating disorders may be associated with a disturbance in the chemistry of the brain involving the neurotransmitters serotonin and norepinephrine.

Family Dynamics. Some clinicians believe that eating behaviors become maladaptive when there are issues of power and control within the family. Perfectionism is expected by the parents for the child to achieve love and affection. Distorted eating patterns may be viewed by the adolescent as a way to gain and remain in control.

How Are Eating Disorders Diagnosed?

Denial (on the part of both the parent and the child) is common in eating disorders. The disorder may progress to a serious condition before treatment is sought. In anorexia nervosa, the individual may be emaciated, not having periods, and a distorted self-image. In bulimia, the diagnosis is made if there are at least two bulimic episodes per week for three months. Lab work is completed: blood count, electrolytes, protein levels, EKG, and chest x-ray. A bone-density test may be administered.

What Is the Treatment for Eating Disorders?

Hospitalization is common for nutritional stabilization is common for anorexia and sometimes for bulimia. For the anorexic person, behavior modification with weight gain is the goal. Cognitive-behavioral therapy, interpersonal psychotherapy, and family therapy are used, along with medication. Medications for eating disorders include antidepressants (the SSRIs) for anorexia, bulimia, and binge eating; appetite stimulants for anorexia; and anorexiants for obesity.

Other Contacts

National Association of Anorexia Nervosa and Associated Disorders, P.O. Box 7, Highland Park, IL 60035, 847-831-3438, http://www.anad.org

Anorexia Nervosa and Related Eating Disorders, Box 5102, Eugene, OR 97405, 541-344-1144 http://www.anred.com

Eating Disorders Awareness and Prevention, 603 Stewart Street, Suite 803, Seattle, WA 98101, 1-800-931-2237, http://www.edap.org

SCHIZOPHRENIA

What Is Schizophrenia?

Schizophrenia is a severe, chronic, and often disabling brain disease. It causes severe mental disturbances that disrupt normal thought, speech, and behavior. It can affect anyone at any age, but most cases develop between adolescence and age 30. Schizophrenia impairs a person's ability to think clearly, make decisions, and relate to others.

What Are the Symptoms of Schizophrenia?

- Delusions (false ideas)
- Hallucinations (hearing, seeing, or feeling things that are not there)
- Confused thinking
- Speech that does not make sense
- Lack of feeling or emotional expression
- Lack of pleasure or interest in life
- Lack of ability to complete activities
- Suspiciousness
- Difficulty socializing with others

What Causes Schizophrenia?

The cause of schizophrenia is unknown. Several theories exist:

Genetics. Genetics appears to play a role, as schizophrenia seems to run in families.

Biochemical. An excess of the neurotransmitter dopamine is thought to play a role in the cause of the disorder. Abnormalities in other neurotransmitters has also been suggested.

Brain abnormalities. Structural and cellular changes in the brain have been noted in people with schizophrenia.

Other. Scientists are currently investigating maternal prenatal viral infections and mild brain damage to the child from complications during birth as contributing to the development of schizophrenia.

How Is Schizophrenia Diagnosed?

To be diagnosed with schizophrenia, a person must have psychotic, "loss-of-reality" symptoms for at least six months and show increasing difficulty in normal functioning. The doctor will rule out other problems that cause psychotic symptoms, such as drugs, mania, major depression, autistic disorder, or personality disorders. Diagnosis should be made by a mental health professional.

What Is the Treatment for Schizophrenia?

Hospitalization is necessary to treat severe delusions or hallucinations or inability for self-care. A combination of psychosocial therapy and medication has been effective in treating schizophrenia. Individual psychotherapy, behavioral therapy, social skills training, and family therapy are appropriate, along with antipsychotic medication. Conventional antipsychotics include chlorpromazine [Thorazine], fluphenazine [Prolixin], haloperidol [Haldol], thiothixene [Navane], prochlorperazine (Compazine), trifluoperazine [Stelazine], perphenazine [Trilafon], thioridazine, loxapine, pimozide (Orap), and molindone [Moban]. Newer atypical antipsychotics have fewer side effects and include risperidone [Risperdal], paliperidone (Invega), clozapine [Clozaril], olanzapine [Zyprexa], quetiapine

[Seroquel], ziprasidone [Geodon], and aripiprazole [Abilify]. Medications must be taken daily for maintenance of symptoms. Certain ones may be taken by injection at one- to-four-week intervals.

Other Contacts

National Alliance for the Mentally Ill, 2107 Wilson Blvd, Ste. 300, Arlington, VA 22201, 1-800-950-6264, http://www.nami.org

World Fellowship for Schizophrenia and Allied Disorders, 19 MacPherson Ave, Toronto, Ontario, M5R 1W7, Canada, http://www.world-schizophrenia.org

ALZHEIMER'S DISEASE

What Is Alzheimer's Disease?

Alzheimer's disease is a type of dementia characterized by a loss of intellectual abilities involving impairment of memory, judgment, and abstract thinking, coordination of movement, and changes in personality. An estimated 4 million people in the United States have Alzheimer's Disease.

What Are the Symptoms of Alzheimer's Disease?

Early Stages

- Forgetfulness (loses things; forgets names)
- Confusion with performing simple tasks
- Confusion about month or season
- Difficulty making decisions
- Increasing loss of interest in activities
- Depression; anger
- Difficulty completing sentences or finding the right words
- Reduced and/or irrelevant conversation
- Visibly impaired movement or coordination, including slowing of movements, halting gait, and reduced sense of balance

Later Stages

- Unable to dress, groom, and toilet self
- Forgets names of close relatives
- Withdrawal; apathy
- Disorientation to surroundings
- Urinary and fecal incontinence
- Wandering
- Loss of language skills

What Causes Alzheimer's Disease?

Genetics. Hereditary factors appear to play a role in the development of Alzheimer's disease.

Biological. Imbalance in the neurotransmitter acetylcholine. Levels of serotonin and norepinephrine may also be affected.

Brain Changes. Twisted nerve cell fibers, called neurofibrillary tangles, and a high concentration of plaques of a protein known as beta amyloid are found in the brains of people with Alzheimer's disease.

Head Injury. Injury to the head can accelerate the development of Alzheimer's in people who are susceptible to it.

Down Syndrome. People with Down syndrome are especially susceptible to Alzheimer's disease.

How Is Alzheimer's Disease Diagnosed?

Family members report difficulties with memory, language, behavior, reasoning, and orientation. The physician then conducts a history and physical examination. Diagnostic laboratory tests are performed. CT scans or MRI may be used to rule out tumors or stroke. The neurologist will perform a mental status exam and possibly other cognitive and functional-ability tests.

What Is the Treatment for Alzheimer's Disease?

Treatment for Alzheimer's disease involves assistance with hygiene, dressing, grooming, toileting, and food preparation. Safety is an important issue, particularly as the individual begins to have difficulty with balance and coordination, and if he or she tends to wander. Individuals with Alzheimer's disease require help with all activities of daily living, and as the disease progresses, usually requires institutionalization. Some medications have been approved for treating the symptoms of Alzheimer's disease. These include memantine (Namenda), tacrine (Cognex), donepezil (Aricept), rivastigmine (Exelon), and galantamine (Reminyl). These medications have been shown to slow the progression of cognitive, functional, and behavioral symptoms in some individuals with Alzheimer's disease.

Other Contacts

Alzheimer's Association, 225 N. Michigan Ave, 1.17, Chicago, IL 60601, 1-800-272-3900, http://www.alz.org

Alzheimer's Disease Education and Referral Center, PO Box 8250, Silver Spring, MD 20907, 1-800-438-4380, http://www.nia.nih.gov/alzheimers

ALCOHOLISM

What Is Alcoholism?

Alcoholism is a disease in which an individual is dependent upon alcohol. About 9 million persons in the United States have this disease. It is a life-long illness, is incurable, and the only cure is total abstinence from alcohol.

What Are the Symptoms of Alcoholism?

Alcoholism may begin with social drinking or drinking to relieve stress and tension. As the individual continues to drink, tolerance develops, and the amount required to achieve the desired effect increases steadily. This progresses to blackouts—periods of drinking time that the individual is unable to remember. The disease has now progressed to the point that the individual requires alcohol to prevent withdrawal symptoms, yet denial of problems is common. Binges occur leading to physical illness and/or loss of consciousness. Abstaining from alcohol at this point can lead to tremors, hallucinations, convulsions, and severe agitation. Chronic alcoholism leads to many serious physical problems involving the heart, brain, and gastrointestinal system.

What Causes Alcoholism?

Genetic. Alcoholism is thought to have a strong hereditary component.

Biological. There may be a connection between alcoholism and certain neurotransmitters that form addictive substances in the brain when they combine with the products of alcohol metabolism.

Social Learning. Drinking alcohol may be learned early in the family of origin, thereby leading to a problem with drinking.

Cultural. The incidence of alcohol abuse and dependence is higher in some cultures than others.

How Is Alcoholism Diagnosed?

Alcoholism is diagnosed when the use of alcohol interferes with any aspect of the individual's life. The individual continues to drink even though he or she understands the negative consequences. When dependence occurs, the individual develops a tolerance and requires more and more of the substance. A syndrome of withdrawal symptoms occurs when the individual stops drinking or drastically cuts down on the amount consumed.

What Is the Treatment for Alcoholism?

Rehabilitation Programs. Help the individual get dry and, through therapy, to work toward achieving and maintaining sobriety.

Alcoholics Anonymous. Self-help support groups made up of alcoholics who work to help each other achieve and maintain sobriety.

Medications. Disulfiram (Antabuse) is a deterrent therapy. Individuals who drink alcohol while taking this drug become very ill. Naltrexone (ReVia) and nalmefene (Revex) have been used with some success in the treatment of alcoholism.

Other Contacts

Alcoholics Anonymous, PO Box 459, Grand Central Station, New York, NY 10163, 212-870-3400, http://www.alcoholics-anonymous.org

National Institutes of Health, National Institute on Alcohol Abuse and Alcoholism, 5635 Fishers Ln, MSC 9304, Bethesda, MD 20892, 301-443-3860 http://www.niaaa.nih.gov

ATTENTION-DEFICIT/HYPERACTIVITY DISORDER (ADHD)

What Is ADHD?

ADHD is a behavior disorder that is characterized by hyperactivity, impulsiveness, inattention, or a combination of these behaviors that are more frequent and severe than would be expected for the age. It is usually not diagnosed before age 4, and is more common in boys than it is in girls. ADHD can also be a disorder in adults.

What Are the Symptoms of ADHD?

There are three subtypes of the disorders:

1. **ADHD, Inattentive type:** has difficulty paying attention; does not listen when spoken to; is easily distracted; does not follow through on instructions; has difficulty organizing tasks and activities.
2. **ADHD, Hyperactive-Impulsive type:** has trouble sitting still; gets up out of seat at times when expected to remain seated; cannot play quietly; talks excessively; blurts out answers before questions are completed; has difficulty waiting turn; often interrupts or intrudes on others.
3. **ADHD, Combined type:** displays a combination of behaviors associated with the above two types.

What Causes ADHD?

Genetics. Hereditary factors appear to be a factor in the development of ADHD.

Biochemical. Abnormal levels of dopamine, norepinephrine, and serotonin have been implicated as a cause of ADHD.

Perinatal factors. Perinatal factors implicated: problem pregnancies and difficult deliveries; maternal smoking and use of alcohol or other drugs during pregnancy; exposure during pregnancy to environmental toxins.

Environmental factors. Exposure to environmental lead may be an influential factor.

Early family life. A chaotic family environment, maternal mental disorder, paternal criminality, and family history of alcoholism, sociopathic behaviors, or hyperactivity may be contributing factors to ADHD.

How is ADHD Diagnosed?

ADHD is difficult to diagnose. A mother's description of her child's behavior can be the most accurate and reliable guide for diagnosing ADHD. A detailed history of the child's behavior will be matched against a standardized checklist used to define the disorder. The physician will inquire about problem behaviors at home and school, about sibling relationships, recent life changes, family history of ADHD, eating and sleeping patterns, and speech and language development. A medical history will be taken of the child, and also of the mother's pregnancy and delivery. A physical examination will be conducted. Screening tests may be used to test neurological, intellectual, and emotional development.

What Is the Treatment for ADHD?

Behavior modification and family therapy, in combination with medication, is used to treat ADHD. Medications include: CNS stimulants, including methylphenidate [Ritalin]; dexmethylphenidate [Focalin]; dextroamphetamine [Dexadrine]; methamphetamine [Desoxyn]; and dextroamphetamine/amphetamine composite [Adderall]. Other medications used for ADHD include atomoxetine [Strattera] and the antidepressant bupropion [Wellbutrin].

Other Contacts

National Institute of Mental Health, 6001 Executive Blvd, Rm 8184, MSC 9663, Bethesda, MD 20892, 866-615-6464, http://www.nimh.nih.gov/healthinformation/adhdmenu.cfm

National Attention Deficit Disorder Association, 15000 Commerce Pkwy, Ste C, Mount Laurel, NJ 08054, 856-439-9099, http://www.add.org

Glossary

A

abandonment. A unilateral severance of the professional relationship between a healthcare provider and a client without reasonable notice at a time when there is still a need for continuing health care.

abreaction. "Remembering with feeling;" bringing into conscious awareness painful events that have been repressed, and re-experiencing the emotions that were associated with the events.

acquired immunodeficiency syndrome (AIDS). A condition in which the immune system becomes deficient in its efforts to prevent opportunistic infections, malignancies, and neurological disease. It is caused by the human immunodeficiency virus (HIV), which is passed from one individual to another through body fluids.

acupoints. In Chinese medicine, acupoints represent areas along the body that link pathways of healing energy.

acupressure. A technique in which the fingers, thumbs, palms, or elbows are used to apply pressure to certain points along the body. This pressure is thought to dissolve any obstructions in the flow of healing energy and to restore the body to a healthier functioning.

acupuncture. A technique in which hair-thin, sterile, disposable, stainless-steel needles are inserted into points along the body to dissolve obstructions in the flow of healing energy and restore the body to a healthier functioning.

adaptation. Restoration of the body to homeostasis following a physiological and/or psychological response to stress.

adjustment disorder. A maladaptive reaction to an identifiable psychosocial stressor that occurs within 3 months after onset of the stressor. The individual shows impairment in social and occupational functioning, or exhibits symptoms that are in excess of a normal and expectable reaction to the stressor.

advance directives. Legal documents that a competent individual may sign to convey to wishes regarding future healthcare decisions intended for a time when the individual is no longer capable of informed consent. They may include one or both of the following: (1) a living will, in which the individual identifies the type of care that he or she does or does not wish to have performed, and (2) a durable power of attorney for health care, in which the individual names another person who is given the right to make healthcare decisions for the individual who is incapable of doing so.

affect. The behavioral expression of emotion; may be appropriate (congruent with the situation); inappropriate (incongruent with the situation); constricted or blunted (diminished range and intensity); or flat (absence of emotional expression).

affective domain. A category of learning that includes attitudes, feelings, and values.

aggression. Harsh physical or verbal actions intended (either consciously or unconsciously) to harm or injure another.

aggressiveness. Behavior that defends an individual's own basic rights by violating the basic rights of others (as contrasted with **assertiveness**).

agoraphobia. The fear of being in places or situations from which escape might be difficult (or embarrassing) or in which help might not be available in the event of a panic attack.

agranulocytosis. Extremely low levels of white blood cells. Symptoms include sore throat, fever, and malaise. This may be a side effect of long-term therapy with some antipsychotic medications.

AIDS. See **acquired immunodeficiency syndrome (AIDS).**

akathisia. Restlessness; an urgent need for movement. A type of extrapyramidal side effect associated with some antipsychotic medications.

akinesia. Muscular weakness; or a loss or partial loss of muscle movement; a type of extrapyramidal side effect associated with some antipsychotic medications.

Alcoholics Anonymous (AA). A major self-help organization for the treatment of alcoholism. It is based on a 12-step program to help members attain and maintain sobriety. Once individuals have achieved sobriety, they in turn are expected to help other alcoholic persons.

allopathic medicine. Traditional medicine. The type traditionally, and currently, practiced in the United States and taught in U.S. medical schools.

alternative medicine. Practices that differ from usual traditional (allopathic) medicine.

altruism. One curative factor of group therapy (identified by Yalom) in which individuals gain self-esteem through mutual sharing and concern. Providing assistance and support to others creates a positive self-image and promotes self-growth.

altruistic suicide. Suicide based on behavior of a group to which an individual is excessively integrated.

amenorrhea. Cessation of the menses; may be a side effect of some antipsychotic medications.

amnesia. An inability to recall important personal information that is too extensive to be explained by ordinary forgetfulness.

amnesia, continuous. The inability to recall events occurring after a specific time up to and including the present.

amnesia, generalized. The inability to recall anything that has happened during the individual's entire lifetime.

amnesia, localized. The inability to recall all incidents associated with a traumatic event for a specific time period following the event (usually a few hours to a few days).

amnesia, selective. The inability to recall only certain incidents associated with a traumatic event for a specific time period following the event.

amnesia, systematized. The inability to remember events that relate to a specific category of information, such as one's family, a particular person, or an event.

andropause. A term used to identify the male climacteric. Also called *male menopause*. A syndrome of symptoms related to the decline of testosterone levels in men. Some symptoms include depression, weight gain, insomnia, hot flashes, decreased libido, mood swings, decreased strength, and erectile dysfunction.

anger. An emotional response to one's perception of a situation. Anger has both positive and negative functions.

anhedonia. The inability to experience or even imagine any pleasant emotion.

anomic suicide. Suicide that occurs in response to changes that occur in an individual's life that disrupt cohesiveness from a group and cause that person to feel without support from the formerly cohesive group.

anorexia. Loss of appetite.

anorexiants. Drugs that suppress appetite.

anorgasmia. Inability to achieve orgasm.

anosmia. Inability to smell.

anticipatory grief. A subjective state of emotional, physical, and social responses to an anticipated loss of a valued entity. The grief response is repeated once the loss actually occurs, but it may not be as intense as it might have been if anticipatory grieving has not occurred.

antisocial personality disorder. A pattern of socially irresponsible, exploitative, and guiltless behavior, evident in the tendency to fail to conform to the law, develop stable relationships, or sustain consistent employment; exploitation and manipulation of others for personal gain is common.

anxiety. Vague diffuse apprehension that is associated with feelings of uncertainty and helplessness.

aphasia. Inability to communicate through speech, writing, or signs, caused by dysfunction of brain centers.

aphonia. Inability to speak.

apraxia. Inability to carry out motor activities despite intact motor function.

arbitrary inference. A type of thinking error in which the individual automatically comes to a conclusion about an incident without the facts to support it, or even sometimes despite contradictory evidence to support it.

ascites. Excessive accumulation of serous fluid in the abdominal cavity, occurring in response to portal hypertension caused by cirrhosis of the liver.

assault. An act that results in a person's genuine fear and apprehension that he or she will be touched without consent. Nurses may be guilty of assault for threatening to place an individual in restraints against his or her will.

assertiveness. Behavior that enables individuals to act in their own best interests, to stand up for themselves without undue anxiety, to express their honest feelings comfortably, or to exercise their own rights without denying those of others.

associative looseness. Sometimes called loose associations, a thinking process characterized by speech in which ideas shift from one unrelated subject to another. The individual is unaware that the topics are unconnected.

ataxia. Muscular incoordination.

attachment theory. The hypothesis that individuals who maintain close relationships with others into old age are more likely to remain independent and less likely to be institutionalized than those who do not.

attitude. A frame of reference around which an individual organizes knowledge about his or her world. It includes an emotional element and can have a positive or negative connotation.

autism. A focus inward on a fantasy world, while distorting or excluding the external environment; common in schizophrenia.

autistic disorder. The withdrawal of an infant or child into the self and into a fantasy world of his or her own creation. There is marked impairment in interpersonal functioning and communication and in imaginative play. Activities and interests are restricted and may be considered somewhat bizarre.

autocratic. A leadership style in which the leader makes all decisions for the group. Productivity is very high with this type of leadership, but morale is often low because of the lack of member input and creativity.

autoimmunity. A condition in which the body produces a disordered immunological response against itself. In this situation, the body fails to differentiate between what is normal and what is a foreign substance. When this occurs, the body produces antibodies against normal parts of the body to such an extent as to cause tissue injury.

automatic thoughts. Thoughts that occur rapidly in response to a situation, and without rational analysis. They are often negative and based on erroneous logic.

autonomy. Independence; self-governance. An ethical principle that emphasizes the status of persons as autonomous moral agents whose right to determine their destinies should always be respected.

aversive stimulus. A stimulus that follows a behavioral response and decreases the probability that the behavior will recur; also called punishment.

axon. The cellular process of a neuron that carries impulses away from the cell body.

B

battering. A pattern of repeated physical assault, usually of a woman by her spouse or intimate partner. Men are also battered, although this occurs much less frequently.

battery. The unconsented touching of another person. Nurses may be charged with battery should they participate in the treatment of a client without his or her consent and outside of an emergency situation.

behavior modification. A treatment modality aimed at changing undesirable behaviors, using a system of reinforcement to bring about the modifications desired.

behavioral objectives. Statements that indicate to an individual what is expected of him or her. Behavioral objectives are a way of measuring learning outcomes, and are based on the affective, cognitive, and psychomotor domains of learning.

belief. A belief is an idea that one holds to be true. It can be rational, irrational, taken on faith, or a stereotypical idea.

beneficence. An ethical principle that refers to one's duty to benefit or promote the good of others.

bereavement overload. An accumulation of grief that occurs when an individual experiences many losses over a short period of time and is unable to resolve one before another is experienced. This phenomenon is common among the elderly.

binge and purge. A syndrome associated with eating disorders, especially bulimia, in which an individual consumes thousands of calories of food at one sitting, and then purges through the use of laxatives or self-induced vomiting.

bioethics. The term used with ethical principles that refer to concepts within the scope of medicine, nursing, and allied health.

biofeedback. The use of instrumentation to become aware of processes in the body that usually go unnoticed and to bring them under voluntary control (e.g., the blood pressure or pulse); used as a method of stress reduction.

bipolar disorder. Characterized by mood swings from profound depression to extreme euphoria (mania), with intervening periods of normalcy. Psychotic symptoms may or may not be present.

body image. One's perception of his or her own body. It may also be how one believes others perceive his or her body. (See also **physical self.**)

borderline personality disorder. A disorder characterized by a pattern of intense and chaotic relationships, with affective instability, fluctuating and extreme attitudes regarding other people, impulsivity, direct and indirect self-destructive behavior, and lack of a clear or certain sense of identity, life plan, or values.

boundaries. The level of participation and interaction between individuals and between subsystems. Boundaries denote physical and psychological space individuals identify as their own. They are sometimes referred to as limits. Boundaries are appropriate when they permit appropriate contact with others while preventing excessive interference. Boundaries may be clearly defined (healthy) or rigid or diffuse (unhealthy).

C

cachexia. A state of ill health, malnutrition, and wasting; extreme emaciation.

cannabis. The dried flowering tops of the hemp plant. It produces euphoric effects when ingested or smoked and is commonly used in the form of marijuana or hashish.

carcinogen. Any substance or agent that produces or increases the risk of developing cancer in humans or lower animals.

case management. A health care delivery process, the goals of which are to provide quality health care, decrease fragmentation, enhance the client's quality of life, and contain costs. A case manager coordinates the client's care from admission to discharge and sometimes following discharge. Critical pathways of care are the tools used for the provision of care in a case management system.

case manager. The individual responsible for negotiating with multiple health care providers to obtain a variety of services for a client.

catastrophic thinking. Always thinking that the worst will occur without considering the possibility of more likely, positive outcomes.

catatonia. A type of schizophrenia that is typified by stupor or excitement. Stupor is characterized by extreme psychomotor retardation, mutism, negativism, and posturing; excitement by psychomotor agitation, in which the movements are frenzied and purposeless.

catharsis. One curative factor of group therapy (identified by Yalom), in which members in a group can express both positive and negative feelings in a nonthreatening atmosphere.

cell body. The part of the neuron that contains the nucleus and is essential for the continued life of the neuron.

Centers for Medicare and Medicaid Services (CMA). The division of the U.S. Department of Health and Human Services responsible for Medicare funding.

child sexual abuse. Any sexual act, such as indecent exposure or improper touching to penetration (sexual intercourse), that is carried out with a child.

chiropractic. A system of alternative medicine based on the premise that the relationship between structure and function in the human body is a significant health factor and that such relationships between the spinal column and the nervous system are important because the normal transmission and expression of nerve energy are essential to the restoration and maintenance of health.

Christian ethics. The ethical philosophy that states one should treat others as moral equals, and recognize the equality of other persons by permitting them to act as we do when they occupy a position similar to ours; sometimes referred to as "the ethic of the golden rule."

circadian rhythm. A 24-hour biological rhythm controlled by a "pacemaker" in the brain that sends messages to other systems in the body. Circadian rhythm influences various regulatory functions, including the sleep-wake cycle, body temperature regulation, patterns of activity such as eating and drinking, and hormonal and neurotransmitter secretion.

circumstantiality. In speaking, the delay of an individual to reach the point of a communication, owing to unnecessary and tedious details.

civil law. Law that protects the private and property rights of individuals and businesses.

clang associations. A pattern of speech in which the choice of words is governed by sounds. Clang associations often take the form of rhyming.

classical conditioning. A type of learning that occurs when an unconditioned stimulus (UCS) that produces an unconditioned response (UCR) is paired with a conditioned stimulus (CS), until the CS alone produces the same response, which is then called a conditioned response (CR). Pavlov's example: food (i.e., UCS) causes salivation (i.e., UCR); ringing bell (i.e., CS) with food (i.e., UCS) causes salivation (i.e., UCR), ringing bell alone (i.e., CS) causes salivation (i.e., CR).

codependency. An exaggerated dependent pattern of learned behaviors, beliefs, and feelings that make life painful. It is a dependence on people and things outside the self, along with neglect of the self to the point of having little self-identity.

cognition. Mental operations that relate to logic, awareness, intellect, memory, language, and reasoning powers.

cognitive development. A series of stages described by Piaget through which individuals progress, demonstrating at each successive stage a higher level of logical organization than at each previous stage.

cognitive domain. A category of learning that involves knowledge and thought processes within the individual's intellectual ability. The individual must be able to synthesize information at an intellectual level before the actual behaviors are performed.

cognitive maturity. The capability to perform all mental operations needed for adulthood.

cognitive therapy. A type of therapy in which the individual is taught to control thought distortions that are considered to be a factor in the development and maintenance of emotional disorders.

colposcope. An instrument that contains a magnifying lens and to which a 35-mm camera can be attached. A colposcope is used to examine for tears and abrasions inside the vaginal area of a sexual assault victim.

common law. Laws that are derived from decisions made in previous cases.

community. A group of people living close to and depending to some extent on each other.

compensation. Covering up a real or perceived weakness by emphasizing a trait one considers more desirable.

complementary medicine. Practices that differ from usual traditional (allopathic) medicine, but may in fact supplement it in a positive way.

compounded rape reaction. Symptoms that are in addition to the typical rape response of physical complaints, rage, humiliation, fear, and sleep disturbances. They include depression and suicide, substance abuse, and even psychotic behaviors.

concrete thinking. Thought processes that are focused on specifics rather than on generalities and immediate issues rather than eventual outcomes. Individuals who are experiencing concrete thinking are unable to comprehend abstract terminology.

confidentiality. The right of an individual to the assurance that his or her case will not be discussed outside the boundaries of the health care team.

contextual stimulus. Conditions present in the environment that support a focal stimulus and influence a threat to self-esteem.

contingency contracting. A written contract between individuals used to modify behavior. Benefits and consequences for fulfilling the terms of the contract are delineated.

controlled response pattern. The response to rape in which feelings are masked or hidden, and a calm, composed, or subdued affect is seen.

counselor. One who listens as the client reviews feelings related to difficulties he or she is experiencing in any aspect of life; one of the nursing roles identified by H. Peplau.

covert sensitization. An aversion technique used to modify behavior that relies on the individual's imagination to produce unpleasant symptoms. When the individual is about to succumb to undesirable behavior, he or she visualizes something that is offensive or even nauseating in an effort to block the behavior.

criminal law. Law that provides protection from conduct deemed injurious to the public welfare. It provides for punishment of those found to have engaged in such conduct.

crisis. Psychological disequilibrium in a person who confronts a hazardous circumstance that constitutes an important problem which for the time he or she can neither escape nor solve with usual problem-solving resources.

crisis intervention. An emergency type of assistance in which the intervener becomes a part of the individual's life situation. The focus is to provide guidance and support to help mobilize the resources needed to resolve the crisis and restore or generate an improvement in previous level of functioning. Usually lasts no longer than 6 to 8 weeks.

critical pathways of care. An abbreviated plan of care that provides outcome-based guidelines for goal achievement within a designated length of time.

culture. A particular society's entire way of living, encompassing shared patterns of belief, feeling, and knowledge that guide people's conduct and are passed down from generation to generation.

curandera. A female folk healer in the Latino culture.

curandero. A male folk healer in the Latino culture.

cycle of battering. Three phases of predictable behaviors that are repeated over time in a relationship between a batterer and a victim: tension-building phase; the acute battering incident; and the calm, loving, respite (honeymoon) phase.

cyclothymia. A chronic mood disturbance involving numerous episodes of hypomania and depressed mood, of insufficient severity or duration to meet the criteria for bipolar disorder.

D

date rape. A situation in which the rapist is known to the victim. This may occur during dating or with acquaintances or school mates.

decatastrophizing. In cognitive therapy, with this technique the therapist assists the client to examine the validity of a negative automatic thought. Even if some validity exists, the client is then encouraged to review ways to cope adaptively, moving beyond the current crisis situation.

defamation of character. An individual may be liable for defamation of character by sharing with others information about a person that is detrimental to his or her reputation.

deinstitutionalization. The removal of mentally ill individuals from institutions and the subsequent plan to provide care for these individuals in the community setting.

delirium. A state of mental confusion and excitement characterized by disorientation for time and place, often with hallucinations, incoherent speech, and a continual state of aimless physical activity.

delusions. False personal beliefs, not consistent with a person's intelligence or cultural background. The individual continues to have the belief in spite of obvious proof that it is false and/or irrational.

dementia. Global impairment of cognitive functioning that is progressive and interferes with social and occupational abilities.

dendrites. The cellular processes of a neuron that carry impulses toward the cell body.

denial. Refusal to acknowledge the existence of a real situation and/or the feelings associated with it.

density. The number of people in a given environmental space, influencing interpersonal interaction.

depersonalization. An alteration in the perception or experience of the self so that the feeling of one's own reality is temporarily lost.

derealization. An alteration in the perception or experience of the external world so that it seems strange or unreal.

detoxification. The process of withdrawal from a substance to which one has become dependent.

diagnostically related groups (DRGs). A system used to determine prospective payment rates for reimbursement of hospital care based on the client's diagnosis.

***Diagnostic and Statistical Manual of Mental Disorders,* 4th ed, *Text Revision* (DSM-IV-TR).** Standard nomenclature of emotional illness published by the American Psychiatric Association (APA) and used by all health care practitioners. It classifies mental illness and presents guidelines and diagnostic criteria for various mental disorders.

dichotomous thinking. In this type of thinking, situations are viewed in all-or-nothing, black-or-white, good-or-bad terms.

directed association. A technique used to help clients bring into consciousness events that have been repressed. Specific thoughts are guided and directed by the psychoanalyst.

discriminative stimulus. A stimulus that precedes a behavioral response and predicts that a particular reinforcement will occur. Individuals learn to discriminate between various stimuli that will produce the responses they desire.

disengagement. In family theory, disengagement refers to extreme separateness among family members. It is promoted by rigid boundaries or lack of communication among family members.

disengagement theory. The hypothesis that there is a process of mutual withdrawal of aging persons and society from each other that is correlated with successful aging. This theory has been challenged by many investigators.

displacement. Feelings are transferred from one target to another that is considered less threatening or neutral.

distraction. In cognitive therapy, when dysfunctional cognitions have been recognized, activities are identified that can be used to distract the client and divert him or her from the intrusive thoughts or depressive ruminations that are contributing to the client's maladaptive responses.

disulfiram. A drug that is administered to individuals who abuse alcohol as a deterrent to drinking. Ingestion of alcohol while disulfiram is in the body results in a syndrome of symptoms that can produce a great deal of discomfort, and can even result in death if the blood alcohol level is high.

domains of learning. Categories in which individuals learn or gain knowledge and demonstrate behavior. There are three domains of learning: affective, cognitive, and psychomotor.

dyspareunia. Pain during sexual intercourse.

dysthymic disorder. A depressive neurosis. The symptoms are similar to, if somewhat milder than, those ascribed to major depression. There is no loss of contact with reality.

dystonia. Involuntary muscular movements (spasms) of the face, arms, legs, and neck; may occur as an extrapyramidal side effect of some antipsychotic medications.

E

echolalia. The parrot-like repetition, by an individual with loose ego boundaries, of the words spoken by another.

echopraxia. An individual with loose ego boundaries attempting to identify with another person by imitating movements that the other person makes.

eclampsia. A toxic condition that can occur late in pregnancy and is manifested by extremely high blood pressure, blurred vision, severe abdominal pain, headaches, and convulsions. The condition is sometimes fatal.

ego. One of the three elements of the personality identified by Freud as the rational self or "reality principle." The ego seeks to maintain harmony between the external world, the id, and the superego.

ego defense mechanisms. Strategies employed by the ego for protection in the face of threat to biological or psychological integrity. (See individual defense mechanisms.)

egoistic suicide. The response of an individual who feels separate and apart from the mainstream of society.

electroconvulsive therapy (ECT). A type of somatic treatment in which electric current is applied to the brain through electrodes placed on the temples. A grand mal seizure produces the desired effect. This is used with severely depressed patients refractory to antidepressant medications.

emaciated. The state of being excessively thin or physically wasted.

emotional injury of a child. A pattern of behavior on the part of the parent or caretaker that results in serious impairment of the child's social, emotional, or intellectual functioning.

emotional neglect of a child. A chronic failure by the parent or caretaker to provide the child with the hope, love, and support necessary for the development of a sound, healthy personality.

empathy. The ability to see beyond outward behavior, and sense accurately another's inner experiencing. With empathy, one can accurately perceive and understand the meaning and relevance in the thoughts and feelings of another.

enmeshment. Exaggerated connectedness among family members. It occurs in response to diffuse boundaries in which there is overinvestment, overinvolvement, and lack of differentiation between individuals or subsystems.

esophageal varices. Veins in the esophagus become distended because of excessive pressure from defective blood flow through a cirrhotic liver.

essential hypertension. Persistent elevation of blood pressure for which there is no apparent cause or associated underlying disease.

ethical dilemma. A situation that arises when on the basis of moral considerations an appeal can be made for taking each of two opposing courses of action.

ethical egoism. An ethical theory espousing that what is "right" and "good" is what is best for the individual making the decision.

ethics. A branch of philosophy dealing with values related to human conduct, to the rightness and wrongness of certain actions, and to the goodness and badness of the motives and ends of such actions.

ethnicity. The concept of people identifying with each other because of a shared heritage.

exhibitionism. A paraphilic disorder characterized by a recurrent urge to expose one's genitals to a stranger.

expressed response pattern. Pattern of behavior in which the victim of rape expresses feelings of fear, anger, and anxiety through such behavior as crying, sobbing, smiling, restlessness, and tenseness; in contrast to the rape victim who withholds feelings in the controlled response pattern.

extinction. The gradual decrease in frequency or disappearance of a response when the positive reinforcement is withheld.

extrapyramidal symptoms (EPS). A variety of responses that originate outside the pyramidal tracts and in the basal ganglion of the brain. Symptoms may include tremors, chorea, dystonia, akinesia, akathisia, and others. May occur as a side effect of some antipsychotic medications.

F

false imprisonment. The deliberate and unauthorized confinement of a person within fixed limits by the use of threat or force. A nurse may be charged with false imprisonment by placing a patient in restraints against his or her will in a non-emergency situation.

family structure. A family system in which the structure is founded on a set of invisible principles that influence the interaction among family members. These principles are established over time and become the "laws" that govern the conduct of various family members.

family system. A system in which the parts of the whole may be the marital dyad, parent-child dyad, or sibling groups. Each of these subsystems are further divided into subsystems of individuals.

family therapy. A type of therapy in which the focus is on relationships within the family. The family is viewed as a system in which the members are interdependent, and a change in one creates change in all.

fetishism. A paraphilic disorder characterized by recurrent sexual urges and sexually arousing fantasies involving the use of non-living objects.

fight-or-flight. A syndrome of physical symptoms that result from an individual's real or perceived perception that harm or danger is imminent.

flexible boundary. A personal boundary is flexible when, because of unusual circumstances, individuals can alter limits that they have set for themselves. Flexible boundaries are healthy boundaries.

flooding. Sometimes called implosive therapy, this technique is used to desensitize individuals to phobic stimuli. The individual is "flooded" with a continuous presentation (usually through mental imagery) of the phobic stimulus until it no longer elicits anxiety.

focal stimulus. A situation of immediate concern that results in a threat to self-esteem.

Focus Charting®. A type of documentation that follows a data, action, and response (DAR) format. The main perspective is a client "focus," which can be a nursing diagnosis, a client's concern, change in status, or significant event in the client's therapy. The focus cannot be a medical diagnosis.

folk medicine. A system of health care within various cultures that is provided by a local practitioner, not professionally trained, but who uses techniques specific to that culture in the art of healing.

forensic. Pertaining to the law; legal.

forensic nursing. The application of forensic science combined with the bio-psychological education of the registered nurse, in the scientific investigation, evidence collection and preservation, analysis, prevention and treatment of trauma and/or death related medical-legal issues.

free association. A technique used to help individuals bring to consciousness material that has been repressed. The individual is encouraged to verbalize whatever comes into his or her mind, drifting naturally from one thought to another.

frotteurism. A paraphilic disorder characterized by the recurrent preoccupation with intense sexual urges or fantasies involving touching or rubbing against a nonconsenting person.

fugue. A sudden unexpected travel away from home or customary work locale with the assumption of a new identity and an inability to recall one's previous identity; usually occurring in response to severe psychosocial stress.

G

gains. The reinforcements an individual receives for somaticizing.

gains, primary. The receipt of positive reinforcement for somaticizing through added attention, sympathy, and nurturing.

gains, secondary. The receipt of positive reinforcement for somaticizing by being able to avoid difficult situations because of physical complaint.

gains, tertiary. The receipt of positive reinforcement for somaticizing by causing the focus of the family to switch to him or her and away from conflict that may be occurring within the family.

Gamblers Anonymous (GA). An organization of inspirational group therapy, modeled after Alcoholics Anonymous (AA), for individuals who desire to, but cannot, stop gambling.

gender identity disorder. A sense of discomfort associated with an incongruence between biologically assigned gender and subjectively experienced gender.

generalized anxiety disorder. A disorder characterized by chronic (at least 6 months), unrealistic, and excessive anxiety and worry.

genogram. A graphic representation of a family system. It may cover several generations. Emphasis is on family roles and emotional relatedness among members. Use of genograms facilitates recognition of areas requiring change.

genotype. The total set of genes present in an individual at the time of conception, and coded in the DNA.

genuineness. The ability to be open, honest, and "real" in interactions with others; the awareness of what one is experiencing internally and the ability to project the quality of this inner experiencing in a relationship.

geriatrics. The branch of clinical medicine specializing in the care of the elderly and concerned with the problems of aging.

gerontology. The study of normal aging.

geropsychiatry. The branch of clinical medicine specializing in psychopathology of the elderly.

gonorrhea. A sexually transmitted disease caused by the bacterium *N. gonorrhoeae* and resulting in inflammation of the genital mucosa. Treatment is through the use of antibiotics, particularly penicillin. Serious complications occur if the disease is left untreated.

"granny-bashing." Media-generated term for abuse of the elderly.

"granny-dumping." Media-generated term for abandoning elderly individuals at emergency departments, nursing homes, or other facilities–literally leaving them in the hands of others when the strain of caregiving becomes intolerable.

grief. A subjective state of emotional, physical, and social responses to the real or perceived loss of a valued entity. Change and failure can also be perceived as losses. The grief response consists of a set of relatively predictable behaviors that describe the subjective state that accompanies mourning.

grief, exaggerated. A reaction in which all of the symptoms associated with normal grieving are exaggerated out of proportion. Pathological depression is a type of exaggerated grief.

grief, inhibited. The absence of evidence of grief when it ordinarily would be expected.

group therapy. A therapy group, founded in a specific theoretical framework, led by a person with an advanced degree in psychology, social work, nursing, or medicine. The goal is to encourage improvement in interpersonal functioning.

gynecomastia. Enlargement of the breasts in men; may be a side effect of some antipsychotic medications.

H

hallucinations. False sensory perceptions not associated with real external stimuli. Hallucinations may involve any of the five senses.

hepatic encephalopathy. A brain disorder resulting from the inability of the cirrhotic liver to convert ammonia to urea for excretion. The continued rise in serum ammonia results in progressively impaired mental functioning, apathy, euphoria or depression, sleep disturbances, increasing confusion, and progression to coma and eventual death.

histrionic personality disorder. Conscious or unconscious overly dramatic behavior for the purpose of drawing attention to oneself.

HIV-associated dementia (HAD). A neuropathological syndrome, possibly caused by chronic HIV encephalitis and myelitis and manifested by cognitive, behavioral, and motor symptoms that become more severe with progression of the disease.

home care. A wide range of health and social services that are delivered at home to recovering, disabled, chronically or terminally ill persons in need of medical, nursing, social, or therapeutic treatment and/or assistance with essential activities of daily living.

homocysteine. An amino acid produced by the catabolism of methionine. Elevated levels may be linked to increased risk of cardiovascular disease.

homosexuality. A sexual preference for persons of the same gender.

hospice. A program that provides palliative and supportive care to meet the special needs arising out of the physical, psychosocial, spiritual, social, and economic stresses that are experienced during the final stages of illness and during bereavement.

humors. The four body fluids described by Hippocrates: blood, black bile, yellow bile, and phlegm. Hippocrates associated insanity and mental illness with these four fluids.

hypersomnia. Excessive sleepiness or seeking excessive amounts of sleep.

hypertensive crisis. A potentially life-threatening syndrome that results when an individual taking MAO inhibitors eats a product high in tyramine. Symptoms include severe occipital headache, palpitations, nausea and vomiting, nuchal rigidity, fever, sweating, marked increase in blood pressure, chest pain, and coma. Foods with tyramine include aged cheeses or other aged, overripe, and fermented foods; broad beans; pickled herring; beef or chicken liver; preserved meats; beer and wine; yeast products; chocolate; caffeinated drinks; canned figs; sour cream; yogurt; soy sauce; and some over-the-counter cold medications and diet pills.

hypnosis. A treatment for disorders brought on by repressed anxiety. The individual is directed into a state of subconsciousness and assisted, through suggestions, to recall certain events that he or she cannot recall while conscious.

hypochondriasis. The unrealistic preoccupation with fear of having a serious illness.

hypomania. A mild form of mania. Symptoms are excessive hyperactivity, but not severe enough to cause marked impairment in social or occupational functioning or to require hospitalization.

hysteria. A polysymptomatic disorder characterized by recurrent, multiple somatic complaints often described dramatically.

I

id. One of the three components of the personality identified by Freud as the "pleasure principle." The id is the locus of instinctual drives; is present at birth; and compels the infant to satisfy needs and seek immediate gratification.

identification. An attempt to increase self-worth by acquiring certain attributes and characteristics of an individual one admires.

illusion. A misperception of a real external stimulus.

implosion therapy. See **flooding.**

incest. Sexual exploitation of a child under 18 years of age by a relative or non-relative who holds a position of trust in the family.

informed consent. Permission granted to a physician by a client to perform a therapeutic procedure, prior to which information about the procedure has been presented to the client with adequate time given for consideration about the pros and cons.

insomnia. Difficulty initiating or maintaining sleep.

insulin coma therapy. The induction of a hypoglycemic coma aimed at alleviating psychotic symptoms; a dangerous procedure, questionably effective, no longer used in psychiatry.

integration. The process used with individuals with dissociative identity disorder in an effort to bring all the personalities together into one; usually achieved through hypnosis.

intellectualization. An attempt to avoid expressing actual emotions associated with a stressful situation by using the intellectual processes of logic, reasoning, and analysis.

interdisciplinary care. A concept of providing care for a client in which members of various disciplines work together with common goals and shared responsibilities for meeting those goals.

intimate distance. The closest distance that individuals will allow between themselves and others. In the United States, this distance is 0 to 18 inches.

introjection. The beliefs and values of another individual are internalized and symbolically become a part of the self, to the extent that the feeling of separateness or distinctness is lost.

isolation. The separation of a thought or a memory from the feeling tone or emotions associated with it (sometimes called emotional isolation).

J

justice. An ethical principle reflecting that all individuals should be treated equally and fairly.

K

Kantianism. The ethical principle espousing that decisions should be made and actions taken out of a sense of duty.

kleptomania. A recurrent failure to resist impulses to steal objects not needed for personal use or monetary value.

Korsakoff's psychosis. A syndrome of confusion, loss of recent memory, and confabulation in alcoholics, caused by a deficiency of thiamine. It often occurs together with Wernicke's encephalopathy and may be termed Wernicke-Korsakoff's syndrome.

L

la belle indifference. A symptom of conversion disorder in which there is a relative lack of concern that is out of keeping with the severity of the impairment.

laissez-faire. A leadership type in which the leader lets group members do as they please. There is no direction from the leader. Member productivity and morale may be low, owing to frustration from lack of direction.

lesbian. A female homosexual.

libel. An action with which an individual may be charged for sharing with another individual, in writing, information that is detrimental to someone's reputation.

libido. Freud's term for the psychic energy used to fulfill basic physiological needs or instinctual drives such as hunger, thirst, and sexuality.

limbic system. The part of the brain that is sometimes called the "emotional brain." It is associated with feelings of fear and anxiety; anger and aggression; love, joy, and hope; and with sexuality and social behavior.

long-term memory. Memory for remote events, or those that occurred many years ago. The type of memory that is preserved in the elderly individual.

luto. In the Mexican-American culture, the period of mourning following the death of a loved one which is symbolized by wearing black, black and white, or dark clothing and by subdued behavior.

M

magical thinking. A primitive form of thinking in which an individual believes that thinking about a possible occurrence can make it happen.

magnification. A type of thinking in which the negative significance of an event is exaggerated.

maladaptation. A failure of the body to return to homeostasis following a physiological and/or psychological response to stress, disrupting the individual's integrity.

malpractice. The failure of one rendering professional services to exercise that degree of skill and learning commonly applied under all the circumstances in the community by the average prudent reputable member of the profession with the result of injury, loss, or damage to the recipient of those services or to those entitled to rely upon them.

managed care. A concept purposefully designed to control the balance between cost and quality of care. Examples of managed care are health maintenance organizations (HMOs) and preferred provider organizations (PPOs). The amount and type of health care that the individual receives is determined by the organization providing the managed care.

mania. A type of bipolar disorder in which the predominant mood is elevated, expansive, or irritable. Motor activity is frenzied and excessive. Psychotic features may or may not be present.

mania, delirious. A grave form of mania characterized by severe clouding of consciousness and representing an intensification of the symptoms associated with mania. The symptoms of delirious mania have become relatively rare since the availability of antipsychotic medications.

marital rape. Sexual violence directed at a marital partner against that person's will.

marital schism. A state of severe chronic disequilibrium and discord within the marital dyad, with recurrent threats of separation.

marital skew. A marital relationship in which there is lack of equal partnership. One partner dominates the relationship and the other partner.

masochism. Sexual stimulation derived from being humiliated, beaten, bound, or otherwise made to suffer.

Medicaid. A system established by the federal government to provide medical care benefits for indigent Americans. Medicaid funds are matched by the states, and coverage varies significantly from state to state.

Medicare. A system established by the federal government to provide medical care benefits for elderly Americans.

meditation. A method of relaxation in which an individual sits in a quiet place and focuses total concentration on an object, word, or thought.

melancholia. A severe form of major depressive episode. Symptoms are exaggerated, and interest or pleasure in virtually all activities is lost.

menopause. The period marking the permanent cessation of menstrual activity; usually occurs at approximately 48 to 51 years of age.

mental health. The successful adaptation to stressors from the internal or external environment, evidenced by thoughts, feelings, and behaviors that are age-appropriate and congruent with local and cultural norms.

mental illness. Maladaptive responses to stressors from the internal or external environment, evidenced by thoughts, feelings, and behaviors that are incongruent with the local and cultural norms, and interfere with the individual's social, occupational, and/or physical functioning.

mental imagery. A method of stress reduction that employs the imagination. The individual focuses imagination on a scenario that is particularly relaxing to him or her (e.g., a scene on a quiet seashore, a mountain atmosphere, or floating through the air on a fluffy white cloud).

meridians. In Chinese medicine, pathways along the body in which the healing energy (qi) flows, and which are links between acupoints.

migraine personality. Personality characteristics that have been attributed to the migraine-prone person. The characteristics include perfectionistic, overly conscientious, somewhat inflexible, neat and tidy, compulsive, hard worker, intelligent, exacting, and places a very high premium on success, setting high (sometimes unrealistic) expectations on self and others.

milieu. French for "middle;" the English translation connotes "surroundings, or environment."

milieu therapy. Also called therapeutic community, or therapeutic environment, this type of therapy consists of a scientific structuring of the environment in order to effect behavioral changes and to improve the individual's psychological health and functioning.

minimization. A type of thinking in which the positive significance of an event is minimized or undervalued.

mobile outreach units. Programs in which volunteers and paid professionals drive or walk around and seek out homeless individuals who need assistance with physical or psychological care.

modeling. Learning new behaviors by imitating the behaviors of others.

mood. An individual's sustained emotional tone, which significantly influences behavior, personality, and perception.

moral behavior. Conduct that results from serious critical thinking about how individuals ought to treat others; reflects respect for human life, freedom, justice, or confidentiality.

moral–ethical self. That aspect of the personal identity that functions as observer, standard setter, dreamer, comparer, and most of all evaluator of who the individual says he or she is. This component of the personal identity makes judgments that influence an individual's self-evaluation.

mourning. The psychological process (or stages) through which the individual passes on the way to successful adaptation to the loss of a valued entity.

multidisciplinary care. A concept of providing care for a client in which individual disciplines provide specific services for the client without formal arrangement for interaction between the disciplines.

N

narcissistic personality disorder. A disorder characterized by an exaggerated sense of self-worth. These individuals lack empathy and are hypersensitive to the evaluation of others.

narcolepsy. A disorder in which the characteristic manifestation is sleep attacks. The individual cannot prevent falling asleep, even in the middle of a sentence or performing a task.

natural law theory. The ethical theory that has as its moral precept to "do good and avoid evil" at all costs. Natural law ethics are grounded in a concern for the human good, that is based on man's ability to live according to the dictates of reason.

negative reinforcement. Increasing the probability that a behavior will recur by removal of an undesirable reinforcing stimulus.

negativism. Strong resistance to suggestions or directions; exhibiting behaviors contrary to what is expected.

negligence. The failure to do something which a reasonable person, guided by those considerations which ordinarily regulate human affairs, would do, or doing something which a prudent and reasonable person would not do.

neologism. New words that an individual invents that are meaningless to others, but have symbolic meaning to the psychotic person.

neuroendocrinology. The study of hormones functioning within the neurological system.

neuroleptic. Antipsychotic medication used to prevent or control psychotic symptoms.

neuroleptic malignant syndrome (NMS). A rare but potentially fatal complication of treatment with neuroleptic drugs.

Index